W9-DFK-663

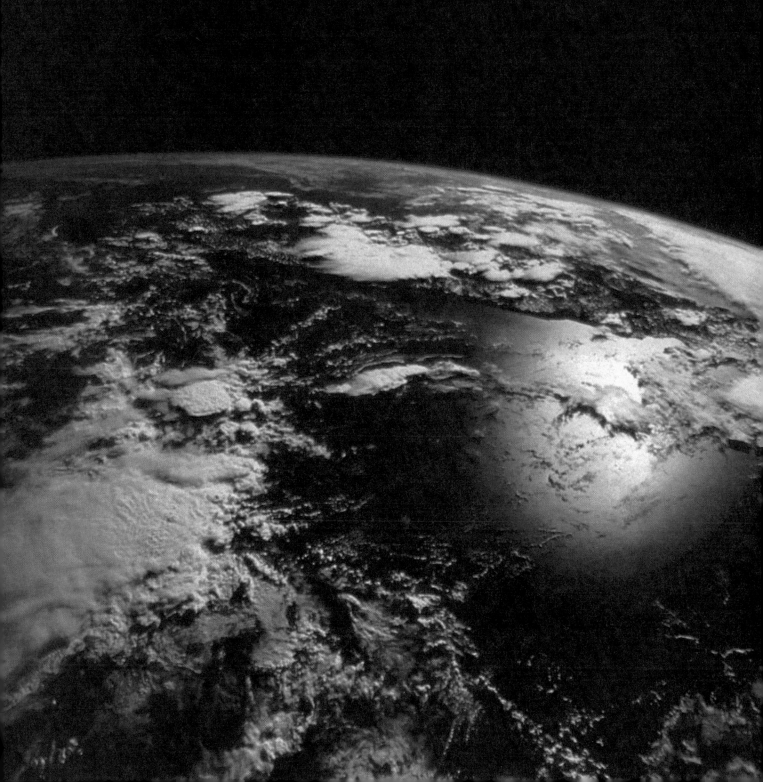

*If you can fill the unforgiving minute
with sixty seconds' worth of distance run,
Yours is the Earth and everything that's in it...*

—Rudyard Kipling

In Memorium

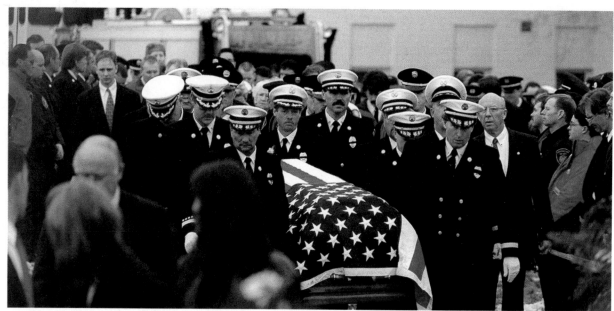

Battalion Chief Tim Hynes was killed in a rescue helicopter flight while working with University of Utah's Air Med. The rescue involved the evacuation of an avalanche victim from Little Cottonwood Canyon to the University of Utah Hospital in a snowstorm.

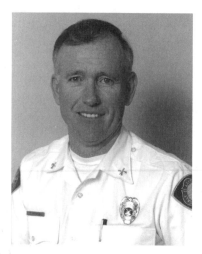

Chief Hynes joined the Salt Lake Fire Department in January of 1976 as a firefighter. In June of 1978 he certified as a Paramedic from Weber State University. In September of 1988 he was promoted to the rank of Lieutenant in the department. In 1990 he received the rank of Captain and served as Director of the Medical Division. Tim reached the rank of Battalion Chief in April 1995 where he served as director of the Research and Project Development Division.

Tim was instrumental in obtaining the Academy Center of Excellence Accreditation for the city's 9-1-1 Dispatch Center. He also served as President and Vice-President of the National Flight Paramedic Association. He was currently working as the Fire Department representative to provide Emergency Medical Services for the 2002 Winter Olympics in Salt Lake, and had plans to attend the Olympics in Nagano, Japan in February. A champion of medical dispatch, he will be greatly missed.

PRINCIPLES

of EMERGENCY MEDICAL DISPATCH

THIRD EDITION

Jeff J. Clawson, M.D.

Kate Boyd Dernocoeur, EMT-P

Library of Congress Catalogue Number: 00-133298

AUTHORS: *Jeff J. Clawson, Kate Boyd Dernocoeur*

CONTRIBUTING AUTHORS: *Geoff Cady, Bob Sinclair*

DESIGN: *Kris Berg, Mindy Blackham, Dustin Pike*

EDITORS: *Gordon W. Cottle, Nancy Hayes, Gary Horewitz, William Lloyd, Robert L. Martin, Harley Pebley III, Bob Sinclair.*

PRINTER: *Liberty Press*
PUBLISHER: *Priority Press*

Patents
The following U.S. patents may apply to portions of the MPDS™ depicted in this manual:

5,857,966; 5,989,187; 6,004,266; 6,010,451; 6,053,864; 6,076,065; 6,078,894; 6,106,459

The National/International Academy of EMD
139 E. South Temple, Suite 430
Salt Lake City, Utah 84111
United States of America
http://www.emergencydispatch.org
email: standards@emergencydispatch.org

Printed in the United States of America
10 9 8 7 6 5 4
ISBN: 0-9658890-2-5
030501

Dedications

To all those who are part of the medical dispatch solution, not part of the problem.

To the expert practice of correct medicine by remote control.

To all telemedics who make it possible.

And, to the wonderful Mouse Kids.

—Jeff J. Clawson

To those EMDs who steadily, patiently, remotely and often bravely give of their talents and souls to faceless strangers.

Also to Alison Taggart, for her steadfast friendship since 1969.

—Kate Boyd Dernocoeur

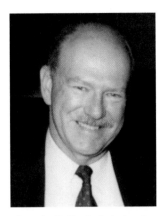

Foreword

Virtually every inch of progress made in the modern era of emergency medical services has required one group or another to change the way they think, perform, or relate to one another. Through human history, in one way or another, expectations or requirements that people alter their beliefs, their behavior, or their relationships have triggered armed conflicts between cultures, religions, and nations. Is it any wonder that so few have survived in positions of leadership in our field of EMS?

Since about 1966, the agents of change have been attending to a long list of people, processes, and things that seemed to be blocking progress in EMS. At various times, some fire chiefs, nurses, hospital administrators, physicians and surgeons, private ambulance operators, and local elected officials have felt the sting of criticism for blocking the path to improvement. Most of these battles are behind us, but many believe that one major obstacle remains in many areas.

All three editions of this book serve as a challenge to what may be the last frontier of EMS. Challenges get big, and frontiers are avoided for the same reason that some children prefer to eat dessert first and avoid spinach altogether. Until the first edition of this book was written, nobody showed an appetite for the last frontier of EMS.

Though there had been minor skirmishes with the topic, nobody had brought forth the necessary intelligence, sense of organization, knowledge of street medicine, and downright courage to fully address the frontier of emergency medical dispatching.

Why is it that this frontier has become the last major change or improvement in the structure of prehospital emergency medical care? Compared to EMT training, or modular ambulances, or advanced skills in the field, or fire department first responders, there is one major difference. That is, most dispatch systems already are well managed and do what they do with commendable precision. It's not a matter of fixing a bad system in most cases. The authors of this book present us with the information and tools to make good dispatching systems even better.

That is the challenge! Some insist that if the system isn't broken, we shouldn't try to fix it. In a discipline where processing information quickly and accurately is paramount, there are many that will resist adding steps and time to the process. Where experienced communicators have learned to distance themselves from the gritty reality of the emergency scene, the suggestion that they get involved with caring for patients—through pre-arrival instructions—may cause discomfort.

It is the nature of the changes that are needed in emergency medical dispatching that have caused the subject to be avoided for so long. At the same time, it is the experience, the integrity, and the communicative talents of Dr. Jeff Clawson and Kate Dernocoeur that have made this book and its predecessor such important hallmarks in our history. A lesser combination would have lacked the credibility that is essential to the book's mission.

In blunt reality, in many cities and communities, there is a gap in the typical emergency medical dispatch and response procedure. At its worst, it provides dying patients and their rescuers with too little help too late. At its least worst, it subjects rescuers and the public to unacceptable risks while delivering excess resources to the patient.

If you've ever arrived at the scene of a non-breathing patient to find you're too late, you've seen the product of this deadly gap. If you've ever seen the outcome of an emergency vehicle collision, you've seen the dangers of dispatching excess resources.

As we look back over the many EMS improvements that have occurred during the past three decades, it's obvious that many gaps in the system have been closed. This book has made it possible finally to close the gap at the front of the emergency care sequence—through which so many patients have fallen. Compared to previous obstacles that have been met and matched, nationwide implementation of the emergency medical dispatching concept can produce major benefits for minor cost and inconvenience.

It's been my privilege to be in contact with Dr. Clawson and Kate Dernocoeur throughout the years that the EMD concept has been developed. Firsthand, I have witnessed the sincerity and thoughtful dedication that has marked this project from the start.

Compared to earlier agents of change who fomented rebellion in their efforts to make things different, the co-authors of this work are gentle people who simply want to make things better for people in peril.

The principles and practices recommended by this book are more than theory. For over two decades, Dr. Clawson has been developing and fine-tuning the concepts of modern emergency medical dispatching. In the meantime, he has provided guidance materials and training to emergency services throughout the world.

Over the years, Dr. Clawson's work has received numerous awards from groups and organizations dedicated to improving emergency services and local government. The accolades have not cooled his passion for improvement, however. That unwavering commitment will be shared by all who venture through these pages.

I hope that readers will gain a feeling of partnership with Dr. Clawson and Kate Dernocoeur as they work to close the final, deadly gap in the circle that comprises a comprehensive EMS system.

—James O. Page, Lifetime Emeritus Member
National Academy of Emergency Medical Dispatch

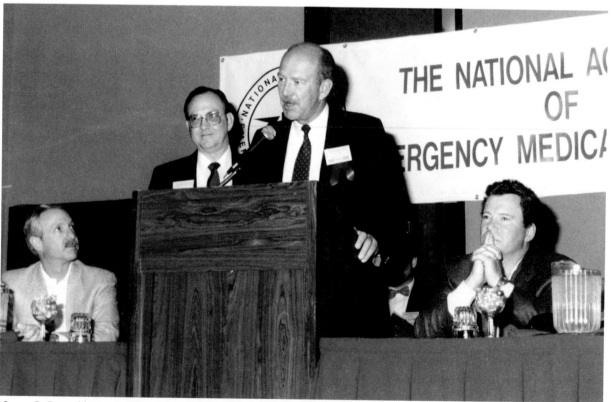

James O. Page addresses the National Academy of EMD. Guests pictured include William Shatner host of the television series "Rescue 9-1-1," the show's creator, Arnold Shapiro, and the current Academy president, Carl VanCott.

Preface 1

We are all agreed that your theory is crazy.
The question which divides us is whether it is
crazy enough.   —*Niels Bohr*

At its inception, the idea of EMD seemed a natural to me. The idea of prioritization probably began years ago with a stern warning from my boss, Gene Moffitt, president of Gold Cross Ambulance in Salt Lake City, as he looked at a fresh, excited EMT and first-year medical student jangling the keys to his expensive Cadillac ambulance. His arresting statement:

"By God, you're trained to know what calls to go
lights-and-siren on, so I better not catch you at it
unless it's really needed!"

After post-graduate work in emergency medicine at Charity Hospital in New Orleans, I returned to Salt Lake City with a strong desire to be active in local EMS. The new paramedic program, led by inexperienced administrators, offered the opportunity. The inappropriate dispatching of paramedic units (each run by a separate agency) was of major interest to me. My first activist letter in EMS, co-signed by seven other emergency physicians, demanded that the closest paramedic unit always be dispatched and not be subject to geopolitics. The letter, naively sent to the Governor and everyone below, caused local fireworks! I was in the city Public Safety Commissioner's office within the week.

Prior to EMD, the practices of dispatch were based on traditional methods. Although these methods probably had a sound basis initially, their application to modern EMS was flawed.

In 1976, as the new medical advisor of the SLC Fire Department, I promised to provide a medical dispatcher training course. But how? And what? EMT-type courses didn't seem appropriate because they were heavily treatment-oriented. More important, they lacked the method of triage needed in the dispatch environment. As a disciple of operating procedures for paramedic field activities, and everyday medicine, I felt that a protocol system could be the ticket. The fact that a dispatcher has significant limitations on time was well known. After formulating the ideas for the key questions, pre-arrival instructions and dispatch priorities, and then writing a few sample "cards," it was evident that the concept would also demand a source of rapid reference. After toying unsuccessfully with a phone number pop-up file one night, I was called to pronounce a patient who had died on the wards. The medication flip-file at the nursing station caught my eye, and the current double-card system idea was born.

The concepts of emergency medical dispatch are rooted in the same fundamental common sense in which I had always prided myself in medical practice. Just because patients have a problem outside the hospital doesn't mean they are going to die. However, the dispatcher, without any comparative medical knowledge of the problems that face him or her on a day-to-day basis, was ill-equipped to decide which of the many requests for medical aid constituted a real threat to life. Also lacking was a clear understanding of which problems might benefit from immediate response, care by advanced life support personnel, or pre-arrival instructions.

EMD was the natural sequel to the training of other emergency medical responders. It is unfortunate that the dispatcher, as the first in the chain of response, was the last to receive this attention. However, this initial EMS and public safety system oversight has proven again the adage that "the last door opened often yields the greatest reward." Appropriateness of response and emergency medical dispatcher intervention can save or improve thousands of lives, not to mention those unknowingly "saved" by response accident avoidance. In the process, EMDs learn the necessary procedures, knowledge and confidence to do the job they have been asked to do for years without training. These are the true rewards gleaned from the discovery of this long-ignored, but vital area of EMS—emergency medical dispatch.

My fortunate collaboration with the exceptionally talented Kate Dernocoeur to write, rewrite, and now version "eleven-ize" this book has fulfilled a very important goal in my professional existence. As my personal motto has been "the creation of meaningful change," I can only hope that these principles will continue to foster such change in emergency medical dispatching.

—Jeff J. Clawson, M.D.

Preface 2

As a circle of light increases, so does the circumference of dark surrounding it.   —Albert Einstein

When I first met Jeff Clawson, I was an overconfident EMS writer/paramedic and he had a great concept that needed to be presented in a book. It seemed a predestined collaboration. Jeff has always been a delight to work with and it has been a true pleasure to watch as his concept has revolutionized EMD.

My pleasure stems from my steadfast support for this carefully-designed and thought-out system. It is easy to do right. It makes consistent possibilities out of the chaos of emergency care. It generates useable data. For the caller, it removes much of the terror from an emergency. For the EMD, it creates a wonderful shield against all the things that can go wrong. It can save lives.

I was a dispatcher years ago. I had dismal training— a week of watching another dispatcher teach me her bad habits. When I was on my own, all sorts of terrible things happened. Shortly into my career, I was completely overwhelmed by a high-speed chase involving three separate radio frequencies and numerous phone calls.

When I heard of a man with a plan for doing dispatch in a sane and orderly manner, I was relieved to know generations of dispatch professionals would be spared my terror.

Many things have evolved since our first edition was written in 1986. The "Clawson system" is now operating in several languages and many countries. People would be amazed if they knew of the incredible attention to detail and compulsive troubleshooting that has gone into each seemingly tiny alteration of the original concept.

The second edition was desperately overdue because Jeff and his team at the Academy in Salt Lake City wanted to ensure that "The Principles" was up-to-date. That edition was stalled primarily by the process of computerization. It's hard to imagine life without computers, but the first edition was written for a system based on flip-file protocols. EMDs have a breathtaking resource in the modern, computerized, priority dispatch system. How lucky you are!

This book explains EMD in detail. It informs you of the background and underlying principles of EMD. No other dispatching process has such a solid foundation and framework as this one, or the benefit of over 20 years of experience gained from multi-site usage and data collection.

As someone who has worked on both sides of the radio, as a dispatcher and as an EMS field provider, I can confidently recommend that the principles of EMD are a vital hub in the overall EMS system. To know and understand them is relevant to EMS dispatchers, field providers, educators and administrators. This is the best resource to gain the information you need to move into the future wisely. Best wishes to you.

—Kate Boyd Dernocoeur, EMT-P, B.S.

About the Authors

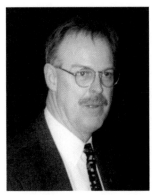

Jeff J. Clawson, M.D., was born and raised in Salt Lake City, where he attended both college and medical school at the University of Utah. His interest in emergency medicine was ignited during his employment at Gold Cross Ambulance. After post-graduate work at Charity Hospital in New Orleans, he returned to Salt Lake, became active in local EMS and worked many years as an emergency physician. In 1977, as the Fire Surgeon of the Salt Lake City Fire Department, he began development of the concepts and protocols described in this book. This protocol system is now used internationally in 20 countries and has been translated into six languages and three English dialects.

Dr. Clawson is the CEO and Medical Director of Research and Standards for Medical Priority Consultants, Inc. (now Priority Dispatch Corporation). He is a past-president of the National/International Academy of Emergency Medical Dispatch and recently retired as the Medical Director of Gold Cross Ambulance in Salt Lake City. As the originator of the Medical Priority Dispatch System™ and medical dispatch training, he is often referred to as the "Father of EMD," and served as medical consultant for the popular television series "Rescue 911."

An avid college sports fan, Clawson is waiting patiently for the Runnin' Utes to "comply with protocol" and win the National Championship in football or basketball. Meanwhile, the "Mouse Kids" have been waiting patiently for him to complete reworking this book!

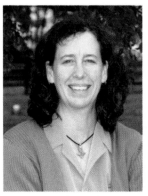

Kate Boyd Dernocoeur received her B.S. in journalism from the College of Communication, Boston University, in 1976. She blended her interests in writing and medicine by working as a volunteer in mountain rescue (Vail, Colorado, 1973-1977), as an EMT for private ambulance companies (Denver, 1977-1978), and as a paramedic for the City and County of Denver (off and on between 1979-1986—long story!). Her brief stint as a Town of Vail Police dispatcher (1976-1977) left her with profound respect for good dispatchers.

Kate has written for the EMS industry and the lay press full-time or part-time since 1979. She has been a popular speaker on a variety of topics for U.S., Canadian, and overseas audiences since 1983. She is also the author of Streetsense: Communication, Safety and Control (third edition), and several other books.

Kate enjoys living with her family in the meadows and woods of rural Michigan, near Grand Rapids.

Acknowledgments

Planning and preparing this edition of the Principles of Emergency Medical Dispatch has been a consuming, long-term effort. The resulting text represents a blending of our career-long experiences, influenced and improved by the inputs of more people than it is possible to list.

Many improvements in the current edition were stimulated by feedback from a number of colleagues and users around the world. Feedback took many forms. For all of these suggestions and criticisms we are most appreciative. In particular, we would like to recognize the helpful contributions of:

The Academy's College of Fellows, for steadfast support in providing excellent data and insight, while maintaining the collective standards of the Academy.

The Academy staff, for managing an ever-growing membership monster, while caring for the little details of each important member.

Alan Fletcher, for supporting the authors in spite of production delays, over-budget excuses and all.

Alexander Kuehl, for providing leadership, encouragement, and an excellent example of what editing a large textbook is all about.

Audra Benson, for dedicated attention to detail in managing the protocol database "monster" in nine languages and dialects.

Bill Lloyd, for always having a positive thing to say no matter what problems faced the writing and production team.

Bob Sinclair, for a detailed and articulate rewrite and edit of the regions of this book impacted by version 11.

Cheryl Collins, for pushing the production staff (and one of the authors) full speed ahead.

The Clawson kids, who have managed to survive in spite of Dad's "EMD."

Council of Standards and the **Board of Curriculum**, for successfully undertaking and completing the Academy's "Manned Mission to Version 11."

Fred Hurtado, personal friend, EMS genius, and tireless warrior, for distilling the "why" of EMD into more understandable and useable doctrine.

Gene Moffitt, and **Jared Miles**—Gold Cross Ambulance Service (Salt Lake City, Utah), for friendship, support, and Jeff's real education in the streets, the basis for the original concept of EMD.

Geoff Cady, whose enthusiasm is only matched by his deep knowledge of "why EMD" and for organizing and writing the Quality Management chapter.

Jim Jensen, aka "Aquaman," for some great data and a great tool.

Jim Page (Solana Beach, California), for his inspiration, ongoing support, review of the manuscript, and legal input.

Harley Pebley, for a thoughtful and masterful edit from the architectural mastermind of ProQA 2000.

The Medical Priority Consultants, Inc. staff, for putting up with all the delays and interruptions of their activities while we alternated between working incessantly and sporadically on the book.

Mike Smith, for several amazing protocol inventions, including the Panel Logic Script structure of the pre-arrival instructions.

Mindy Blackham and **Kris Berg,** for graphically orchestrating the publishing of the third edition and the EMD Manual. "Sleep's for wimps!" should have been their motto.

The Research & Standards Division—the "Bell Laboratories of EMD," for technical support, direction, and help.

Richard Saalsaa, for keeping the software ship afloat and providing the software CAD integration genius resulting in tremendous data from many MPDS users.

Richard Warburton and **Jan Buttrey** and the Utah State Bureau of EMS (Salt Lake City, Utah), for their initial foresight and hard work in making EMD a functioning reality in Utah.

Robert Martin, for editing, and being a right-hand man during the firestorm of Academy projects that never paused just because we "had to do the book."

The Salt Lake City Fire Department and Communication Center, for "walking the walk" of EMD.

Steve Gustavson, **Dave Hudson**, and **Rein Kauffmann** for countless laughs, memories, and true friendship.

Suzie Cozakos, for doing just about anything asked, including psychological support for one of the authors.

Tim Cohane, Journalism Professor, New Hampshire (deceased), for his knowledge and excellence in teaching journalism.

Tor Langlo, the "mad" Norwegian genius behind the protocol database and the new version 11 "holodeck" software project.

About this Book

This is the official textbook of the National Academy of Emergency Medical Dispatch. Founded in 1988, the Academy is a non-profit, certification and standard-setting organization for emergency medical dispatchers. With more than 32,000 currently certified emergency medical dispatchers in 20 countries, the Academy is the largest independent EMS registry in the world.

This text defines the principles, practices, and standards of care which the Academy (as well as several national standard-setting organizations) has set for practitioners of Emergency Medical Dispatch (EMD). Professional EMDs should understand and be able to effectively use the tools and information provided in this book. Academy training, testing, and certification is based on the principles contained in this text.

As this Book goes to Press...

The MPDS™ is an evolving system. The National Academy of EMD continually reviews and evaluates proposals for change from a user group that comprises over 32,000 people in 20 countries. The Academy also responds to changing standards from the medical community as research continues to improve medical practices. The Academy also introduces new features and tests improved wording. Add to this the significant number of language variants and you have a very complex set of documents.

In this book we have tried, wherever possible, to reflect the language used in the North American English version 11 of the MPDS (released June 2000) and the version 11.1 update (released April 2001). However, as this book goes to press there still may be some minor wording changes that have yet to be fully ratified by the various councils and committees that have the ultimate control of the protocol's wording. There are also numerous examples included in which call transcripts are quoted that contain wording from previous versions of the MPDS. The EMD should therefore, treat the exact wording used in this book as an illustrative example only. When you are using the MPDS in the dispatch environment you should use the precise wording that is on the current (up-to-date) cardset or screen in front of you. It is very important to be sure you are using the most current version of the protocol.

About Authors' Notes

The authors have added comments (called Authors' Notes) to shed light on trends and patterns in EMD, changes anticipated in standards and protocol, and to share their insight and opinions on certain controversial issues. These opinions and clarifications do not necessarily represent the official opinion of the National Academy of EMD or of other medical or public safety experts associated with the Academy.

SPECIAL NOTICE

Authorized Training and Certification

The Academy maintains a cadre of trained and certified instructors who are qualified to teach the proper use of the Medical Priority Dispatch System™ (MPDS). These instructors are continually updated as to new curricula and MPDS version updates. Academy approved EMD courses use the MPDS EMD Course Manual and audiovideo materials.

Any MPDS instruction without such materials is not authorized, accepted, or approved by the Academy.

Trainers not currently certified by the Academy as EMD Instructors are not qualified to safely instruct dispatchers in the proper and effective use of the MPDS. Using this book and associated manual to teach the use of alternative protocols or guideline-based systems is neither advised nor authorized by the authors or the Academy.

These textbooks are to be kept by the individual EMD student and are not allowed or authorized by the Academy to be archived or collected by any agency or individual for future courses or resale. This textbook may not be resold or provided to anyone not currently certified or licensed by the Academy.

Use of this textbook for teaching or any non-personal use may not occur outside of a currently licensed training organization or agency.

THE NATIONAL ACADEMY EMD PROTOCOLS

0. Case Entry
1. Abdominal Pain/Problems
2. Allergies (Reactions)/Envenomations (Stings, Bites)
3. Animal Bites/Attacks
4. Assault/Sexual Assault
5. Back Pain (Non-Traumatic or Non-Recent Trauma)
6. Breathing Problems
7. Burns (Scalds)/Explosion
8. Carbon Monoxide/Inhalation/HAZMAT
9. Cardiac or Respiratory Arrest/Death
10. Chest Pain
11. Choking
12. Convulsions/Seizures
13. Diabetic Problems
14. Drowning (Near)/Diving/SCUBA Accident
15. Electrocution/Lightning
16. Eye Problems/Injuries
17. Falls
18. Headache
19. Heart Problems/A.I.C.D.
20. Heat/Cold Exposure
21. Hemorrhage/Lacerations
22. Industrial/Machinery Accidents
23. Overdose/Poisoning (Ingestion)
24. Pregnancy/Childbirth/Miscarriage
25. Psychiatric/Abnormal Behavior/Suicide Attempt
26. Sick Person (Specific Diagnosis)
27. Stab/Gunshot/Penetrating Trauma
28. Stroke (CVA)
29. Traffic/Transportation Accidents
30. Traumatic Injuries (Specific)
31. Unconscious/Fainting (Near)
32. Unknown Problem (Man Down)
33. Transfer/Interfacility/Palliative Care

A. Airway/Arrest—Infant (<1 year old)
B. Airway/Arrest—Child (1 to 7 years old)
C. Airway Arrest—Adult (≥ 8 years old)
D. Choking—Infant/Child
E. Choking—Adult
F. Childbirth/Delivery
X. Scene safety, 1st and 2nd-Party Caller routine or urgent disconnect, patient reassurance and observation, danger awareness, bleeding control, cooling and flushing directions, and scene preparation for responders.
Y. Tracheostomy (Stoma) Airway/Arrest
    Ya. Infant—Airway/Arrest
    Yb. Child—Airway/Arrest
    Yc. Adult—Airway/Arrest
Z. AED Support

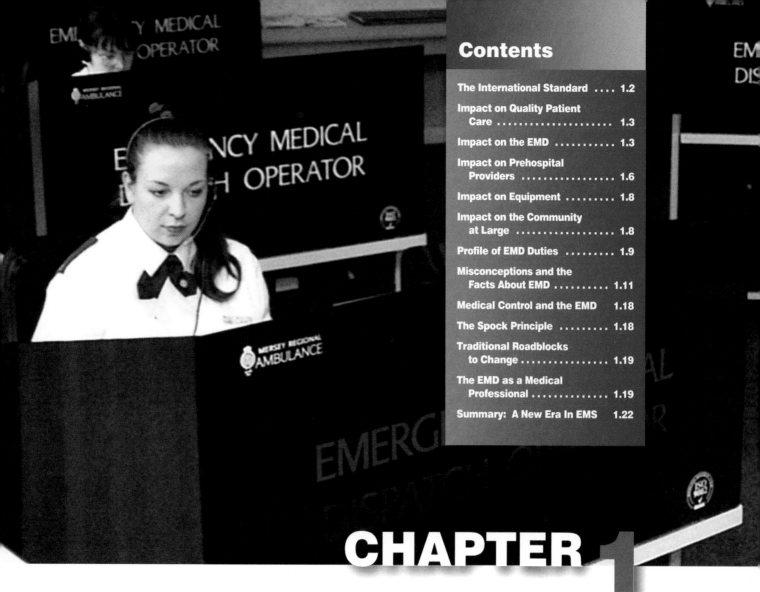

Contents

CHAPTER 1

The First, First Responder

Chapter Overview

This chapter lays the groundwork for understanding the complex role of the emergency medical dispatcher (EMD) as the "first, first responder." EMDs have the potential to make the difference, literally, between life and death, through proper application of the principles described in this book. The EMD's specialized skills and equipment can minimize the risks faced by field personnel and enhance the quality of patient care.

This chapter describes the many purposes of emergency medical dispatch. It includes the broader historical and anecdotal perspective and research collected since this book's first edition. It also summarizes the reasons the EMD system has become the national standard for emergency medical dispatchers.

Emergency medical dispatch is the jewel upon which the watch movement of public safety turns.

—F. Hurtado

The team approach to emergency medicine is well-established. As patients traverse the medical system, they generally encounter prehospital life support providers—first basic, then advanced. Then come the healthcare providers in the emergency department, followed typically by in-hospital personnel. Within the process, though, there is one group of people well-insulated from the sights, sounds, and activities of hands-on emergency assistance: the dispatchers. Because of their isolation, they have not traditionally been regarded as members of the emergency medical team.

When **emergency medical services** (EMS) were modernized, beginning in the late 1960s, development of the people in the *alarm office* or *radio room*, as it was called, was overlooked. If anything, these people were maligned and misunderstood. Fortunately, the intervening years have been kinder. Increasingly, **emergency medical dispatchers** (EMDs) are recognized as the spearhead of the emergency medical services team.[1] EMDs know what to do and how to help in their own special way. Instead of being the weak link in the chain of medical care (the historical perception), they are increasingly the hub of a worthwhile community service.[2]

The purposes of **emergency medical dispatch** are numerous and impact many aspects of emergency medical care.[3,4] A properly trained EMD utilizing a fully implemented **Medical Priority Dispatch System™** has a significant and positive influence in the following areas:

> **Properly trained EMDs can positively influence all aspects of EMS.**

- The quality of patient care
- The performance of prehospital EMS providers
- The cost effective allocation of EMS equipment
- The professionalism of individual EMDs
- The community's EMS experience

The International Standard
Before the advent of the EMD concept and the Medical Priority Dispatch System™ (also known as priority dispatch), much of the information gathered by dispatchers was unclear, incomplete, or distorted. A critical purpose of priority dispatch is to create for the EMS system the same benefit that a lens creates for a camera. Priority dispatch is the *lens* of EMS. All initial information comes through it. Priority dispatch provides the capability to focus clearly on each situation, eliminating inconsistency and vagueness through its standard, precise approach to each call.

The calltaker has the ability to have a profound effect on all patients. This is why dispatch is the hub of the EMS circle of care. The chance to give CPR, deliver a baby, or use an automatic defibrillator happens on a case-by-case basis for field crews but these situations may be happening all at once for the EMD. Thus the EMD has an impact on 100 percent of emergency medical calls. A system that promotes EMD excellence—focusing the EMD's efforts and talents on customer service to the caller, patient care to the victim, and on the rational, informed dispatching of EMS responders—improves the quality of service to the entire community.

Numerous factors identify the EMD and priority dispatch as the international standard of care. Since their initial development in 1976, the concepts described in this book have been refined and disseminated to thousands of municipalities in every U.S. state and Canadian province, 25 of 33 ambulance trusts in the United Kingdom, and 18 other countries. As cases of successful telephone instruction have been increasingly reported in the media, public expectations have changed.

Industry use of EMDs tends to follow a generally accepted format. Position papers from influential organizations (see references) plus other supportive documentation of the principles of EMD have solidified

> **Educating EMDs can save emergency agencies money, resources, and time. It can even save lives.**

its place in the evolution of EMS. Administrative rules and regulations concerning dispatch roles and procedures have been bolstered, in many places, by legislation. Finally, certain cases have been brought to the judicial system for resolution, and legal outcomes have universally supported proper implementation of a priority dispatch system.

It is a human characteristic to resist change. But dispatchers with no previous medical training can certainly learn to make informed decisions, using priority dispatch when properly trained.

The EMD is the sole authority over an emergency scene until the first responding crew can make initial assessments and establish scene control. (In essence, the "scene commander" until someone physically reaches the scene.) Until that moment, the EMD knows more

! Authors' Note

Since the methodology of EMD became accepted as the U.S. national standard of dispatch care and practice, EMS systems that have lagged behind appear to be in mounting jeopardy; a trend being copied internationally. The success of EMD as the standard of care in the U.S. and the U.K. has prompted other countries to adopt EMD, to the point that the science of EMD is now generally accepted as the international standard of care and practice.

about the scene than anyone else in the emergency care pipeline. Through telephone interrogation, the EMD can continually access patient information. This is then used to select the appropriate response for each call. Unsafe situations can be identified and relayed almost instantly to responding crews. Additionally, the EMD can provide directions to the caller about what to do, or not to do, on the patient's behalf.

EMS and public safety systems place themselves at risk if they fail to appropriately develop and support their communication specialists.

All these actions can help avert unnecessary tragedy. EMS and public safety systems place themselves at risk if they fail to appropriately develop and support their communication specialists.

Impact on Quality Patient Care

The welfare of the patient is of primary importance to the EMS system. The mission of EMS is to help others, not just to save lives. One of the finest examples of how EMD benefits each patient is by considering the concept of Zero-Minute Response™.

Much attention has been placed on the importance of quick response times by emergency medical crews. People in life-threatening circumstances need immediate help. Yet a certain amount of response time always exists. In general, studies have shown that there is a delay of about two minutes—even after a cardiac arrest—before anyone calls for help. Excellent call processing time (how long it takes to answer the call, evaluate, and get responders' wheels turning) is 60 to 90 seconds.

An excellent **average response time** once wheels are rolling to the address would range from five to ten minutes. Then, additional time (average 1½ minutes) ticks by while crews leave the emergency vehicle and make actual patient contact (see fig. 1-1).

Thus, the best to-the-patient time often exceeds eight minutes during which time the patient may not be receiving any care.

A properly-trained EMD can effectively eliminate this time gap for many situations. Willing bystanders can provide first aid via telephone instructions. In fact, callers increasingly expect to be coached in this way. If oxygenated blood can be pumped to a clinically dead brain within one minute because of the combined efforts of an EMD and the people at the scene, that is obviously better than waiting seven—and sometimes 10 or more—minutes for *trained* people to arrive at the patient's side. This concept, trademarked as the Zero-Minute Response, is changing the complexion of emergency care.

Impact on quality patient care also stems from sending the appropriate EMS response. A prime objective of priority dispatching is to send the right resources to each call. The positive impact on patients is obvious when an EMD can differentiate minor from possibly severe situations. Someone with a cardiac emergency gets advanced life support help, and someone with a cut finger gets a perfectly suitable **basic life support** provider. Or, in a differently designed EMS system, the whole volunteer squad is toned out for a three-car crash with multiple injuries—but only the two volunteers on first call need to drop everything to respond to a single-car accident with minor injuries. Appropriate resource allocation depends on a proper interrogation-based evaluation, which depends on knowing the necessary questions to ask.

Impact on the EMD

Historically, many public safety administrators believed all it took to be a dispatcher was the ability to push buttons and talk on the phone; anybody (literally) could do it. The dispatch office and those stuck there were not well-respected.

EMD education has now given dispatchers a new lease on their professional life.[2,7] A cycle of improved pride among EMDs raises morale, which naturally makes the dispatch office a more appealing place to work. The increased appeal draws in employees of increasing quality and ability. The communication center is no longer an EMS dumping ground; rather, it is a proving ground

Time Interval: Vehicle-at-Scene to Patient Access

The vehicle-at-scene to patient-access interval is the time between the ambulance arriving at the scene and responder arriving at the patient's side. This time period is not normally distributed, so it is best presented as a median value and interquartile range rather than mean and standard deviation.

Using third-party observers on 216 ambulance responses, Campbell[5] reported the median arrival-to-patient time was 1.33 minutes, with an interquartile range of 0.67 to 4.13 minutes (the interquartile range defines the 25th and 75th percentiles).

Further research[6], using the **CAD** clocks rather than direct observation, gave similar estimates of the vehicle-at-scene to patient-access interval: a median of 1.3 minutes with an interquartile range of 0.8 to 2.6 minutes.

The 216 responses that were observed by a third party could be divided into two classes: those where barriers were present and those where the responder's access to the patient was unhindered. There were 122 responses (56.5 percent) with barriers present and 94 responses without.

In those responses that were hindered by barriers, between one and seven barriers were encountered. Major barriers included doors (25 percent, locked 14.8 percent), stairways (19.9 percent), and crowds or bystanders (7.4 percent). Police secured the scene in 12 percent of incidents; police scene security contributed to the longest recorded patient access time (38.7 minutes).

For responses that encountered barriers, the median patient access time was 2.29 minutes (interquartile range of 1.01 to 4.82 minutes). For responses that were free of barriers, the median patient access time was 0.82 minutes (0.37 to 1.96 minutes). The differences between the barrier and no barrier data are statistically significant (p <0.001).

It should be remembered that it is often the ambulance's arrival at the scene which provides the time stamp that is used to determine the response time. When this is the case, the vehicle-at-scene to patient-access interval is often not accounted for. Although in the 216 responses Campbell studied, the median vehicle-at-scene to patient-access time was only 1.33 minutes, in 25 percent of those responses it took over four minutes for the responder to arrive at the patient's side after the ambulance had "arrived" at the scene.

Fig. 1-1. Vehicle-at-Scene to Patient Access Time Intervals.

of its own—and only an elite group qualify for the job. A commensurate increase has been noted in dispatcher pay and benefits, with bottom-line actual savings occurring because of this improved capability.

The result is a skyrocketing sense of professionalism. No longer the bottom rung of the ladder, EMDs are proud of their work. They are eager to share their stories and to learn yet-better ways to do their job. They have the air of confidence that stems from knowing that coordinating the entire EMS system is something only a few people can do well.

The opportunity to make a difference has increased dispatcher morale. Stories are abundant of over-the-phone lifesaving intervention. Impacting lives, not pushing plastic buttons, is the name of the EMD game, and the result is tremendously improved job satisfaction. No longer does an EMD simply obtain the address and callback number and hang up. EMD (versus unqualified dispatcher) enthusiasm is justifiable and common.

News clippings from throughout the world share the joy of EMD success in providing post-dispatch first aid instructions to lay persons. For example:

[EMD] is the greatest thing that ever happened to dispatching," said Ann Marie Cartwright, an EMD formerly with Sacramento Regional Fire-EMS Communication Center in California. An 11-year

veteran of EMS dispatching at the time, she said, "I can't help but think of how many lives could have been saved if we had had the education, the ability and the permission to do this earlier.[8]

Another part of increased professionalism and improved morale lies with the recognition by field personnel that communication specialists are an important part of the EMS team. Few would question that a definite sense of separation long existed between field providers and the voice on the radio. The norm in many places was for dispatchers to indulge in power-trips whenever possible, as retaliation for various antics and disrespectful behavior leveled at them by the field personnel. The "Us versus Them" cold-war relationship is being gradually replaced by a more professional alliance between these groups now seen as members of the same team (see fig. 1-2).

> **EMDs, using dispatch life support, are the life-saving link which has been missing from "dispatch."**

Being part of the team also means occasionally being part of the hurt. Some calls are tragic. Formerly,

---

My First Experience with Emergency Medical Dispatch

I received the call on 9-1-1 at approximately 0255. The victim was a 7 year-old girl. The girl's mother is the one who called. She told me "my little girl has stopped breathing." I immediately paged the ambulance, while trying to calm the mother.

At this time I radioed Bob Hawley, who was working with me and had him return to the station. I asked the mother to not hang up the phone, and if there was anybody else there with her. She told me that her husband was with the girl. I established that the girl was not choking because she had been sleeping for a few hours. The mother told me that the girl couldn't breathe at all and was starting to turn blue.

I asked if anyone there knew how to do mouth-to-mouth resuscitation or CPR, and she responded "no." I told her to relay instructions to her husband, because he would have to breathe for her. He then started to breathe for her, but couldn't get a pulse.

About this time the ambulance crew left the station. The house is in the community of Heath, about 20 miles in the mountains. I began relaying directions to the house and informed the crew of what was happening.

After the ambulance left, Hawley came into the dispatch room. I told him what we had. He then talked with the mother. Hawley was teaching an EMT class and one of the people in the class is a neighbor to these people. Hawley had the lady hang up and call this neighbor. Hawley also told her to call us back after she contacted Gregory. When she called back, Hawley began talking them through CPR. After a few minutes Gregory arrived and began doing CPR. This entire time span since beginning to this point was about 4 to 5 minutes.

Gregory and the girl's father continued doing the CPR until the ambulance arrived, which was just about 30 minutes after I first received the call.

As the ambulance got there the girl still had no pulse and was not breathing. Her pupils were fixed and dilated also. The ambulance continued the CPR until they arrived at the hospital. The girl was pronounced dead on arrival.

Even though the girl died, the training I had received through the Dispatch RT school on Emergency Medical Dispatch was invaluable. I was able to control my own emotions and also control the mother's emotions. We learned in the school to keep the party on the phone and relay instructions to another person. The procedure worked exactly as it is planned. It is amazing how effectively it worked.

I only wish the parents had called us quicker. The mother said that it had been 10 to 15 minutes since the girl had quit breathing before we were called. Maybe we could have helped to save the girl's life if she had called sooner. ✦

Fig. 1-2. "My First Experience with Emergency Medical Dispatch" by Don McCoy, Lewiston P.D., Montana, 1982.

dispatchers had no idea what field personnel went through; now, the EMD is more present, by phone. When the gun goes off, when a beating continues, or when the choking worsens, the EMD is still listening. Appropriate follow-up is obviously important; the EMD needs to manage the stress as detailed in Chapter 10: Stress Management in Dispatch.

Finally, EMD has been responsible for some good news in the communication center that has been a long time coming. Keller reported in JEMS that:

> One of the most encouraging trends demonstrated in this analysis is the marked improvement in dispatcher salaries. It is hoped that this is due to recognition of the importance of these individuals in the performance of modern EMS systems.[9]

Impact on Prehospital Providers

EMD also provides demonstrable benefits for field personnel. These include safety, minimization of stress, increased knowledge about a situation before arrival, and improved interagency cooperation.

From a safety perspective, positive public perception of emergency services is created when the initial telephone interaction has a confident, helpful tone. A good EMD knows how to be the vocal salve to calm callers and help them through the first frightening minutes of an emergency. This paves the way for field personnel to arrive to a more receptive welcome. A reputation for helpfulness from the outset of a medical crisis has a ripple effect throughout the community; an "everything that could be done, was done" feeling is often relayed to scene personnel; callers tell others of an experience that, despite its unhappy nature, was positively handled.

Safety is enhanced when the EMD can provide responders with information about potential scene hazards. An increased sense of control and cooperation emerges among bystanders who have been "put to work" providing first aid, making them easier to work with. And EMDs can readily distinguish levels of severity for emergency calls and send field personnel without lights-and-siren; making it safer for everyone on the roadway.

> **Positive perception of emergency services is created when the initial telephone interaction has a confident, helpful tone.**

The archive of **Emergency Medical Vehicle Collisions (EMVCs)** is full of stories about collisions that have killed or permanently injured people. In Richfield, Utah, a headline read: "Seven Injured as Ambulance, Truck Collide." A grain truck tried to turn left while the ambulance, running with lights-and-siren (depicted in this text as HOT), was next to it, passing.[10]

In Bloomington, Illinois, a young lady riding in a pickup truck was hit broadside by an ambulance running HOT on a sprained ankle call. Sharron Rose Frieburg—then 18 and an honors student—is permanently disabled (physically and mentally).[11] It is now costing this city $5 million in cash payments, including $2,000 per month for 10 years and $3,000 per month after that.[11] Such stories are far from unique. A study done by the **National Academy of Emergency Medical Dispatch** (the Academy) in 1990, through subscription to a national press-clipping service, counted 298 emergency medical vehicle collisions, resulting in 537 injuries and 62 fatalities. That equates to one death every 5.9 days in North America involving EMS responses (see fig.1-3).

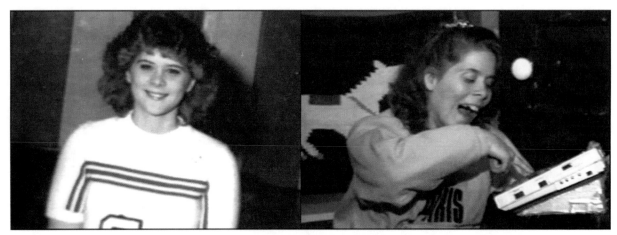

Fig. 1-3. Sharron Rose Frieburg, before and after the emergency medical vehicle collision that seriously disabled her.

Another way the EMD can positively impact the lives of field personnel is in the rational allocation of resources. On many calls, the EMD can safely send fewer responders.[3] This is true in any type of EMS system, from rural volunteer to inner-city, complex, tiered systems. The result is a more efficient use of resources and less wear-and-tear emotionally and physically on personnel—without jeopardizing patients. Fewer responders have to disrupt off-call activities, which is particularly relevant to volunteers or 24-hour shift workers, who may be trying to sleep, train, or perform other duties.

It is also helpful to field personnel to know certain details about the scene ahead of time. Several protocols have questions relating to scene safety, such as whether a fire is still burning, whether there are known weapons, or whether an assailant is still present. Answers to these questions help minimize high stress levels common to field personnel, which, in turn, improves morale. Increased contentment among employees tends to reduce attrition. A long-term field provider knows the layout of the district better (resulting in improved response times) and has better street sense. Field personnel tend to be more compassionate and professional when they know their skills and energy will be suitably matched to each situation.

Once the medical decision-making professionalism of well-trained EMDs becomes apparent to responders, an

---

```
                                           Fire Station #5
                                           October 28, 1983

        Peter O. Pederson, Chief
        Fire Department

        Sir:

             On October 19, 1983 at 2010 hrs. we were dispatched to 450
        Williams Avenue on a choking woman.  Upon our arrival at 2012 hrs.
        we found Minnie Orr lying on the kitchen floor.  The report that
        we received was that she was choking and not breathing.  She had
        choked on a marshmellow which lodged in her throat.  When we arrived
        we found her breathing normally.

             Her son informed us that she had stopped breathing and was
        turning blue.  He also stated that he felt that she would have died
        had he not received the instructions that he did from the dispatcher
        for the Fire Department.  Patricia Holt had instructed him over the
        phone in the action of the Heimlich Maneuver.

             We feel inclined to agree with him and wish to commend Patricia
        for her excellent actions in handling the emergency.  If you would be
        kind enough to pass on this letter of commendation to the proper parties
        we would appreciate it.

             For the crew at #5 station "A" platoon!

                                           Respectfully,

                                           Kirk Arnold, Captain
```

Fig. 1-4. Earliest known document of field personnel praising an EMD.

> **Estimates indicate that total annual emergency medical vehicle collisions and less evident wake effect collisions exceed 50,000.**

> ### ! Authors' Note
>
> A revealing joke circulated within EMD circles following the local release of the letter of praise (fig.1-4). As it went, the fire department retains only a copy of the letter at headquarters. The original is on display in the rotunda of the State Capitol Building under bullet-proof glass. Obviously, these welcome events are much more common today.

And to expensive equipment! Reducing HOT responses obviously reduces equipment wear and maintenance. More subtle reductions in this area derive from a reduction of equipment abuse by over-tired, over stressed employees. It is not a coincidence that ambulance services often have difficulty maintaining their equipment. Breakage increases, predictably, when those using it suffer elevated levels of physical and emotional exhaustion. Poor maintenance and handling is a common cause of equipment failure and damage. Someone exhausted by a badly designed EMS system will not be as careful with expensive equipment as someone who knows each call was carefully scrutinized and appropriately dispatched. This translates directly into cost savings for budget-conscious managers.

increase in teamwork becomes evident between the dispatch center and the field. What has been described as the public safety version of the "cold war" between dispatch and the field slowly yields to a more synergistic harmony of colleagues.

Figure 1-4 is the earliest known written document both recognizing and, more importantly, praising the actions of an early EMD's efforts to help via phone (see Choking on a Marshmallow, Chapter 8: Time-Life Priority Situations for full transcript).

Impact on Equipment

Any program that decreases the rate of EMVCs has a beneficial impact on equipment. One letter to an industry journal describes three goals held by the EMS system when choosing to implement priority dispatch: post-dispatch instructions, accurate pre-arrival instructions, and reducing HOT responses.

> **We have reduced HOT responses by 35 percent, and now on minor medical calls, the closest basic life support engine is dispatched without advanced life support back up.**

By far, the third goal... has been the most obvious improvement in our service. We have reduced [HOT] responses by 35 percent, and now on minor medical calls, the closest basic life support engine is dispatched without advanced life support back up...We have had 325 medical incidents during this period [the first two months of the program], and no patients have had a delay of necessary attention. The staff... feels the reduction of [HOT] responses increases the safety of both citizens and personnel, and decreases the city's liability. We believe... emergency medical dispatch is one proactive way to reduce risk to our personnel.[12]

—Deputy Chief Darrel Willis, Prescott, Arizona

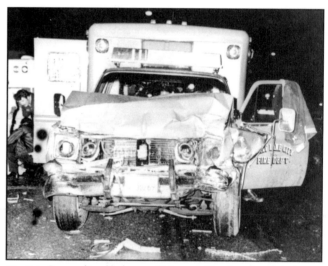

Fig. 1-5. Paramedic ambulance collision resulting in serious injuries.

Impact on the Community at Large

Examined from the point of view of the overall community, the EMD positively impacts a number of lives. The decrease in lights-and-siren responses alone results in diminished disruption of traffic flow in the community. This decreases emergency-related accidents. Estimates indicate that total annual emergency medical vehicle collisions and less evident **wake effect** collisions exceed 50,000. Wake effect collisions are those that appear to be caused by the passage of an emergency vehicle, but do not involve the emergency vehicle itself.[13]

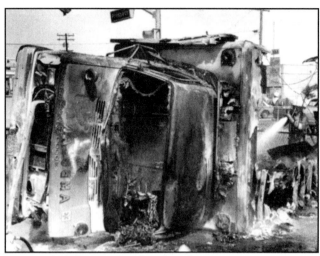

Fig. 1-6. Ambulance crash and resultant fire.

In fact, there may be as many as five citizen crashes for each one involving an ambulance. By minimizing lights-and-siren responses, EMD has a clearly beneficial impact on these figures. All too often, what seems to be a senseless death is blamed on the community's failure to look out on the highway. However, it is not reasonable to expect to educate the entire population of a given nation regarding what to do when approached or startled by a rapidly approaching emergency vehicle. Diminishing death and damage is truly the responsibility of emergency system designers.

> The EMD will have more comprehensive knowledge about the situation than anyone responding until emergency personnel arrive at the scene.

Increased quality of dispatchers also has positive impact on the community. Imagine the fear callers experience when confronted by a medical crisis. And imagine how much many people dislike having to admit the need for help. Historically, there have always been outstanding dispatchers. But others have been disgruntled, unfriendly, gruff, and sometimes downright rude and unhelpful to callers. When a caller encounters an EMD with a higher degree of job satisfaction, who has mastered basic telecommunication techniques, and who knows how to maintain a positive tone, the beneficial impact is obvious.

In addition, increased standardization of the dispatch process has increased predictability of what to expect. For anxious callers, this removes some fear of the unknown that is inherent to their responses to an emergency. If the community can rest assured that those in the emergency services ranks are likely to respond in a consistent and helpful manner, the public trust is increased and everyone shares the advantage.

Profile of EMD Duties

For the EMD to have the impact described, he or she must be a multi-task specialist. There are four general functions:

1. To receive and process telephone calls. These often come in batches, as multiple phone lines are used at once. The public-access lines may light up at the same time as the direct lines to other emergency agencies or the hospital.

2. To dispatch and coordinate EMS resources. The EMD coordinates radio traffic, often over several frequencies. There may be several EMS teams on different calls at once, radioing with various needs to be addressed by the EMD. Or, several EMS teams may be isolated at the same situation, requiring the EMD to act as central coordinator.

3. To provide medical instructions to callers and scene information to EMS crews. The public typically has come to expect dispatchers to help them with their emergencies. Post-dispatch and pre-arrival instructions are an important cornerstone of the EMD process. In addition, the EMD can prepare responding crews by informing them of relevant medical and safety information.

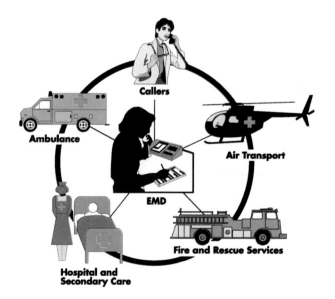

Fig. 1-7. EMD as the hub of the prehospital information wheel and circle of care.

4. To coordinate with other public safety agencies. This may be via a special telephone, a different radio frequency, or both. It may be to summon help or to hand off a situation that should properly be handled by another local emergency provider. Some situations are even handed over to other public service providers, such as the electric or water company.

Any one of these four main functions is demanding in itself. When they are all happening at once, the challenge of maintaining a clear head and calm demeanor intensify. Clearly, it is a job designed only for a select few specially talented people.

The actual role of a professional medical dispatcher can be summarized as follows:[14]

Telephone Interrogation (input). Notification of a problem in the community comes to the dispatcher first. Input to the entire EMS system begins here, with the *first*, first responder. Obtaining the appropriate information routinely can be demanding, but professional EMDs are expected to do it. The EMD will have more comprehensive knowledge about the situation than anyone responding until emergency personnel arrive at the scene.

Triage. The EMD allocates system resources to their most appropriate use. This is done by differentiating life-threatening situations from those where fewer units (or EMS personnel of more basic-level education) can safely be sent, often without using lights-and-siren. Savings in both physical and emotional terms are both measurable and substantial.

> **The EMD knows how to use resources that are inevitably limited so they can serve for the good of the many.**

Dispatch Allocation and Field Communication (output). Field communication completes the input-output loop. Important information is delivered succinctly to personnel. Responders traveling to the scene can receive continually updated information about scene hazards, violence, exact location, and changing patient condition.

Logistics Coordination. The dispatcher maintains sight of the "big picture." The EMD knows where all emergency crews are at all times. Resources can be allocated based on the immediate needs of the system, balanced by the requirements for district-wide

coverage. This allows field personnel to concentrate on their individual tasks without having to worry about the overall state of the EMS system.

Resource Networking. The EMD knows how to access support resources. These may be backup ambulances (from within the system or through mutual-aid agreements with neighboring services), police coverage, the regional poison control center, hazardous material information, child-abuse caseworkers, power companies, and anything else needed by on-scene EMS personnel. The dispatch center is the hub of the information wheel, and a professional EMD knows what is available and how to find it.

Life-Impacting Via Telephone Instruction. This part of the dispatch role is most well-recognized, thanks to media coverage of success stories. The first recorded efforts at "medical self-help" (as it was called) occurred in 1974 in Phoenix, Arizona.[15] Since then, hundreds, if not thousands, of accounts of positive results from pre-arrival telephone instruction have joined the EMD track record. Even when a life is not threatened, the EMD has the opportunity to impact lives positively through telephone intervention.

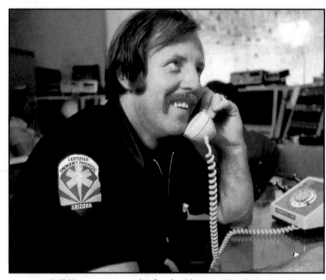

Fig. 1-8. Bill Toon, a paramedic for the Phoenix Fire Department, gave the first recorded pre-arrival instructions in 1974.

The listed roles and functions depict the EMD as much more than someone who simply answers the telephone and radio. EMDs know how to continually handle radio and telephone traffic promptly and professionally.

To consider a broader view of the EMD, this professional is a *system* advocate. The EMD knows how to use

Bill Toon Recalls Giving the First Recorded Pre-Arrival Instructions

In 1973 the Phoenix Fire Department was just getting into the emergency medical service business. In fact the term EMS was not in use at that time. Phoenix Fire began by putting twelve volunteers, of which I was one, through what some considered at the time, "Advanced First Aid" training.

We were sent to Maricopa County Hospital for 30 days to get hands on training in obstetrics, orthopedics, burn injuries and other emergency related injuries. We were also put through some limited mountain rescue training. The Department had just purchased Hurst™ extraction tools which were to be placed on the ladder trucks and also on the first rescue truck which at that time had not been acquired by the Department yet.

We began by responding to calls as Rescue One and remained in this capacity for approximately eighteen months as "Rescue Medics." Following this period we were put through paramedic training.

We were the first paramedic class in Phoenix so the entire curriculum had to be established. For several weeks after we graduated we were unable to use our newly acquired skills because the Paramedic Bill had not been passed into law by the Arizona State Legislature. After the law was passed we were required to have a nurse from our base hospital ride along with us to provide the legal link between ourselves and the hospital, since at that time we still did not have telemetry in place. Without it we were unable to send EKG strips to our base hospital.

It wasn't long before our Alarm Headquarters began to get more and more requests for medical help everyday. The dispatchers had little or no training in this area at this point in time so we were asked to work extra duty on our days off to answer the phones and give medical advice until we could get a unit on the scene.

While working in this capacity I received a call on a child drowning. At that time in Phoenix we had only one paramedic unit and the rest of the Department had very little training. Even to get the closet unit on scene was going to be of limited value. I began to give the caller a crash course in CPR because the only real chance the child had of surviving was with his family doing the saving. The person on the other end of the line was able to remain calm and follow directions. He described the child as "blue and lifeless and still out by the pool" I had him bring the child closer to the phone so we could communicate better. I talked him through the resuscitation process and in a few minutes I heard the child begin to cry. That was a pretty sweet sound for everyone involved.

The tape of this call was used around the country for several years to help pass paramedic legislation (see Phoenix Call—Baby Fell in Pool, Chapter 5: Caller Management Techniques for a full transcript of this call). ✳

Fig. 1-9. Bill Toon's description of giving the first recorded pre-arrival instructions.

resources that are inevitably limited so they can serve for *the good of the many.*

Misconceptions and the Facts About EMD

From its inception, EMD has grown, through healthy skepticism, into what is now considered the standard of care and practice in many countries. During this evolution (to some, more of a revolution), various misconceptions which blocked initial progress, were debated, and finally laid to rest.[16] An examination of the eight most common misconceptions about EMD can help overcome traditional resistance to change:

1. The caller is too upset to respond accurately.

2. The caller doesn't know the required information.

3. The dispatcher is too busy to waste time asking questions, give instructions, or flip through card files.

4. The medical expertise of the dispatcher is not important.

5. Phone information from dispatchers cannot help victims and may even be dangerous.

6. More personnel and more units at the scene are always better.

7. It's dangerous not to maximally respond or to not respond lights-and-siren.

8. Protocol and training is all that's needed to "do EMD."

Misconception One. The caller is too upset to respond accurately.

The Facts. One of the most universal notions encountered in public safety dispatching is that emergency callers are "hysterical" and "uncooperative." This is simply untrue. Most callers are calm. In fact, about 96 percent of callers are able to work effectively with the EMD. Although some callers may initially need help calming down or focusing, a professional EMD knows the telecommunication tactics to try and has the patience to use them. The misconception that the caller is too upset to respond accurately may be the dispatch equivalent of what is called the "Campfire Story Syndrome." An interesting psychological process, this term stems from the ritual of recounting (or remembering) around the campfire, stories of hunting and fishing, of accidents and encounters that involve the best or worst, the most bizarre, most extreme or intense experiences. This same process contributes to the "too hysterical" misconception in EMD; recollection of events experienced in dispatch may be skewed so that only those situations that were particularly challenging, or unusually colorful and interesting, are recounted. No one wants to admit that the nature of their job is easy or uneventful, especially in public safety professions.

The impression that most callers are out of control is statistically incorrect. A 1984 random case study by the Salt Lake City Fire Department's Medical Dispatch Review Committee classified only 4 percent of their callers as hysterical. An independent State of Utah EMD Instructor, reviewing the same cases, validated this finding. In 1986, Eisenburg, et al., studied 640 calls to a communication center in the U.S. Pacific Northwest, using a simple emotional scale to describe the caller's emotional content.[17] The scale ranged from normal, conversational speech (1) to

> **Thinking is easy, acting difficult, and to put one's thought into action, the most difficult thing in the world.**
>
> **— Johann Wolfgang von Goethe**

extreme emotional distress (5). The average score for 146 non-cardiac arrest callers was 1.4, and for 494 cardiac arrest callers was just 2.1. The Academy uses the following, similar scale during routine quality assurance case review to assign each caller an **emotional content and cooperation score (ECCS)** at the beginning and end of each call:

5 Uncontrollable, hysterical
4 Uncooperative, not listening, yelling
3 Moderately upset but cooperative
2 Anxious but cooperative
1 Normal conversational speech

Using this scoring process, a 6,400-case study was performed and published in 2000 (Jeff J. Clawson, M.D. and Robert Sinclair, PhD, *The Emotional Content and Cooperation Score in Emergency Medical Dispatching; Prehospital and Emergency Care*).[165] Data collected from British Columbia included 3,019 cases. The overall ECCS was 1.05.

1st party callers — ECCS was 1.02 (n=277)
2nd party callers — ECCS was 1.07 (n=1941)
3rd party callers — ECCS was 1.02 (n=511)
4th party callers — ECCS was 1.0 (n=290)

An analysis of 3,430 cases from Monroe County, New York, showed remarkably similar results. With the majority of callers exhibiting an ECCS of only slightly over 1, maybe the important question should be "Who's calmer—the caller or the calltaker?"

An interesting (although equally incorrect) corollary to this misconception is that the EMD can use the level of emotion to determine the level of the emergency. This has been reinforced by the misguided notion that the worse the emergency, the more hysterical the caller will be. Using this as a rule will get the calltaker into trouble on either side of this minefield.

The 3,019 British Columbia calls were subdivided into calls that could be reasonably expected to involve cardiac arrests (MPDS protocol 9) and all other calls. There were 358 protocol 9 calls, with an average ECCS of 1.22; the remaining 2,661 non-protocol 9 calls had an average ECCS of 1.03. Again, very similar results were obtained using the 3,430 Monroe County calls. While relationships can be identified between the ECCS and the caller party and nature of call, the overall scores are very low and the differences are too small to be of practical value.

Some callers are upset by little things and some are remarkably calm in the light of tragic events. Most callers, however, keep their emotions under strict control when requesting 9-1-1 emergency assistance. In 1981, legal expert James George commented:

> Without a unified system, one dispatcher may decide that a crucial situation exists primarily on the level of emotion he detects in the caller's voice, while another may depend on his own "gut" reaction, without being able to articulate a clear reason for his decision.[18]

The data show that most callers are, in fact, remarkably calm, but regardless of the caller's emotional state, the calltaker must dispatch based on the information and priority symptoms reported, not based on the caller's emotional content.

Misconception Two. The caller doesn't know the required information.

The Facts. Most callers know at least some, if not all, of the information required by the EMD. Case review at hundreds of dispatch centers worldwide has shown that the majority of callers (even some third-party callers who are not even near the patient), can provide the EMD with enough information to allow appropriate prioritization. Not asking the right questions in third-party situations is more often the cause of incomplete information than the lack of caller knowledge. As the saying goes, "If you don't ask the right questions, you can't get the right answers."

A very instructive call reviewed several years ago demonstrates the central issue here (see fig. 1-10).

Now, what did the EMD *want* to know versus what did the caller *think* the EMD wanted to know? The EMD actually just wanted to know *what* happened, while the caller thought the EMD wanted to know *why* the patient was in cardiac arrest (stroke, heart attack, seizure, overdose, etc.) As they say in the military, "What we have here is a failure to c-o-m-m-u-n-i-c-a-t-e."

Most callers should know something about the victim. Theoretically, more than 70 percent of callers are first- and second-party callers and therefore can provide information and some help, although some, unfortunately, still focus on the 30 percent who are third-party callers—yet even these callers can often provide critical information. Should some callers be denied the opportunity to help just because some professionals are

---

A Failure to Communicate

Dispatcher:	**Nine-one-one, what is your emergency?**
Caller:	We need the paramedics over to the Fashion Place Mall right away.
Dispatcher:	**What seems to be the problem there, ma'am?**
Caller:	(brief pause) Ah, I don't know what's the matter with him. I'm not a doctor.
Dispatcher:	**(longer pause) Well, does he have any medical identification tags or bracelets or anything?**
Caller:	Look, I don't know. I'm not a doctor.
Dispatcher:	**(somewhat despairingly) Okay then. You say you don't know?**
Caller:	Like I said, I'm not a doctor.
Dispatcher:	**(typing into the CAD and resigned to send now) Okay.** *[The EMD can faintly make out muffled noises in the background, becoming clearer as she stops typing: One, two, three, four, five, whooo... one, two, three, four, five, whooo... one, two... at which point the EMD nervously blurts out:]* **What's that noise? What's that... counting? What are they doing?**
Caller:	(matter-of-factly) Oh, they're doing CPR.
Dispatcher:	**I thought you said you didn't know what happened?**
Caller:	I don't ma'am. I'm not a doctor. 🌿

Fig. 1-10. This call, received from the security office of a large shopping center, demonstrates the, "If you don't ask the right questions..." problem.

unable or unwilling to believe they can? Prioritizing EMS resources properly because the caller can answer basic questions serves the system. And if the caller is calm enough (or calmed enough) and follows the EMD's lead in providing pre-arrival first aid, so much the better. In fact, many callers now expect to be told how to assist properly.

> **! Authors' Note**
>
> In actual QA case review, it has been our universal experience that dispatchers functioning on their own (even if aided, as they say, by an infinite number of monkeys provided with an infinite number of typewriters) will never replicate the questions listed on Protocol 32: Unknown Problem (Man Down).

Misconception Three. The dispatcher is too busy to waste time asking questions, give instructions, or flip through card files.

The Facts. The uninitiated have previously complained that dispatchers should not waste precious seconds asking all these questions. The priority dispatch process does demand more of the EMD, but the information needed to do the job properly can usually be obtained in the same or less time than the freestyle methods of yesteryear.

The time required to interrogate is not a factor in most cases. Call-processing time was carefully observed in Los Angeles in 1988, before and after implementation of priority dispatch.[19] The average time required to process a call before initiating use of the system was 72 seconds. At the beginning of priority dispatching, this average time increased to 80 seconds, but after less than one week, total call-processing time had returned to 72 seconds—even allowing for the new provision of post-dispatch and pre-arrival instructions. Not only was the overall call processing time the same, but the

information obtained was more usable and complete. In fact, further evaluation indicated that interrogation time was actually decreased, since the added time of occasionally providing CPR or other extended pre-arrival instructions did not increase call processing time overall. And, of great importance to the system's managers, the number of EMDs required to process calls both before and after priority dispatch implementation remained the same!

Overall, this saves the system time in the long run, because the key questions assist the EMD in gathering the information necessary to establish the correct level of medical response.

Remember that a full interrogation is not always necessary before sending help. There are two regular points at which the priority dispatch protocol directs the EMD to send assistance. The first, which is nearly immediate, simply allows for early recognition of time-critical situations where the patient is not breathing or where breathing is uncertain. A full-blown EMS response is made at that point. The difference is that for the other cases—the vast majority—priorities are objectively sorted out before resources are sent. A good maxim to remember is that, "It takes the same time to ask the right questions as it does to ask the wrong questions," and if you ask the right questions, you get the right answers.

Misconception Four. The medical expertise of the dispatcher is not important.

The Facts. The medical expertise of the EMD is certainly important. This misconception is largely dead as it pre-dated the EMD standard and was essentially the old excuse, "They don't need any medical training, they're just clerks." However, a form of this improper thinking that still persists is that those in medical dispatch positions should have various types of field training—such as EMT or paramedic. Such issues

> **If you ask the right questions, you get the right answers.**

Does it take more time, or more control staff?			
	Before	**During**	**One Week After**
Average time in queue	7 sec.	8 sec.	7 sec.
Total call-processing time	72 sec.	80 sec.	72 sec.

Fig. 1-11. City of Los Angeles Implementation, 1988; Population 3.2 million (1,200 calls per day). Total staffing before and after implementation remained the same (approximately 70 EMDs).

are often raised by centers that have traditionally utilized these training curricula or by previous field personnel with these training levels, when a move is made to switch to professional EMDs who have no other medical training. This often confuses the issue. The official position of the Academy is that no matter what the previous training or experience of the dispatcher might be, they must be trained and certified as EMDs—there are no exceptions. As the old saying goes, "If you want someone to function as an apple, don't train them to be an orange, and just because they are round and a fruit, then think they can do the same job."

In 1989, the National Association of EMS Physicians (NAEMSP) directly confronted this issue by stating:

> *In order to prioritize calls properly, the EMD must be well-versed in the medical conditions and incident types that constitute their daily routine. Training in these priorities must be detailed and dispatch-specific (not EMT or paramedic training per se). Since, much of the knowledge and many of the skills required by the EMD are dispatch-specific, a curriculum for their training differs substantially from those used in the preparation of EMTs or paramedics. Training as an EMT or paramedic does not adequately prepare a person for the role of an EMD. Much of the required EMD curriculum cannot be found in standard EMS training curricula. It consists of content and emphasis which differ significantly from that used for the training of all other health professional and public safety dispatchers. The unique teaching forum necessary to provide this essential training requires unprecedented cooperation between the diverse disciplines of telecommunications and prehospital and emergency medicine. Essentially, EMD training is required for all dispatchers functioning in medical dispatch agencies, and contains significant content and competence which differs substantially from that ordinarily provided to EMTs and paramedics.[20]*

> **The unique teaching forum necessary to provide this essential training requires unprecedented cooperation between the diverse disciplines of telecommunications and prehospital and emergency medicine.**

An EMD should always receive medical dispatch-specific training and then, under quality management evaluative and feedback mechanisms, be entrusted with the power necessary to effectively use that training. It is important that this training be specific to the EMD's understanding of, and ability to use, the central tool of their practice—the protocol. Hundreds of medical dispatch centers staffed by thousands of EMDs with no other medical training effectively and admirably do just that for the number-one employer of EMDs in North America. And that employer is not ambulance services, hospitals, or fire departments—it is rural law enforcement.

Misconception Five. Phone information from dispatchers cannot help victims and may even be dangerous.

The Facts. This was initially the most widely stated misconception, but in the twelve years since the first edition of this textbook, it has become the most thoroughly debunked misconception in the industry. Hundreds, and more likely today thousands, of cases involving effective telephone-directed formal care take place every day in myriad communication centers that have embraced this very important facet of priority dispatch. The additional fact remains that while, historically, dozens of lawsuits have been initiated against medical dispatch centers, an increasing number of these have been directed at what plaintiff's attorneys have now called "dispatcher **abandonment**"—the failure to provide pre-arrival instructions. Universally these have involved those *not* utilizing priority dispatch. Indeed, the provision of pre-arrival and post-dispatch instructions is clearly considered the standard of care and practice in North America and the U.K. Two statements in the NAEMSP Position Paper on EMD seem to sum things up from any potential patient's viewpoint, "Pre-arrival instructions are a mandatory function of each EMD in a medical dispatch center," and, "Standard medically approved telephone instructions by trained EMDs are safe to give and in many instances are a moral necessity."[20]

Misconception Six. More personnel and more units at the scene are always better.

The Facts. It is possible to send an appropriate emergency response without utilizing multiple vehicles. An *appropriate* response is nearly always better than a *maximal* response. Overkill does not equal adequate handling of the job and it is simply not wise to react this way at dispatch when non-critical and non-life threatening situations are clearly identified. Prioritization of response has been the method of reasonable management of valuable and often scarce pre-hospital resources. The article, *Medical Priority Dispatch—It Works,* described the early experience of the Salt Lake City Fire Department's

1990 EMVC Study, Statistical Information

	Fatal EMVCs	Non-Fatal with injuries	Non-Fatal without injuries	Total EMVCs
To scene	16 (37%)	75 (46%)	37 (40%)	128 (43%)
From scene	18 (42%)	43 (27%)	25 (27%)	86 (29%)
Other or Undetermined	9 (21%)	44 (27%)	31 (33%)	84 (28%)
Total	43	162	93	298

Fig. 1-12. 1990 EMVC Study Statistical Information, October 1, 1989 through September 30, 1990.

prioritization of response.[3] They reported a 50 percent reduction in total responding vehicles, a 50 percent reduction in lights-and-siren (referred to in this text as HOT) responses, and the elimination of 33 percent of calls run by the fire department due to referral of non-urgent basic life support cases to the private ambulance service, Gold Cross. These experiences have been reproduced in many other systems. The management of response and personnel is the central premise of priority dispatching whose mission can be summed up by the goal of "sending the right thing, to the right patient, at the right time, in the right way, and doing the right thing for the patient through the caller until the troops can arrive."

Misconception Seven. It's dangerous not to maximally respond or to not respond lights-and-siren.

The Facts. Unfortunately, HOT responses are not without significant risk. Each year thousands of accidents occur as the result of extreme response and transport practices. Thousands of people are injured and dozens are killed. In 1990, the Academy funded a revealing press clipping data collection of emergency medical vehicle collisions in the U.S.[21] The following figure is a partial depiction of the raw data obtained.

Of the 298 EMVCs documented in the study, 205 resulted in injury or death—injuring 537 people and killing 62.

The more appropriate use of warning lights-and-siren will make the First Law of Medical Practice more relevant to emergency medical services and medical dispatch: "First, do no harm."

HOT responses do not save enough time to affect outcome in most cases. Much of EMS response

rationale has evolved from long-standing, public safety practices.[22, 23, 24, 36] But medical emergencies are not the same as fires (see fig. 1-13). A fire usually gets worse as the seconds tick by. In most cases it is considered to be escalating until proven otherwise. However, the great majority of medical situations are not getting worse as time passes. Many patients who receive a HOT ride to the hospital wait from 30 minutes to several hours for complete diagnostic workup and treatment. Are the few seconds saved running HOT worth it? Probably so in choking, respiratory failure, cardiac arrest, or severe bleeding situations. But not most others. An EMD using priority dispatch protocols will properly determine when the few seconds or minutes shaved off by a HOT response will make no difference, such as in chronic, unchanging, stable, or improving situations.

Regular use of lights-and-siren is a bad habit in emergency services generally. They should not be used simply because they are there.[24] Through proper caller interrogation and pre-arrival instructions, those with minor—even moderate—injuries can safely await emergency responders who travel in the much safer non-emergency mode (referred to in this text as COLD). Because relatively sophisticated medical expertise goes to the problem, it is almost always possible to travel to the medical treatment center COLD as well. The rapidly mounting evidence that COLD responses, as well as COLD transports, can be reliably and appropriately selected, as well as being significantly safer, is presented in Chapter 2: Basic Telecommunication Techniques.

Many services now run significant numbers of their calls COLD. The seminal position paper by NAEMSP titled, "Use of Warning Lights and Siren in Emergency Medical Vehicle Response and Patient Transport," has set an appropriate standard of practice with an emphasis on medical dispatch processing as central to the proper management of responses.[25]

Misconception Eight. Protocol and training is all that's needed to "do EMD."

The Facts. Appropriate resource allocation can be accurately determined by EMDs using the priority dispatch system correctly. Unfortunately, many EMS managers have decided to try incomplete and partial forms of EMD without thorough research, education, and compliance based on quality management principles. Some systems misinform their communities that they are using EMD when they are, in fact, only providing ad-lib (not scripted) telephone aid and only utilizing partially or untrained dispatchers. Others try to use resource prioritization without fully understanding the concepts and underlying principles. This is called "the illusion of priority dispatch." Failure to be thorough at dispatch can have disastrous repercussions.

Response prioritization is the most fundamental concept of priority dispatch. To "be doing EMD" correctly, dispatch centers and their dispatchers must be reproducibly, and closely, using the protocol in order to safely match pre-determined response modes to caller situations. We have simplistically defined priority dispatching as, "sending the right thing, to the right patient, at the right time, in the right way, and doing the right thing for the patient through the caller until the troops arrive." EMD managers, and EMDs, must understand what the "right thing" actually is (i.e., advanced or basic life support unit), how long "the right time" is, and what mode "the right way" implies (i.e., HOT or COLD response). They must also understand, and use, the pre-arrival and post-dispatch instruction sequences in the protocol appropriately and correctly.

There is more to this than simply purchasing a protocol and initially training dispatchers to use it.

The protocol (and therefore the entire EMD system) can only function correctly when the EMD's compliance to the protocol (strictly following it) is high or absolute.[26] In order for EMDs to achieve these levels of compliance, management must be prepared to honestly, regularly, and impartially provide them with feedback regarding past performance; if EMDs are not told when they make a mistake, they cannot correct that mistake in the future. Provision of this information to the EMDs, as part of an ongoing "total quality management" process requires unbiased review of recorded cases by a trained reviewer. If EMDs are regularly provided with information pertaining to how well they are doing (rather than only being told when they are doing something wrong as a punitive measure), compliance to the protocol can skyrocket. In centers (and only in centers) where these ongoing quality management processes are in place, we routinely see overall compliance above the 95 percent level.[26] Complete understanding of this principle of EMD is a moral obligation, since the lives of field personnel, their patients, and members of the general public might be at stake.

To practice incomplete EMD is risking the consequences of poor patient care at a time when a much more informed and demanding public has grown to expect services that are often demonstrated to them graphically and convincingly on primetime television. Priority dispatch must be properly understood by those with the power to initiate and manage its use. Responsible public safety systems must resist taking shortcuts. By plugging all the holes that the misconceptions represent in the fabric of pre-arrival and pre-hospital care, a safer, more efficient, and effective medical dispatching system has emerged.

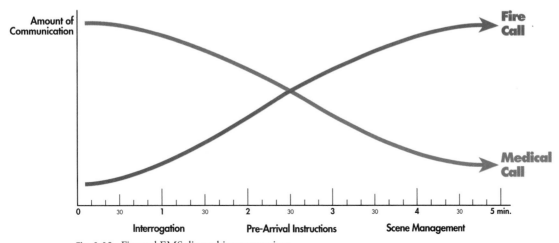

Fig. 1-13. Fire and EMS dispatching comparison.

Medical Control and the EMD

Success has spawned additional responsibilities for EMDs, now that they are more widely acknowledged to be members of the EMS team and the first professional link in the chain of survival. Because the EMD is interacting daily with people in medical crisis, there is a clear need for medically attuned input to the appropriateness of those actions. Thus the dispatch process comes under the watchful eyes of medical control.

Until recently, physician oversight of dispatchers lagged significantly behind other areas of pre-hospital care. The "out-of-sight, out-of-mind" physical existence of the EMD has been identified as a contributing factor to this evolutionary dawdling. The National Association of EMS Physicians published its position paper in 1989 that helped create the needed national-level emphasis on EMD:

> *Medical direction and control for the EMD and the dispatch center… constitutes part of the prescribed responsibilities of the medical director of the EMS system. The functions of emergency medical dispatching must include the use of predetermined questions, pre-arrival telephone instructions, and pre-assigned response levels and modes.*[20]

NAEMSP advocates thorough and correct implementation of emergency medical dispatch. The process of implementation must be regularly reviewed by impartial, objective people who understand the nature of the changes that have occurred. This includes those within the medical control structure who oversee the medical expertise and performance of EMDs.

> **Until recently, physician oversight of dispatchers lagged significantly behind other areas of prehospital care.**

As already stated, an EMD does not need to be an EMT or a paramedic. The curriculum and education needed for communication center activities are very different from those needed for hands-on care.[20] This means EMDs are increasingly recognized as medical colleagues in their own right. Although the way medical care is given differs, the EMD is as responsible as anyone who physically touches the patient. Imagine correctly helping a father deliver his child by telephone! Or knowing how to obtain and give the information necessary to provide correct, useful first-aid suggestions via telephone. When appropriate, the EMD should provide a brief telephonic hand-off report to field personnel when they arrive at the scene, just as other medical colleagues do face-to-face.

By both national and international standards, EMDs perform their duties under the guidance of medical control. Because of increased ex-posure to intervention opportunities, their actions should be properly and consistently reviewed through a management-based quality assurance and improvement process. This closely parallels the risk management programs established as a normal part of the practice of other allied health professionals.

> **The man who has never made a mistake will never make anything else.**
> **—George Bernard Shaw**

Who controls dispatch policy and practice? Many medically oriented participants in the process of developing EMD have hesitated because their medical connection to dispatch seems less tangible. The element of quality improvement and medical direction is presented in Chapter 12: Quality Management.

The Spock Principle

The advocacy of system versus patient is a dilemma continually facing the EMD in appropriately balancing the importance of one call with all potential calls. Managers and supervisors responsible for medical dispatch programs are also forced to deal with similar issues.

We have simplified the understanding of this aspect of medical dispatch from the ethical viewpoint of the "Spock Principle."[27, 28] At the end of the motion picture, Star Trek II, the Starship Enterprise faced certain destruction from a runaway fusion reactor. The logical Vulcan, Mr. Spock, placing personal safety aside, entered the main reactor area unprotected. Now exposed to lethal radiation, he repaired the engine, and saved the Enterprise and all on board. When asked by an emotional Captain Kirk why he did it, he gave the memorable reply, "The good of the many outweighs the needs of the few or even the one."

While the EMD is the caller's personal advocate during single call episodes (the one), the EMD must also maintain the continuous role of advocate of the system (the many). The process of safe and effective prioritization of calls, and even the activities within a call, allows the EMD to balance these competing responsibilities while adhering to this important principle.

Traditional Roadblocks to Change

In many cases, the hardest part in the local advancement to EMD is making the transition happen in the first place. Changing from an archaic system that has a weak link at the very spot where coordination and control ought to be strongest requires the support and encouragement of all levels of authority within a public safety or EMS system. The effect of resistance to change, especially by those in power, can be daunting! But the appeal of a well-rounded team that uses a system that can save money has enticed even hard-core bureaucrats to modify their thinking about EMD. With increased recognition as the international standard for medical dispatch, the arguments for implementation of priority dispatch are even more compelling.

It is said that the only person who likes change is a wet baby. The change process requires effort, enthusiasm, and energy. The status quo is usually much more appealing, particularly when implementation is going to be disruptive. Perhaps it would be more effective to focus on how to minimize the difficult aspects of change.

Change requires recognizing that humans are bound by habits. If a dispatcher is in the habit of hanging up on callers after getting the address and callback number, new behaviors must be learned. Fear is another common impediment to change. It is much easier to continue a familiar, if outdated, routine whether or not the old system is in the best interests of the community. Education maximizes the acceptance of the change process. Those convinced that priority dispatch is the best system must help those who resist by explaining the benefits of implementation, and the risks of not doing so. This becomes easier in an environment of support, particularly when the supporters are those with the power to mandate change.

The EMD as a Medical Professional

There is probably no medical profession other than emergency medical dispatching in which the core time for patient evaluation and decision making is routinely around one minute, and where more is potentially at stake on a case-by-case basis.[29] Unfortunately the EMD has not been generally accepted as a professional by EMTs, paramedics, and other members of the medical team. Thus, EMDs in many places, occupy somewhat ambiguous roles within the medical profession and public safety agencies.

One of the difficulties EMDs have had in gaining acceptance as medical professionals is that the rest of the medical profession isn't clear on the EMD's role and whether the EMD's tasks are truly medical. Most prehospital care providers are directed and regulated by medical control physicians and some form of governmental authority. In contrast, EMDs are typically hired, trained, managed and paid by law enforcement, fire, or ambulance agencies. In many areas, the EMD's practice lacks adequate medical control and management. No quality improvement is undertaken, and the dispatchers lack professional certification. However, properly-trained EMD performance is based on medical protocols similar to other medical professionals except in two ways; a lack of direct patient contact and the abbreviated decision-making time frame.

> **Education maximizes the acceptance of the change process.**

Practice Dissimilarities. EMDs essentially practice their profession via remote control, dealing nonvisually with someone who is generally not the patient. The lack of direct access requires EMDs to rely heavily on interrogative skills.

However, with tested protocol-driven questioning, EMDs can successfully elicit the necessary information to dispatch appropriate personnel with adequate information.

Unfortunately, in addition to the physical constraints, there exists system-imposed time limits on emergency medical dispatching. "The 60-second dilemma" was a phrase coined several years ago to emphasize that in today's high performance EMS systems, the EMD has only 60 seconds to interrogate (i.e., evaluate the situation) and render a decision (i.e., provisional diagnosis). Very few, if any, medical professionals are required to consistently perform the evaluation and decision-making part of their patient care process in 60 seconds. Even more astounding is that there is no scientific rationale for the 60-second time frame for dispatching.

The 60-second time interval should be used as a goal or objective to strive for in most situations—*not* a rule or absolute upper limit. In most medical situations, the time to dispatch should not be treated as a ticking time bomb, since the majority of incidents are not escalating in any appreciable way, whether life-threatening or otherwise. With this in mind, 75 to 90 seconds is a more reasonable goal for most calls of a non-time-life priority basis, and some places are instituting just that. As Thera Bradshaw, past-president of the National Emergency Number Association stated, "It's time we start doing it right, not just fast."

Patient Care Routines for EMD and EMS

EMD	Emergency Physician/Paramedic
Call receipt	Patient introduction
Case Entry interrogation	Primary survey
Four Commandments/questions	Vital signs
Immediate dispatch (when necessary)	Call for MD specialist
Pre-Arrival Instructions	Support ABCs
Key Questions interrogation	Secondary survey
Dispatch code selection	Working diagnosis/action plan
Routine dispatch (send mobile evaluators)	Further evaluation of patient (order lab tests, ECG, X-rays, etc.)
Post-Dispatch Instructions	Routine treatments
Case Review	Morbidity/mortality conferences
QA/QI processes	QA/QI processes
Total quality management	Professional review organization

Fig. 1-14. Comparison of similar roles and routines between EMDs and paramedics or emergency physicians.

Practice Similarities. Fortunately, the similarities between EMDs and other medical professionals are more prominent. In fact, the individual practice of a physician-managed EMD closely resembles the emergency medical model.

As is evident from the above comparison, the elements of medical care cross over easily and are equally relevant to both groups. For example, the primary survey must be as consistent and complete for the EMD as for the hands-on medical provider. No one can afford to abort or supersede this evaluation, no matter if these initial findings seem obvious. The importance of this is reflected in the "Four Commandments," the EMD's term for the dispatch primary survey. Like an inconsistent EMT who checks the airway, but not breathing and circulation, an EMD who does not always ask these four questions risks missing essential information. As with an EMT's secondary survey, these answers provide relevant information regarding patient care, scene safety and response choices. Omissions in the information-gathering process can result in sending the wrong response and providing the wrong treatments.

> **EMDs cannot assume answers to questions they never asked.**

Perhaps this point can be made by asking yourself, "When you or a family member are taken to the emergency department, do you want the emergency physician to perform a *complete* or an *incomplete* evaluation?" Keeping in mind that each of the interrogation questions may lead to a different evaluative conclusion, different treatment, different information relay, or different advice, EMDs cannot assume answers to questions they never ask. It is true that, "a thing not looked for is seldom found."

Compliance to the EMD protocol ensures all essential elements will be "found," and clarification or enhancement of the protocol will be accomplished only when necessary. In fact, EMD training directs that, "dispatch personnel will follow all protocols per se, avoiding freelance questioning or information unless it enhances not replaces, the written protocol questions and scripts."

The EMD as an Advanced Life Support Professional. It is widely believed a trained EMD is essentially a basic life support-level provider. Reacting to this notion, an EMD once stated in a self-mocking tone, "That's right, we're sub-basic life support life forms." This belief, however, is incorrect. The basis of the core curriculum for EMD training, specifically the "dispatch priorities" is, in fact, *advanced* life support-level.

What has confused most casual observers is that the EMD appears to perform basic life support-type tasks, such as **CPR**, the **Heimlich maneuver**, and airway control. However, the EMD is not required to *perform* the basic life support skill but *instruct* it on the fly. In fact, the majority of the information in the EMD curriculum is derived from the knowledge base of emergency physicians and nurses. For example, the commonly taught dispatch rule, "A healthy child (or young adult) found in cardiac arrest is considered to have a foreign body airway obstruction until proven otherwise," cannot be found in standard publications such as: Karren and Hafen's EMT text, Nancy Caroline's paramedic text, or the basic text by the American Academy of Orthopedic Surgeons. Most paramedics eventually learn this "rule" from emergency department physicians.

This level of knowledge is why it is necessary for **ALS**-level personnel (paramedics, RNs, and MDs) to train EMDs. No EMD training program should use non-ALS personnel as instructors. The use of specific EMD protocols to aid in the provision of a complete and comprehensive "remote" assessment of the patient in combination with on-the-fly bystander training requires that the EMD process information or "think like" ALS personnel.

The Medical versus the Protocol Models of Practice. With all this knowledge, then why shouldn't EMDs routinely practice their medical routines as doctors do—without a formal protocol in hand? After all, the practice of medicine by physicians appears to be safe without the use of well-defined protocols. The answer lies in a very important distinction between physicians and "paramedical" practice methods, which can be illustrated by comparing the "medical model" of medical practice with the "protocol model" of evaluation and care.

Physicians are allowed by law to deliver medicine in the way they deem best because of years of rigorous education and training and even more years of supervised post-doctoral practice. The seasoned practitioner in his or her office working from years of experience perhaps best illustrates the medical

> **Such "peripheral brains" are commonly used by medical professionals. They are called protocols.**

model of practice. In contrast, the new physician or intern with approximately 10,000 hours of medical training and experience on his or her first official day of practice is hardly an amateur, but a professional who relies on routine access to pertinent additional information. Pockets are stuffed with all kinds of

helpers: *The Harriet Lane Pediatric Handbook*, the *Washington Manual of Therapeutics*, the *Surgical Manual*, and a plethora of drug company-provided neonatal and gestational plastic calculators. Such "peripheral brains" are commonly used by medical professionals to ensure complete and accurate medical treatment under demanding time constraints. They are called protocols.

Compare to that, the typical paramedic who has 1,000 to 1,500 hours of training and the EMT who has 120 to 200 hours of training. The current minimum amount of training for an EMD is 24 hours. Thus, it's easy to see why an EMD may need a "peripheral brain." It need not be a big peripheral brain but simply well-designed, medically sound, and up-to-date.

The EMD and other out-of-hospital providers, therefore, use the protocol model of medical practice. The protocol model is the backbone of the EMD's permission from responsible medical authority to "practice" **dispatch life support** medicine. As such, compliance to the protocol model significantly enhances the EMD's method of practice by:

- Executing the basic rules of dispatch medicine.

- Standardizing patient and situational evaluations.

- Permitting the EMD to concentrate on processing obtained information.

- Reducing dispatcher bias by formalizing interrogation question structure.

- Structuring medical pathways to further evaluations, verifications, and necessary treatments.

- Reducing the time required for evaluation through optimization of interrogation and decision processes.

- Enabling rapid, consistent evaluation and treatment within a time-restricted environment.

For example, physicians and nurses use a protocol model for resuscitations and trauma codes. The whiteboard found in every major trauma room lists an orderly series of actions, tests, and treatments that must be accompanied in rapid but standardized resuscitative efforts—in essence, a protocol.

The EMD–EMS Partnership. The time has come when we must think of EMDs as medical professionals and, in every sense of the word, medical colleagues, who care for the patient when other medical professionals can't. They must receive the tools, training, and time to perform their jobs well. Doing it right is even more important than doing it fast. This fact should be understood and embraced by public safety management and medical control.

Rather than de-cry the formal use of protocol as somehow demeaning, punitive, robotic, or even non-medical, it is important to understand that it is the tool of *both* field practitioners and EMDs. It speeds up and improves the evaluation and decision-making in both EMD and traditional medical practice.

> **EMDs must receive the tools, training, and time to perform their jobs well.**

Non-EMDs can help the professionalization process in a number of ways. Ask about EMDs in prehospital care surveys. Recognize them as part of the EMS team in papers and articles. Routinely list them as part of the medical control span of responsibility. Include them in consideration of EMS funding issues as well as for reasonable parity in pay.

EMDs can demonstrate their professionalism to their medical colleagues by seeking on-going medical dispatch education to keep current as their relatively new profession and protocol evolve: certifying and re-certifying; being customer service-oriented, rather than complaint-driven and reactive in attitude; and maintaining and demonstrating a high respect for the human conditions entrusted to them, whether minor indecision on the part of the caller, or outright terror at the scene. Such actions by those in responsible positions within public safety, EMS, and the medical community, as well as by EMDs themselves, will ultimately place the label of "medical professional" on the EMD, where it should have been all along.

> **Include EMDs in consideration of EMS funding issues as well as for reasonable parity in pay.**

Summary: A New Era In EMS

In response to the growing acceptance of priority dispatch, the standards of acceptable system design for communication centers have been redefined. No longer is it tolerable for the dispatch office to be the receptacle of marginal or disciplined field providers. Once viewed as a good location for organizational dumping of sick or injured personnel, the up-to-date communication center now enjoys increased levels of respect and professionalism.

Selective prioritization of calls does not equal downgrading of service. True, it may reduce the thrill and the drama associated with seeing several emergency units roar by. But in the end, it upgrades the quality of care in the community in many ways: fewer accidents, better understanding of the problem before arrival, better preparation by the crews as to what to expect, and more enthusiastic crews. They know chances are good that their skills are what is needed at a particular scene.

> **No longer is it tolerable for the dispatch office to be the receptacle of marginal field providers.**

Pressures to hold down the cost of municipal services will increase in coming years. Traditional medical care has been replaced by a more cost-conscious process of managed care. Priority dispatch allows the EMS team to not respond reflexively, but with the informed, trained capability now within reach of the medically trained telecommunication specialist—the Emergency Medical Dispatcher.

Change is the way the future reveals itself.
                    —Unknown futurist

6 BREATH...
7 BURNS (SCALDS) / EXPLOSION
8 CARBON MONOXIDE / INHALATION/HAZMAT
9 CARDIAC OR RESPIRATORY ARREST / DEATH

KEY QUESTIONS
1. Did you see what happened?
   a. **(Yes)** Did s/he **choke** on anything first? _____update code to 11-E-1
      Yes
2. **(Appropriate ≥ 8)** Is there a **defibrillator** (AED) available?
3. **(Suspected death)** Tell me please, **why** does it look like s/he's **dead?**
   a. **(OBVIOUS DEATH)** Do you think s/he is **beyond** any **help** (resuscitation/CPR)? ✪
   b. **(EXPECTED DEATH)** Are you **certain** we should **not** try to **resuscitate** her/him? ✪

POST-DISPATCH INSTRUCTIO...
a. **(Suspected Workable Arrest)** (ambulance) to help you now. **Stay on the line** and I'll tell y...
b. **(OBVIOUS or EXPECTED DE...** to assist you. Is there anyt...

* (OBVIOUS or EXPECTI...

DLS   * Link to ☎ A...
Danger or Contamination
Suspected Workable Ar...
AED available (age ≥ 8)
Choked first _____
                                    CODE...

LEVELS # DETERMINANT DESCRIPTORS

E 1 Suspected Workable Arrest
         (NOT BREATHING/INEFFECTIVE BREATHING)
   a. **Not breathing** at all
   b. **Breathing uncertain** (agonal)
   c. **Hanging**   * (to be selected from Case Entry only)
   d. **Strangulation**
   e. **Suffocation**
   f. **Underwater**

D 1 INEFFECTIVE BREATHING (discovered during Key Questioning only)
      * (select only when bridging from other **Chief Complaint** protocols

B 1 OBVIOUS DEATH (unquestionable)

Ω 1 EXPECTED DEATH (unquestionable)

This protocol system for use under MPDS™ license agreement only. U.S. Patent 5,857,966. © 2000 Medical Priority Consultants...

Contents

EXPECTED DEATH
Local Medical Control must define and authorize (DS) any of the patient conditions below before this determinant can be used. Situations should be unquestionable and may include:
☐ Cold and stiff in a warm environment
☐ Decapitation
☐ Decomposition
☐ Explosive gunshot wound to the head
☐ Incineration
☐ **NON-RECENT** death
☐ Severe injuries obviously incompatible with life
☐ Submersion (> 6hrs)

NON-RECENT
Six hours or more have passed since the incident or injury occurred.

INEFFECTIVE BREATHING
The following, when volunteered at any point during Case Entry
• "Barely breathing"
• "Can't breathe at all"
• "Fighting for air" (agonal respirations)
• "Gasping for air" (agonal respirations)
• "Making funny noises" (agonal respirations)
• "Not breathing"
• "Turning blue or purple"

Rules
Often, when faced with a dying **DNR** patient, **callers just want reassurance** that doing the right thing...

3. An unconscious person in whom breathing cannot be verified by a 2nd party caller (with the patient) is considered to be **in cardiac arrest until proven otherwise.**
4. When the initial **Chief Complaint appears to be seizure,** use Protocol 12 regardless of consciousness and breathing status.

Axioms
1. "Funny noises" reported by the caller generally means the patient is unconscious with an uncontrolled airway and often represents agon... (dying) respirations at the beginn... **cardiac arrest.**
2. Agonal respirations can be co... with "still breathing" before away during an arrest.
3. Automated external defibr... might also be called "sh... Other local names may...

CHAPTER 2

Basic Telecommunication Techniques

Chapter Overview

Few people are really talented at telecommunication. Even for those who are, it requires practice and dedication to organize and process multiple simultaneous tasks. The basic roles and responsibilities of an EMD include telephone interrogation, radio dispatch, prioritizing responses to emergencies that compete for time and resources, logistics coordination among crews at various settings, resource backup, and long-distance lifesaving via pre-arrival telephone instructions.

Dispatch centers vary. Some assign different people to each function; others have only one person to perform all functions. Some centers are handled by volunteers. Regardless of the setup, the EMD must always strive to behave in the most professional manner possible. This chapter outlines basic telecommunication techniques for radio and telephone operations. It includes tips for beginners and experienced dispatchers. After all, a professional knows there is always more to learn.

Remember not only to say the right thing in the right place, but, far more difficult, to leave unsaid the wrong thing at the tempting moment.

—*Benjamin Franklin*

There is a misconception among many people that all it takes to be an emergency telecommunication specialist is to sit down in front of a lot of equipment and push buttons.[169] But the ability to talk does not necessarily equal the attribute of communicating. And just because a person is raised using telephones does not mean anybody can dispatch. The nature of emergency medical telecommunication has changed, just as field care has. The difference is education. Field providers aren't just ambulance drivers anymore. They are EMTs and paramedics; their titles signify role sophistication. In the communication center, the familiar term may still be "dispatcher," but pity the person who does not understand the demands and extent of an ETC's (certified Emergency TeleCommunicator) and EMD's responsibilities.[169]

Being a good dispatcher requires many quick-witted skills. Numerous telecommunication techniques can make a major difference in dispatcher effectiveness. These attributes are even more admirable when seasoned with experience. It is an incorrect (but, in places, enduring) perception that the dispatch office is the *weak link* in the helping chain.

> **The provision of customer service during the difficult and challenging situations facing EMDs every day is the mark of an excellent telecommunicator in action.**

While mastering the time-driven tasks discussed in this text, the essence of superior telecommunicators are not always the things they accomplish, but, more importantly, how they are accomplished. The provision of *customer service* during the difficult and challenging situations facing EMDs every day is the mark of an excellent telecommunicator in action.

Dispatching does not occur in the spotlight. Since it is a somewhat obscure activity, it has not been perceived traditionally as glamorous or prestigious. However, the difference between a case handled and a case handled *well* often stems from the abilities of the person overseeing the event from the hidden realm of the communication center. Emergency medical dispatch is finally getting the *respect* it has long deserved.

The EMD attends to six basic areas of activity.[14]

• Telephone Interrogation (input)

• Dispatch Allocation (field communication)

• Triage

• Logistics Coordination

• Resource Networking

• Life-Impacting via Telephone

These roles are discussed in detail in this chapter. Additional topics addressed are: specific telephone techniques, mechanics of good telecommunication, special situations (such as elderly and very young callers), inappropriate activities, coordination with other agencies, and ways of coping with dispatch overload.

Six Roles of Telecommunication

Telephone Interrogation (input): Telephone interrogation can be one of the dispatcher's greatest challenges but it's crucial to the success of a call. As if it is not difficult enough by itself, telephone interrogation must often be done in conjunction with other tasks. The EMD's focus is constantly switching from the telephone to the radio to the computer to other demands of a dispatch office. The variety can be entertaining, but it occasionally makes the communication center a hotbed of activity—with the EMD on the coals!

> **The caller can clearly perceive the EMD's professionalism (or lack of it).**

Most emergency responses originate with a telephone conversation. Seldom does a field unit stumble across an emergency situation, and relatively few calls are referred from affiliated emergency agencies. The dispatcher must first control the telephone conversation, thereby setting the tone for managing the situation. Through appropriate interrogation, the EMD obtains the information needed to begin the next part of the emergency care process.

Interrogation is generically referred to as the "input" function of the EMD. Since dispatch is a non-visual world, a lot of verbal psychology is used by those professional EMDs who have mastered the art of culling the right information from the caller. It has been said that understanding this process in-depth could involve enough study, learning, and practice to achieve a minor degree in college.

For some reason, the term calltaker does a disservice to this aspect of telecommunicating. You are not just "taking" a call. That implies gathering the address and pointing in the direction of the smoke, commotion, or pile of bodies. The ability to obtain useful information is worth its weight in gold. Anybody can "ask a bunch of questions." But the ability to successfully evaluate a situation is core to the professional nature of dispatching. As the old saying goes, "garbage in, garbage out."

The EMD is the first link between the caller and the emergency care system—the first helping hand in a crisis. When the beginning goes well, it can make a profound difference in the progress of a call. First impressions do matter. The caller can clearly perceive the EMD's professionalism (or lack of it). Dispatcher sarcasm, disinterest, cynicism, or disdain can impact the entire call. These attitudes, if present, are often apparent to a caller even if they are not openly expressed. Arriving prehospital crews may suffer negative repercussions that the EMD never knows about. In potentially violent situations, the result of the EMD's mis-actions on the telephone can even be tragic.

On the other hand, if the EMD's voice is warm, caring, polite, interested, sympathetic, non-judgmental, and otherwise indicates a positive approach to the caller's sense of emergency, the setting may be entirely different for arriving crews. A positive tone of voice is an excellent way to begin interacting with strangers, especially those in crisis.

> **The professional EMD would never make independent, biased, or prejudicial decisions about the resources to send on a call.**

The professional EMD must take care to *never* make dispatch decisions or judgments based on a caller's demeanor. The EMD should never bypass the fail-safe mechanisms built into the priority dispatch protocol, particularly the Four Commandment questions and key questions. It may be a normal human reaction in non-professionals to respond in kind to how others treat them; to be angry with angry callers, snide with snide callers, or profane with profane callers. It is tempting to apply derogatory labels to some callers. Such reactions, however, are neither normal nor acceptable for the professional EMD, who would never make independent, biased, or prejudicial decisions about the resources to send on a call.

Many EMS calls sound bizarre, questionable, or plain funny. The EMD hears everything from, "There's been a terrible explosion!" to, "I can't zip up my pants," or, "Just send the *@#$&% paramedics right now!" In the first case, the EMD can easily sense a really bad situation. Anyone would react to it right away. In the second, the call may sound phony, or at least minor.

The second example led crews to a patient who had a serious cardiac arrhythmia, causing his legs and groin to swell to an unbelievable degree! In the third case, the professional EMD must allow the profanity to pass without comment, and instead focus on working with the caller on the *facts* of the case—no matter how unpleasant the conversation may be. Even when a caller's honesty or integrity is questionable, the EMD must take the caller's information at face value and proceed accordingly.

> **Even when a caller's honesty or integrity is questionable, the EMD must take the caller's information at face value and proceed accordingly.**

EMD's First Rule of Judgment
The EMD is never allowed to judge the integrity or honesty of the caller.

The right to judge the caller or patient's intent is *always* left to in-person professionals: law enforcement, firefighters, EMTs, ambulance officers, or paramedics.

In both telephone and radio work, it is natural to recall situations similar to the one at hand and to assume that similar circumstances will produce similar results. They may not. Apply personal lessons of experience judiciously. Experience helps build a basis for decision-making, but be careful about being influenced inappropriately. Be patient with each new situation. All drunken people are not alike (and all "drunks" are not really drunk).

EMD's Second Rule of Judgment
The caller is not the patient.

Avoid stereotyping parts of town, types of people, or times of day. Some violent and unmannerly people live in the poshest part of town. It is demonstrably not true that, "nothing ever happens at 5 a.m." Build on the experiences of the past, but do not depend on stereotypes to hold true in every case. Apply this concept to both good and bad experiences.

Some callers abuse the EMS system.[30] They make phony calls for help or get angry when *the system* does not provide instantaneous results. The difference between those callers and the professional EMD is that the EMD is aware of the complexity of human emotion and motivation. An EMD can wipe the emotional slate clean between each new call for help. Professional EMDs seldom, if ever, let the obnoxious aspects of dispatch get under their skin—and they know how to cope with it *appropriately* if it does happen.[60]

Dispatch Allocation and Field Communication (output): Also known as radio "dispatch," once pertinent information has been obtained, it must be quickly and succinctly shared with the responders. The ability to synthesize variously useful piles of *data* into *information* is key to this specific role of dispatching. As an apparent carry over from law enforcement dispatching, the constant cry to minimize "air time" has been overused and over-emphasized in EMS. Saying it right is more important than saying it short or fast (although no one is arguing with "short, right, *and* fast").

The allocator (an emerging term for radio dispatch) must also select and approve the unit assignment recommended by the calltaker (or CAD program). Depending on local setup, the EMD may also be responsible for opening a telecommunication channel between field EMS providers and medical care and control facilities. This may include radio, telephone patch, **telecommunication device for the deaf (TDD)**, **biomedical telemetry**, or other high-tech capabilities.

Intimate familiarity with the technology is paramount. Good training is essential. It is unacceptable for dispatch training to consist of watching another dispatcher do the job for a week or two. The British call this "sitting with Nellie" and many a trainee has merely learned the mistakes of the old-timer by just observing. The neophyte then goes to work, perhaps without a clear understanding of the equipment and without even having experience with some of it. Nothing is as uncomfortable as being turned loose at the console without feeling prepared to respond correctly to each button and alarm. Worse, there may be few subsequent opportunities to remedy the situation—or even recognize that certain dispatch behaviors are inappropriate.

> **Many a trainee has merely learned the mistakes of the old-timer by just observing.**

Experience is one of the best trainers of all, but that takes time. Dispatch novices can strengthen their capabilities by studying maps, asking questions, getting as much training as possible, and familiarizing themselves with the various rapid-reference resources available.

It helps to review seldom-used options frequently, such as telephone patching or phone traces. Instead of slipping into the complacency that seldom used capabilities will never be needed, invite field personnel to practice phone patches and other unusual telecommunication maneuvers regularly. This has two benefits: the EMD can use the equipment readily, and the various communication options are highlighted for field personnel. With the increased prevalence of computerization, much of this information is now accessible literally at the touch of a keyboard.

> **Any time there is a question of access, the EMD must work carefully with the caller to ensure prompt arrival of emergency crews.**

Triage: The EMD's main task is to determine the relative importance of each call and which emergency crew can best handle it according to various factors (such as location or severity). Someone with a broken leg on a quiet day may get a response that could not be duplicated during a mass casualty situation. **Triage** (from the French language) means to "sort out."

EMD's First Law of the Courtroom

If you didn't write it down, you didn't do it.

The EMD must record information as soon as it is gathered, usually on standard forms or through computerized procedures. (Computerized systems greatly facilitate long-needed data collection and analysis.) Complete documentation is very important for legal purposes. For example, recording times should be second nature to every dispatcher. Do not rely on memory, or even on the back-up taping systems. Each fails sometimes. For dispatch systems not using CAD, all call times and EMD actions should be written down or time-stamped.

Logistics Coordination: An obvious task is to maintain up-to-date knowledge of the status of available EMS resources. Without knowing where all the prehospital personnel are, the EMD cannot dispatch the closest crew. A thorough knowledge of the district, and of the best routes of response from place to place, must be adjusted according to changing geographic constraints such as rush hour. For example, perhaps a time-critical emergency comes in near where the EMD knows a crew is handling a minor call. If the first call is not a transport situation, that crew might be able to handle the time-critical call sooner than another crew could arrive. No one knows staffing patterns better than the EMD. Logistics coordination includes making it as easy as possible for responding crews to access the scene. Any time there is a question of access, the EMD must work carefully with the caller to ensure prompt arrival and interface of emergency crews. Prehospital personnel already face numerous obstacles:

- Few homeowners realize that emergency providers may not be able to see their house numbers from the street, especially in the dark or in inclement weather.

- In cities, skyscrapers may have numerous entrances and different elevator banks. Waiting for an elevator takes time, as does a ride to the top when others are stopping it to enter and exit. Arriving at a high-rise and getting to the patient are two distinctly different events!

- Some apartment or condominium complexes use a code number instead of the dweller's name on the buzzer. Responders must know the code to avoid access delays. Access may also be held up by fences at the street entry that require special keys or codes to open.

- Some communities paint house numbers along the curb. This system works well—until some one parks in front of the number, leaves collect in the gutter, or it snows.

- In rural areas, the challenge of address access may be alleviated somewhat by familiarity with "Farmer Connor's red barn" and other prominent landmarks. However, landmarks often disappear, especially when real estate developers come in. The EMD must be ready to help responding crews with the logistics of access.

EMD's First Rule of Scene Command

Until field responders arrive, no one can know more about the scene than the EMD.

There are various ways to enlist the help of someone at the scene with access. If someone is available, that person can turn on outside lights, or open the garage door and turn on the light. Blinking those lights might help when access is difficult. Relay a description of the house or apartment, or of vehicles in the driveway. Easily identified landmarks can greatly assist emergency crews.

Residents of high-rise buildings can also assist field personnel in reaching the patient. They can notify building security that an emergency exists. Security personnel can reserve an elevator, meet the crews at the entrance, unlock the front gate to the driveway (if necessary), and guide them to the apartment or office involved.

> **Easily identified landmarks can greatly assist emergency crews.**

Other access situations can be yet more confusing. In some apartment complexes, Building "F" is next to Building "M" (and the building letters may be nearly impossible to see anyway). The EMD can suggest that someone meet the crews at the complex entrance. In rural areas, it might be helpful for someone to meet the ambulance crew at the turnoff from the main road; or to advise them to use a flashlight at night.

There are other logistical services that the EMD can provide. Imagine that a shooting occurs on the east side of town, warranting a maximum response of closest first responders, advanced life support, and transport unit. The trauma center is three minutes away. The only available advanced life support unit is 15 minutes away, and the basic life support crew arrives in one minute. The EMD can advise the basic life support providers that it will take longer for the advanced life support crew to

> **Wisdom is knowing when to speak your mind and when to mind your speech.**
> **—Evangel**

get to the scene than it would for them to take this patient to the trauma center themselves. This logistical advice may be lifesaving in such time-critical instances. What to do is ultimately a field decision, but without the EMD's logistical input, field crews may have no way to weigh the options. The ability to perceive the "Big Picture" and relay it appropriately is a great attribute of a good EMD.

The EMD also facilitates mutual aid. Coordinating and linking the involved public safety services (e.g., fire, police, EMS, helicopters, hazardous materials, extrication, rescue, etc.) requires good communication and multi-tasking skills. Finally, the EMD must balance the flow of information so enough is said without saying too much. Do not waste others' time trying to satisfy curiosity about what is going on out there.

Resource Networking: The dispatcher is the ultimate resource person for the EMS system. The EMD must know the resources that can give prehospital personnel the best chance to cope successfully with each case. For example, field personnel are usually in no position to call the electric company to turn off power to a certain area or to send a lineman to assist. But the EMD can.

One resource that may be needed occasionally is telephone number tracing. However, with the addition of enhanced 9-1-1 systems this need is being reduced. The EMD must know how to implement the procedures for requesting telephone traces. Until the address is known, no one but the dispatcher can help. These procedures should already be clearly defined. If they are not, a good starting point is to call the security department at the local telephone company. The process may vary from place to place.

> **The EMD must balance the flow of information so enough is said without saying too much.**

As soon as the EMD recognizes the need trace the call, the proper individual at the telephone company may be contacted on another telephone line. Traces are easier in areas with enhanced 9-1-1 capability, since permanent traps have been included in the system for tracing caller addresses. In areas without enhanced 9-1-1, the procedure involves keeping the telephone connection long enough to trace the call through the system.

The time needed to do a phone trace varies depending on the equipment. In areas with electronic switching, an answer may be available rapidly. In areas with mechanical switching, a person must be sent to the switching station (if it is normally unmanned), and the call traced manually. This obviously takes time, especially if a telephone company employee has to be awakened in the middle of the night to go to the switching station.

Because there are a number of agencies and groups who would like phone traces (such as various crisis lines, annoyance-call recipients, and others) telephone companies may have a policy of releasing addresses only to local law enforcement. Be prepared to tell them whom to call at the police department if alternative arrangements have not been made. The more recent advent of caller ID (like enhanced 9-1-1) can provide caller phone number identification for non-emergency links.

Resource networking also extends to the media. Many dispatch centers have specific protocols for dealing with the press. Know the policy and stick to it. If official protocols do not exist, the EMD must be careful what information is shared with the media. At the same time, do not play unnecessary games with reporters. They have a job to do too. Certain information is within their *right to know*, and it should be given readily; this includes the EMD's name and title, and generalities about what has occurred.

Above all, the EMD must guard patient **confidentiality**, especially when discussing names or patient status on the air. This can be very difficult in smaller communities where names are more familiar and many people have scanners, citizen-band radios (CB), or are just eavesdropping. Others around the radio at the scene can often hear what you say. Patient name and status should not be disclosed until next of kin have been identified (see figure 2.4).

> **The EMD must guard patient confidentiality, especially when discussing names or patient status on the air.**

As a resource person, the EMD also integrates information. The opportunity to provide continuity from day to day and hour to hour is obvious. For example, if something about a caller reminds the EMD of a similar call a couple of weeks ago, and that call resulted in the use of a deadly weapon, the EMD can alert the crew. Certain addresses become familiar over time. Occasionally, individuals learn to work the EMS system to their advantage and know the right buzz words to generate a big response. Luckily, this problem is quite rare and has not appeared to increase over time. Again, take care not to judge. Send first, *then* advise.

In some jurisdictions, system policies, and even public ordinances,[30] have evolved for handling people who call for emergency medical attention frequently and frivolously (see Salt Lake City EMS Abuse Ordinance, Appendix C). The EMD can advise on-coming crews, for example, that false calls have been coming in all day long from the neighborhood to which they are responding. An attentive EMD provides this sort of continuity as field staffing changes.

> **An attentive EMD provides continuity as field staffing changes.**

Knowing how to provide resource information quickly for unusual situations can be a uniquely challenging part of the job. It is easy to be complacent with the status quo. This increases the risk of a rude awakening when something out of the ordinary happens. Be ready to use all the various resources available in the dispatch office. Even those that are seldom used are familiar to a professional EMD.

Finally, field personnel may not know about the resources available to them through the EMD. It might benefit everyone to speak about communication resources at continuing medical education meetings.

Life-Impacting via Telephone Instructions: The EMD has a real chance to impact the ultimate outcome of sick and injured people. This is done via post-dispatch and pre-arrival instructions.

It is important, however, to understand the limitations of the system. Almost all callers, with the help of the EMD, are willing to intervene and provide first aid. But offers to assist with pre-arrival first aid may be refused. A few callers have no interest in getting involved. This is their choice. Others have physical limitations, such as age or physical disability.

Even if the EMD offers and is refused, a subtle message is still given. Because a caller now knows that pre-arrival assistance is available, he may be more emotionally prepared to use it another time. The strategy of avoiding even the appearance of asking the caller's permission to give pre-arrival instructions is discussed in Chapter 11: Legal Aspects of EMD.

Specific Telephone Techniques

There are specific techniques and strategies which can help the EMD handle the volume and types of calls that come in. These can make both telephone and radio interactions more positive and rewarding.

EMD's First Rule of Incoming Calls

Expect each call to be an emergency until proven otherwise.

Even though most emergency calls—especially in urban areas—turn out to be relatively minor, each new encounter represents the chance that a true emergency exists. This automatically places the EMD in an attitude that promotes quick thinking, instead of having to gear up on those occasions when close attention is immediately needed.

Remember, any call you receive is now *your call* and remains so legally and morally until properly transferred

EMD's Second Rule of Incoming Calls

Accept all emergency calls (even if they are from the wrong area).

to the correct public safety agency. Obtain complete information and forward it to the proper jurisdiction. Never make a caller redial in an emergency. Imagine how it must feel for someone in crisis, confronted by an emergency, to be told to redial and explain the situation all over again! Some people put in that position will just say, "Ah, to heck with it" and try driving the victim quickly to the hospital in the family car. During the stress of an emergency, untrained drivers exhibit poor driving techniques, endangering innocent people along the way. Emergency callers should never be expected to understand jurisdictional boundaries and other EMS system parameters. That remains our job.

EMDs must answer each call promptly. To the caller, each ring feels like an eternity. Also, ring cycles can differ from one end of the line to the other. If the EMD hears two rings, the caller may have heard three (or more) ring signals at the other end. Try to answer within two rings (the retail business standard is three). Handle emergency lines first, business lines next. (It is important, however, to answer business lines promptly, since emergencies sometimes come in on non-emergency lines as well.) This is particularly true in areas where night and weekend dispatchers answer municipal telephones after business hours.

The EMD can reassure callers that they have dialed correctly and accessed a source for help. This is imparted nonverbally when the EMD can *smile* with their voice. In fact, if a person actually smiles when hearing the telephone ring (but before contact with the caller), it is surprising just how much difference this makes in removing the stress and strain from the tone of voice. Although emergency medical dispatching is a high-pressure job, it is possible to sound helpful to encourage and reassure the caller. After all, the caller is simply obeying the rules for handling an emergency that have been drilled in time and again, "Dial 9-1-1! Don't try to handle things yourself!" Callers do not care, or even understand, that the EMD may be juggling several situations at once.

Keep in mind the caller's feelings. Visualize the caller and imagine being in that person's situation. There is a balance between becoming too emotionally invested in callers and not invested enough—but it is okay to have some human concern. Even if the Chief Complaint does not sound too terrible, remember that people in

> **There is a balance between becoming too emotionally invested in callers and not invested enough.**

EMS handle emergencies daily; the general population does not. It is easier to remain empathetic when the EMD can stay in tune with the caller's likely emotions (such as anxiety, fear, confusion, or panic). Remember, the telephone is the caller's only link to assistance until field responders arrive.

Use the caller's name often. This is very reassuring. It humanizes the situation, shows special interest in the call, and can help calm antagonistic callers. However, be sensitive about how a caller wishes to be addressed; using a stranger's first name can impart unintended familiarity. The best clue to how the caller prefers to be addressed is obtained in response to the question, "What is your name?"

When in doubt, it is best to use a formal title, such as, "Mr. Smith" or, "Ms. Russell." This can contribute to a sense of control for the caller at an important time. It is generally okay to use first names when dealing with children, or adolescents, or during the provision of pre-arrival instructions.

When multiple calls happen, the EMD has a responsibility to other callers too. If it becomes necessary to put a caller on hold, explain what is happening and why, "Ma'am I need to talk to the paramedics, I'll put you on hold for a minute. Please stay on the line. Don't hang up." Juggling radio traffic plus the emergency phone lines is a frequent dilemma. But after about 17 seconds someone on hold begins to feel forgotten. Avoid making a caller wait longer than that.

> **Use first names when dealing with children, adolescents, or during the provision of pre-arrival instructions.**

A common trap among dispatchers, especially in quiet EMS systems or on quiet shifts, is to become lethargic or bored. Snapping into an appropriate frame of mind instantly is hard. Guard against this by being prepared and staying alert for calls. Scrambling for a pen or pencil or having to get feet, newspapers, schoolwork, or food off the console quickly to be in the correct position to handle the computer keyboard or other technology can lead to unnecessary mistakes. It might even lead to the unforgivable sin of showering sensitive equipment with a spilled drink.

Another form of being unprepared stems from preoccupation with outside events. EMDs are susceptible to worrying about the same things that concern other people: mortgage payments, relationships with loved ones, finagling time off for an upcoming conference or sports event, and watching soap operas, etc. Learn to mentally compartmentalize those preoccupations quickly when the phone rings, to give undivided attention to the caller and the situation at hand. Mental alertness and the ability to adapt quickly counts.

Strategies for Good Telecommunication

Good telecommunication abilities are important to both telephone and radio communication. For example, certain vocal mechanics can expedite the process. Speak clearly, distinctly, and with adequate volume. People who mumble, or who have very breathy voices need to adjust these characteristics. No one likes to waste valuable air time repeating unintelligible messages.

Speak at a reasonable rate. The pace within the dispatch office can be very fast, so the EMD usually needs to slow down. One dispatcher had a habit of delivering *all* of the information about a call in the first transmission, "Ambulance Seven, Code Three, 9464 Conservation, on a fall from a tree." (This was in a system not using the EMD model.)

> **Always speak clearly, distinctly and with adequate volume when sending information over the radio.**

To a crew that has slipped into the lethargy of several hours of waiting for a call, this is an overwhelming amount of information. That crew cannot be expected to absorb so much information so fast, especially if it is the middle of the night or if they have a handful of fast food.

That dispatcher invariably had to repeat himself. At the same time, he made it abundantly clear by his tone of voice that the paramedics must be morons for not catching the entire message the first time. This is poor interpersonal communication. Better to accept that, whereas the EMD has to remain alert to function as the initial public contact, field personnel have some cushion. In fact, many EMS responders expect to sleep on the job since their shift structure may consist of 24- or 48-hour tours of duty.

Another common error is wordiness. Avoid it. Be efficient when choosing words. Compare the following:

Bad: "Attention Ambulance 508, we need you to respond Code Three as quickly as possible on an elderly, unconscious, not breathing man with a chief complaint of possible cardiac arrest, at 2159 Hannibal Street. We are starting to give telephone CPR instruction to his wife. That's all the information we have right now."

Good: "Ambulance 508, 9-ECHO-1a on a suspected cardiac arrest. 2159 Hannibal Street. Elderly male, unconscious, not breathing. Phone CPR in progress."

That is 51 words versus 22 words. The words "attention" and "possible" are wordy; the tone alert preceding the transmission brought the crew to alertness. "We need you to respond," and, "as quickly as possible," are both inherent within the context of a time critical message. "That's all the information we have right now" is implied when the transmission stops. *Listen to radio reports and to tapes of phone conversations.* Notice wordy habits and work hard to minimize them.

Note whether the person at the other end of the radio or phone can hear. Ask about it. Perhaps the EMD's rate of speech is too fast, or the volume too soft. Mechanical interference may stem from food, gum, or smoking a cigarette. These activities can prevent one from speaking directly into the mouthpiece or headset. In addition, be aware of the positioning of the speaker or headset. Something as minor as dropping the telephone receiver an inch or two below the chin can muffle one's voice and make it difficult for others to hear. Conversely, *eating* the microphone can over-resonate the voice.

It's also valid to check whether messages have been received accurately. On first verification, have the caller repeat the address and call-back telephone number. Nicely ask, "Please repeat your address *for verification.*" Verify the telephone number in the same way. Then, if there is any question, repeat the information back to the caller. Radios sometimes transmit in broken patches, so technology can even interfere with the transmission of information. Always clarify whenever there is any doubt.

> **Nicely ask, "Please repeat your address for verification."**

At times it is necessary to get to the caller's level to get the information needed. The voice necessary to reach and comfort a child may not please the chairman of the board. People are individuals and do not fit a single mold. Rather than forcing a stranger to fit the EMD's style, the EMD should fit the caller's needs. The result is greater success at penetrating the haze of excitement that can surround calls for emergency help. Know how to rephrase messages, if not initially understood. Be as kind and empathetic as the situation warrants.

For example, one dispatcher was having a very difficult time with an inebriated caller one night. "Where are you?" he asked repeatedly. "Right here," the caller kept saying. He and the other dispatcher tried different ploys to discover the caller's location. Finally, the dispatcher had a thought, "Hey, if we wanted to send you a pizza right now, where would we send it?" This was a very creative solution to a difficult situation!

Using precise English, French, Italian, German, Spanish, or Finnish—whatever the case may be—also minimizes obstacles to effective telecommunication. Avoid jargon, slang, codes, medical terms, and other confusing semantics except when they are appropriate and understandable to the listener. The term, *code three* to a lay person may be impressive, but she will not understand your message as readily as the term *lights-and-siren.*

> **Avoid jargon, slang, codes, medical terms, and other confusing semantics except when they are appropriate and understandable to the listener.**

How to judge what usage of the language is appropriate is a minute-by-minute decision, depending on who is on the line: a child, a caller not using the primary language, a doctor, a paramedic, the media, your mother, or others. The term *en route*—while common responder jargon—may be misunderstood by callers outside of French-speaking areas.

On the other hand, be aware of the various local slang terms for medical problems and situations. To *fall out* in some U.S. cities means to lose consciousness, not a fall from a height. Slang terms come and go; stay current with local street terms to avoid embarrassing misperceptions about the nature of a call.

> **Slang terms come and go; stay current with local street terms to avoid embarrassing misperceptions about the nature of a call.**

For example, in the U.K., *collapse* is used as a noun, "We have a woman in collapse." An interesting phrase used in some areas of England is *off his legs*. This is roughly equivalent to what North Americans mean by *man down*.

Once the EMS response has been sent, collect further information about additional scene hazards, or specifics about the patient's condition. Relay pertinent findings to responding units. If the caller is able to provide initial emergency care, proceed into Dispatch Life Support (DLS: PAIs, PDIs, and the Exit–X–sequence) as directed by the protocol.

Instructions on the X-protocol include:

• Gathering patient's medications

• Writing down the doctor's name

• Turning on an outside light

• Unlocking the front door

• Locking up the dog in the bathroom (see Authors' Note)

• Having someone meet the ambulance

These and other useful activities are especially good when the caller is unable to do first aid. Purposeful activity helps people stay calm, just as its equivalent of "deputizing bystanders" works for field personnel.

> **! Authors' Note**
>
> The bathroom is a preferred location to temporarily place dogs and cats since if everyone leaves the scene and the animal is left in a room, an open (flushed) toilet is a water source.

The EMD does not always stay on the telephone with the caller after giving post-dispatch instructions. Thus, there is an all-important final tactic: encourage callers to follow the universal post-dispatch instruction given here.

> **The Universal Post-Dispatch Instruction**
>
> If s/he gets **worse** in any way, **call** me **back immediately** for **further instructions**.

Special Caller Situations

Some situations cause particular challenges (especially in telecommunication) because the only way to touch the person at the other side is by voice. Populations that tend to require special communication efforts include elderly people, children, people who do not speak the primary language well, people who have difficulty speaking (dysphonia) or use an augmentative communication device.

Elderly people tend to process sensory input more slowly than younger people. The problem is related more to rate than to volume. EMDs may ask too much, too fast. To communicate with elders effectively, the EMD should use a slower-than-normal rate of speech, keep sentences short and to the point, and ask one question at a time. Some older people are also hard of hearing. It is not necessary to shout; this only distorts those words that do penetrate. Enunciate clearly, without exaggeration. Rate often counts more than volume.

Many people encountering the acute stress of a medical emergency regress to a more childlike state. Someone may seem all right outwardly, yet be in knots inside. When this happens in elderly people, they may experience memory blocks. The caller may be unable to provide even familiar data such as the address they have lived at for decades. Be patient. Rather than becoming increasingly demanding, try to reassure the caller. ("It's okay. I'll stay on the line with you until you remember... don't worry.") Reassurance may calm an elderly person enough to reduce the anxiety to manageable levels, so the needed information becomes available.

> **Chazal's First Law of Adults**
>
> Extreme terror gives us back the gestures of our childhood.

In one amazing case, an EMD receiving a call from a man who could not speak (and had collapsed) because of a stroke, could obtain nothing but grunts in response. After he determined that the caller could understand him, the EMD concocted a "code." He asked the caller to identify the quadrant of the city, starting with the north, then south, east and west. He told the man to tap the phone twice whenever he was correct. He rapidly narrowed down the area to the street, then guided the ambulance by listening to the increasing volume of the siren over the phone! Interestingly, the patient turned out to be a grateful city alderman.

Five Tips for Working with Children

1. **Ask to speak to an adult.** Get as much information from the child as possible, then ask to speak to an adult if one is present.

2. **Get to the child's level.** Options will expand the older the child is, but keep in mind the tendency for people to regress in crisis. This is true in children as well. Keep the conversation elementary.

3. **Does the child know her home address, or last name?** Be exact, and assume nothing. Is the child calling from her own home? If a child goes out to look at the house number, understand that the child may not read from left to right or from top to bottom. Sometimes a child can look for addresses on letters or bills that are near the telephone. Still, the child may read the return address instead of the correct one. Another method is to inquire whether there are any easily recognizable landmarks nearby such as a school, store, or playground.

4. **Does the child know the phone number?** Asking the child to read the phone number off the phone may work, assuming the child does not read the numbers next to the push buttons. Unfortunately, as people more commonly own their own phones, the telephone number may be located anywhere on the telephone—or may not have been put on it at all.

5. **Tell the child not to hang up and to always come back to the phone.** Be specific. Anticipate that the child may not realize it is necessary to return to or stay on the phone, and giving them specific instructions to return to the phone may keep the situation under control. ⚜

see also: EMD for Children position paper on page A.58

Fig. 2-1. Five tips for working with children.

Hearing a child on the telephone asking for help raises anxieties in practically everyone. Adults *want* to help children. It is natural to feel bothered by circumstances that indicate missing adult supervision. In one dramatic case, a 2½ year-old child called 9-1-1 because the baby sitter was unconscious and bleeding from the head. The dispatcher worked with the child for about 20 minutes before the right combination of information led to discovery of the address.

EMD's First Law of Children

The children will be calmer than their parents.

Some children sound suspiciously calm in the face of crisis. Perhaps they do not fully appreciate the gravity of a serious medical emergency, or perhaps they have not learned to be as anxious as older people. A true emergency may exist regardless of how calm a child sounds during the telephone interrogation.

When faced with a caller unable to answer all the EMD's questions, it may be justifiable to select a higher level of response if key information is missing. In some instances, a DELTA-level response may be warranted as an "unknown" default when the nature of the information requested is of life-threatening importance (i.e., "I don't know if he's disconnected from the power source.").

Second Law of Medical Dispatch

When in doubt, send them out. (Always err in the direction of the patient safety.)

There are several approaches which may be helpful in these types of situations. For example, when a language barrier presents a problem, is anyone in the dispatch center able to speak the caller's language? Ask the caller if there is someone at that end of the line who can speak the language. Perhaps the people on the scene called without thinking to ask the predominant language-speaking family members or neighbors for help. Certain telephone companies now offer on-line interpreters for various foreign languages; check on local availability and languages offered.

The relationship between the dispatch office and the crews in the field is that of people on the same team who play different positions.

The EMD's voice must remain clear, slow, distinct, and patient. People in crisis are excited; when they have the additional anxiety of struggling with a language barrier, the last thing they need is a mean-sounding, demanding person they cannot see who is talking too fast. Stick to protocol, but clarify by asking "Yes" or "No" questions as a last resort. Put the power of reassurance to work; once they feel calmer, they may display a better command of a secondary language. *The EMD may be able to successfully prioritize such calls after all.*

Inappropriate EMD Activities

Some dispatchers think that the extended responsibilities of EMD imbue them with dictatorial power. Professional EMDs, however, view themselves as members of a team helping others in crisis. They may not go to the scene; they also do not run the show. The EMD may tell crews where to go, but only in the respect that the dispatch determinant and response assignment is being communicated and followed.

EMDs who view this as a power trip are taking inappropriate advantage of their position. The relationship between the dispatch office and the crews in the field is that of people on the same team who play different positions.

> ### EMD's Law of Teamwork
> Team players are essential, "star" players are not.

The EMD does not control what field personnel should do at a scene. The EMD, even if a veteran of years in the field, does not tell those who are in the field how to do their jobs. The EMD is the scene commander until field personnel arrives at the scene, but once they do, the on-scene providers take command.

The EMD (at the hub of the system) then works to accommodate their needs, channeling information and linking them with any resource they need. The EMD can make field personnel aware of options. Information that may help them successfully handle a problem should be articulated in a way that gives the field personnel the option and ultimate responsibility for choosing the actions they take.

An Example of Second-Guessing the Caller

Dispatcher: Fire Department Emergency.
Caller: Yes, I see some smoke.

Dispatcher: Yes ma'am, can I have your address?
Caller: 13 Bobolink Road.

Dispatcher: Okay, and you see smoke.
Caller: Yes.

Dispatcher: Can you tell me what direction it's coming from?
Caller: What?

Dispatcher: The smoke, what direction is it coming from?
Caller: I don't know.

Dispatcher: Can you see out your front window from the phone?
Caller: Yes.

Dispatcher: Okay, looking out the window, which way does the sun rise? In front of you, in back, to the left or right?
Caller: It rises in front of me.

Dispatcher: Okay, that's east. Okay, looking in that direction, which direction is the smoke coming from?
Caller: What?

Dispatcher: Looking out the window, which way is the smoke coming from, left, right, or what?
Caller: Well, it's coming from the right.

Dispatcher: Okay, that's south. Can you give me a landmark?
Caller: What?

Dispatcher: Well, is the smoke near a PG&E tower or water tank or something? *(Pause.)*
Caller: Mister, the smoke is coming out of my closet!

Dispatcher: Oh! We'll be right there!

Fig. 2-2. An example of second-guessing the caller.

EMD's First Law of Arrival

The EMD is the scene commander until field personnel arrive at the scene.

Second-guessing is beyond the domain of the EMD. There are two tempting kinds of second-guessing. One is with field personnel, the other with callers. Wait until field personnel express their needs; be prepared to respond to those requests, but do not interfere with their work by pestering them with over-eager suggestions. To second-guess callers is to risk making dangerous, incorrect assumptions.

An amusing anecdote to illustrate this point happened one summer in an area where there had been a rash of wildland arson fires. The dispatcher reported that several times a day calls would come in from nervous residents who saw barbecue, fog, or water evaporation. The problem was pinpointing the smoke without driving all over the district, so a greater than average burden was placed on the dispatcher to get complete directions. An example of one of these infamous calls is shown in figure 2-2.

Another, less amusing anecdote occurred in a well-known dispatch situation in Dallas, Texas, mentioned in Chapter 11: Legal Aspects of EMD. In that case, the triage nurse refused to believe the caller's mother was too incoherent to speak on the telephone. In other words, she tried to second-guess the caller with fatal results. One must rely on the face value of the words spoken and let responding field crews validate the caller's honesty.

> **The EMD is the member of the EMS response team with the broadest view of the entire emergency system's current status and capabilities.**
> **—ASTM F 1258-00-5.5**

One last inappropriate behavior for the EMD should be obvious: Never leave the console without being sure there is someone ready to answer the phones and radio. This may be easy to say but difficult to justify when the EMD is the only person in the office at 0200 and the needs of the bladder exceed the needs of the EMS system. Humane dispatch systems should have policies to help EMDs avoid such dilemmas. Those that do not are overdue for administrative revamping.

Communication and Coordination Between Agencies

Dispatchers are accustomed to having most emergency calls come in via the public emergency access phone lines, either 9-1-1 or local seven-digit emergency numbers. Requests for help from other emergency agencies can be disconcerting, since they tend not to come through normal channels. When an EMS system implements priority dispatch, dispatchers from other agencies and field personnel who might make requests for EMS over the radio must change along with the needs of the EMD. They need to supply the additional information needed. This requires administrative collaboration and tact (see SEND, Chapter 3: Structure and Function of Priority Dispatch).

> ### Cocteau's Corollary of Tact
> Tact consists of knowing how far to go too far.

Also, EMDs often use a different communication style with colleagues at other agencies than they would with the general public. Each knows the lingo, the challenges, and the frustrations of life in emergency services. Nevertheless, it is important to retain a strong standard of professionalism, such as shielding confidentiality for patients or extraordinary situations. In the U.S., a lawsuit based on allegedly inappropriate dispatch agency communications with the press was filed in connection with a deadly federal assault on a religious compound in Waco, Texas. Careful management of communication between emergency agencies is fundamental to good telecommunication. Be careful not to spread rumors, gossip, or even what may appear to be "innocent" information with relatives or friends.

Above all, there is never room for rudeness or apathy. Be professional, efficient, and helpful to everyone, but particularly to colleagues in other dispatch centers (whether public or private). If requested, clarify and repeat vital information with an attitude of respect. If advised to cancel an emergency unit or asked to relay information, identify the requesting authority to the field crew. Do not argue with that request. Transmit the cancellation reason for proper documentation. Relay no more than the pertinent information to medical care

> **Never assume that the patient "has left" until proven otherwise.**

facilities. Be prepared with such information as patient vital signs and the ambulance's ETA (estimated time of arrival).

It is recommended that associated communication centers synchronize their time-keeping mechanisms at least once a month because of the routine and intertwined activities. Accurate times are easily found within the emergency call system and caller ID systems of most phone companies.

First Party Gone-On-Arrival Situations

First party callers are usually easier to deal with than other callers who often are more remote from the patient. First party (patient) callers constitute approximately 10-15% of all EMS callers. However, one challenge to dealing with these usually straightforward patients is the fact that there may be no one to watch over them during the response interim or to come to the door on arrival. Every patient has the potential to do three things after their evaluation by the EMD. They can get better, get worse, or stay the same. First party callers are no exception. If they get worse and suffer a decrease in level of consciousness, become too weak to shout or ambulate, or just outright collapse, the situation is dramatically altered for the EMD and the responders. What should the EMD do if the arriving crews report back to dispatch that nobody appears to be at home, the doors and windows are locked, and a call back from dispatch goes unanswered? Only breaking in will answer the question of whether the patient is actually "gone-on-arrival" versus incapacitated or dead. What to do?

Several recent legal cases have pointed out the problems that exist when contact is lost with first party callers. Since so many of these cases have been reported and resulted in lawsuits, this new type of EMS and dispatch "Danger Zone" needs to be addressed.

Case in Tennessee: On March 24, 1993, a 45-year-old male called 9-1-1 from home to report he was having "real bad chest pains." The dispatch case transcript revealed the following interrogation and advice:

Calltaker: 9-1-1

Simmons: Uh, yes... uh... this is Tony Simmons. I'm in... uh... uh... Concord Hills.

Calltaker: Uh, huh.

Simmons: I'm having these real bad chest pains...

Calltaker: **Okay, you need an ambulance?**

Simmons: ... and I'm here by myself. And I don't know if it is... this is indigestion or what.

Calltaker: **Well, it doesn't pay to... to wonder. Okay, I'm gonna connect you down to the ambulance service so... a... they can talk to you about it. Okay, so we're gonna get somebody started.**

Calltaker: **(unintelligible) answers the paramedics, so they can put you on the phone, too.**

EMS: **Emergency Medical Services.**

Simmons: Yes, I'm Tony Simmons. I'm up in Concord Hills.

EMS: **Uh, huh.**

Simmons: I'm here by myself and I started just a little while ago having these real bad chest pains. And I don't know if it is some indigestion or what. But I'm not feeling very good.

EMS: **Okay. How old are you?**

Simmons: I'm 45.

EMS: **45. Okay, and you're at (address on screen verified)?**

Simmons: That's right.

EMS: **Okay. I'll get somebody out there. Have you ever had any chest pain or a heart attack before?**

Simmons: No. Never have.

EMS: **Okay, I'll get somebody out there to you.**

Simmons: Thank you.

Simmons then called his secretary at work to let her know he wasn't coming in and asked her to notify his wife. The paramedics arrived to find no one apparently at home. After a walk around check of the residence revealed no signs of an occupant except a dog barking in the house, the dispatcher was requested to call back and reported to the crew, "Patient probably went by POV" (privately owned vehicle). Dispatch also tried calling a local hospital to determine the possible whereabouts of the patient, to no avail. Simmon's wife came home half an hour later to find him dead. A lawsuit resulted.

Case in Chicago, Illinois: About 8 a.m. in October, 1995, a 26-year-old female called 9-1-1 to report a severe asthma attack:

Kazmierowski: I need help.

Calltaker: What happened?

Kazmierowski: I'm having an asthma attack.

Calltaker: What?

Kazmierowski: It's so bad.

Calltaker: What?

Kazmierowski: Is this 9-1-1?

Calltaker: Do you need an ambulance?

Kazmierowski: Yeah.

Calltaker: I'll connect you. Hold the line.

[After two rings, a fire department dispatcher takes the call. Kazmierowski can be heard wheezing and struggling to breathe.]

Fire Dispatcher: Fire Department.

Kazmierowski: Oh, God. I need an ambulance.

Fire Dispatcher: Fire Department.

[Dispatcher repeats, "Fire Department," seeming not to hear the caller.]

Kazmierowski: I need an ambulance—forty-five twenty Greenview.

Fire Dispatcher: Forty-five two oh Greenview?

Kazmierowski: Forty-five two oh. I can't breathe.

Fire Dispatcher: What floor are you on?

Kazmierowski: I'm on the third floor. Please come up.

Fire Dispatcher: Yeah, we'll be over. What's your phone number?

Kazmierowski: I think I'm going to die—hurry!

Fire Dispatcher: Just let me read it out.

The dispatcher read back the telephone number to the caller and the call was disconnected. The paramedic ambulance crew entered the apartment building and knocked on the front door; they also heard a dog barking. After the paramedics failed to get an answer, a neighbor opened his apartment to let them knock on her back door. Still no answer. A call back to the residence went to an answering machine. After 15 minutes the crew left having never attempted to open the door, which was unlocked at the time. Kazmierowski's boyfriend found her lifeless on the bed later that afternoon. At a recent EMS conference, a former employee of the City defended their performance in this case on the premise that the paramedics had no legal responsibility to attempt to open the door if the patient didn't open it on request. After an initial Appellate Court ruling that the City was immune from damages, in an unusual move the Illinois Supreme Court narrowed significantly the interpretation of the fire department's immunity and remanded the case back to the trial court whose action is pending as of this printing.[167]

Case in Texas: On July 25, 1996, a 55-year-old female with post-recurrent polio syndrome was in her motorized wheelchair gardening in a field adjacent to her house when she hit a depression in the dirt and the cart overturned. The caller historically had trouble breathing when not sitting up. She called 9-1-1 from a mobile phone on the cart, obviously in distress and vaguely stating what was later interpreted as, "Help. I'm… I'm…a field, I'm dying." The initial calltaker thought she said, "Help. I'm… I'm… ill, I'm dying," after which the caller did not speak. Five minutes later the line went dead. The calltaker, using enhanced 9-1-1, called back but only got the answering machine. They immediately called the fire/ambulance department to respond and had also sent a deputy sheriff. Interestingly, the sheriff's calltaker stated in a very caring tone to the ambulance EMD, "When people say that [I'm dying], they usually are." Another call was received from the residence but no one spoke and the line went dead again.

After multiple searches inside the house failed to locate the patient, a multi-person circumferential search (of a disputed distance) around the caller's semi-rural residence was also unsuccessful. After law enforcement's inquiry of a neighbor, no one was found and the patient was assumed to have left with her husband. Later he came home and found her dead, 50 yards from the house and partially hidden in some relatively tall weeds.

In the resulting lawsuit the jury found for the various dispatch and public safety defendants, based partially on the fact that a reasonable attempt to locate a patient cannot be defined by how much further out an unsuccessful search should be extended. We call this the "just a little further would be better" philosophy, which seems nice on the surface but would obviously be difficult to use as the basis for an objective standard of practice. In this case, while the parties agreed the search was not optimal, the jury determined that a reasonable effort had been made before leaving the scene.

Case in Georgia: On July 6, 1986, the following call was received at a large public safety dispatch center. Obviously this case involved a first-party caller who only produced grunting noises throughout the entirety of the call. The calltaker apparently did not recognized the caller had a major problem and on several occasions threatened the caller (judgment danger zone). The following is a partial transcript:

Dispatcher: Hello?

Caller: (grunting)

Dispatcher: Hello? What's your address?

Caller: (grunting)

Dispatcher: Hello? What's your address?

Caller: (grunting)

Dispatcher: Do you need a police out? Cause if you're playing on the ph... if you're playing on the phone, officer's gonna come and take you to jail.

Caller: (grunting) Time passes as the dis patcher continues to ask caller for information.

Dispatcher: Do you need an ambulance out?

Caller: (grunting)

Dispatcher: Do you need a police out?

Caller: (grunting)

Dispatcher: Hello? I'm gonna hang up if you don't tell me what's the problem.

Caller: (grunting)

[For a more complete transcript of this case, see Hendon Case, Chapter 8: Time-Life Priority Situations.]

Creating a Policy for Gone-on-Arrival

In the absence of a national standard policy, it is imperative that every communication center has a written local policy regarding what to do, who to call, and when to leave the scene in first-party, possibly "gone-on-arrival" cases. Law enforcement notification and response is the norm in these situations. Never assume that a first-party caller patient "has left" until that has been reasonably established based on an in-place policy. In such a policy the following should be considered for inclusion:

1. **Call-back several times on the verified callback number.** Establish a minimum number of call backs. With call waiting and call messaging, what appears to be a "not home" may be a "non- (or can't) answer" for a variety of reasons.

2. **Verify that any callback number that is not answered is indeed a correct number.** Even enhanced phone systems may contain errors that can be corrected by a standardized tape or digital playback procedure.

3. **Crews should not be advised to break in unless a clear policy** is in place and/or they have **legal authority** or the **approval of law enforcement.**

4. **Responders have a responsibility to exercise due regard in determining that a first-party caller is indeed gone.** A well-articulated policy statement to this effect will set forth a reasonable process, as well as a reasonable limit, to such searches.

5. **Animals impeding (or apparently impeding) entry or access should not alter the responsibility to locate the patient.** When it is obvious that additional help in the form of law enforcement or animal control is required, do not hesitate to request it. Again, a reasonable attempt to isolate or bypass the animal is required. Leaving because of hearing barks or howls without actually seeing the animals may add the embarrassment of learning later that the pet was a miniature poodle named "Fluffy."

6. **Certain critical determinant codes that are to be given an extra level of regard,** or that warrant a legal break-in, should be explicitly listed (i.e., 10-C-2, Chest Pain with abnormal breathing). Essentially, the clinical ranking of a dispatch determinant code can strongly suggest (or discourage) that a patient who appears to be initially stable, could later deteriorate.

Fig. 2-3. Creating a Policy for Gone-on-Arrival.

This call, an amazing 55 minutes long, had an equally amazing ending. Upon successfully tracing the call, the fateful decision to only send a police unit was made. According to case depositions, on arrival the police team found a car in the driveway, but after a careful walk around the outside could see no evidence of anyone in the locked house. The older, more experienced officer mentioned enroute that he had responded to this location in the past and that the occupant was an alcoholic. He then recommended leaving. The rookie officer, however, insisted that more be done, even suggesting they break in. The older officer then called dispatch and asked, "Do you still have the RP [reporting party] on the line?" The dispatcher replied, "Yes, but he's refusing to come to the phone." Upon hearing the dispatcher's misinterpretation of the facts, the officers drove away. Nearly a day later, the patient's son found him lying in the house, critically ill from a massive stroke. Upon regaining some ability to speak the caller recounted how he had actually called 9-1-1 several hours before the call transcribed here, but was hung up on. The patient apparently was not currently a drinker nor a derelict, but was a recently retired superior court judge for the region. Not surprisingly, a lawsuit followed.

It is always wise to exercise caution in ruling out a serious problem that may be preventing the patient from answering the door. Retrospectively, calls resulting in a non-answering patient at a residence likely involve first-party callers (otherwise someone else would have answered the door). This should be a warning sign that increases the responsibility to rule out serious patient deterioration before giving up. In any first-party case involving a reasonable chance of patient deterioration, such as the patient with chest pain, it is advisable to stay on the line with the patient. Any subsequent inability of the patient to meet the arriving units would then be clearly known.

Dispatch Overload

The potential for dispatch overload always exists, whether one works in a state-of-the-art, high-tech dispatch system with separate personnel to take calls and do the radio work, or as the sole operator of a quiet rural center. It has to do with relative volume. In the former, a large plane crash in conjunction with a subway fire (plus the normal call volume) might constitute overload. In the latter, a second one-patient emergency call may send the system into overload. One fact is universally true: there will never be enough equipment and personnel for the worst possible scenario.

Koenig's Maxim for Disasters
There will never be enough equipment and personnel for the worst possible scenario.

Dispatch overload is also relative according to the experience of the EMD. For example, one rookie was left to cope with a one-person office (radios and telephones for fire, police and ambulance, the computer, plus walk-in counter complaints). A supervisor across the room was there for backup. A high-speed chase involving a Porsche and several law enforcement units from different agencies erupted about midday. The police officers were on two different radio frequencies, and could not speak directly to each other. Community-minded citizens started calling in the Porsche's location as it sped through residential areas. Everything had to be relayed through dispatch. The whole console was ablaze with flashing lights. The rookie was entirely overwhelmed almost immediately.

The supervisor, on the other hand, viewed it as a refreshing change of pace. Nothing so exciting had happened in that town for months. She gave the rookie a splendid example of doing many tasks simultaneously, expertly demonstrating the ability to evaluate and respond to several nearly concurrent calls at a fast clip.

Although every EMD evolves methods for managing dispatch overload, here are a few tips that may help. Always be sure to answer emergency lines first. Asking, "Where is your emergency?" identifies the location for response immediately and subtly indicates to the caller that the EMD is in charge. Many callers also quickly recognize that their sprained ankle is a minor problem and not an emergency while providing needed address verification.

When multiple lines are ringing, if the caller says, "Well, it's not really an emergency," the EMD should tell the person not to hang up, that he or she will get back on the line quickly, and then put that line on hold and screen the other emergency lines, which should be handled in order, starting first with the most time-critical, life-threatening situation.

EMD's First Law of Relative Value
Threats to life have a higher priority than threats to property.

Often, when the entire communication panel lights up at once, the same situation has generated more than one call. After asking, "Where is your emergency?" if the caller says, "There's an accident at 1184 First Ave.," ask for the address verification immediately. "The accident is at 1184 First Ave." If it is exactly the same address as a call already receiving a response, tell the caller you know of the incident, say thanks, and clear the phone line. Be absolutely sure, however, that the call involves the same *exact* incident. Secondary callers may be reporting additional, more remote victims from the same wandering assailant or high speed crash (two real cases) that were initially disregarded by the calltaker.

Most calls require only a few seconds to get the address, callback number, and answers to the Four Commandment questions (see A Real Tough Time Breathing, Chapter 12: Quality Management). When volume is flooding the communication center, the EMD must make decisions more quickly than usual, but never take shortcuts in gathering data. Inaccurate call evaluation at initial dispatch can be catastrophic, jeopardizing the patient and the responding crews. Ask *all* the questions in the priority dispatch process, and dispatch at the *appropriate* point in the case.

> ## Bradshaw's Law
> It's time we start doing it right, not just fast!

Although it may not always be possible, try to avoid carrying on two conversations at once. This may be easy to say but is admittedly very difficult to do in real life. When the radios are going and the phone rings, the EMD must sometimes integrate more than one item of attention at once—thus the success of the experienced supervisor versus the overwhelmed rookie during the high-speed chase example. With more practice in the art dispatch, the more adept the EMD becomes at attending to many details simultaneously.

Mass Casualty Incidents

Mass casualty incidents are among the most intense challenges an EMD can face. Juggling such a situation requires a great deal of presence and balance on the part of the EMD. One fact about mass casualty incidents is certain: normal,

> **Normal, everyday calls do not suspend themselves for the EMD's benefit during the course of handling other incidents.**

everyday calls do not suspend themselves for the EMD's benefit during the course of handling other incidents. One must still apply the principles of emergency medical dispatch to the full spectrum of complaints coming to the communication center that day.

In a mass casualty incident, avoid unnecessary use of the radio. Air legitimate transmissions but otherwise curb the temptation to satisfy curiosity about non-essential details. Field personnel have enough tasks demanding their attention; they do not need to talk on the radio unnecessarily.

A mass casualty incident need not be equated solely with the "Big One." A crippling blizzard can be a logistical nightmare that creates a form of mass casualty incident, as can the traffic-flow impediments of earthquakes, floods, and hurricanes. A citywide epidemic may critically drain resources. A five-car crash with several critical injuries in the middle of a large bridge at the height of rush hour may constitute a mass casualty incident due to scene access challenges.

The best way to handle this type of incident depends mainly on local system design. This book deals with the routine activities that more commonly challenge the EMD, not mass casualty, because such instruction is outside its scope and purpose.

Summary

It takes time and effort to become a really good EMD. Increasingly, people are dedicating their professional careers to this new medical niche. The tips in this chapter are meant as a springboard for establishing or improving the capabilities of emergency medical dispatchers. Trained, experienced dispatchers can share numerous other tips; anyone well-practiced at the art of dispatching should share that expertise freely with those who follow. New EMDs are wise to listen. Veteran EMDs can make wonderful mentors.

Being an excellent EMD comes with practice, especially to those cultivating the necessary talents. Regard this achievement with respect. As the main spearhead of the EMS response, and as the logistician and coordinator, the EMD is in a position of considerable trust and power. The EMD should do his or her best to earn that trust and use that power wisely. Be proud of the humanitarian impact of this important role!

Courage is the first of human qualities because it is the quality that guarantees all the others.

—*Winston Churchill*

Confidentiality in Emergency Medical Dispatching

Confidentiality is an essential concept to understand and practice as a professional EMD. In this world of instant communication and information exchange, the possibility of serious violation of the confidence entrusted to public safety personnel is not only great but predictable.

Confidentiality is defined as the need to be kept secret or private; in EMD it implies the necessity to not release or broadcast certain information about patients' situation, conditions, names, and illnesses unless approved by supervisors or by policy.

General communication center functions expose EMDs to intimate information concerning patients, their families, and bystanders. EMDs are morally, and in many cases legally obligated to ensure confidentiality with regard to such information. Legislation mandates such confidentiality in many communities and communication centers should consider such legislation when enacting related policies. Strict policies that ensure confidentiality are necessary because of the social implications associated with the inappropriate disclosure of personal information, particularly with regard to infectious diseases. Communication center policies should consider what information is shared among EMS personnel and limit the exchange of information to what is in the best interest of the patient and the responders. How information is exchanged should be considered as well as what information exchanged. It is helpful to construct policies with the input of organizations that advocate patient rights, such as the American Civil Liberties Union and local AIDS organizations. Policies aside, it is never appropriate to discuss personal patient information outside the context of necessary and appropriate workplace communication.

An event in Waco, Texas reaffirmed the need for absolute confidentiality at dispatch. On February 28th, 1993, various special law enforcement arms of the United States government, including the FBI and ATF (Alcohol, Tobacco, and Firearms) were staged outside the now infamous Branch Davidian religious group complex. With a planned raid by the federal agents imminent, the local dispatch center was alerted to have several ambulances ready at an predetermined time. No mention of a raid was made. It was reported that a dispatcher who had a personal relationship with local television newsreporter, mentioned to him the request for the ambulance call-up. The newsreporter, sensing an impending action, arrived on a road near the edge of the complex before the reported time. Seeing a mailman, he asked the apparent postal worker if he new of anything happening that morning. The mailman, a follower of the Davidian group, reported the information immediately back to the sect's leader, David Koresh.

With the Davidian's now reportedly alerted to the impending raid, government sources alleged that the breach of confidentiality was the cause of four agent's deaths. A lawsuit was initiated by the U.S. government against the communication center but was apparently never litigated in the turmoil following this widely criticized event.

Certainly, all breaches in confidentiality do not result in such serious or loss-of-life outcomes. And just as certainly, it is impossible to know just how any breach in the chain of confidential information control may ultimately play out. All information entrusted to dispatch personnel should be respected at the highest level of required confidence—nothing less. ⚜

Fig. 2-4. "Confidentiality in Emergency Medical Dispatching," by Brett Patterson, 2001.

Contents

CHAPTER 3

Structure *and* Function *of* Priority Dispatch

Chapter Overview

This chapter describes the theories and concepts underlying the Medical Priority Dispatch System.™ It is the basic anatomy and physiology, the underlying machinery, of priority dispatch.

The goal is to provide a clear map of priority dispatch to anyone involved in system implementation, on-line use, and management. These people need to understand what EMDs do and why.

Everything should be as simple as possible, but not simpler.
—Albert Einstein

The Medical Priority Dispatch System™ is designed to draw the EMD through a predictable, repeatable, verifiable process. This means that every caller can rely on consistent assessment and EMS response. It means that patients will receive the same level of assistance sent to other, similar situations. And if something on the call should go wrong, it is possible to verify that the assistance sent was, indeed, appropriate. In today's climate of accountability, these are valuable protective mechanisms against certain legal liability issues.

To understand how such a statement is true, one must first understand the anatomy and physiology of priority dispatch. Years of evolution and refinement have resulted in a misleadingly simple-looking structure that has been tested in the real-life lab of thousands of EMD centers on tens of millions of calls. It is characterized by a rigorously defined and time-proven order for doing things throughout each interaction with callers in crisis. Despite what may appear to be a strict framework, the EMD has to be able to think and make decisions in the heat of the moment. Priority dispatch is the safety net that allows EMDs to craft the best solution to each caller's problem, balanced with the needs and capabilities of the rest of the EMS system.

> **It has been said that laws make one free. In the same way, the structure of priority dispatch frees the EMD to concentrate on the call, rather than concentrating on what comes next.**

Basic Priority Dispatch Anatomy

At the core of the system are 33 priority dispatch protocols. Each of the protocols is carefully standardized, containing consistently partitioned information, with separate sections for Key Questions, Dispatch Determinants, Response Codes, Additional Information, and Post-Dispatch Instructions and Pre-Arrival Instructions. With proper education, the EMD knows how to flow through the system with appropriate ease.

Case Entry Protocol. Before turning to one of the 33 priority dispatch protocols, the EMD must always ask certain essential questions. The Case Entry protocol serves as a universal starting point for priority dispatch. From here, the EMD can select the appropriate dispatch protocol each time. Earlier versions of priority dispatch called this element the invisible protocol, since it was not written out. Today, a detailed

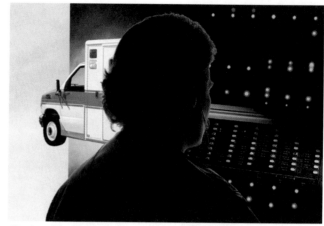

Fig. 3-1. The EMD has been called the "Air Traffic Controller" of the ground.

protocol exists for the purpose of gathering essential logistical information, including the classic "**Four Commandment**" questions familiar to many early users of priority dispatch.

Key Questions. There is an average of 4.4 required key questions per protocol. As the caller answers each question the EMD establishes the correct medical response (see Appendix B).

Dispatch Determinants. These are the six different dispatch coding choices. The EMD selects the most appropriate determinant based on the answers to the key questions. The different dispatch determinants are known as OMEGA-, ALPHA-, BRAVO-, CHARLIE-, DELTA-, and ECHO-level (Ω-A-B-C-D-E). Each reflects a different response group option.

ECHO Code. In version 11.0, an important feature—the ECHO code was added to the Case Entry protocol. In previous versions of the MPDS, the EMD was allowed to send only at the end of all Case Entry questioning—in essence after consciousness and breathing were determined. However, this process was not optimally structured, and became a safety issue on some protocols. The ECHO determinant provides EMDs with a way to get a response moving quickly. But ECHO goes much further than that, allowing mobilization of unusual resources and maintaining tight integration with v11's increased focus on scene safety. ECHO is discussed in more detail later this chapter.

OMEGA Code. A vital principle in priority dispatch is that the caller receives someone at their door to evaluate the situation firsthand—with just three exceptions. On three standard dispatch protocols there is an added response possibility called the OMEGA code.

These are actually pre-planned referrals. On protocol 9, in cases of unquestionable expected deaths (for example, long-term and terminal cancer patients) it is not necessary to send an EMS response (unless the caller appears to need medical support). In these cases, the call is referred to the proper authorities who will take over, and an EMS response will not be mobilized. On protocol 17, the concept of non-injury "public assist" is now incorporated to aid (in a non-emergency way) a caller in situations where someone has fallen but is not injured or accutely ill and needs help getting the patient returned to a comfortable resting place. On protocol 23, certain ingestions and poisonings are transferred by telephone to a regionalized Poison Control Center, the best resource for specific well-defined poisoning situations. (In some centers, other OMEGA "responses" have also been developed to accommodate different EMS systems.)

Post-Dispatch Instructions. These are a list of caller instructions relevant to each Chief Complaint but not necessary to each patient. They should be given *whenever possible and appropriate.* Each protocol contains a universal statement that should be read to the caller: "I'm sending the paramedics (ambulance) to help you now. Stay on the line and I'll tell you exactly what to do next." Some protocols also contain special treatments (see protocol 2: if snakebite "Keep her/him from moving around. Keep the bitten area below heart-level if possible. Do not apply ice or a tourniquet. Do not giver her/him any alcohol to drink."), warnings (see protocol 3: "Avoid further contact with the animal"), or advice (see protocol 4: if sexual assault "Do not change clothes, bathe, shower, or go to the bathroom.")

Critical EMD Information. Immediately following PDIs are vital reminders to the EMD regarding hazard warnings, non-scripted advice for callers, special notifications, and directions for when to stay on the line with callers. This information is contained in a blue-shaded area and preceded by a blue asterisk symbol (see protocol 10: "Stay on the line with caller if her/his condition seems unstable or is worsening").

DLS Links. The post-dispatch instructions panel is followed by links to various DLS protocols. These are generally ordered with scene and caller safety issues first, extreme patient problems next, and patient-support issues last. Each DLS link leads the EMD to the appropriate starting point for dispatch life support on protocols A, B, or C for airway and CPR, protocols D and E for choking, protocol F for childbirth, protocol Z for AED support, protocol Y for tracheostomy (stoma) airway/CPR, and protocol X for safety warnings, bleeding, burns, general patient support, and call termination techniques.

The post-dispatch instructions, guided by the DLS links to the appropriate pre-arrival instructions, have five basic goals:

1. Prevent the caller or others at the scene from causing further harm to the patient.

2. Facilitate scene safety.

3. Enable the caller to provide basic first aid.

4. Calm undirected, possibly uncooperative callers.

5. Provide follow-up and callback instructions.

Card Title Bars. There are two special types of protocol that serve unusual purposes, called SHUNT and BRIDGE protocols. These are easily identifiable from their title bars. Two other title-bar conventions identify protocols that contain ECHO determinants and protocols that are used for pre-arrival instructions.

The SHUNT protocols are designed to assist the EMD in selecting the best protocol to use when callers cannot, for some reason, provide a clear or useable Chief Complaint. There are two types of SHUNT protocols: those

> **SHUNTS help the EMD select the best protocol to use on calls lacking a definitive Chief Complaint.**

that are "shunted from" and those that are "shunted to." The SHUNT-from protocols have questions that are designed to evaluate a relatively non-specific complaint (such as back pain) and to redirect the EMD to other protocols for some patients (recent fall SHUNTS to protocol 17, recent trauma to 30, and so forth). The title bar on SHUNT-from protocols is colored yellow, the SHUNT-to protocols have the protocol number highlighted in a similarly colored box. This allows the EMD to rapidly and efficiently move from the start to then end of the SHUNT. (In software the SHUNT happens automatically, but the different protocols are still labeled "SHUNT.") Protocols 5, 17, 21, 22, 25, and 26 are "shunt from" protocols, and protocols 2, 6, 8, 10, 11, 15, 17, 21, 23, 24, 26, 27, 30, and 31 can be "shunted to."

The BRIDGE protocols are designed to lead the EMD smoothly into the telephone first aid known as dispatch life support. There are three BRIDGE protocols in MPDS v11: protocol 9: Cardiac or Respiratory

> **BRIDGES move the EMD smoothly from prioritizing dispatch to providing dispatch life support.**

Arrest/Death; protocol 11: Choking; and protocol 24: Pregnancy/Childbirth/Miscarriage. One key purpose of these protocols is to direct the EMD, via the DLS links, to the appropriate panel in the correct pre-arrival script. Another key purpose is to verify the initial problem prior to committing to a particular line of DLS treatment.

The Case Entry protocol has a purple title bar indicating that it is the only place in the MPDS where an ECHO determinant can be selected. Each ECHO determinant, however, refers to a specific Chief Complaint, so chief complaint protocols that contain ECHO determinants have a similarly-colored purple box around the protocol number. The ECHO-containing protocols are 2, 6, 9, 11, 15, and 31. Remember, the ECHO determinant is selected and sent only from Case Entry, but the EMD must then complete the Case Entry key question sequence and then turn to the appropriate Chief Complaint protocol. This ensures scene safety issues are correctly handled and directs the EMD to the panel for the most appropriate Pre-Arrival Instruction script. Pre-Arrival Instruction scripts have their titles highlighted in blue and are found on the far right side of the title bar.

Additional Information. This is rapid reference information for the EMD. The EMD often relies on information included here while making a dispatch decision. Specialized lists, categories, and dispatch definitions aid the EMD—in a standardized and efficient way. All the protocols include certain relevant **Axioms, Rules,** and **Laws** in the Additional Information section. Axioms are important features that are actually the basis of many of the decision-making processes in priority dispatch. They are self-evident truths that need no proof. They differ from rules in that they tell us *why*—rather than *how*—we do things. Rules are more definitive action statements. They convey specifically how Axioms are used and provide many of the do's and don'ts of priority dispatch. The Rules contained within a particular protocol are to be considered always true in the medical dispatch environment, without exception. Laws set forth general medical and medical dispatch principles in an interesting and catchy form. In general medicine, they are referred to as "the pearls." These Rules, Axioms, and Laws form "the pearls" of priority dispatch thinking.

> **These Rules, Axioms, and Laws form "the pearls" of priority dispatch thinking.**

Pre-Arrival Instructions. These are in-depth scripts used to work closely with callers involved in the

---

Medical Miranda—Extending Priority Dispatching to Law Enforcement

"Dispatch, Patrol Car 15. Call City Fire and have them send their paramedics over here right away." How do most paramedic providers respond? They send over the paramedics, of course. And why not? The police ordered it. But how did they assess the need for paramedics? If this is a trauma case, what will ALS personnel add to the victim's definitive care? Do they really mean they need advanced life support?

Since the advent of dispatch priority protocols, the practice of sending paramedics on request is finally disappearing. It makes sense. Often law enforcement officers don't clearly understand that paramedics aren't just better EMTs, but that they offer specific additional treatment adjuncts. That they add little to the treatment of most non-critical trauma is not usually perceived.

We now instruct EMDs that a request for "paramedics" means that "emergency help is needed." Tell us what you've got and we'll apply dispatch protocol and send the appropriate medical personnel. Unless every police officer carries a set of protocols in their pocket, they can't possibly request, on a consistent basis, the correct personnel and response configuration in a multi-unit, tiered response system. Yet the "ham-on-rye" practice of ordering paramedics happens every day throughout the world of public safety.

This is not an ill-thought out slap at "police mentality." Let's illustrate. Suppose police arrive first at the scene of a car vs. tree accident in which it is obvious that a woman is pinned in the wreckage. The officer immediately radios his dispatcher to request the fire department to "send the paramedics."

(continued on 3.5)

Medical Miranda—Extending Priority Dispatching to Law Enforcement

(continued from 3.4)

The officer attends to the victim while awaiting the arrival of a nearby paramedic unit. As it pulls up a few minutes later, the officer yells, "She's trapped in the car. Bring your jaws-of-life." minutes later, the officer yells, "She's trapped in the car. Bring your jaws-of-life."

Everything's okay so far you say? Not quite. Ask the bewildered paramedics who reply, "We don't have the 'jaws.' They're on Rescue-12 near the freeway entrance four miles from here." Access to the victim is delayed an additional seven minutes. To the officer in this case, "paramedics" meant "extrication"—not advanced life support. Had the officer indicated to dispatch *what* the problem *actually was,* Rescue-12 would have been initially dispatched to extricate.

Even if every unit has heavy extrication capability, how many police officers were told at their morning report that your "jaws" were down for repair or that your MAST suit had not been returned yet by Life Flight? This "what if" case actually happened and it helped to make a very important point with the City Police administration who likewise want the best, most efficient care for their citizens.

From our experience we can suggest some relatively simple solutions. If law enforcement doesn't understand new necessities and capabilities based on this evolution in medical dispatching they can't possibly be expected to mysteriously adapt to our needs.

We have to rationally explain our improved methods to them. And knowing the caliber and professionalism of the majority of law enforcement agencies, they'll come through. But not until you make the effort to meet, discuss, and plan with them—not just sit back and complain about "the cops."

The seminal meeting with the City Police administration was, to their credit, generated by them to ask about what they referred to, not comically, as our "Twenty questions game."

During that meeting, we described the priority card system and the necessity to ask a minimal number of questions to ascertain the nature of the problem and therefore the appropriate response, whether paramedic/engine, EMT/engine, private BLS ambulance, or HOT and COLD combinations of the above.

It wasn't surprising to us that the "cops" understood the first time. They merely stated, "What specifically do you want our scene officers to relay to you on each case?"

What would you want the EMD to know if the answers to a generic set of questions could be relayed from each first arriving scene officer? Simply start with the Four Commandments of medical dispatch:

1. Chief Complaint

2. Age (approximate)

3. Status of Consciousness

4. Status of Breathing

"Anything else?" the police major asked.

If the case is medical, do victims age 35 and over have chest pain? If the case is trauma, is severe bleeding present? "No problem," he replied. "Is that all?" If any additional information or special circumstances are appropriate or apparent, such as the need to respond lights-and-siren, or not, relay them please. End of meeting.

To accomplish this, we initiated a two-part program. First a mandatory four-hour in-service was presented to all patrol personnel. This required three sessions to catch all 375 City Police officers. Each four-hour training session included a description of the fire department's tiered response system, and how the response mode and configuration are determined through interrogation. Copies of the priority dispatch protocols were given to each officer and the important priorities on appropriate protocols common to law enforcement experience were reviewed. Pre-arrival instruction example tapes were played.

(continued on 3.6)

Medical Miranda—Extending Priority Dispatching to Law Enforcement

(continued from 3.5)

A brief explanation of a specific area of EMS directly applicable to police activities, Salt Lake City's unique EMS Abuse Ordinance, was given. In addition, a number of very interesting questions were posed by some very street-savvy officers.

The second phase of the solution involved the introduction of the "generic" questions plus three additional "optional" questions for either medical or trauma printed on a wallet-sized card to be carried by all City Police officers.

This card we affectionately nick-named, "Medical Miranda." The subsequent result has been better initial information and fewer relays of questions between police and EMS. The problems have not disappeared but some important ground has been broken.

We also found out that "the other guys," in this case the "cops," were just as interested in good citizen service and patient care as we were. As it usually happens, the solution was found in direct communication and rational discussion followed by a game plan involving a definitive method to effect the necessary instruction and, as a result, the desired change.

We feel that the simple introduction of the SEND program to extend the concept of priority dispatch to law enforcement has significant potential to improve information secured from the professionals at scene and to effect appropriate allocation of our medical response resources in every case possible. ❦

Fig. 3-2. "Medical Miranda–Extending Priority Dispatching," revision of an article originally published in JEMS, 1985.[32] Reprinted by permission.

---

following potentially life-threatening situations: cardiac and/or respiratory arrest, choking, and childbirth. In the manual system, these dispatch life support protocols are found at the back of the flip file. In the early days of priority dispatch, they were known as "**Treatment Sequence Protocols.**" This important element of priority dispatch is described and explained in full in Chapter 4: Dispatch Life Support.

SEND™ (Medical Miranda). People from other emergency agencies need to be educated about priority dispatch so they can facilitate its proper use.[32] This need gave rise to the **"SEND"** card concept. (The term

"Miranda Rights" is universally familiar to U.S. law enforcement personnel and most of North America through television. It stems from a 1966 U.S. Supreme Court ruling—Miranda v. Arizona—which stated that people must be advised of their legal rights when they are taken into police custody.)[33] The SEND card has resulted in better initial information and fewer relays of questions between police and EMS.

When priority dispatch was first introduced in Salt Lake City, police calling from a scene for the paramedics resisted providing adequate information. A credit-card-sized, plastic protocol was developed to help remind law enforcement personnel exactly what information was needed so the most appropriate prehospital response could be dispatched. It was originally called the "Medical Miranda" card to provide a sense of familiarity to those using it. As priority dispatch spread into other countries, where the term "Miranda" was not recognized, SEND, the generic name of the card was used. SEND stands for "Secondary Emergency Notification of Dispatch".

Following consolidation of two fire-based medical dispatch centers in the Salt Lake metropolitan area, we recognized a unique opportunity to evaluate possible differences in the information obtained from two

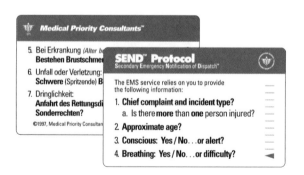

Fig. 3-3. SEND cards, NAE and EUG. © 1984-2002 MPC.

external law enforcement dispatch centers.[164] [Jeff J. Clawson, MD. and Robert Sinclair, PhD. *Medical Miranda–Improved Medical Dispatch Information from Police Officers,* Prehospital and Disaster Medicine]. Medical Miranda (SEND) training had been provided to all patrol-division personnel of the Salt Lake City Police Department (approximately 375 field officers) in the previous year while the program was not scheduled for the Salt Lake County Sheriff's Office (approximately 400 field officers) for several months. It was believed that there was a general equivalency in previous medical training and general law enforcement experience between the two groups of law enforcement personnel, and that pronounced differences in the Fire Central Dispatch EMDs' perceptions of the dispatch information collected from the two groups would likely be a consequence of the Medical Miranda protocol.

We developed a brief study questionnaire which asked the emergency medical dispatchers at Salt Lake Central Dispatch to indicate their perception of the level of understanding of the two center's law enforcement personnel. The questionnaire asked the dispatchers to indicate which of the two departments provided the most useful information and which of the two departments' officers and dispatchers had the best apparent understanding of EMD, to indicate an overall level of satisfaction with the two departments, and to say whether they felt the "Medical Miranda" program had improved their interaction with the City's law enforcement agency.

The results showed that nine of the eleven emergency medical dispatchers claimed they got better initial medical information from the City Police, ten of the eleven claimed the City Police dispatchers have a better understanding of EMD than the County Sheriff's dispatchers, and all eleven claimed the City Police officers themselves had a better understanding of EMD than the County Sheriff deputies. On average the emergency medical dispatchers were approximately twice as satisfied with their interaction with the City Police as with their interaction with the County Sheriff, and seven of the eleven dispatchers believed their increased satisfaction was a result of the Medical Miranda program.

The MPDS is available as both hard-copy and expert-system computer software The hard-copy is organized within the framework of a flip chart. The protocols are tabulated so the EMD can see the title of each protocol easily for quick reference after obtaining the Chief Complaint from the caller.

ProQA. ProQA™ is a computerized version of the priority dispatch protocols. It has all the components that have been described, together with automated data collection and reports for case analysis. Benefits of the computerized model are that it saves time, provides easy-to-generate EMD performance and medical case statistics for quality improvement, medical study, and resource planning, and is already integrated into many popular **CAD** systems.

Conventions. Both models of the protocols have consistent stylistic cues, known as **conventions**, to help the user find needed information. The conventions consist of a combination of font (the shape and look of the letters), color, background, upper and lower case, and the use of symbols, bold and italic fonts, and parentheses. Each convention indicates certain things and has particular meaning within the protocol. These cues, colors, and connectors all have meaning. There may be a relationship to another area of the protocol, or to the activities of the EMD.

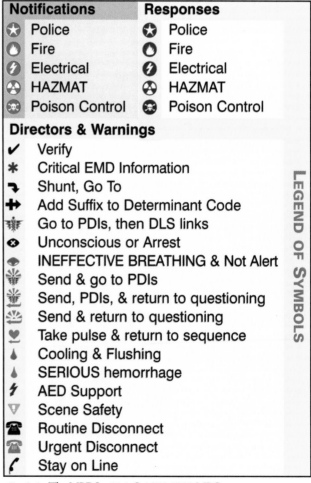

Fig. 3-4. The MPDS, v11.1 © 1978-2003 MPC.

The purpose of conventions is to provide the EMD with a consistent and more meaningful document. The result is greater ease-of-use and reliability.

Principles for Getting Started

There are different kinds of callers, so the EMD must be emotionally prepared to use a host of telecommunication strategies to project professionalism and command over the situation. This builds the caller's trust in the system. Using the Case Entry protocol, the EMD determines what has happened, and, for a select few types of situations, dispatches resources within 20 to 30 seconds. In most cases, the EMD chooses a dispatch protocol—perhaps using a SHUNT or BRIDGE protocol along the way—to gain more information before sending the necessary response. Sounds easy, and it usually is if the important principles surrounding this part of the protocol system are understood.

> **Callers often have valuable and detailed information necessary to perform a complete assessment.**

Types of callers. Who calls for emergency medical assistance? There are actually four basic types.

First-party callers. The caller is the person with the actual problem. For example, a first-party caller is reporting his own chest pain or asking for help with a burn sustained while cooking.

Second-party callers. The caller is directly involved with, and in close proximity to the person having the problem. A second-party caller may be the friend who was with the patient when she collapsed, or someone who was in an auto accident and is unhurt, but is calling to report someone else who was injured.

Third-party callers. These people are not directly involved with or in close proximity to the incident, but are helping by calling. They are the people who heard a crash, glanced out the window, and saw that an accident had occurred, but did not actually go to the scene. They are the ones who work as security guards and can only tell you that someone rushed up to the desk yelling, "Call an ambulance!" and then rushed off. Third-party callers tend to know less specific things (but rarely nothing) about the situation.

> **Third-party callers tend to know less specific things (but rarely nothing) about the situation.**

Fourth-party callers. Sometimes, reports of emergencies are relayed from other public-service agencies. These are known as fourth-party callers and may (or may not, depending on cross-agency education) have a notion about priority dispatch. One significant limitation of fourth-party callers is that the EMD cannot speak with the primary caller, and the fourth-party caller may not have obtained correct, dispatch-significant information.

About 75 percent of all callers are either first-party or second-party callers. Third-party callers constitute almost all the remaining telephone population. First- and second-party callers are almost always able to provide the information required to implement priority dispatch. Third-party callers may be able to report only the call location and a callback number. Priority dispatch may not be fully used in all instances, such as when callers do not know the needed information. But statistics indicate that most callers do have valuable and detailed additional information.

Breakdown of Caller Party			
Caller Party	**Monroe County (U.S.)**	**British Columbia**	**Melbourne**
First	14 %	9 %	15 %
Second	63 %	63 %	80 %
Third	20 %	17 %	3 %
Fourth	2 %	9 %	0 %
Unknown	2 %	2 %	2 %
Total Cases	3515	3109	2374

Fig. 3-5a. Percent of callers that fall in first, second, third, fourth, and unknown party, 1996-97. Data obtained from random case review AQUA™ statistics.

Analysis of Caller Party in Traffic Accident Cases		
Caller Party	**Percent of Total Cases Reviewed**	**Number of Total Cases Reviewed**
First	0.6	1
Second	16.5	26
Third	82.1	129
Fourth	0.6	1

Fig. 3-5b. Caller-party percentages in 157 randomly selected traffic accident cases from South and East Wales, U.K. 1996.

Experience has shown that the majority of callers are able to perform well. Although they tend to be good reporters of what has happened, they often use lay terms to interpret the events. This can be confusing to dispatchers used to codes or precise medical terminology, but priority dispatch has been crafted to protect the EMD from making false assumptions based on unclear interpersonal communication. And when the EMD begins to describe ways to help, callers are, not surprisingly, able to perform. A review of 157 randomly-selected protocol 29: Traffic Accident cases from South and East Wales, U.K., reveals a predictable finding (see figure 3-5).

This sample shows a very high percentage (82.1) of third-party callers. A special feature on Case Entry, the "fast track" link, occurs when traffic accident is the chief complaint and after the number of patients is asked, the EMD then bypasses patient-specific Case Entry questions and begins the secondary survey interrogation on protocol 29: Traffic/Transportation Accidents (see fig. 3.5b below). High percentages of third-party callers support this pathway.

Rule 4	PROTOCOL **29**

A traffic accident in which injury to a **NOT DANGEROUS** Body Area is **reported but not verified by a 1ˢᵗ party caller**, should be classified as injuries (29-B-1) because of the mechanism of injury.

Case Entry Protocol Theory. It is impossible to judge the severity of a situation on the basis of the caller's tone, rate, and volume of speech. Sometimes the most distraught callers seem to have the most minor problems, and the least desperate-sounding, the worst. A formal study of the emotional content and cooperation scores (ECCS) of over 6,000 callers showed that while the emotional content of some callers does correlate with the caller's relationship to the patient and

> ! **Authors' Note**
>
> Variations in "random" selection practices affect the direct extrapolation of these data sets to full populations. The inclusion of most or all cardiac arrest, choking, and childbirth cases would enrich second-party percentages, while exclusion of traffic accidents (because of their third- and fourth-party nature) would also increase second-party findings.

the nature of the incident, the actual differences are too small to be of any value in prioritizing the call[165] [Jeff Clawson, MD. and Robert Sinclair, PhD., *The Emotional Content and Cooperation Score in Emergency Medical Dispatching*, Prehospital Emergency Care, 2001.] The answers to the Case Entry protocol questions are a far more reliable source to use in assigning priority to a call for help.

The Case Entry protocol is the starting point for each call. It is the equivalent of the field provider's "initial assessment" commonly called the **primary survey**. That is, just as hands-on emergency care providers begin all medical intervention by checking the "**ABCs**" (airway, breathing, and circulation), the EMD always begins with the Case Entry protocol. The information elicited from Case Entry sets the stage for the remainder of the call.

Of highest priority is the location of the call and the telephone number being used by the caller. If for any reason the conversation is cut off at this point, the EMD has enough information to send an emergency response.

1. The location: "What's the address of the emergency?"

2. The phone number: "What's the phone number you're calling from?"

One crucial aspect of the Case Entry protocol is verification. Verification of the caller's location and telephone number should come from the caller, not the EMD, to minimize errors. For example, if the caller says "2555 Oakwood," and the EMD repeats the address for verification, but says "255 Oakwood," the distraught caller cannot be expected to catch the slip-up—which could put rescue units many blocks off course. The EMD should always verify the location and call-back telephone number by asking the caller to repeat it. (Example: "Please repeat the address for verification," has been observed to work well in several centers and does not irritate or confuse callers.) Enhanced 9-1-1 systems automatically provide location and call-back number, eliminating the need to initially obtain them, but not the need to verify.

The EMD should always verify the address and phone number even if the first presentation of these items seems correct initially. A recent case in Illinois resulted when a caller with a name familiar to the calltaker appeared on the ANI/ALI screen. The caller, having a heart attack at the time, was asked if he was at a tavern the calltaker recalled that he owned. Having extreme difficulty breathing, he correctly gave the address of his actual location at his residence several miles away. Similar numbers were present in both addresses and the calltaker sent the paramedic crew to the location she thought she

> **The EMD should always verify the location and callback telephone number by asking the caller to repeat it.**

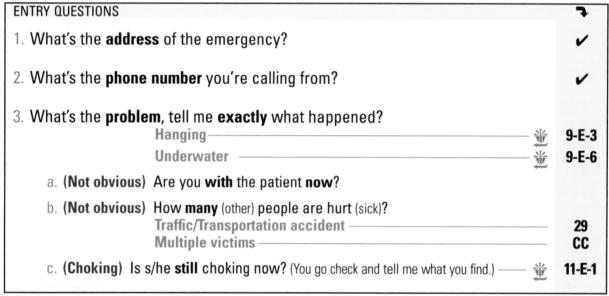

ENTRY QUESTIONS   ↱

1. What's the **address** of the emergency?   ✔

2. What's the **phone number** you're calling from?   ✔

3. What's the **problem**, tell me **exactly** what happened?

        Hanging ———————————————————————— 9-E-3

        Underwater —————————————————————— 9-E-6

  a. **(Not obvious)** Are you **with** the patient **now**?

  b. **(Not obvious)** How **many** (other) people are hurt (sick)?

        Traffic/Transportation accident ——————————— 29

        Multiple victims ——————————————————— CC

  c. **(Choking)** Is s/he **still** choking now? (You go check and tell me what you find.) —— 11-E-1

Fig. 3-6. The MPDS, v11.1 protocols. © 1978-2003 MPC.

Complaints vs. Chief Complaints

The following are assorted complaints received by dispatch. Identify which are *Chief Complaints* that can be categorized and which are not:

1. He's dying, come quick.

2. She's got really bad chest pain.

3. Baby come now.

4. It's really bad, hurry, hurry, hurry.

5. He's making funny noises breathing.

6. She needs an ambulance.

7. Her stomach pain made her pass out.

8. We need the paramedics here now!

9. She's turning blue.

10. The baby needs oxygen.

Answer: Only 2, 3, 5, 7, and 9 are Chief Complaints. (Items 5 and 9 are Chief Complaints for ECHO dispatch purposes but, it is still necessary to determine *why* she is turning blue, or "making funny noises"— choking, electrocution, drowning, heart attack, overdose, etc.)

Fig. 3-7. Complaints vs. Chief Complaints.

recalled seeing on the screen initially (his tavern) without verifying it visually. ALS arrival was delayed 8 to 10 minutes and the patient was found in cardiac arrest and died. Any notification by a crew that the patient can't be located should result in a verification of the address on the ANI/ALI device or via direct callback.

Next on the protocol are four questions known as the "Four Commandments." (The name stems historically from efforts by the developers of priority dispatch to instill complete and reverent appreciation for their universally vital importance.) These questions serve as the springboard for accessing the proper dispatch protocol within priority dispatch. They relate specifically to selection and use of the appropriate dispatch protocol. They are:

1. **The Chief Complaint:** "What's the problem, tell me exactly what happened?"

2. **Patient's Age (or approximation):** "How old is s/he?"

3. **Status of Consciousness:** "Is s/he conscious?"

4. **Status of Breathing:** "Is s/he breathing?"

Pivotal to success in using the system is discovering a usable chief complaint (see fig. 3-7). The EMD must routinely ask, "What's the problem, tell me exactly what happened?" just as it is written.

But what constitutes a true Chief Complaint? "He's dying!" is certainly a complaint! But it is not a Chief Complaint. The EMD must inquire as to what the patient seems to be dying of. The answer, which may perhaps be something like, "He's had terrible chest pain for an hour and is really sweaty," provides a useable Chief Complaint such as protocol 10: Chest Pain. The definition of a Chief Complaint is the reason the patient or caller is seeking emergency medical care. In some instances, this may only be the mechanism of injury such as a long fall or a car accident. A Chief Complaint must contain sufficient information to allow categorization into one of the 33 defined Chief Complaints. A Chief complaint, then, provides the EMD with enough information to access a specific priority dispatch protocol; vague complaints do not (fig. 3-7).

Some callers may seem specific in their description of the complaint: "He's having a heart attack!" yet the EMD can still generate a more accurate chief complaint. The question, "Tell me exactly what happened?" might result in this answer: "While he was eating he suddenly couldn't talk and then fell over"

(suggesting choking, a clearer Chief Complaint). Or "He can't talk or move his left arm" (suggesting stroke). Callers should obviously not be expected to have sophisticated medical knowledge, or to use medical terms. Ask all listed questions which ensures obtaining usable answers. The EMD can always access something—even if only protocol 32: Unknown Problem (Man Down).

Improved responder safety is another by-product of getting an accurate Chief Complaint. When a caller reports a person is bleeding, the EMD should ask what happened. If the answer is, "Because I shot him! He was trying to beat me again!" the EMD can initiate the more specific Stab/Gunshot/Penetrating Trauma protocol, warn responding crews of a volatile situation, and send the police.

A new feature in v11 is to ask (when not obvious) "Are you with the patient now?" This will set the stage for appropriate patient condition verifications such as "Is s/he still choking now?" and "You go check and tell me what you find." In the computerized program, this helps determine the party of the caller which allows instant conversion of questions and treatment scripts into first vs. second or third-party format (you vs. s/he).

The second of the Four Commandment questions is "Is s/he conscious?" There are three possible answers: "Yes," "No," or "I don't know." Even if the caller is unsure of consciousness, the EMD then asks the third of the Four Commandment questions: "Is s/he breathing?" There are four possible answers: "Yes," "No," "I'm not sure," (uncertain) and "I don't know" (unknown).

Axiom 1	CASE ENTRY PROTOCOL

Uncertain breathing status indicates a **2nd party** caller who has seen the patient and is still unsure. **This is considered NOT BREATHING until proven otherwise.**

Axiom 2	CASE ENTRY PROTOCOL

Unknown breathing status indicates a **3rd or 4th party** caller who cannot personally verify the patient's status.

The age of the patient is included in the Four Commandments because age is often a pertinent factor in prioritization. The EMS response may be more urgent for some situations than others solely on the basis

> ### ⚠ Authors' Note
>
> Age is useful as a delineator of urgency in Chief Complaints types such as: Abdominal Pain/Problems, Back Pain (Non-traumatic or Non-recent), Chest Pain, Convulsions/Seizures, Overdose/Poisoning (Ingestion), and Sick Person (Specific Diagnosis). Chest pain is an example of where age is an important clinical divider. Obviously, children are not having heart attacks.
>
> The actual age range established is based on clinical data and medical standards of care and practice already in place. There is no justification for the use of age across all Chief Complaint types to determine a higher level of response. For example, sending a delta-level response for all children under three years of age is not clinically supportable by the current medical literature (see The Age Factor in Chest Pain, Chapter 6: Medical Conditions).

of age within certain Chief Complaints. For example, with chest pain and abdominal pain in females, age is statistically relevant when considering the likely severity of the situation. Also, there are age-dependent instructions when providing Dispatch Life Support, with differences in technique for infants (less than 1 year), children (ages 1-7), and adults (age 8 and over).

> ### Rule 8   CASE ENTRY PROTOCOL
>
> The patient's **age does not need to be determined initially in multiple-patient events.** If individual patient assessment is possible, age should be determined.

> ### Rule 10   CASE ENTRY PROTOCOL
>
> Ask, "Is the patient **male** or **female**?" if the patient's gender is not obvious.

Additional questions on the Case Entry protocol help the EMD refine the available information. The EMD must occasionally inquire (if it is not already obvious) whether the patient is male or female, so that Key Questions can be appropriately customized according to gender to the caller's situation. Gender is unofficially referred to as the "fifth commandment" for software systems. When applicable, the EMD asks for the approximate number of patients. This is actually a sub-question of the Chief Complaint having to do with further determining exactly what happened.

Obviously, an ambulance can handle more than one patient, if both are not seriously injured, although this can be difficult to determine at times. Remember that multiple victims triggers a DELTA response on several protocols, so try to distinguish "occupants" from "patients" in traffic accidents whenever possible. If the caller knows nothing (cannot report state of consciousness, status of breathing, or even a Chief Complaint), the EMD uses protocol 32: Unknown Problem (Man Down).

The only time an EMD turns to a priority protocol before finishing all questions on the Case Entry protocol is when the caller reports multiple patients. In these situations the Case Entry guides the EMD to turn directly to the appropriate Chief Complaint protocol. There, the remaining Four Commandment values are included in the Key Questions.

> ### Rule 7   CASE ENTRY PROTOCOL
>
> If traffic/transportation accident, determine the **number of patients**, then go to Protocol 29.

The age, status of consciousness and breathing are considered the vital signs of EMD, and, as such, are never optional in assessment. They are to be asked, and the answer relayed to responding units, without exception. If the answer to a particular commandment question is "unknown," then that is what is relayed. For example, "Engine 13, Ambulance 512, you are responding on an unknown problem at Pioneer Park. The patient is a male adult, age unknown. The status of consciousness and breathing are not known. No further details. Advise caution, no police backup." From this method of information relay, the responders know what is known—and what is not. Four commandment status is not left to their imagination. These four questions clearly constitute the medical dispatch standard of care and practice.

When to dispatch prehospital responders. There are only two standard times that dispatch of prehospital personnel occurs within priority dispatch: during the Case Entry protocol, or at the conclusion of the key questions on the priority dispatch protocol selected. For most calls, the patient will be conscious and breathing. Traffic/Transportation Accidents and other situations with multiple victims are an exception to this. Rule 7 explains how to handle these cases. In these situations, determine the number of people injured (not the number of people present, only those actually injured) and then go to the appropriate protocol.

> **Only on traffic accident calls does the EMD turn to a specific protocol before completing all questions on Case Entry.**

The other (rarer) situation that the EMD will encounter is the patient who is not breathing or conscious and who needs an immediate and urgent response. The ECHO determinant was designed for these patients.

Understanding ECHO Determinant Practice

Essentially, ECHO can be considered an extended subset of the DELTA-level codes similar to how OMEGA has evolved as subset of ALPHA—but in the reverse acuity direction. An example of the functionality of the ECHO is demonstrated by the capability of public safety systems that have a variety of response-capable units, to be able to more easily delineate and *mobilize crews that normally would not respond on typical EMS problems,* to be "ethically" sent when true obvious critical time-life situations exist. Most metropolitan and/or fire-based EMS systems have special response vehicles staffed with trained first responder or EMT-level personnel on ladder trucks, snorkels, and platform apparatus. Supervisor vehicles, HAZMAT, heavy rescue, and special extrication teams may also be available for special, limited ECHO response. An increasing number of systems utilize police with AEDs. The dilemma is *when* to send these non-standard and sometimes less-than-economical and/or more ponderous responding crews to people actually in the process of expiring. This problem has surfaced on several occasions in the history of EMD evolution and was once addressed during a large system implementation in the late 1980s by creating a DELTA-1 versus DELTA-2 division in the version 9.0 protocol prior to the introduction of the diverse sub-determinant codes first contained in version 10.

It is important to understand that the ECHO level *does not require* a different response from DELTA, but only suggests that one is, at times, *ethically* appropriate. This will move agencies with the capability to formally consider (once approved) such special response vehicles *at their own* (clinical and local availability*) discretion.*

> ### ECHO Determinant Practice
>
> The **ECHO** level allows **early recognition** and **closer response initiation** based on **extreme conditions of breathing**.
>
> Such coding is separated from **DELTA** to encourage **local** assignment of the **absolute closest** response of **any trained crew** (i.e., police with AEDs, fire ladder or snorkel crews, **HAZMAT** or other specialty teams).

ECHO coding has a great potential advantage in certain systems. It can allow a closer response on critical time-life events as well as an earlier response without requiring the EMD to "fudge" the point of response while attempting to adhere to protocol. The automated version of the protocol, ProQA™, will benefit as well. In many critical cases, the problem with incorrect chief complaint selection is minimal since the terrible state of the patient is known at, or even before, the "what's the problem" stage. Further delineation of the chief complaint is still necessary to provide the correct PAIs, not just the correct response. Detection of an ECHO-level problem early on does not preclude the correct use of the Case Entry process, but in critical time-life situations enhances it.

The ECHO-level process is designed to allow early recognition and closer response initiation, based on extreme conditions of breathing in obvious cases of specific time-life situations. Such coding is separated from DELTA to encourage the special local assignment of the absolute closest response of trained crews (i.e., police with AEDs, fire ladder or snorkel crews, HAZMAT, heavy extrication, or other specialty teams) that are not routinely utilized in the standard medical assignment choice grid.

It is important to note, that ECHO should not be construed as being a just a higher time-based problem list. Because of safety issues, many DELTA clinical codes are time sensitive but are not, at this time, identified as ECHO. The use of ECHO as a time delineator would not be a correct understanding of the objectives on which it was organized.

The MPDS v11 Case Entry protocol has a number of points where an answer to a Key Question leads to the "send, PDIs, and return" symbol. These are the points where and ECHO response can be correctly coded. The Critical EMD Information, printed along side the Case Entry questions panel, explains the use of this symbol.

CRITICAL EMD INFORMATION

✻ For **NOT BREATHING** situations or **INEFFECTIVE BREATHING**, code as **ECHO** on Protocols 2, 6, 9, 11, 15, 31 **only**, initiate **dispatch**, give **PDIs**, and **return** to question sequence when directed by 🌿 symbol.

After the ECHO response has been initiated and the PDIs given, the "and return" part of this symbol leads the EMD back into the Case Entry question sequence. Rule 4 explains that even after an ECHO response has been mobilized, it is important to always continue with the Case Entry sequence.

Rule 4   CASE ENTRY PROTOCOL

Case entry questioning **must always be completed**, even when an **ECHO** determinant has been selected.

The reason the EMD must complete the key question sequence is that it will provide more detailed information relevant to the safety and patient issues of that chief complaint. Therefore, it is imperative that the EMD carefully comply with protocol and complete ALL listed questioning. This will insure that the proper knowledge regarding safety issues and the appropriate warnings and/or advice is always passed on to the responders and potential scene helpers.

The following is an example of Case Entry ECHO use (in an enhanced system):

Caller: (Yelling) He can't breathe at all, he's turning blue!

EMD: What's the address of the emergency?

Caller: 442 Glenwood Avenue.

EMD: What's the phone number you're calling from?

Caller: 466-9376.

EMD: What's the problem, tell me exactly what happened?

Caller: He's dying from an asthma attack. Send someone quick!

EMD: How old is he?

Caller: I don't know.

EMD: Tell me approximately, then.

Caller: He's about 30, hurry!

EMD: Is he conscious?

Caller: Barely.

EMD: Is he breathing?

Caller: He's fighting to breathe.

[Send Dispatch Code: 6-E-1 INEFFECTIVE BREATHING. Tell the caller, "I'm sending the paramedics to help you now. Stay on the line." Return to question sequence.]

Axiom 3   CASE ENTRY PROTOCOL

After an **ECHO** response, **completing all Case Entry and Chief Complaint** key questions ensures that the proper knowledge regarding **safety** issues and the appropriate warnings and/or advice are immediately and always **passed on** to the responders and potential scene helpers.

Rule 5   CASE ENTRY PROTOCOL

Chief Complaint key questioning must **always be completed** to cover scene **safety** issues, even when an **ECHO** determinant is selected.

Since each ECHO-containing Chief Complaint protocol has only one ECHO determinant, correct coding from Case Entry is greatly simplified. Protocol 9, however, allows several sub-determinants to be coded. The Additional Information section adds more details regarding the use of protocol 9 and 11 ECHO determinants.

When an emergency response is dispatched directly from the Case Entry protocol, the EMD still turns to the appropriate dispatch protocol Case Entry after questioning is completed. In many cases, this selected protocol will be a BRIDGE protocol. There are BRIDGE protocols for:

- Cardiac/Respiratory Arrest
- Choking
- Childbirth

It may seem that, for the patient who appears to warrant the "send in the cavalry" ECHO response, it might make most sense to go directly from Case Entry to Dispatch Life Support protocols A, B, C, D, E, Y, or Z. Under

NOT BREATHING Situations

The following, when **offered** in response to "What's the problem" or any listed Entry Question:

- **Choking** (verified)   **11-E-1**
- **Not breathing** at all   **9-E-1**
- Breathing **uncertain** (agonal) **9-E-2**
- **Hanging**   **9-E-3**
- **Strangulation**   **9-E-4**
- **Suffocation**   **9-E-5**
- **Underwater**   **9-E-6**

INEFFECTIVE BREATHING

The following, when **volunteered** at any point during Case Entry (code as **ECHO** on 2,6,9,11,15,31):

- "Barely breathing"
- "Can't breathe at all"
- "Fighting for air"
- "Gasping for air" (agonal respirations)
- "Making funny noises" (agonal respirations)
- "Not breathing"
- "Turning blue or purple"

Rule 11   CASE ENTRY PROTOCOL

Do not advise callers to perform any PDIs or PAIs **until all safety key questions are completed** (those in red).

POST-DISPATCH INSTRUCTIONS

a. **(ECHO)** I'm sending the **paramedics** (ambulance) to help you now. **Stay on the line**.

b. **(Hanging and not OBVIOUS DEATH)** **Cut** her/him **down** immediately, loosen the noose and see if s/he's **breathing**.

c. **(Underwater)** **Do not go in the water** unless it's **safe** to do so. ▽

d. **(Critical Caller Danger)** (If it's too **dangerous to stay** where you are, and you think you can leave safely,) **get away** and **call me** from somewhere **safe**. ▽

Rule 9   CASE ENTRY PROTOCOL

When the initial **Chief Complaint appears to be seizure, go to Protocol 12** regardless of consciousness and breathing status.

no circumstances is this appropriate. Completing the question sequence on Case Entry and then turning to the appropriate Chief Complaint protocol is a critical part of correct use of the MPDS. Only by turning to the appropriate Chief Complaint protocol and asking its Key Questions is the EMD able to evaluate scene safety issues (Rule 5, Axiom 3). Scene safety questions will lead the EMD to the correct Post-Dispatch Instructions and then to the correct—appropriate and safe—DLS links. Going directly from Case Entry to Pre-Arrival Instructions misses these important steps and, in many situations that have already led to an ECHO-requiring response, will place the caller (and later the responder) in danger. Callers should not be advised to perform any PDIs or PAIs until all safety Key Questions (those listed in red) are completed.

ECHO does, however, have its own set of Post-Dispatch Instructions, which should be followed (see Post-Dispatch Instructions following).

There is one exception to the ECHO determinant for the patient who is not breathing: convulsions and seizures. The seizure patient who is not breathing is a unique situation as once the seizure stops—in most instances—breathing will resume. For this reason, if the caller provides information that the not-breathing patient has actually suffered (is currently suffering from) a seizure, the EMD should complete Case Entry questioning and then turn to protocol 12: Convulsions/Seizures.

Titles of the Dispatch Protocols. The titles of the dispatch protocols vary according to the type of call being dispatched (see fig. 3-8). This subtle principle stems from something that developers noticed during early formulation of priority dispatch. That is, in medical situations, callers are far more likely to base their report of a Chief Complaint on signs and symptoms. "He's having chest pain!" "She's having trouble breathing!" "My son's having a seizure!" Therefore, medical protocols are titled "Chest Pain," "Breathing Problems," "Convulsions/Seizures," and so on. In cases of injury, however, callers are more likely to describe *what* has happened. "There's been a terrible accident!" "Our nephew is drowning!" "I've been raped." Thus, incident-type protocols are titled in those terms, for example, as "Traffic/Transportation Accidents," "Drowning (Near)/Diving/SCUBA Accident" and "Assault/Sexual Assault."

Chief Complaints by Protocol Type

Medical Incident Protocols

1. Abdominal Pain/Problems
2. Allergies (Reactions)/Envenomations (Stings, Bites)
5. Back Pain (Non-Traumatic or Non-Recent Trauma)
10. Chest Pain
12. Convulsions/Seizures
13. Diabetic Problems
18. Headache
19. Heart Problems/A.I.C.D.
20. Heat/Cold Exposure
23. Overdose/Poisoning (Ingestion)
25. Psychiatric/Abnormal Behavior/Suicide Attempt
26. Sick Person (Specific Diagnosis)
28. Stroke (CVA)
33. Transfer/Interfacility/Palliative Care

Traumatic Incident Protocols

3. Animal Bites/Attacks
4. Assault/Sexual Assault
7. Burns (Scalds)/Explosion
16. Eye Problems/Injuries
17. Falls
21. Hemorrhage/Lacerations
22. Industrial/Machinery Accidents
27. Stab/Gunshot/Penetrating Trauma
29. Traffic/Transportation Accidents
30. Traumatic Injuries (Specific)

Time-Life Incident Protocols

6. Breathing Problems
8. Carbon Monoxide/Inhalation/HAZMAT
9. Cardiac or Respiratory Arrest/Death
11. Choking
14. Drowning (Near)/Diving/SCUBA Accident
15. Electrocution/Lightning
24. Pregnancy/Childbirth/Miscarriage
31. Unconscious/Fainting (Near)
32. Unknown Problem (Man Down)

Fig. 3-8. Chief Complaints by protocol type. The MPDS, v11.1 protocols. ©1978-2003 MPC.

The reason people calling to report medical problems tend to use symptoms to describe what is happening is because they are usually either first- or second-party callers. People calling in injury cases tend to be less close to the incident. They may be second- or even third-party callers, who know very little about the details of the incident. Even if they can describe specific symptoms, people calling to report injuries are still likely to focus on the type of incident that has occurred. For example, a caller is less likely to report, "He's unconscious" than, "He fell off his roof and was knocked out."

The Chief Complaint protocols in MPDS v11 have further refined the distinction between medical and traumatic incidents. "Snakebite", for example, has a consequence that is medical (poisoning) as well as a consequence that is traumatic (the physical bite). The medical consequence is far more important than the generally trivial traumatic puncture wounds, so snakebite is now handled on protocol 2 which is a medical protocol—Allergies (Reactions)/Envenomations (Stings, Bites)—rather than protocol 3 which is a trauma protocol—Animal Bites/Attacks. Rules 1, 2, and 3 outline the basic directions for selecting the correct chief complaint.

Rule 1   CASE ENTRY PROTOCOL

If the Chief Complaint includes scene **safety** issues, choose the protocol that best addresses those issues.

Rule 2   CASE ENTRY PROTOCOL

If the Chief Complaint involves **TRAUMA**, choose the protocol that best addresses the **mechanism of injury**.

Rule 3   CASE ENTRY PROTOCOL

If the Chief Complaint appears to be **MEDICAL** in nature, choose the protocol that best fits the patient's **foremost symptom**, with **priority symptoms** taking precedence.

Remember, lay people usually do not speak in medical terms. The caller may say, "He's jerking all over the place and his eyes are rolled back..." when the EMD asks, "What's the problem?" When asked if the person is breathing, the response may be, "Yes, but he's making a snoring sound." Is he conscious? "Well, not really. He's just kind of out of it." The trained, thinking EMD will know that the caller just described a seizure, even though the caller did not know the medical term. A situation that sounded horrendous a moment ago can now be prioritized; the EMD turns to protocol 12: Convulsions/Seizure.

Rule 9	CASE ENTRY PROTOCOL

When the initial **Chief Complaint appears to be seizure, go to Protocol 12** regardless of consciousness and breathing status.

Rule 6	CASE ENTRY PROTOCOL

If the Chief Complaint and status of **consciousness and breathing are unknown** initially (3rd party caller), **go to Protocol 32.**

There is one other situation that might arise during Case Entry questioning. Question 5 (Is s/he conscious?) and/or question 6 (Is s/he breathing?), as well as the Chief Complaint question 3, can elicit "I don't know" responses. In this situation, the EMD should initially select protocol 32: Unknown Problem (Man Down) as indicated in Rule 6.

Principles Related to the Dispatch Protocol

Based on the answers to the Case Entry protocol, the EMD selects the *most* appropriate of the priority dispatch protocols. The EMD then asks all the key questions. Then, perhaps after consulting the **Additional Information** section for help in categorizing an injury or area, the EMD chooses the determinant code most closely linked with what the caller has reported. Once the determinant code has been identified, the EMD matches it with the prehospital response that has been assigned by the local Medical Dispatch Review Committee (see Chapter 12: Quality Management). Designated resources are then sent. In some cases, resources were already sent when the caller reported absence of (or second-party doubt about the status of) breathing. This is the other standard time field providers are dispatched. Finally, the EMD provides post-dispatch instructions to the caller.

> **Asking all the key questions leads to a more appropriate field response and more effective dispatch life support.**

Working with priority dispatch requires mental flexibility and complete familiarity with the system. It requires an intelligent, thinking EMD to be able to function in the hot seat of dispatch, sometimes juggling several emergency calls at once. The Medical Priority Dispatch System provides the framework to keep all the "balls in the air" at once without dropping anything or letting anything slip through the cracks. What seems to some a cut-and-dried process, is as alive and as much an art form as any emergency procedure.

Key Question Theory. The Key Questions are to the EMD what the secondary survey is to field providers. Whereas the Four Commandments established "The Big Picture," the Key Questions provide the answers that depict the situation more precisely. The increase in an EMD's base of information is similar to

Medical Call is Received

Case Entry protocol (primary assessment)

Shunt (identify Chief Complaint) (19, 22, 26)

Key Question-Dispatch protocol (secondary assessment)

Dispatch Units (life-threat—maximal response)

When no other Chief Complaint is identified

Dispatch Units (appropriate response)

Alternate Care Referral (OMEGA)

Bridge (verify life-threat) (9, 11, 24)

Post-Dispatch Instructions (ensure ABCs) (X)

Pre-Arrival Instructions (A, B, C, D, E, F, Y, Z)

Fig. 3-9. Priority dispatch flow chart (the most common pathway is shown in blue).

what a field provider gains by doing a head-to-toe survey. Despite the intensity and urgency of an evolving emergency, asking these specific questions creates a more accurate, useable understanding of each situation. This leads to a more appropriate field response and better pre-arrival instructions.

The schematic in figure 3-9 demonstrates the orderly functioning of a priority dispatch protocol and helps to put to rest a common misconception about the name "priority dispatch." This misconception stems from the protocol's initial successful use in tiering responses within the Salt Lake City EMS system. Because of this association, it was often heard, "We don't need priority dispatch because we aren't going to prioritize any of our calls." While the protocol does, as one of its four main functions, prioritize response (if that is desired), this was not the reason it was titled priority dispatch in the first place. The higher application of the term prioritization is recognized in the EMD's First Law of Prioritization:

EMD's First Law of Prioritization

The MPDS prioritizes the actions of the dispatcher, not just the response.

Corollary to the 1st Law of Prioritization

Therefore, the MPDS is an action plan, not a menu.

Key Question Objectives. Priority dispatch assessment is comprised of four specific objectives that drive interrogation. Just determining the response is a commonly encountered, but completely inadequate, interrogation practice. These are essential reasons why the EMD must take time to ask all the Key Questions.

1. **Determine the proper response configuration.** Only with answers to the Key Questions can an EMD best determine the proper field response for that situation.

2. **Determine the presence of conditions requiring Pre-Arrival Instructions.** The Key Questions help EMDs determine how best to assist the caller: with simple, basic Post-Dispatch Instructions (found on each protocol) or with the more intensive, scripted Dispatch Life Support instructions.

3. **Help the responders address the call.** The answers to the Key Questions also provide more definitive information for responders about what (exactly) is happening at the scene; informed responders can

select their equipment more carefully and mentally prepare for the case at hand.

4. **Provide for the safety for all those at the scene.** Certain Key Questions help the EMD determine whether there are any hazards or threatening situations. This promotes the safety of field responders as well as those there already.

The average number of Key Questions per dispatch protocol is 4.4 (see Appendix B) with the potential for an additional 1.5 optional questions based on previous answers. In some cases these include refinements to one or more of the Four Commandments to gain a clearer idea about the patient's status. For example, two common key questions are

> **A question used without a clear objective, is just that, a question—not an evaluation.**

"Is s/he breathing normally?" and "Is s/he completely awake (alert)?" These differ subtly from "Is s/he breathing?" and "Is s/he conscious?" They ask the caller to examine the *quality* of breathing and consciousness, and act as essential verification of this important assessment of the body's vital status.

The level of emergency response may be affected if a person is making strange noises while breathing, or is conscious but not alert. For example, in a choking situation in which the person is not breathing, a maximal (ECHO) response will have already been dispatched while the EMD was on the Case Entry protocol. The EMD then completes the questions on Case Entry and turns to protocol 11: Choking. Here, the first line: "Choking verified/INEFFECTIVE BREATHING (per Case Entry) directs the EMD to the DLS panel. However, if the person was conscious and breathing, the EMD now asks the Key Questions on protocol 11 to determine the appropriate response. The key questions on that protocol are:

1. **Is s/he completely awake (alert)?** The progression from conscious to unconscious in a completely obstructed person occures in approximately 2-4 minutes. If the patient is losing consciousness it indicates a high probability that the patient's airway is completely obstructed.

2. **Is s/he breathing normally?** The emphasis is on normally. If the patient is able to breathe at all, the situation is a partial obstruction, not a full choking. This is important as performing the Heimlich maneuver is not entirely without risk. The EMD should pay attention to the caller's answer to this question, as comments about the caller talking,

wheezing, or coughing will indicate that some air is getting into the lungs.

3. **What did s/he choke on?** If known, the EMD can relay this information to the responding crews. This can be important when considering the best way to cope with the obstruction.

Key Questions should always be asked completely and in sequence so that DELTA-level, or maximal problems (known as "DELTA-driver" situations) are determined before those of lesser degrees of severity. Yet all the key questions must be asked. Even if the EMD "hits" on a DELTA-level situation, the other Key Questions can still provide important information and satisfy other objectives of dispatch. Early adopters of priority dispatch were concerned that asking the complete sequence of key questions took longer than doing it on-the-fly. Such is not the case. The Los Angeles Fire Department is a good example. During implementation of priority dispatch, they discovered that interrogation time actually dropped enough to allow the inclusion of all Pre-Arrival Instructions, making the new average of call processing times equal to their previous 72 second average.[19]

"Sick Person" Call (2:19 elapsed time)

EMD:	**Fire Department, how can I help you?**
Caller:	I hope I have just a very bad case of food poisoning.
EMD:	**Okay, what's the address, sir?**
Caller:	(gives address)
EMD:	**Okay, it is a house or an apartment?**
Caller:	It's a house on the corner. I'll go ahead and turn the outside porch light on.
EMD:	**Okay, and what did you say what was wrong with you?**
Caller:	Um, woke myself up out of a sleep. I went to the bathroom throwing up. I'm weak in my arms. I'm able to get back and forth to the bathroom. I'm hoping it's just like a food poisoning or something.
EMD:	**Okay, um… how's your breathing right now?**
Caller:	Um, it's short, but it's not…
EMD:	**Is it labored?**
Caller:	A yeah, a bit.
EMD:	➡ **Okay, you're not having trouble breathing are you?**
Caller:	Not particularly, no.
EMD:	**How old are you, sir?**
Caller:	I'm 36.
EMD:	**Do you have a history of heart problems?**
Caller:	I don't, but my father had a heart attack…

EMD:	**Do you have any chest pain or anything like that?**
Caller:	There is some, yeah.
EMD:	**And you said this is… um… you think possibly food poisoning?**
Caller:	Well, like I say, I've just been vomiting from some doughnuts I had at Smiths.
EMD:	**And you're more or less linking that to…**
Caller:	I'm hoping.
EMD:	**Okay, um, are you vomiting any kind of blood or anything like that?**
Caller:	No sir.
EMD:	**Okay, and you said this was, um, (repeats address).**
Caller:	(confirms address)
EMD:	**What's the telephone number you're calling from?**
Caller:	(gives telephone number)
EMD:	**Okay, and you said this is at the corner?**
Caller:	Yeah.
EMD:	**Um, corner of. . . which corner?**
Caller:	(confirms address again)
EMD:	**Okay, sir. Well I'm going to go ahead and send the rescue out there to check you out, okay?**
Caller:	Thank you, sir.
EMD:	**We'll be out there shortly.**
Caller:	Uh huh.
EMD:	**Okay, bye.** ⚜

Fig. 3-10. "Sick Person" call, 1992.

The wording of Key Questions is carefully considered to discourage "ad-lib" efforts by the EMD. In earlier versions of priority dispatch, protocols simply indicated what sort of question the EMD might like to ask—paraphrases like "chest pain?" were standard. Now, the entire sentence is written on the protocol, and should be read verbatim by the EMD. For example, on protocol 2: Allergies (Reactions)/Envenomations (Stings, Bites), one key question asked "When was the exposure?" But the word "exposure" is easily misunderstood; now, the question is asked, "When did this start (happen)?" Once EMDs began reading carefully-scripted questions exactly, much of the confusion and inconsistency that was occurring with ad-lib and paraphrase questioning was eliminated.

> **The information to do the job properly can usually be obtained in the same or less time than the "freelance" style of yesteryear.**

Without compliance to the protocol, freelance dispatchers often get off the track, and lose focus on the issues at hand. For example, in one U.S. city in 1992, an apparently non-urgent call was received. The new EMD did not yet understand that compliance was important as can be seen in the "Sick Person" call figure 3-10.

Several problems are evident in this case of clear noncompliance to protocol 26: Sick Person (Specific Diagnosis). The EMD did not understand that using the exact wording on each question is important (see Protocol 26, Chapter 6: Medical Conditions). "How's your breathing right now?" is not "Are you breathing normally?" In addition, it is an open-ended question that can generate a myriad of answers. However, his answer, "Um, it's short, but it's not..." led the dispatcher to cut the caller off in mid-sentence, and, even though he now had a clear answer to his first question, continued to ask suggestively, "Is it labored?" At this

point the second positive answer to the rephrased question, "Yeah, a bit." was apparently not believed, or, more likely, was not considered *enough* difficulty breathing to be important. The third form of this same question is now a complete reversal of question polarity resulting in the very leading syntax, "Okay, you're not having trouble breathing are you?" At this point the caller appears to have given up and submits stating, "Not particularly, no."

This is a common pattern of unstructured interrogation that reveals not only a structural flaw in protocol compliance but a profound misunderstanding that is unfortunately observable in call after call in many centers. That is, in this case the EMD's role is not to determine the quality of signs and symptoms. Their role is to only quantify their existence. They are either present or they are not. The acceptable answers to the correctly posed key question, "Are you breathing normally?" should be interpreted only as "Yes" or "Everything else" (everything else equaling "No"). Just a little trouble breathing is trouble breathing. Just a little chest pain is still chest pain. Dispatchers like the one in the above case have not properly understood this basic tenet of interrogation at the outset. Adding qualifying words such as, "bad" or "a lot" or vague open-ended questions like "how's your breathing?" demonstrate the problems with ad-lib questioning and adding the words to paraphrases to complete a full question. This is poor medical dispatch practice and results in a predictably confused interpretation of the resulting answers by the EMD.

The dispatcher in this case, because of his "quality of symptoms" filtering, then became intent on verifying the caller's diagnosis of "food poisoning" even though to the experienced quality management reviewer (and medical armchair Monday morning quarterback), the caller was exhibiting signs of denial stating, "I'm hoping it's just like a food poisoning or something." The EMD's completely extraneous question of, "And you're

---

Chest Pain Call: Quantity vs. Quality

EMD:	**Are you breathing normally?**		*[In MPDS version 10.1—removed by the College of Fellows in version 10.2, 3/95.]*
Caller:	Well, I just can't quite... I don't know.		
EMD:	**Do you have any heart problems?**	Caller: ➡	Well, that's the problem... It's gone now.
Caller:	No.		
EMD:	**Where exactly is the pain?**	EMD:	**Oh!**

Fig. 3-11. "Chest Pain" call, Montreal, Quebec 1992.

more or less linking that to..." received the sad and fateful reply, "I'm hoping."

The fact that the EMD here coded the call as a 26-A-1 (sick person without priority symptoms) reveals what was subjectively evident in his interrogation. He believed the symptoms weren't "serious enough" to warrant a higher level of concern.

The rest of the story is literally a coffin nail. About 3 minutes after arrival of an **advanced life support** equipped crew, this calm, very cooperative caller collapsed in cardiac arrest and was not resuscitated. The appropriate review and quality assurance feedback of this case resulted in a sudden and significant increase in general compliance to protocol within this center which later became an Academy **Accredited Center of Excellence.**

Quantity vs. Quality: A Lesson in Understanding Priority Symptoms

On August 13th, 1992. The City of Montreal implemented the MPDS at 4:00 am. The second call received was memorable. A 50 year-old male reported the complaint of being "awakened from sleep with a real strong pain in my chest." Obviously conscious, breathing, and alert, the new EMD handling her first official call continued the interrogation in fig. 3-11.

After coding the call and forwarding the determinant code to the dispatch room (separate union, separate room then) she rapidly gave the appropriate post-dispatch instructions, asking the caller to call back if his condition worsened in any way for further instructions.

At this point the new (and a bit self-conscious) EMD looked up at the 10 or so QIU personnel, implementation consultants, and dignitaries from the Ministry of Health, who had gathered around her desk and said, "Well, how did I do?" To which a consultant replied, "By the numbers." Noting that she still looked like all wasn't quite well, he asked her if she felt there was a problem with her coding of the call. She replied, "Oh no, it was a 10-C-2 (chest pain with abnormal breathing). You guys taught us that." "What's the problem then?" She sheepishly replied, "Well, it's 4:30 in the morning. When the ambulance gets there (HOT) they're going to find a 50 year-old with indiscernible difficulty breathing and no chest pain," adding firmly, "They're going to kill me!" The consultant quickly replied, "It's absolutely irrelevant what they find when they get there." "Irrelevant?" asked a distinguished physician present at the time. "Irrelevant!" he affirmed.

The fact that this caller had reported any chest pain at all was of dispatch significance, regardless of the amount. The fact that his subtle abnormal breathing pattern would be "indiscernible" to the arriving personnel did not lessen the fact he had some.

An extremely important point about the difference between dispatch and field evaluation must be learned here. The EMD "sees" the patient at the earliest point in time in the public safety chain of events. This occurs several minutes (from five up to sixty minutes in rural areas) before responders have the luxury of an in-person visual as well as manual evaluation of the patient. In this time interval the patient can do one of three things:

1. They can get **better;**

2. They can get **worse;** or

3. They can **stay the same.**

Changes may be due to physiological events occurring within the patient, external environmental forces around the patient, or even caller EMD-directed care of the patient that is appropriate—or undirected bystander "help" which may not be.

With this in mind, arriving field personnel would be wise to consider that this "physiologic/time gap" might explain observed differences between the EMD's patient description and their own. The inevitable presence of this interval also makes the comparative study of patient outcomes based on dispatch assessments hard to accurately assess.

A very important similarity exists between the 50 year-old male in Montreal and the 36 year-old male in the "Sick Person" case transcript just reviewed.

In dispatch reality, these patients are identical—males in the cardiac age range with chest pain and abnormal breathing. The difference exists only in the eventual outcome—which is a statistical constant within this group of patients, but not predictable from patient-to-patient. A certain number of these patients will arrest and many that do will die. The famous Clint Eastwood film character, Dirty Harry Callahan summed up the core dilemma of basing response and treatment on such qualitative differences in symptoms demonstrated by these two patients when he asked "Do you feel lucky today?" As a colleague once stated, "Only the 'Big Paramedic in the Sky' knows which one will live and which one will die."

The comment by the consultant in Montreal that, "It is irrelevant what the responders find when they get there," is supported by the fact that, until the standard of care regarding chest pain changes, any male within the cardiac age range complaining of chest pain should receive an advanced life support (ALS) level response to evaluate, apply a cardiac monitor, and transport this type of patient—anywhere, in any system.

Safety Features

In addition to giving patients what they need, the EMD has a chance to discover safety hazards for responding emergency crews. For example, on the Stab/Gunshot/Penetrating Trauma protocol, the first key question is "Is the assailant still nearby?" Responding crews need this information. Later in the key questions, "When did this happen?" should be asked. Even if Key Question 1 suggested the assailant had left the scene, if the answer to this question indicates it was a very recent event there is more chance the assailant could suddenly return.

Similarly, on the Burns (Scalds)/Explosion protocol, the first questions ask whether (if not obvious) the burn was caused by a building fire, and whether anything is still burning or smoldering. Once that has been established, Key Question 3 asks, "Is everyone safe and out of danger?" Next, question 4 determines exactly how the patient was burned (or injured): electrical, explosion, HAZMAT, heat/fire, or household chemical. This is all scene safety information that is crucial to preventing injury to the caller. It also allows the most appropriate responders to be sent and alerts them to act in an appropriately cautious manner. Only

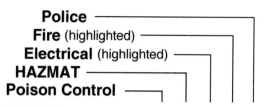

| **Police** ———————————————— |
| **Fire** (highlighted) ———————————— |
| **Electrical** (highlighted) —————————— |
| **HAZMAT** ——————————————— |
| **Poison Control** ————————————— |

POST-DISPATCH INSTRUCTIONS

a. **I'm sending the paramedics** (ambulance) **to help you now. Stay on the line** and I'll tell you **exactly** what to do next.

b. **Beware** of electrical **risks** and electrified **water**. ▽

c. If it's **safe** to do so, **turn off the power**. ▽

d. (≥ **8**) If there is a **defibrillator** (AED) available, **send** someone to get it **now** in case we need it later.

✳ **Stay on the line** with caller until **breathing** can be **safely verified**.
✳ Advise caller and responders of **potential hazards**. ▽

Fig. 3-12. The MPDS, v11.1 protocols. ©1978-2003 MPC.

once that information is gathered can the EMD begin to assess the actual patient, and questions 5, 6, and 7 deal with consciousness, breathing, and the extent of any burns.

On protocols that typically involve dangerous situations, the MPDS makes recommendations to notify the appropriate agencies as determined by local policy. Symbols—that occur in the same place on every card—are highlighted (turned "on") when it may be appropriate to notify them. For example, protocol 4: Assault/Sexual Assault, has the police symbol highlighted indicating the EMD should notify the police department to respond to an assault; protocol 7: Burns (Scalds)/Explosion, has both police and fire symbols highlighted, indicating a potential need to notify the police (following an explosion) or the fire department (if something is still burning or smoldering); protocol 8: Carbon Monoxide/Inhalation/HAZMAT, has police, fire, and HAZMAT symbols highlighted because a HAZMAT response team may be called for; protocol 15: Electrocution/Lightning, has the electrical symbol highlighted, indicating the possibility that the power company may need to be contacted to disconnect the power; and protocol 23: Overdose/Poisoning (Ingestion), has the police symbol highlighted—to notify the police if the overdose patient is violent—and the poison symbol highlighted to indicated a possible necessity for contacting the regional poison control center.

The fact that notification symbols are highlighted does not require that, in all cases, notifications must occur. They are unique reminders that local policy likely

> ### ❗ Authors' Note
>
> Extensive case review in Accredited Centers has strongly substantiated that following carefully scripted questions exactly significantly reduces the confusion and inconsistency present in ad-libbing situations. In addition, the control of the call clearly rests with EMDs who follow the protocol question sequences "by the numbers." The brief gaps that occur when ad-libbers are contemplating the next question often allows the caller to interject anxiety, questions, and, at times, essentially take control of the call.

requires this be done. Local policy is the ultimate rule for all notifications.

While safety is of primary importance to responders, it is also a significant issue for callers and bystanders who may become potential rescuers. On many caller instructions, a qualifier which cautions "If it's safe to do so," is a prompt to the EMD to advise reasonable (and informed) care to those facing difficult choices far away at the scene.

The "Go To" Function. Sometimes, an answer to one of the Key Questions generates a shift to more relevant protocol than the one the EMD initially chose. This is known as the GO TO function. For example, on protocol 1: Abdominal Pain/Problems, the first question asks "Does she have chest pain also?" If the answer is "Yes," a line with a green "Yes" points to the GO TO column, which refers the EMD to protocol 10: Chest Pain for a more relevant set of questions. On other protocols, especially SHUNT protocols, a line with a grey answer condition (see protocol 5) drives the EMD to the protocol listed in the GO TO column. On one protocol, 26, a line with a red "No" sends the EMD to protocol 6 via the GO TO column if the patient is not breathing normally (see figure 3-13).

SHUNT Protocols. If the caller cannot provide a chief complaint, perhaps because the caller is third party or has a language barrier, the EMD turns to the appropriate SHUNT protocol. Predictably, these protocols make liberal use of the GO TO function, since

the goal is to SHUNT the EMD to the most relevant priority dispatch protocol.

SHUNT protocols help the EMD contend effectively with the various ways people respond to their medical crises. Although most people describe what they see ("He's bleeding!" or, "She can't breathe!"), others are vague or unclear. The SHUNT protocols prompt the EMD to dig deeper and gather more useable information.

The first question on protocol 17: Falls, demonstrates the shunting mechanism. A caller might initially report a Chief Complaint of a "fall." The EMD turns to the Falls protocol. The first question asks "What caused the fall?" If the caller describes an electrocution followed by a fall (quite a common cause of a long fall) the EMD is directed to protocol 15: Electrocution/Lightning. If the fall was a ground-level fall caused by a faint or near faint, the EMD is directed to GO TO protocol 30: Unconscious/Fainting (Near). The GO TO feature works effectively as a fail-safe mechanism to help the EMD clarify sometimes convoluted reports from callers.

Sometimes, the EMD cannot gather enough information to SHUNT to a more specific protocol. An appropriate determinant (and EMS response) based on the answers to the key questions can be selected directly from each SHUNT protocol. Remember, everyone should receive an in-person field evaluation (except certain specific poisonings and other approved OMEGA responses, as previously discussed).

Key Questions on the SHUNT protocols also elicit other specific information. On the Sick Person protocol, for example, the EMD is seeking cardiac history. On the Industrial/Machinery Accidents protocol, the EMD seeks information about the mechanism of injury, as well as whether the patient will need extrication from machinery. If the EMD discovers that the situation stemmed from a medical cause, such as fainting, the information can help field EMS providers select the most appropriate equipment to carry in.

The Sick Person (Specific Diagnosis) protocol was developed for cases involving chronic illness. Words such as cancer, leukemia, meningitis, and dehydration sound serious, and can elicit an emotional response in dispatchers. The terminology

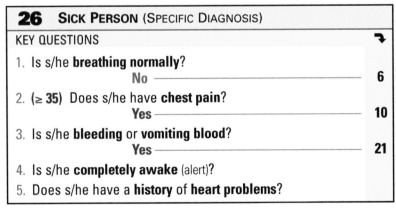

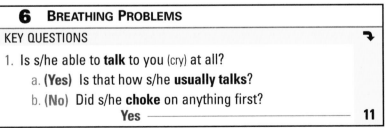

Fig. 3-13. The MPDS, v11.1 protocols. ©1978-2003 MPC.

simply sounds bad. However, the chronic illness may have nothing to do with the actual reason why the patient needs emergency assistance. Much more relevant to these cases is whether the patient has chest pain, trouble breathing, bleeding, abnormal level of consciousness, or certain specific heart problems. A diagnosis of cancer is not as relevant in the emergency context as is the presence of a priority symptom. However, cancer patients (who may survive for years) can have heart attacks, too.

Additional Information Sections. The priority dispatch protocols were described earlier in this chapter as having two parts. The first part is the priority dispatch protocol itself, containing Key Questions, Post-Dispatch Instructions, Critical EMD Information, dispatch determinants and customized responses. The second part is Additional Information. It includes a potpourri of useful information for the EMD. Some of it is useful background review of the situation pertinent to the protocol and is helpful to read occasionally.

> **The Additional Information contains definitions, classifications, and other quickly accessed relevant information.**

However, on some protocols, the EMD uses the Additional Information section during decision-making. For example, on protocol 16: Eye Problems/Injuries, additional information includes a classification list that delineates whether a reported injury is SEVERE, MODERATE, MINOR, or MEDICAL. On protocol 30: Traumatic Injuries (Specific), the Additional Information section includes lists of areas of the body where an injury would be considered NOT DANGEROUS, POSSIBLY DANGEROUS, or DANGEROUS. The EMD uses such lists when selecting a dispatch determinant. Additional Information often contains decision-enhancing definitions and other relevant information.

Axioms, Rules , and Laws also appear in the Additional Information section. These important features are actually the basis of many of the decision-making processes in priority dispatch. They are the expression of how medical science and scene management (especially safety) fits together with dispatch function.

- **Axioms:** are important features that are actually the basis of many of the decision-making processes in priority dispatch. They are self-evident truths that need no proof. They differ from rules in that they tell us *why*, rather than how we do things.

- **Rules:** are more definitive action statements. They convey specifically *how* axioms are used and provide many of the do's and don'ts of priority dispatch. The rules contained within a particular protocol are to be considered always true in the medical dispatch environment, without exception.

- **Laws:** set forth general medical and medical dispatch principles in an interesting and catchy form. In general medicine, they are referred to as "the pearls."

These conventions of priority dispatch help explain the reasoning behind some of the dispatching decisions which, to untrained people, may not seem evident.

For example, one Axiom on protocol 26: Sick Person (Specific Diagnosis) is, "When the caller gives dispatch a previous disease or current diagnosis, it may be because they do not know what is actually causing the patient's immediate problem." This Axiom helps EMDs remember that callers do not try to confuse the system on purpose. They simply may not know the best way to help the EMD help their loved ones. With the trained EMD's assistance and focused evaluation, a good outcome can result despite the caller's confusion. The rules that appear in the Additional Information section may have a medical basis, or they may relate specifically to the priority dispatch process. For example, on the Drowning (Near)/Diving/SCUBA Accident protocol, the second rule is:

Rule 2	PROTOCOL **14**
A submerged patient, regardless of time underwater (≤ 6hrs), is considered **resuscitable by definition until proven otherwise**, especially in a cold-water situation.	

Rule 1	PROTOCOL **15**
All electrocution and lightning strike patients are **assumed to be in cardiac arrest until breathing is verified**. Stay on the line with caller until breathing can be safely verified.	

This information has no bearing on the Dispatch Determinant or the Key Questions. However, it helps the EMD remember that a situation like this must be treated in a different way than other, apparently obvious deaths. Rule 1 on the Electrocution/Lightning protocol provides a good example.

Dispatch Determinant Theory. Once the EMD determines the level of concern using the answers to Key Questions and the Additional Information, the proper Dispatch Determinant can be selected. There are six Dispatch Determinant categories:

E = ECHO-level

D = DELTA-level

C = CHARLIE-level

B = BRAVO-level

A = ALPHA-level

Ω = OMEGA-level

A vital principle is that the names—ECHO, DELTA, CHARLIE, BRAVO, ALPHA, and OMEGA—of the Dispatch Determinant levels do not change. EMS systems implementing priority dispatch must understand that the system can design responses to each determinant as best fits their needs (see Response Theory and Local Development in this chapter). Each EMS system must decide which resources the six levels best require. For example, ALPHA-level may mean basic life support COLD and DELTA-level mean advanced life support HOT.

The E-D-C-B-A-Ω determinant levels are vital for meaningful data collection and quality assurance. The ability to gather meaningful statistical data with this standard coding system allows performance comparisons between cities, regions, and even countries. In this sense, priority dispatch is the first EMS data collection system with more than a local meaning— it has an international scope. The capacity to participate in a broad-spectrum priority dispatch database using this system is useful in an era where procedures, outcomes, and, more recently, payments for emergency services are increasingly scrutinized.

> **The ability to gather meaningful statistical data with this standard coding system allows performance comparisons between cities, regions, and even countries.**

Use of the statistics generated through use of the dispatch determinant codes can demonstrate accurately what types and severity of calls an EMS system has spent its resources handling. For example, there is a perception within EMS that about 5 to 10 percent of calls are of a life-threatening nature, but no one really knows if this is accurate. Priority dispatch allows for

evaluation and verification that the system is being used appropriately and effectively.[166]

Dispatch determinants do not indicate the severity of a situation. That is, the E-D-C-B-A-Ω levels are not related in a linear sense of becoming progressively worse. Rather, they have to do with how many responders will go and (when there are tiers of capability), which levels of expertise are needed, and how rapidly they are needed. The system operates as a two-dimensional, non-linear matrix (see figure 3-14).

The vertical axis on the grid relates to response time. Could responders travel COLD, or are they needed HOT? The horizontal axis relates to rescuer ability. Could basic life support providers handle this or are advanced life support providers needed?

> **Priority dispatch promotes the concept of using the most appropriate resources.**

Priority dispatch has replaced the traditional "more is better" concept. When a crew's training and manpower is matched to a particular situation, that crew can more efficiently handle it. For example, basic-level EMTs are experts at splinting, bandaging, and other basic skills. There is no reason they cannot be trusted to handle basic-level situations, freeing advanced life support providers (who are invariably fewer in number) for advanced-level situations.

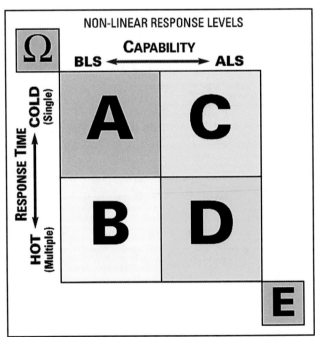

Fig. 3-14. Non-Linear Response Level Theory. The MPDS, v11.1 protocols. ©1978-2003 MPC.

In a study of the Long Beach, California system published in the *Journal of Prehospital and Disaster Medicine* in 1992, Stratton, et al., concluded:

> *Emergency Medical Dispatchers, medically controlled and trained in a nationally recognized dispatcher triage system, were able to provide medical triage to incoming emergency medical 9-1-1 calls with minimal error for under-triage of ALS runs and high selectivity for non-emergency situations.*[34]

Understanding Determinant Terminology

First-time users of priority dispatch are sometimes confused by the terminology, especially in the determinant response section of the protocol where terms such as "determinant," "determinant code," "determinant level," "response code" and "response mode" sound so similar. The following discussion will help take the mystery out of the determinant response section of the protocol.

Determinant Coding Components. First, consider the E,D,C,B,A (and in some instances Ω) classifications. These letters correspond to the determinant levels ECHO, DELTA, CHARLIE, BRAVO, ALPHA, and OMEGA as discussed earlier in this book. Within each determinant level there can be a number of determinant descriptors, listed roughly in order of decreasing significance. The Determinant Descriptors within a determinant level have a medical relationship to each other, which suggests a similarity of response. Put the two together (dispatch level and determinant number) with the protocol number (e.g., 12) and the Determinant Code is the result. For example, after interrogating the caller on protocol 12, the EMD determines that the most appropriate classification is the "continuous or multiple seizures" determinants. This is the first (and in some instances the most critical) of the determinants listed in the DELTA-level, and results in a "12-D-2" Determinant Code (see figure 3-15).

Response Assignment Components. Next comes the Response Assignment, which is where the dispatching agency determines what resources should be assigned, whether mobile or referral, and their mode of travel to the scene. Each agency, through its Medical Control and EMS administration, establishes which Response Assignment best fits each Determinant Code as most appropriate—given the agency's available resources, geography, and political mandates prior to using priority dispatch on-line.

The Response Level is the *type* of responders—specifically, their training or certification level (advanced life support versus basic life support in North America; Paramedics versus Qualified Ambulance Officers in Australasia; or Paramedics versus Ambulance Officers in the United Kingdom).

LEVELS	#	DETERMINANT DESCRIPTORS	CODES	RESPONSES
D	1	**Not** breathing (**after** Key Questioning)	**12-D-1**	
	2	**CONTINUOUS** or **MULTIPLE** seizures	**12-D-2**	
	3	**Irregular** breathing	**12-D-3**	
	4	Breathing regularly **not** verified ≥ 35	**12-D-4**	

Fig. 3-15. The MPDS, v11.1 protocols. ©1978-2003 MPC.

Determinant Coding Components

Protocol Number	Determinant Level	Determinant Number	Determinant Descriptor		Determinant Code
12	D	2	**CONTINUOUS** or **MULTIPLE** seizures	=	12-D-2*

*Note: Several protocols contain additional code-type differentiator letters at the end of the full code called suffixes (see figure 3-22).

Fig. 3-16. Determinant coding components diagram.

Response Assignment Components

Response Level	Mode		Response Assignment
Advanced Life Support (Amb)	HOT	=	ALS Amb HOT

Fig. 3-17. Response assignment components diagram.

Finally, comes the Response Mode, which is what the dispatching agency determines the urgency of response travel to the scene to be. This is done by designating a HOT (lights-and-siren) or COLD (routine) response. Remember, of course, that the EMD always has the option to override the recommended Response Assignment and send a higher level of response if circumstances warrant it. Sending a lower response is not allowed unless patient symptoms or situations are determined to have subsequently improved.

Defining Response Assignments is the responsibility of each agency's Medical Director, Medical Dispatch Review Committee, and Steering Committee. Using the 12-D-1 Determinant Code as an example, the Medical and Dispatch Oversight Committees may decide that an advanced life support unit responding with lights-and-siren is typically the most appropriate response.

The Response Assignment (an advanced life support unit) may be shown as "Amb" and the Response Mode as "HOT," thus generating the Response Code of "ALS Amb HOT" (see figure 3-17).

Priority dispatch has two very important coding systems. The first, the Determinant Codes, are determined and maintained by the Academy's College of Fellows, according to current medical practices, user feedback, and on-going evaluation. The second, the Response Assignment is determined and maintained by each agency according to its available resources, user feedback and on-going evaluation. In a properly established priority dispatch environment, the code and response areas of the system work together to ensure that EMDs choose the most appropriate clinical determinant and assign the most appropriate responses. Figure 3-18 is an example of one particular system's baseline response assignments to each level (but not necessarily to each Chief Complaint). This would be this system's starting point for developing responses to match the codes.

Avoiding Response Code Confusion

The Academy has received requests asking for clarification of how to assign priority dispatch determinant response codes; or more specifically, how to properly assign system resources to the determinants. Typically, an agency requests to make changes in the determinant section of the protocols in an effort to match them to local field responses.

Frustration results when EMDs or their managers confuse the determinant *codes* with unit *response*

assignments. Each determinant code is just that—a code. These clinical codes have no response value as such. In essence, these codes are the dispatch equivalent to a type of medical coding system called diagnosis-related groups (DRGs) used by most hospitals and clinics to bill patients. While these groups are universal (like priority dispatch codes worldwide)

> These baseline response assignments are, in essence, the most commonly used response modes for each level.

the specific amount billed for each code by one hospital may differ from that billed by another (just like different agencies may respond differently to the same determinant code). It is unnecessary to change or move the determinants in either case, as they only represent the medical (clinical) classification determined by the system, and not a response assignment per se. Changing determinant code numbers or positions is not allowed by the Academy. **Changing responses to them is.**

In the case of priority dispatch, each locality's responses are always selected by their responder agency, approved by the agency's medical director, and then listed in the Responses-Modes section. On the printed protocols these are located to the right of the determinants

Baseline Response Example All actual response assignments are decided by local Medical Control and EMS Administration		
Level	**Response**	**Mode**
ECHO	Closest Apparatus–Any (includes Truck Companies, HAZMAT, or on-air staff)	**HOT**
DELTA	Closest BLS Engine Paramedic Ambulance	**HOT** **HOT**
CHARLIE	Paramedic Ambulance	**COLD**
BRAVO	Closest BLS Engine BLS Ambulance (alone HOT if closest)	**HOT** **COLD**
ALPHA	BLS Ambulance	**COLD**
OMEGA	Referral or Alternate Care	

*Note: This is **not** to be considered the Academy's official recommendation for Baseline Responses.

Fig. 3-18. Example of one system's baseline response choices for each level. The MPDS, v11.1 protocols. ©1978-2003 MPC.

LEVELS	#	DETERMINANT DESCRIPTORS	CODES	RESPONSES	MODES
D	1	**Unconscious** or **Arrest**	3-D-1	Priority 1	
	2	**Not** alert	3-D-2	Priority 1	
	3	**DANGEROUS** body area	3-D-3	Priority 1	
	4	**Large** animal	3-D-4	Priority 1	
	5	**EXOTIC** animal	3-D-5	Priority 2	←
	6	**ATTACK** or **multiple** animals	3-D-6	Priority 1	
B	1	**POSSIBLY DANGEROUS** body area	3-B-1	Priority 2	
	2	**SERIOUS** hemorrhage	3-B-2	Priority 2	
	3	**Unknown** status (3rd party caller)	3-B-3	Priority 2	
A	1	**NOT DANGEROUS** body area	3-A-1	Priority 3	
	2	**NON-RECENT** injuries (≥ 6hrs)	3-A-2	Priority 3	
	3	**SUPERFICIAL** bites	3-A-3	Priority 3	

Fig. 3-19. Example of an intra-level locally chosen response variation. The MPDS, v11.1 protocols. ©1978-2003 MPC.

LEVELS	#	DETERMINANT DESCRIPTORS ✚ A	CODES	RESPONSES	MODES
E	1	**INEFFECTIVE BREATHING** ∗ (to be selected from **Case Entry** only)	6-E-1	Closest Staff (any) HOT Paramedics HOT	
D	1	**SEVERE RESPIRATORY DISTRESS**	6-D-1	Closest BLS/Paramedics HOT	
	2	**Not** alert	6-D-2	Closest BLS HOT/Paramedics COLD	
	3	**Clammy**	6-D-3	Closest BLS/Paramedics HOT	
C	1	**Abnormal** breathing	6-C-1	Paramedics HOT	
	2	**Cardiac** history	6-C-2	Paramedics COLD	

Fig. 3-20. Sample of response assignments. The MPDS, v11.1 protocols. ©1978-2003 MPC.

> **! Authors' Note**
>
> Version 11.0 contains the results of over 400 submitted proposals for change recommendations, as well as a roughly equivalent number of Academy-initiated changes.

(numerals). It is not necessary to assign the same response (or approved referral for OMEGA) to all determinants within a determinant level (ECHO, DELTA, CHARLIE, BRAVO, ALPHA, or OMEGA).

By virtue of their medical relationship to one another, determinants are grouped into one of the six levels. On a local response basis however, it is not necessary to adhere to this grouping concept by assigning the same response to all determinants within a given level.

For example, if an agency wishes to assign a response group to the "EXOTIC animal" determinant (3-D-5)" that is different from the baseline response group assigned to the five remaining DELTA determinant

codes, they should not attempt to move the determinant text to another level, rather they should assign the desired response assignment to that code where it lies (see figure 3-19).

The Academy recommends initially assigning a baseline response to each different determinant level—ECHO DELTA, CHARLIE, BRAVO, ALPHA, and OMEGA. ECHO responses, as discussed earlier, may involve different resources on different protocols (refer to fig. 3-18).

These baseline response assignments are, in essence, the most commonly used response modes for each level. They represent the four basic responses for each determinant level and are initially agreed to independent of any chief complaint. This forms a common starting point from which to specifically examine if each Chief Complaint's individual determinant codes can be appropriately handled by the baseline response type.

With these initial baseline responses in mind, each protocol should then be carefully reviewed by local medical control, with special attention given

LEVELS	#	DETERMINANT DESCRIPTORS	CODES	Correct RESPONSES	Incorrect MODES
D	1	**Not** alert	1-D-1	Zulu HOT	~~Delta HOT~~
C	1	**Fainting** or **near fainting** ≥ 50	1-C-1	Yankee COLD	~~Charlie COLD~~
	2	**Females** with **fainting** or **near fainting** 12-50	1-C-2	Yankee COLD	~~Charlie COLD~~
	3	**Males** with **pain above navel** ≥ 35	1-C-3	Zulu HOT	~~Delta HOT~~
	4	**Females** with **pain above navel** ≥ 45	1-C-4	Yankee COLD	~~Charlie HOT~~
A	1	Abdominal pain	1-A-1	X-ray COLD	~~Alpha COLD~~

Fig. 3-21. Sample of "correct" vs. "confusing" response assignment localizations. The MPDS, v11.1 protocols. ©1978-2003 MPC.

to any determinant code whose optimal response type (from the agency's perspective) doesn't exactly fit the baseline response for that level. Such special resource assignments are therefore *exceptions* to the base-line. From a legal stand point, it is essential to document the rationale for why each exception to the baseline response was preferred. This documentation then becomes the agency's self-defined standard of practice for responding.

Each agency, therefore, may define specific responses for any one of the 296 separate determinant codes that are found in priority dispatch. Theoretically, it is conceivable that an agency could have up to 296 different response assignments in a single protocol set, although the average agency appears to only use approximately three. For example, the CHARLIE-level determinants on protocol 10: Chest Pain could appear as shown (see figure 3-20).

> From a legal standpoint, it is essential to document the rationale for why each exception to the baseline response was preferred.

Additional confusion may occur if an EMS agency uses the same names or letters for their response groups that are used within the protocol for its codes—e.g., ALPHA, BRAVO, CHARLIE, DELTA, or ECHO. When this is the case, baseline exceptions to response assignments can be extremely confusing (i.e., "send a BRAVO response for an ALPHA determinant code"). The Academy recommends that agencies choose response group terms such as numerals, proper names, or unused letters of the phonetic alphabet such as X-RAY, YANKEE, and ZULU to avoid this inevitable confusion (see figure 3-21).

In accordance with the Academy's scientific process, individual users are not to make changes to, or deletions from, the Academy-approved protocols. Such revisions are properly implemented only through the Academy's College of Fellows and may be requested by a user submitting a formal "Proposal for Change" form (see Appendix A) with appropriate rationale, case studies, data, or research to the Academy as outlined in the appendix of each EMD Course Manual and this book.

Certain protocols (4, 6, 15, 23, and 27) also have determinant code **suffixes**. These suffixes are used to aid in the computerized relay of specific sub-types within a Chief Complaint to CAD systems which need to identify these differences for add-on responses such as scene security by police in violent situations. For example, it is important to differentiate a stabbing situation from a shooting for responder safety reasons. Safe distance for knives is obviously different than for guns. You can shoot a gun a lot farther than you can throw a knife. A 27-D-3s (stab) versus a 27-D-3g (gunshot) makes this distinction possible to relay electronically (see figure 3-22).

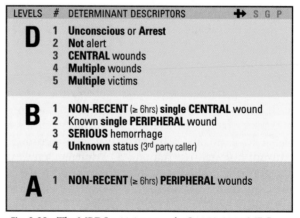

LEVELS	#	DETERMINANT DESCRIPTORS	➡ S G P
D	1	**Unconscious** or **Arrest**	
	2	**Not alert**	
	3	**CENTRAL** wounds	
	4	**Multiple** wounds	
	5	**Multiple** victims	
B	1	**NON-RECENT** (≥ 6hrs) **single CENTRAL** wound	
	2	Known **single PERIPHERAL** wound	
	3	**SERIOUS** hemorrhage	
	4	**Unknown** status (3rd party caller)	
A	1	**NON-RECENT** (≥ 6hrs) **PERIPHERAL** wounds	

Fig. 3-22. The MPDS, v11.1 protocols. ©1978-2003 MPC.

Well-delineated determinants allow for even more accurate information. For example, note that the CHARLIE-level determinants for protocol 12: Convulsions/Seizures, are numbered one through three (see figure 3-23).

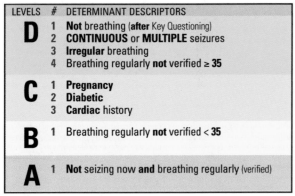

LEVELS	#	DETERMINANT DESCRIPTORS
D	1	**Not** breathing (**after** Key Questioning)
	2	**CONTINUOUS** or **MULTIPLE** seizures
	3	**Irregular** breathing
	4	Breathing regularly **not** verified ≥ **35**
C	1	**Pregnancy**
	2	**Diabetic**
	3	**Cardiac** history
B	1	Breathing regularly **not** verified < **35**
A	1	**Not** seizing now **and** breathing regularly (verified)

Fig. 3-23. The MPDS, v11.1 protocols. ©1978-2003 MPC.

There are various benefits to knowing which of the conditions (pregnancy, diabetes, or cardiac history) was present during a convulsion or seizure. For example, a 12-C-3 determinant means the caller reported a person with a cardiac history who was having a seizure. Field crews receive more accurate information. The patient theoretically receives the benefit of helpers carrying the correct equipment. The data collected is more useful. And the quality improvement manager has better information.

Response Theory and Local Development. At a certain point during initial priority dispatch implementation, a committee including medical directors, field personnel, managers, and administrators faces the task of defining the response assignments to each protocol. The goal of response configuration is to match local EMS capability with the dispatch determinant codes on each protocol. It does not change the protocol; rather, it allows for each community to choose what resources to send for each of the determinant levels—ECHO, DELTA, CHARLIE, BRAVO, ALPHA, or OMEGA.

The political element of establishing localized responses for the dispatch determinants is probably the biggest hurdle an EMS system faces when implementing priority dispatch. Different EMS services within a region (each possibly a bit protective of its territory), different hospital base stations, and different medical directors, may initially complain to priority dispatch advocates that "this concept may work elsewhere, but won't work here."

The more relevant point is to look at what these somewhat diverse entities have in common: a desire to serve the public, and a commitment to emergency patients, and the safety of responding crews. They must eventually sit together and objectively assess the purpose and structure of priority dispatch. Implementation may be an initial challenge, but it is has been accomplished successfully in the full range of EMS system designs and community sizes around the world.

> **! Authors' Note**
>
> So-called American "ingenuity" in this regard has at times been a detriment to system design by creating regionally fragmented response methodologies. The "commonly organized" U.K. system, by design, has limited their response chaos. However, the fear of "prioritization" which conjures up visions of patient care "rationing" as it is referred to in the U.K. has briefly delayed the movement nationally from a time-based response standard (ORCON) to a more useful clinical one.

Not every EMS system is like the example shown. Currently the diversity of response capability from system to system is amazing. But each EMS system, with its unique characteristics, can maximize the efficiency of their response with correct use of priority dispatch.

Not usually understood, nearly every volunteer service can benefit from priority dispatch because it is no longer necessary for every available volunteer to respond on every call. Volunteer time and talent can thus be used more appropriately. Busy volunteer systems might configure their responses as shown here:

ECHO:	Police HOT on-call EMTs HOT Back-up crew HOT
DELTA:	On-call EMTs HOT Backup crew HOT
CHARLIE:	On-call EMTs HOT Backup crew COLD (for extra man power if needed)
BRAVO:	On-call EMTs HOT Backup crew stand-by at home
ALPHA:	On-call EMTs COLD

An Example of Response Configuration—How One System Does It.

Take, for example, a not so mythical EMS system where a private ambulance company provides basic life support-level transport services for a fire department-based EMS system. Each fire station has EMT-level first responders. Advanced life support is provided by firefighter/paramedics at a few of the strategically placed fire stations. Since the ambulance always responds, there are five tiers available to the system and six response-group options. With this sort of configuration, the response section next to the determinants truly demonstrates the user-defined flexibility of priority dispatch.

ECHO-level

Closest apparatus of any kind HOT, ALS responders HOT.

Local rationale: The correct use of ECHO now allows this system to implement reasonable use of non-standard EMS responders such as truck companies, the HAZMAT unit, and other approved on-air staff to immediately aid patients who are literally dying right now. ECHO-initiated crews must be at minimum BLS trained and understand scene safety entry procedures. For 9-E-1 patients, several police units that now carry AEDs are dispatched as "first in."

DELTA-level

Maximal response (both basic and advanced life support providers).

Local rationale: While advanced life support providers would always go HOT, the basic life support transport unit may respond HOT to cases of critical trauma where rapid transport is essential, or they may respond COLD when a medical cardiac arrest patient will be worked for 20 to 30 minutes at the scene. There will always be situations that warrant having every appropriate responder travel HOT to the scene.

CHARLIE-level

Closest advanced life support unit COLD (occasionally HOT), basic life support transport COLD.

Local rationale: Facets of the caller's interview have identified a need for the expertise, judgment, and skills of advanced life support providers. Also, the need for patient transport is likely, so basic life support transport is dispatched COLD, since advanced life support crews will take a few minutes to evaluate and treat the patient at the scene.

BRAVO-level

Closest basic life support unit HOT (occasionally COLD).

Local rationale: Something about the situation merits a rapid response, but the entire system does not need to be mobilized. Since there are inevitably more basic life support providers than advanced life support, they are usually not only closer, but also more available. Depending what the "first-in" crew finds, BRAVO-level calls may result in occasionally discovering a patient who needs advanced life support evaluation or care, and they can request an such a response while providing on-scene basic life support.

ALPHA-level

Closest basic life support transport unit COLD.

Local rationale: Basic EMTs are educated to handle anything that appears in this category. Since the transport company has EMTs driving their ambulances, the fire department does not need to respond at all, leaving that resource available in case of other emergencies. The Salt Lake City Fire Department decreased the need for its EMS fire apparatus at 33 percent of its calls in the first year of full implementation. The private ambulance company handling basic life support (fortunately under the same medical control as the fire department), was able to handle the majority of ALPHA-level calls without any compromise to patients.

OMEGA-level

Special referral and special response as approved.

Local rationale: This system's high compliance to protocol assures that patient situations identified as OMEGA can be safely and more effectively handled by non-traditional response means. An appropriate joint policy with the regional Poison Control Center allows caller transfer for in-depth evaluation and handling of certain types of asymptomatic poisoning and ingestion cases. Carefully evaluated EXPECTED deaths are more correctly and tactfully handled without EMS responders. Customer service to callers in need of physical help for people who are uninjured but have fallen or need aid returning to their usual resting place can be aided by various crews sent non-urgently under their PUBLIC ASSIST assignment program. This system is seeking Accredited Center of Excellence designation so that it can implement the full 21 OMEGA protocol determinant levels in the near future, many safely handled in conjunction with an established nurse advice line service.

Fig. 3-24. One example of an individual system's response configuration thinking.

Priority dispatch responses can also be configured for rural BLS services. In some cases, there are so few calls per year that everyone is more than willing to drop everything to respond. The main issue is whether they should drive HOT or COLD.

For this example, let us also say this group has distant ALS backup, such as a helicopter:

ECHO: Police HOT on-call
          EMTs HOT
          Back-up crew HOT

DELTA: Everyone HOT
          Helicopter dispatched

CHARLIE: EMTs HOT in EMS unit
          EMT COLD with personal vehicle
          Helicopter on stand by

BRAVO: EMTs HOT in EMS unit
          EMT COLD with personal vehicle

ALPHA: EMTs COLD in EMS unit

Knowing that priority dispatch is being used to determine an ECHO- or DELTA-level situation would increase the flight services comfort-level with an "early" dispatch command.

There are five rules for system planners to remember when assigning field responses to the dispatch determinant codes.[24]

1. **Will time make a difference in the final outcome?**
   In other words, is the patient's problem one of the few true time/life priorities requiring the fastest possible response time, with a goal of less than five minutes? Most systems identify the most time critical calls as cardiac or respiratory arrest, airway problems (including choking), unconsciousness, severe trauma or hypovolemia, and true obstetrical emergencies. The early identification of these chief complaints means a maximum response is sent. For the majority of other problems planners need to carefully consider using a less than all-out response.

   For example, situations that tend to generate a misdirected sense of urgency (in both the EMD and in field personnel) are those involving "dispatcher hysteria." One classic case is abdominal pain. Unexplained abdominal pain is frightening, yet true abdominal pain, except in rare instances, is not a prehospital medical emergency. The great majority of patients with abdominal pain face a lengthy workup in the emergency department.

! Authors' Note

The State of Pennsylvania has currently before it proposed EMS rules for the use of lights-and-siren. Pending official approval, their draft 4 includes:

Operators of EMS vehicles have the privilege of using emergency warning lights-and-siren to decrease their response times to life-threatening or potentially life-threatening conditions. Operating emergency vehicles with lights-and-siren has potential for emergency medical vehicle crashes which would not have occurred during non-lights-and-siren responses. Studies have shown that the use of lights-and-siren may only decrease transport time by a couple minutes in most systems and by less than one minute in many systems. Every decision to use lights-and-siren must be based upon the patient's clinical condition, the estimated time saved by a lights-and-siren response/transport, and the increased risk of an emergency medical vehicle collision during such response/transport.

Lights-and-siren may only be used when responding to or transporting a patient with a life-threatening or potentially life-threatening condition.

Dispatch centers and EMS regions are encouraged to have medically approved EMD protocols that differentiate emergency (for example, emergency, code 3, red, CHARLIE, etc...) responses from a lesser level of response (for example, urgent, code 2, yellow, ALPHA, etc...) based upon medical questions performed by the dispatcher.

Each licensed EMS service must assure that every EMS vehicle driver reads and signs a copy of this policy. This applies to all advanced life support, basic life support, and quick response service units.

Through careful use of the Key Questions, the EMD can determine whether a person is within the parameters of those rare situations that might be time-critical. To have an ambulance crew, or worse yet, a full-tiered response, running HOT to any but those rare cases is unnecessary and hazardous (see Authors' Note).

2. **How much time leeway is there for this problem?** That is, what range of time is appropriate for the problem? In medicine, this ranges from seconds to minutes to hours to days. The trained EMD knows that time can make a difference in life-threatening situations, so there is little time leeway; emergency crews must arrive at the scene as quickly as possible. However, the majority of calls lie in a range from those warranting prompt (but not breakneck) responses to those where there is significant time leeway for minor problems.

3. **How much time can be saved by responding HOT?** Accurate information about HOT vs. COLD response times is uncommon but increasing.[36, 37] Response times from time of call to patient contact (vs. pulling up at the address) have not been well-reported. Typical local traffic patterns, time of day, how fast local ambulances actually roll, typical roadway conditions such as stoplights, roads that demand frequent deceleration or acceleration, and local speed limit laws for emergency units should be some of the committee's concerns. If an EMS unit has to respond a mile or two, are the very few seconds saved running HOT worth the disruption to traffic and pedestrians, not to mention the safety of the motoring public and prehospital crew?

New studies published regarding whether time is actually saved running HOT reflect clinically minimal time differences between responding HOT and COLD—yet the relative safety of a COLD response is well-demonstrated and also medically appropriate (see figure 3-25).[25, 36, 38]

The collective perception of lights-and-siren is that their use indicates a real emergency situation. The principles of priority dispatch have resulted in a redefining of emergency. Reducing the use of lights-and-siren is, in itself, a concept that can save lives.[11, 38] When a person's life clearly depends on quick action and rapid motion, lights-and-siren is an important tool. However, there are many times when a situation that appears urgent in the field will not be helped by the use of lights-and-siren. The time saved using them (either going to the patient or to the hospital) is long gone before the patient benefits from definitive care. An ever-increasing number of public safety agencies are adopting a more responsible approach in limiting lights-and-siren use to potentially critical emergencies.

4. **What time constraints are present in the system?** Each system design has its limitations. In some areas, the crews are all-volunteer, and it routinely takes 10 minutes or more to get to the ambulance shed. There is a greater inherent time constraint there than a setup in which prehospital personnel await calls from inside an ambulance stationed on a street corner when the posting selection is done through use of a well-designed system status plan fluidly redeploying available units based on call-frequency predictive analysis.[40] Their departure is immediate and their arrival significantly shortened overall.

5. **When the patient gets to the hospital, will the time saved using lights-and-siren be significant compared to the time spent awaiting care?** This is the most ignored rule. When the critical needs of the patient do warrant the fastest possible response time to the hospital, proper advance notification of the emergency department staff results in immediate, continuing definitive care after arrival.

However, except for the most critical cases, patients do a great deal of waiting. Each usually first sees the ward clerk (who has to generate paperwork), and the health aide (who dresses the patient in proper emergency department attire). Only then might a nurse or a doctor enter the room.

Tualatin Rural Fire Protection District Priority Dispatch Implementation Study			
Period	**Before Implementation**		**After Implementation**
Cases	905		1057
Lights-and-Siren	905	(100%)	406 (38%)
No Lights-and-Siren	0	(0%)	651 (62%)
Response Time	4:31		4:58 (10% increase)
	Time difference after implementation = 27 seconds		

Fig. 3-25. Tualatin Rural Fire Protection District study shows a 27-second response time difference after implementation of priority dispatching in 1985. (Courtesy of Diane Brandt and Pat Southard.)

Non-critically ill or injured people in an emergency department wait for their turn with the doctor, then for transport for X-rays, for the person who will take blood for lab tests, for test results, for the doctor's decision, and for finalization either of admission to the hospital or subsequent release. This process can take many hours and requires much endurance. Did the HOT ride in really help? In essence, was it medically ethical?

Assigning response configurations to all determinant codes is also a political process. No one can expect to sit at a meeting table and hammer out every possible contingency. Something normally handled COLD may—due to weather, traffic, or other unusual circumstances—someday at some particular time warrant a HOT response. The EMD can be provided with the flexibility to choose other options as clearly defined in locally written dispatch policies. The process should obviously be backed up by strong, attentive medical control (see Chapter 12: Quality Management).

Telephone Instruction Theory

Telephone instruction in priority dispatch comes in two styles. The difference rests in how precisely the EMD must relay information, and when. The two styles are Post-Dispatch Instructions and Pre-Arrival Instructions:

Post-Dispatch Instructions. These contain specific advice and warnings to callers specific to each Chief Complaint. They generally involve lower-level situations the caller can handle without the EMD remaining on the telephone, see figure following. When warranted, then, the EMD may sometimes hang up—but never without telling the caller, "If s/he gets worse in any way, call me back immediately for further instructions."

Post-Dispatch Instructions are relayed after appropriate emergency units have been dispatched. (Formerly lumped in with and termed "pre-arrival instructions," these special instructions were separated and given a different name to more accurately reflect when they are given to the caller.) They consist of general instructions relevant to each Chief Complaint, but not necessarily to each patient situation. This must be determined by the EMD through a complete interrogation.

Post-Dispatch Instructions may range from very basic, simple advice for mild or minor situations to extremely important information that can make the difference between life and death. The EMD relays these instructions based on information gathered from the

> ### ! Authors' Note
>
> An interesting difference in nomenclature exists between the name of pre-arrival instructions in English and that used in German. At an early age, the German public is taught that special first aid actions are necessary to help victims at the scene of an accident. These treatments are referred to as *Sofortmassnahmen* meaning literally, "to take immediate action."
>
> The term pre-arrival instructions did not translate well directly, therefore this term was used by the European German Standards Subcommittee to impart the importance of this type of help to EMDs functioning in applicable German-speaking countries.

answers to the Key Questions. In some cases, the instructions tell the caller what not to do, or they address the caller's safety as a primary issue. They are quick to provide, yet can lend immense relief to callers.

The positive public relations of these simple instructions is widely appreciated. The EMD must not confuse this area of the protocol, however, with the full-blown assistance provided by "Pre-Arrival Instruc-

> **Which Post-Dispatch Instructions are given is dependent on the circumstances of each specific incident.**

tions" described briefly below, and fully in Chapter 4: Dispatch Life Support. Post-Dispatch Instructions are designed to be read out loud by the EMD. Some advice depends on the circumstances of a specific incident. For example, on protocol 12: Convulsions/Seizures, the Post-Dispatch Instructions that are specific for convulsions and seizures are listed. Other instructions, which are often less Chief Complaint specific, are listed on protocol X, and are accessed via the DLS links on the individual Chief Complaint protocols.

Critical EMD Information. In v11 the information that is directed to the EMD is now separated into a distinct section between PDIs and DLS Links. This information is considered "critical" because is contains essential directions for EMDs to consider and follow

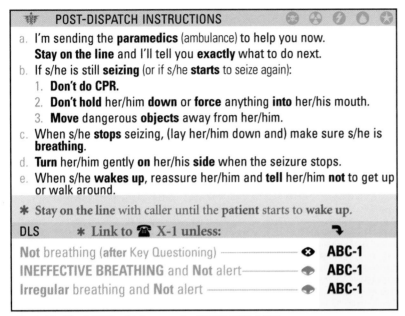

Fig. 3-26. The MPDS, v11.1 protocols. ©1978-2003 MPC.

where appropriate. There are five specific objectives of the CEI:

1. To provide general, non-scripted instructions to callers and responders regarding safety in potentially hazardous situations.

2. To advise the EMD when special notifications (such as Animal Control on protocol 3).

3. To improve the ability of responders to locate the scene or patient.

4. To advise the EMD when it is appropriate to remain on the line with the caller.

5. To give the EMD special directions for protocol navigation.

Once the CEIs are considered, the EMD selects the most appropriate DLS link.

DLS links. These provide a mechanism for the EMD to transition from Post-Dispatch Instructions to Pre-Arrival Instructions. The DLS links often direct the EMD to have the caller ensure the patient's airway. This refers to the universally-applicable initial action of all emergency care providers, which is to be sure the patient has an open pathway for air to enter the lungs (airway) and is breathing. When the patient is not breathing, or when the patient may not be able to maintain an airway due to being not alert and breathing abnormally, the EMD is directed to protocol A, B, or C. These protocols present clear and concise

instructions spelling out the appropriate steps required to assess the patient's airway, open it if it is not adequate, and proceed with mouth-to-mouth breathing and CPR if necessary. This eliminates avoidable ad lib and caller interpretation confusion and reduces the chance of inadvertent omissions.

On protocols where significant hemorrhage is a possibility, the EMD is referred to protocol X-5, to control the bleeding.

Pre-Arrival Instructions. These are listed as protocols A through F, Y, and Z. They are for critical situations in which the caller must act while responders are in transit, for patient observation and reassurance, and for preparing the scene prior to responder arrival. When the nature of a situation is grave and precise instructions are vital, the DLS links of priority dispatch system guide the EMD rapidly to the pre-arrival instructions. Formerly known as "Treatment Sequence Protocols,"[41] these have been revised extensively from earlier versions and are now much more user friendly. These protocols are also used after appropriate field responders have been dispatched, but their structure is different from post-dispatch instructions. Pre-arrival Instructions are scripted in precise language intended to be read verbatim by the EMD.[42] This maintains the proper order of care and eliminates unintentional but critical errors that can occur otherwise. Dispatchers working without scripts can too easily forget to have the caller check to see if the chest is rising or the air is going in before starting chest compressions in CPR. Regrettably, this has happened.

Pre-Arrival Instructions appear in numbered panels. Each panel contains a title, instruction text, an operative question, and a "yes/no/special answer" director telling the EMD which panel to access next (see figure 3-27).

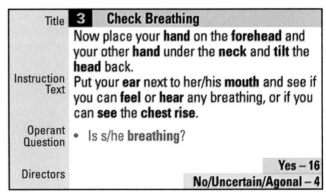

Fig. 3-27. The MPDS, v11.1 protocols. ©1978-2003 MPC.

There are specific instruction series for the following situations:

A   Arrest—Infant (<1 year old)

B   Arrest—Child (1 to 7 years old)

C   Arrest—Adult (≥8 years old)

D   Choking—Infant/Child

E   Choking—Adult

F   Childbirth/Delivery

X   Scene safety, patient reassurance and observation, bleeding control, cooling and flushing, scene preparation for responders, caller disconnect.

Y   Tracheostomy (Stoma) Arrest

Z   AED Support

See Chapter 4: Dispatch Life Support for an explicit description of how to use these protocols.

It is an important theoretical principle to understand that telephone instructions alone do not mean an EMS system offers full EMD service. Yet many EMS systems still declare, "we don't need all that other stuff; we just do pre-arrivals." Unfortunately, providing remote first aid—although a step ahead of doing nothing at all—is not enough.[42] Telephone instructions do not "stand alone." They must be based on a full interrogation evaluation. Primary surveys must be done before secondary surveys and complete evaluation before treatments. Safe and effective instructions do not occur out-of-the-blue, but as a result of a structured, prioritized action plan.

Partially implemented or partially used priority dispatch is counter to the international standard. EMS systems doing this will ultimately provide inconsistent and substandard patient care.

Case Completion Theory

During hands-on emergency medical care, the caregiver provides a "hand-off" report to those assuming care of the patient. This may be when the first responder turns the patient over to the arriving EMT or paramedic. It occurs again when the transporting caregiver turns the patient over to the nurse or physician at the emergency department. Similarly, now that the EMD is clearly regarded as a member of the response team, it makes sense to hand off the situation appropriately to arriving crews (see figure 3-28).

18   Arrival Interface

When you **hear** the paramedics (EMTs) arrive, **don't** stop **CPR** (Mouth-to-Mouth) until they **take over** from you.

• (Is the door **unlocked**?)
(Send someone to **open** it now.)

Tell me **when** they're **with** her/him.

End of Sequence

Fig. 3-28. The MPDS, v11.1 protocols. ©1978-2003 MPC.

An EMD who has stayed on the telephone during prehospital response knows the most about the situation until field providers arrive. At that time, when appropriate, the EMD can provide a quick verbal hand-off report to the prehospital professionals. A simple "goodbye" and "good luck" to the caller can also provide for the EMD an important element of closure to the relationship while strengthening the customer service aspect of daily call management.

Summary

No single component of priority dispatch occurs in a vacuum. Each depends on the others to link into a chain of assistance for people needing emergency help. The flow of priority dispatch, from start to finish, is carefully designed using often subtle but proven principles. Just as a single part of the human anatomy is difficult to appreciate in isolation from the whole body, priority dispatch is best appreciated when the overall anatomy and physiology of its structure is understood. In many cases, problem and case-specific elaboration will occur in subsequent chapters of this book. The purpose of this chapter has been to introduce all its parts, some of their functions, and the fundamental understanding of their interactions. The architecture of an EMD's successful learning requires a sound foundation of priority dispatch structural understanding.

Don't rely on words or equations, until you can picture the idea they represent.

—*Lewis Epstein and Paul Hewitt*

Contents

CHAPTER 4

Dispatch Life Support

Chapter Overview

Dispatch life support is the body of information and methods used by EMDs to help callers deal with a wide range of patient and scene circumstances. The scripted protocols enabling this crucial exchange of information lead the EMD through a verifiable, comprehensive process that eliminates the chance of inadvertent omissions of vital information.

The procedures include some variations from hands-on cardiopulmonary resuscitation. These have been carefully modified and approved by the Academy's Council of Standards to enable the EMD to transmit material safely via the unique telephonic setting.

The Pre-Arrival Instructions found in the current Medical Priority Dispatch System™ represent a quantum leap in development and design over those described in the first edition of this book.

I get by with a little help from my friends.

—Lennon and McCartney

Dispatch Life Support (DLS) is the EMD's version of basic life support. It is geared toward the unique challenges associated with providing crucial instructions via the telephone to strangers in crisis. It is carefully crafted to work in these unusual circum-stances, and is not simply basic life support in disguise. It incorporates many advanced life support "rules" within its fundamental structure.

Interestingly, the first words uttered on a telephone were a cry for medical aid. In 1875, Alexander Graham Bell said, "Mr. Watson, come here. *I need you,*" after spilling a caustic substance on himself. But even Bell could not have had the foresight to see how far telephonic first aid has since developed.

It took nearly 100 years, but the era of pre-arrival instructions was launched in 1974 when the Phoenix, Arizona, Fire Department began its innovative telephone self-help program. By 1980, a few more agencies had begun official programs. Since then, there has been a virtual explosion in the use of formal telephone care instruction protocols, given before EMTs, ambulance officers, and paramedics arrive at the scene.

When Dispatch Life Support is needed, the EMD uses Post-Dispatch Instruction protocols and Pre-Arrival Instruction scripts. Think of DLS as a brain transplant for onlookers. It allows a medical professional to practice their life-sustaining skills via remote control, using onlookers as hands.

> **Think of dispatch life support as a brain transplant for onlookers. It allows a medical professional to practice their life-sustaining skills via remote control, using onlookers as hands.**

Using such a system demands practice, but once familiar with it, the EMD can assist callers through a series of relatively sophisticated tasks. Pre-Arrival Instructions, which are presented as specially designed logic algorithms, are different from the Post-Dispatch Instructions which are found on each of the priority protocols. Pre-Arrival Instructions represent structured care for high-level emergencies in which the exact order of critical evaluation and task completion can be crucial. While field responders are on their way, the EMD uses these important protocols to maximize the patient's chances of survival by prompting bystanders to provide appropriate aid.

Dispatch Life Support is different from basic life support. EMDs are different from EMTs or ambulance officers—not better or worse, but different. Dispatching is not a matter of putting an EMT or **QAO** behind a dispatch console. You don't get apples by training people to be oranges, and you won't create a tasty apple pie by using the recipe for peach cobbler.

Dispatch Life Support

The knowledge, procedures, and skills used by trained EMDs in **providing care through pre-arrival instructions** to callers. It consists of those basic and advanced life support principles that are appropriate to application by medical dispatchers.

Dispatch Life Support

The known art and science of giving non-visual, verbal assistance, and leadership via the telephone. It consists of the knowledge, procedures, and skills used by trained EMDs in providing care through pre-arrival instructions to callers. It consists of those BLS and ALS principles that are appropriate to application by EMDs.

ABCs

Brief scripted instructions directly applicable to the mission of the first responder—verify, maintain, and monitor the Airway, Breathing, and Circulation of all patients if possible and appropriate. This is an important responsibility of the first, first responders.

Post-Dispatch Instructions

Important basic-level instructions that are always given when possible and appropriate. Realistically, they may be possible but not appropriate or appropriate but not physically possible. These constitute caller directions that are relevant to this chief complaint, but no necessarily to this particular patient or situation.

Critical EMD Information

Vital reminders to the EMD regarding hazard warnings, non-scripted advice for callers, special notifications, and directions for when to stay on the line with callers.

Pre-Arrival Instructions

Scripted advanced-level instructions given in time-critical situations where correct evaluation, verification, and advice is essential. These are medically approved, written instructions given by trained EMDs to callers that help provide necessary assistance to the patient and control of the situation prior to the arrival of EMS personnel. Pre-arrival instructions are read word-for-word by the EMD.

Fig. 4-1. Relationship between the components of Dispatch Life Support.

Standards That Work

The core of BLS, CPR, and ACLS revolves around the standards and guidelines developed and adopted by the American Heart Association (AHA), Canadian Heart and Stroke Foundation, European Resuscitation Council, Australian Resuscitation Council, etc., which are tailored for EMS providers. Unfortunately, difficulties arise when these guidelines are applied directly to medical dispatching.

The consistency of care and acceptance brought about by these much-needed standards created order from the chaos that previously existed in these areas of EMS. However, to some extent, blind acceptance of the standards, coupled with their limitations in certain situations, has caused significant difficulties when the standards are applied directly to pre-arrival instructions given by EMDs.

> **The EMD must teach the caller a physical procedure in a matter of seconds, without visual aids of any kind or even any opportunity to practice.**

These "problems" surface when medical control physicians adopt and review pre-arrival instruction protocols, and find that they appear to deviate from current guidelines, such as those of the AHA. Actually, the medical director's true dilemma is in attempting to understand the special limitations that are inherent in the dispatch situation, not in the pre-arrival instruction itself.

Since the AHA changed its recommended airway control maneuvers to the chin-lift and jaw-thrust methods in 1987, some believe that continuing to include the head-tilt method in dispatch protocols is incorrect. However, from a dispatch perspective it is not, which reveals the problem of direct application of these standards to dispatch.

The National Association of EMS Physicians (NAEMSP) stated in its 1988 Consensus Document on Emergency Medical Dispatching that, "Training and recertification [of EMDs] in basic life support, as is appropriate to application by medical dispatchers, is necessary to maintain and improve this unique, and at times, lifesaving, non-visual skill." NAEMSP's more recent position paper on EMD makes this distinction more specific by defining this area as Dispatch Life Support.

The AHA's **BLS** standards are designed for the teaching of physical procedures in person to a willing student, often over many hours with lots of "do-overs" and practicing until a certain level of excellence is achieved. Although the creators of these standards could not have foreseen the limitations placed on dispatching, their guidelines currently do recognize the need for some flexibility.

Still, certain obstacles present themselves to dispatchers when applying these standards. Thrust in the role of "instructor," the dispatcher must teach the caller (an unwilling student) a physical procedure in a matter of seconds, without visual aids of any kind or even any opportunity to practice.

Obviously, this means there is no in-person verification that the procedure is properly performed or that it was performed at all. If the limitations of a given process are understood up front, the procedure can be molded to effectively meet the needs of the user while still creating the desired results. This, unfortunately, has not yet been done; no currently published BLS standards have been designed with the dispatcher's situation in mind.

> **No currently published BLS standards have been designed with the dispatcher's situation in mind.**

Although the chin-lift method of airway control is not difficult to perform, EMDs must recommend that callers use the most simple method of securing a patent (meaning open) airway, as long as it is safe and effective. Since most cardiac arrest situations require that airway management (as instructed by the EMD) only briefly precede mouth-to-mouth resuscitation as a precursor to CPR, the more complicated chin-lift instruction is not as feasible in a dispatch setting. The jaw-thrust method is also not practical when conveying instructions to callers who have no assistance and has been shown to be particularly confusing to instruct via telephone in both real and video-taped situations.

The head-tilt method of airway control, however, can be easily taught to an untrained caller in the following manner: "Now place your hand on the forehead and your other hand under the neck and tilt the head back." There is nothing basically wrong with the head-tilt method. In fact, any street practitioner has probably personally experienced its effectiveness. Of course, EMDs are taught to be aware of the hazards of neck manipulation if the patient has sustained a significant mechanism of injury and several protocols have a rule describing how to modify the basic head tilt for trauma patients.

| **Rule 1** | PROTOCOL **30** |

The **head-tilt is the prefered method of airway control** in the dispatch environment. When a neck injury is likely, an attempt should first be made to open the airway without moving the neck. If this is unsuccessful, then advise to **gently tilt the head back,** a little at a time, until the air goes in and the chest rises.

For example, Rule 1 on protocol 30 (above).

Callers need simple, easy to understand "verbal pictures" to follow. During the evolution of citizen CPR, it was discovered that, if training instructions were too complicated and confusing as to the sequence of CPR actions, people might hesitate and delay the procedure. This concern first surfaced many years ago when the initial process for doing CPR differed in witnessed versus unwitnessed arrest situations. One might think that people would, if confused, decide immediately that either method was better than doing nothing at all. But this is not always the case, as people would sometimes hesitate or, even worse, give up.

Although this cannot be observed firsthand at the scene of an actual citizen CPR case, the fact that it occurs in practice on mannequins supports the contention that it occurs in the confusion of a real crisis. This delaying mental trap has been appropriately termed "paralysis by analysis."

> **This delaying mental trap has been appropriately termed "paralysis by analysis."**

There are several other examples that illustrate the problems of applying BLS training taught in a controlled environment directly to medical dispatching. The following are important concepts that are not present in BLS guidelines, but are essential to dispatch life support:

- A seizure or convulsion may be a symptom in the onset of cardiac arrest. Any patient 35 years or older who presents with a seizure as the chief complaint should be assumed to be in cardiac arrest until proven otherwise. This is a statistical probability that occurs with some regularity.

- Cardiac arrest in a previously healthy child or youth should be considered to be caused by a foreign body obstructing the airway until proven otherwise.

- EMDs should be trained to identify obvious death situations (as defined by medical control), mobilize the response accordingly and give limited PAIs.

- If the patient is unconscious and breathing cannot be verified by a second-party caller, the victim should be assumed to be in cardiac arrest until proven otherwise.

- EMDs should assume that bystanders have inappropriately placed a pillow under the head of an unconscious victim until proven otherwise, and ensure that it is removed.

- BLS protocols for choking victims should be modified to reflect that EMDs recommend a specific number of thrusts rather than stating a range of six to ten thrusts. The present guidelines contain no basis for deciding during the crisis how many to use. This simplification will eliminate any confusion and subsequent hesitation on the caller's part.

Most of this information is not directly taught to the majority of EMTs and paramedics and is not covered in the current EMT and paramedic textbooks. Addressing these omissions highlights the need for "dispatcher-specific training." There is no question that DLS is different from BLS just as EMDs are different from EMTs—not better or worse, but different.

In 1992, the American Heart Association stated in their guidelines for Adult Basic Life Support:

> *EMDs have been identified as a vital but often neglected part of the EMS system. All communities should provide formal training in emergency medical dispatch and require the use of medical dispatch protocols, including pre-arrival instructions for airway control, foreign-body airway obstruction, and CPR by telephone.*

> *By following a written protocol, the dispatcher can rapidly assess the patient's condition and activate the necessary emergency service.*[43]

Who Should Give Pre-Arrival Instructions?

Differing evolution and composition of communication centers, problems with maintaining adequate staffing levels, and misconceptions about the effect of pre-arrival instructions have led to this question of who should give pre-arrival instructions being posed in several different forms. Should the caller be transferred

Seeing the AHA "Standards" from a Medical Dispatch Perspective

The following are excerpts from the American Heart Associations "Standards and Guidelines for Cardiopulmonary Resuscitation and Emergency Cardiac Care," published in the Journal of the American Medical Association on June 6, 1986.

1. **Emergency Cardiac Care:** Basic life support is that particular phase of ECC that either (1) prevents circulatory or respiratory arrest or insufficiency through prompt recognition and intervention, early entry into the EMS system, or both, or (2) externally supports the circulation and respiration of a victim of cardiac or respiratory arrest.

2. **Standards and Guidelines:** The 1980 standards and guidelines were intended (1) to identify a body of knowledge and certain performance skills that are commonly necessary for the successful treatment of victims of cardiorespiratory arrest or of serious or life-threatening cardiac or pulmonary disturbance.

3. **Standards and Guidelines:** The 1980 standards and guidelines were intended (2) to indicate that the knowledge and skills recommended or defined do not represent the only medically or legally acceptable approach to a designated problem, but rather an approach that is generally regarded as having the best likelihood of success in view of present knowledge.

4. **Standards and Guidelines:** The standards and guidelines were not intended to imply (1) that justifiable deviations from suggested standards and guidelines by physicians qualified and experienced in CPR and ECC under appropriate circumstances represent a breach of a medical standard of care, or (2) that new knowledge, new techniques, or clinical circumstances may not provide sound reasons for alternative approaches to CPR and ECC before the next definition of national standards and guidelines.

5. **Basis for Changing Recommendations:** In some subject areas, sound data had accumulated, and changes were recommended on that basis. In other areas, while the experimental data were not conclusive, changes were recommended on the basis of clinical evidence or in order to improve educational efficacy.

6. **Standards and Guidelines:** "Loose constructionists," while realizing the need for uniformity and consistency, have believed that more flexibility is needed, for two principal reasons: (1) New knowledge and innovation are ongoing, and failure to permit flexibility can result in delay of potentially lifesaving advances; (2) The physician prerogative for discretionary action may be threatened by overly rigid standards, particularly because the term has important legal, as well as medical, overtones.

7. **Emergency Cardiac Care:** Emergency cardiac care is dependent for it success on lay persons' appreciation of the critical importance of activating the EMS system as well as their willingness to initiate CPR promptly and their ability to provide it effectively.

8. **Basis for Changing Recommendations:** Final decisions took into account not only which technique or adjunct or therapy was the most correct, but also how the public could best be served, which brought into the decision-making such factors as safety, effectiveness, teach ability and ease of sequencing into related maneuvers.

9. **Public Education:** Other changes for improving retention should include simplification of the sequences of BLS and inclusion of only one method of managing foreign body obstruction in the adult.

10. **Public Education:** There are many reasons why lay individuals do not become involved in performing CPR. These include lack of motivation, fear of doing harm, inability to remember exact sequences and poor retention of psychomotor skills.

11. **Reasons to Withhold CPR:** Few reliable criteria exist by which death can be defined immediately. Decapitation, rigor mortis and evidence of tissue decomposition and extreme dependent lividity are usually reliable criteria. When they are present, CPR need not be initiated.

Fig. 4-2. Seeing the AHA "Standards" from a Medical Dispatch Perspective. Excerpts from the Journal of the American Medical Association on June 6, 1986.

from the original calltaker to someone else, potentially someone at a completely different location? Examples of some caller-transfer variations that have been proposed are:

1. Transfer the caller to the hospital and have nurses at the emergency room give the instructions;

2. Transfer the caller to a cell phone link in the responding vehicle and let the EMT or paramedic give the instructions;

3. Transfer the caller to an advice line and have the nurse give the instructions;

4. Transfer the caller to another agency that routinely gives instructions;

5. Transfer the caller to another person in the communication center who is better trained or more available (or willing) to give the instructions.

The central issue here should not be system convenience but patient care. And better patient care is evident in situations that ensure the continuity of that care directly from the evaluation that led to it. Just as "no one can know more about the scene than the calltaker until someone arrives," no one knows more about the patient (and the caller) than the EMD interrogator.

> **The central issue here should not be system convenience but patient care.**

For the same reason that "shift change" is dreaded in medicine and other public safety circles, transferring a caller is fraught with potential problems:

1. The caller becomes disconnected;

2. The caller becomes frustrated and hangs up;

3. The information upon which correct treatments are based, gets "lost in the translation" and therefore subsequent treatment or advice doesn't quite match the situation at hand;

4. There is a waiting interval to achieve the completed transfer (time in the queue);

5. New information realized by the "new" pre-arrival instruction-giver cannot be easily transferred back to the dispatcher;

6. The caller perceives differences in pre- and post-transfer "customer service" demeanor or competence.

Obviously, behind many of these potential problems lurk mechanical "difficulties" with caller transfer. An excellent analogy exists in Olympic relay races. World class sprinters in the four-by-100 relay must pass a baton three times during this famous event. Time after time, the best teams are disqualified or lose significant time (and the gold medal) because of errors in simply transferring a baton from one runner to the next—no history, no information, no subtle rapport—just a piece of wood.

A colleague once advised against the concept of transferring calls using a play on words from a well known U.S. television advertisement for laundry detergent—"Don't ring around the caller."

An early relative of this caller transfer problem evolved in several dispatch centers in the early 1980's. Since pre-arrival instructions were given sporadically in the absence of sound quality management, maybe one or two EMDs on a given shift felt confident enough, or were moved by the spirit, to give instructions. As a well known early 1980s CPR transcript from Aurora, Colorado revealed:

> *Kathy, you're better at this than me. He's turning blue. Why don't you talk to her?*

This practice became so evident in another center that one of the EMDs who was "really good at this" became known as "the designated hitter," after the controversial American baseball situation in which a better hitter can bat for the pitcher—a traditionally weak batter. Several EMDs in this center later complained that this internal transfer was inappropriate, comparing it to the EMS field situation of weak paramedics always gravitating to radio duties and leaving their stronger partners to intubate or start IVs. This practice was eventually ended by official policy.

> **The most effective argument against caller pre-arrival instruction transfer is that the evaluator should always be the caregiver.**

The most effective argument against caller pre-arrival instruction transfer is that the evaluator should always be the caregiver. This has been a valued concept in medicine for centuries, with good reason. Each evaluation and caller interaction is unique.

It contains subtle personal rapport and empathy that cannot be transferred or even well described. This relationship with the caller sets the stage for caller acceptance and subsequent performance of the advice and treatment appropriate to each situation. A transfer clearly breaks that chain of evaluation, rapport, and caring, leaving the new caregiver to start "cold" or start over—either of which is clearly not optimal.

This was felt to be such an important issue that the ASTM Subcommittee creating the Standard Practice for Emergency Medical Dispatch unequivocally stated:

There must be continuity in the delivery of EMD care. To safely and effectively provide correct medical care, the EMD that is medically directing, evaluating, and coding must maintain direct access to the calling party and must use a medically approved emergency dispatch priority reference system. The person giving the medical instruction to the caller must be the same person that asks the systematic interrogation questions.[54]

This has clearly established the correct standard of care and practice regarding this issue.

Pre-Arrival Instructions

The procedure for using Dispatch Life Support begins with the same tasks as any priority dispatch situation: identifying the Chief Complaint. The EMD may already know that a patient is not conscious and not breathing (and has thus already sent the maximal response). This condition is generally classified as protocol 9: Cardiac (Respiratory) Arrest/Death. Or the caller may have said, "Quick! My grandfather is choking!"—which is protocol 11: Choking. Or "Help! My wife's baby is coming too fast! We don't have time to get to the hospital"—protocol 24: Pregnancy/Childbirth/ Miscarriage. Each of these is additionally designed as a BRIDGE protocol, meaning that the EMD uses it as a bridge between Case Entry and dispatch life support. On each BRIDGE protocol, the key questions help the EMD quickly assess scene safety, confirm (verify) the need for dispatch life support, and move to the most appropriate panel of the correct DLS protocol.

For example, on protocol 9: Cardiac/Respiratory Arrest, the first key question is: "Did you see what happened?" followed by the qualified second Key Question (If yes) "Did s/he choke on anything first?" A "Yes" answer tells

> **The EMD must identify the presence of conditions requiring pre-arrival instructions before any treatment begins.**

the EMD to update the dispatch code to 11-E-1 (from 9-E-1) and to go to the DLS links via the appropriate Post-Dispatch Instructions. First-aid instructions are different for a person who can still breathe or cough than for someone who cannot, and the DLS links refer the EMD to the correct place in the pre-arrival scripts. Distinguishing the difference is crucial. The goal is to verify the existence or absence of cardiac arrest and choking before beginning "dispatch-invasive" procedures that may not be totally benign in actual application.

In essence, the EMD must identify the presence of conditions requiring Pre-Arrival Instructions before any treatment begins.

On the pregnancy protocol, the Key Questions help the EMD discover exactly how far along the childbirth is, and whether there are obvious complications: "Is the baby completely out yet?" "Can you see any part of the baby yet?" has the sub-qualifiers "Breech or Cord" and "Head visible/out." Other questions establish the length of the pregnancy and the spacing of the contractions. These, too, are vitally-important distinguishing particulars, the answers to which lead the EMD to specific DLS links that ensure the correct panel of the childbirth pre-arrival scripts is used.

After asking all the Key Questions in a critical emergency (which is still completed, even though a maximal response was sent during the Case Entry protocol), the EMD confirms that the appropriate field response was sent. Then the Post-Dispatch Instructions link the EMD to a Pre-Arrival Instruction sequence. There are nine:

A   Arrest—Infant (less than 1 year old)

B   Arrest—Child (1 to 7 years old)

C   Arrest—Adult (8 years old and over)

D   Choking—Infant/Child

E   Choking—Adult

F   Childbirth/Delivery

X   Scene safety, patient reassurance and observation, bleeding control, cooling and flushing, scene preparation for responders, caller disconnect

Y   Tracheostomy (Stoma) Arrest (all ages)

Z   AED Support

What's Wrong With "Telephone Aid" (excerpt from NIH position paper on EMD)

Telephone aid, as defined herein, consists of "ad libbed" instructions provided by either trained or untrained EMDs. Telephone aid differs from dispatch life support in that the instructions provided to the caller are based on the dispatcher's previous training in a procedure or treatment but are provided without following a scripted Pre-Arrival Instruction protocol. This method exists because either no protocols are used in the medical dispatch center or protocol adherence is not required by policy and procedure (e.g., the dispatcher is "trained" in CPR and thus describes to the caller, to the best of his or her verbal ability, how to do CPR).

As noted previously, dispatchers must carefully adhere to written protocols. Unfortunately, coupled with a growing interest and effort within public safety agencies to provides some type of telephone instructions to callers, many agencies are "allowing" dispatchers to ad lib instructions. There appears to be a significant difference between Dispatch Life Support-based Pre-Arrival Instructions and telephone aid. Telephone aid may only ensure that the dispatcher has attempted to provide some sort of care to the patient through the caller but does not ensure that such care is correct, standard, and medically effective or even necessary in the first place.

Telephone aid often causes the following predictable errors:

1. Failure to correctly identify conditions requiring telephone intervention andtherefore pre-arrival instruction in the first place (e.g., "saving" an infant having a febrile seizure who was incorrectly identified as needing CPR due to failure to follow protocols that are medically designed to verify need—verify breathing, pulse, etc., before potentially dangerous dispatcher-invasive treatments such as compressions are initiated).

2. Failure to accurately identify the presence of interim symptoms and signs (or lack of them) during the in-progress provision of telephone intervention (e.g., dispatchers who ad lib CPR sequences often miss important patient verifiers that cannot be seen by the dispatcher, such as watching for the chest to rise).

3. Failure to perform (describe or teach) multiple step procedures, such as CPR care, in a consistent and reproducible fashion regardless of which dispatcher in a center provides such help (e.g., quality assurance review of these types of cases often reveals that dispatchers in the same center [or even the same dispatcher] perform care differently each time if they are not following scripted pre-arrival instruction protocols closely).

Telephone aid, as defined, often provides only the illusion of correct help via telephone without predictably ensuring consistent and accurate instructions to all callers. **Telephone aid, therefore, is usually considered an inappropriate and unreliable form of dispatcher-provided medical care.**

Medical dispatch practice must be safe, competent, and effective. The systematic use of medically pre-approved protocols will help to ensure that the dispatcher performance is structured and reproducible and can be objectively measured.

In light of the important differences between pre-arrival instructions and telephone aid, and to improve standardization of EMD training and practice, it is recommended that:

- Dispatch life support be adopted nationwide as an essential concept of emergency medical dispatch

- Dispatch life support be standardized

- Pre-arrival instructions be provided from written protocols scripts for all medical emergencies.

Fig. 4-3. Excerpt from the U.S. National Institutes of Health position paper on EMD—DLS vs. Telephone Aid.[42] (See Appendix I for complete text of the paper.)

Pre-Arrival Instructions are configured in panels. Each panel contains four sub-sections.

- On the top line is a number (for reference purposes) and a title explaining the basic activity on that panel.

- In the middle is the scripted instruction text that the EMD reads verbatim to the caller.

- The third section consists of a color-text phrase that either asks a follow-up question to the task just done such as "Can you see any part of the baby coming out yet?" or informs the caller what the EMD will do. This is called the operant question or phrase. In some cases, the caller has to put down the telephone to check or do something; Protocol X contains some universal instructions that should be used whenever there is the possibility the caller will put down the phone: "Don't hang up. Go do it now and tell me when it's done."

- The bottom section contains the director, which, like a GO TO, directs the EMD to the next appropriate panel. The EMD is not necessarily directed to the next adjacent panel, since traversing the system depends on the answers to the EMD's follow-up questions.

In all cases, EMDs must resist the temptation to paraphrase or ad lib the instructions, no matter how well they know the hands-on procedure. A dispatcher may know CPR, the Heimlich maneuver, and how to deliver babies—but this does not mean it is possible to teach these things comprehensively and efficiently over the phone.

> **It's easy to forget a minor detail in a stressful situation, especially when you have no visual clues.**

It's easy to forget a minor detail in a stressful situation, especially when you have no visual clues. That is why having and using scripted Pre-Arrival Instructions is absolutely essential.

The telephone is a non-visual medium. Imagine trying to tell someone who doesn't know how, how to tie a shoe over the phone! The error rate with paraphrasing or ad libbing can be very high, and the EMD's actions are indefensible if something goes wrong. However, this does not preclude the careful practitioner from *enhancing* or *clarifying* (a different concept than replacing) the pre-arrival instructions when common sense or caller confusion requires it.

When pilots relay course information to an air traffic controller, their message can arrive garbled. To ensure the information is received, pilots repeat the course information in two ways, in the clear (as normal speech), and using a special code where each number and letter has a unique sound. Similarly, the caller may not understand the questions or scripted instructions, and the EMD must choose other (but equivalent) words.

Each pre-arrival instruction is carefully designed with cues and colors. There are consistent reasons why certain words appear in bold face or capital letters, in parentheses, or in certain colors. These are referred to as the conventions of the MPDS and are learned in Academy EMD certification courses.

Certain elements of intervention occur on each protocol, the first being to get the patient as close to the telephone as possible. In the early years of pre-arrival instructions, the EMD sometimes discovered late in the call that the poor caller was running quite a distance between the patient and the telephone (wasting precious time) or was yelling to another room (with the risk of miscommunication).

---

1   Patient to Phone

Listen carefully and I'll tell you how to help her/him.

Get her/him as **close** to the **phone** as possible. Don't hang up.
Do it now and tell me when it's done.

(If I'm not here, stay on the line.)

- **Where** is s/he now?

_– 2_

Fig. 4-4. The MPDS, v11.1 protocols. ©1978-2003 MPC.

---

2   Check Airway

Listen carefully.

(**Not breathing**) **Lay** her/him **flat** on her/his **back** on the **floor** (ground) and **remove** any **pillows**.

(**Breathing**) **Lay** her/him **flat** on her/his **back** and **remove** any **pillows**.

Kneel next to her/him and **look** in the **mouth** for **food** or **vomit**.

- Is there **anything** in the mouth?   Yes – 13 / No – 3

Fig. 4-5. The MPDS, v11.1 protocols. ©1978-2003 MPC.

The first panel on all Pre-Arrival Instructions introduces the caller to the concept that help is available. In childbirth, for example, the instructions begin: "Listen carefully and do exactly as I say. Where is she now? (Get her as close to the phone as possible.) Lay her on her back in the center of a bed or on the floor. I'm going to tell you how to help deliver the baby." Similar scripts begin the instructions for CPR and the Heimlich maneuver.

Each of the treatment scripts have been refined and repeatedly field-tested. Still, someone with previous experience in emergency medical care may not initially understand the rationale that explains the differences between telephone-directed and hands-on care.

> **When a neck injury is likely, an attempt should first be made to open the airway without moving the neck.**

For example, although the chin-lift method of airway control is not difficult to perform, trying to teach it to an unprepared student in seconds, without visual aids, and without a chance to practice first, has been shown to be unrealistic.[45]

Therefore, the EMD uses the most simple-to-describe method of securing an open airway: the head-tilt method of airway control. It can be taught easily to an untrained caller as described in A-3, B-3, or C-3 (fig.4-6)

Unless there is a question of spinal injury, there is basically nothing wrong with this method. A warning rule occurs on several protocols where neck injuries are possible (Rule 1).

Callers need the simple, easy-to-understand verbal pictures that occur with the careful wording of the pre-

3   **Check Breathing**
Now place your **hand** on the **forehead** and your other **hand** under the **neck** and **tilt** the **head** back.

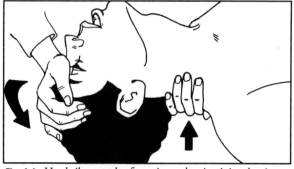

Fig. 4-6. Head-tilt example of opening and maintaining the airway.

> | Rule 1   Protocol **30** |
> | :--- |
> | The **head-tilt is the prefered method of airway control** in the dispatch environment. When a neck injury is likely, an attempt should first be made to open the airway without moving the neck. If this is unsuccessful, then advise to **gently tilt the head back,** a little at a time, until the air goes in and the chest rises. |

arrival instruction protocol scripts. This is embodied in the concept of dispatch life support.[45] When there is a question of spinal injury, the EMD needs to decide what would be a reasonable action, as stated in "Airway Management in Difficult Situations" from the *The National EMD Journal*:

Although the protocol states quite plainly that patients [with airway problems and suspected spinal injuries] should not be subjected to aggressive airway management, there is a need to explore the possibilities. Is there room to enhance the protocol if ventilation without tilting the head is not working? If the patient is in cardiac arrest, could they be made worse? Is the patient going to die anyway from airway obstruction and hypoxia with the ambulance still several minutes away? The key here is "reasonable." What would be a reasonable action? The EMD must decide. In the U.K., medical experts feel that if all efforts to ventilate according to protocol is not working then it would be advisable to enhance the protocol by placing the head in a neutral position initially, then, if still not working, go ahead with tilting the head.[46]

Unique Concepts of Dispatch Life Support

There are several concepts and premises that are unique to dispatch life support. One is that the EMD should never ask if the caller would like to provide aid. Instead, the EMD should assume that the caller would like to help. After all, simply by dialing 9-1-1, the caller indicated a willingness to help. Essentially, the EMD has the caller's *implied* consent to continue helping. In reality the caller has no *legal* right to determine whether the patient gets care. The patient has the right, if they are capable, of accepting or refusing care, and the caller can easily exercise the same right.

If the EMD asked callers whether they'd like to help, there is a subtle suggestion that there might be a reason *not* to help. With that question raised in their minds, some callers might say "no" without any good reason. Instead, with a take-charge approach, the EMD tells the caller that, together, they might be able to help the patient: "Sir, if you stay calm, we can help your friend while you're waiting for help to arrive." The caller receives a subtle message to cooperate. (Callers who are limited by a physical disability will usually mention it at this point.) Remember, we can't *make* them do anything over the phone. It is ultimately the caller's choice to continue their involvement—or not.

> **Never ask if the caller is willing to help. The caller has already implied consent by making the call in the first place.**

Certainly safety and physical or environmental constraints must be factored by the EMD. However, the majority of choking, childbirth, or CPR cases do not involve these considerations. The "permission" issue has been observed to be an easy way out of helping—both by the caller *and* the dispatcher.

The Dispatch Life Support scripts make it possible for the EMD to provide simple, easy-to-understand verbal pictures for callers to follow. One reason meticulous use of the scripts is so strongly emphasized relates to the trap known as *paralysis by analysis*.

Being told too much too fast sometimes overwhelms and literally paralyzes people cognitively, especially in an emergency. They are already embroiled in unusual, often frightening circumstances.

If instructions are too confusing or complicated, people hesitate, or worse, do nothing at all. And delays are something patients in critical circumstances can ill afford.

Dispatch Life Support, which takes a dispatch-oriented view of prehospital care, incorporates certain important tenets that emergency physicians know well. That is, certain clinical situations command an interaction by the EMD that is different from what a field provider might do.

For example, there are multiple reasons for a seizure to occur. A generalized seizure is a self-limited event involving total-body convulsions that last typically about 60 seconds. The worst reason for a seizure is cardiac arrest as blood pressure drops suddenly to zero in the brain. As a result, many people, when they go into cardiac arrest, have an even shorter seizure lasting only a few seconds. This occurs with a reasonable statistical probability, and is therefore medically predictable.

However, coronary heart disease is much less likely in people younger than age 35. Age becomes a determining factor in what sort of response is sent. Calls involving seizures are considered cardiac in origin until proven otherwise—in all patients 35 or older. And, for every patient, breathing must be verified when the seizure stops as noted by the last, but essential, set of questions on protocol 12: Convulsions/Seizures. If breathing is absent, after the jerking stops, a DELTA determinant is selected, and the EMD turns to the age-appropriate dispatch life support protocol for cardiac arrest.

Another statistical probability is that cardiac arrest in a previously healthy child or teenager must be considered a foreign body airway obstruction until proven otherwise. It does not change the fact that the EMD will send ann ECHO- or DELTA-level response or that the appropriate dispatch life support protocol will be quickly accessed and used. However, it serves as a red flag for the EMD about the probable underlying cause of the situation and subsequent correctly chosen telephone treatment.

Sometimes, getting a clear picture whether the patient is breathing can be difficult. If breathing in an unconscious patient cannot be verified by a second-party caller, the EMD must presume cardiac arrest until proven otherwise.

> **Rule 2**   PROTOCOL 9
>
> A healthy child (or young adult) found in cardiac arrest is considered to have a **foreign body airway obstruction until proven otherwise.**

Nothing in the EMD's actions changes: A ECHO-level code is generated from the Case Entry protocol in the first 20 to 30 seconds. The EMD then proceeds through the system by accessing the appropriate BRIDGE protocol based on the Chief Complaint. The EMD, guided by proper initial evaluations and verifications, provides appropriate Pre-Arrival Instructions, but the time-critical situation places the EMD on red-alert for a potentially intense interaction.

For example, say the caller said, "He's in the garage! I think he's been electrocuted!" In answering Case Entry questions, the caller indicates that the patient is unconscious, but is unable to tell for certain whether he is breathing. An ECHO-level determinant is selected, and then the EMD turns to protocol 15: Electrocution/ Lightning to determine the safety of the situation prior to beginning any PAIs.

Dispatch Invasive Procedures

While the EMD can't physically touch the patient via the Pre-Arrival Instructions given to the caller, certain instructions could result in physical harm, and are considered "dispatcher invasive" procedures. These procedures must be medically controlled dispatch life support treatments (administered strictly according to protocol). Dispatcher invasive procedures include: inappropriate chest compressions (CPR); improperly applied head-tilt actions (airway control); and unnecessary Heimlich maneuver abdominal thrusts (choking relief).

Nothing in the Key Questions will change the response (although the EMD can report safety factors and clinical information to responding crews). But in the DLS links the EMD is referred to protocol A, B, or C (depending on the patient's age) to verify the status of breathing. If the patient is not breathing, the EMD starts the CPR Pre-Arrival Instruction.

In situations of reported choking, developers of EMD and dispatch life support concepts originally avoided what has been a major international debate about the best approach to begin a choking-relief sequence—back blows or the Heimlich maneuver. The initial DLS method adopted was reinforced by then U.S. Surgeon General C. Everett Koop's proclamation in 1985:

Millions of Americans have been taught to treat persons whose airways are obstructed by a foreign body by administering back blows, chest thrusts, and abdominal thrusts. Now they must be advised that these methods are hazardous, even lethal. A back slap can drive a foreign object even deeper into the throat. Chest and abdominal thrusts, because they refer to blows to unspecified locations on the body, have resulted in cracked ribs and damaged spleens and livers, among other injuries…

The best rescue technique in any choking situation is the Heimlich Maneuver. I urge the American Red Cross, the American Heart Association, and all those who teach first aid to teach only the Heimlich Maneuver. Manuals, posters, and other materials that recommend treating choking victims with slaps and chest thrusts should be withdrawn from circulation.

The Heimlich Maneuver is safe, effective, and easily mastered by the average person. It can be performed on standing or seated victims and on persons who have fallen to the floor. It can be performed on children and even on oneself.[47]

This issue has remained one of the most controversial in EMD.[48] A lack of definitive science has resulted in what are often subjective, and, at times, emotional arguments about which methods to use. What is unquestionable is that callers need simplicity and clarity. For this and other reasons, priority dispatch instructs callers in the Heimlich maneuver for choking in adults and children. The Council of Standards and Council of Research approved modifications to the instructions for choking infants (age < 1) for the use of chest thrusts (without back blows). These modifications appeared in version 10.3.

The EMD departs from hands-on convention (of 6 to 10 thrusts) by prompting the caller to initially perform the described procedure five times (repeated 5 times if unsuccessful).

This avoids the paralysis by analysis that occurs when the caller is asked to make decisions. Neither the EMD nor the caller should ever have to arbitrarily choose how many thrusts to do.

> **A critic once suggested that since the Heimlich maneuver has been known to occasionally cause an internal injury, it should not be used by the EMD.**
>
> **A physician made the reply, "Isn't the patient choking to death worse than living with an injury?"**

> **! Authors' Note**
>
> The authors consider the use of a range (6 to 10 thrusts in choking relief treatment) an error in basic life support standards development unless a method such as size, age, or other delineator is provided for applying this range. This example demonstrates another problem with the use of guidelines in critical care settings.

A final aspect of the unique nature of Dispatch Life Support is that EMDs should be trained to identify situations where death is absolutely obvious. If the caller says the patient is not breathing, not conscious, and reports a situation where the fact of death is unquestionable, there is no reason to send in the same resources that would be sent if even a remote chance of resuscitation existed. In the Additional Information section of protocol 9: Cardiac (Respiratory) Arrest/Death, an OBVIOUS DEATH situation is defined and approved by Medical Control as shown in figure 4-7.

Addressing these unique aspects of priority dispatch highlights the need for strong, involved medical control and dispatcher-specific training. A regular reinforcement of these protocols is essential.

National Standard of Practice

A woman visiting a friend in another region needed help and dialed 9-1-1. When the dispatcher had taken her address and phone number, she was told that help would be there shortly. The caller said, "Aren't you supposed to tell me what to do?" Priority dispatching, with its element of Pre-Arrival Instructions, was already present in her hometown. The dispatcher's answer: "No, we don't do that here." It was a surprise to the caller (but not the authors) that Post-Dispatch Instructions were not universally available.

Since the inception of EMD, a steadily increasing number of people have assumed that they will receive telephone instructions while awaiting the arrival of field personnel. They have seen it on television, heard about it on the radio, and read it in magazine and newspaper accounts.[8, 49, 50, 51, 52, 53]

> It was a surprise to the caller that post-dispatch instructions were not universally available.

In addition, a growing number of position papers (seven by 2000) by prominent organizations have solidified dispatch life support as the modern national standard.[20, 42, 43, 54, 55, 56]

For example, in 1989, the National Association of EMS Physicians published its position paper on priority dispatching stating that:

> *Pre-arrival instructions are a mandatory function of each EMD in a medical dispatch center… standard medically approved telephone instructions by trained EMDs are safe to give and in many instances are a moral necessity.*[20]

The same document denotes Dispatch Life Support as consisting of the basic and advanced life support principles that are *appropriate* to application by medical dispatchers—freeing those in this unique environment from the constraints of certain less effective hands-on methods for applying these skills.

Another document in the *Annual Book of ASTM Standards*, also states that one of the functions of the EMD is to provide PAIs:

> *To the caller, the EMD is the contact with the emergency response agency and must be prepared to provide emergency care instructions to callers waiting for an EMS response. These instructions should enable the caller to prevent or reduce further injury to the victim and to do as much as possible under the circumstances to intervene in any life-threatening situation which exists.*[54]

The American Heart Association has recommended support for medical dispatch protocols, EMD training, dispatch life support standards, pre-arrival instructions, and quality improvement:

> *As is evident from an existing body of medical and EMS literature… there is a broad national consensus that EMD protocols, practices, training, certification, and program management should be standardized nationally. There is also general agreement that such national standards should not be static, but should evolve and be maintained by lead medical dispatch*

OBVIOUS DEATH

Local Medical Control must define and authorize (☒) any of the patient conditions below before this determinant can be used. Situations should be unquestionable and may include:

☐ Cold and stiff in a warm environment
☐ Decapitation
☐ Decomposition
☐ Explosive gunshot wound to the head
☐ Incineration
☐ **NON-RECENT** death
☐ Severe injuries obviously incompatible with life
☐ Submersion (> 6hrs)
☐ _____
☐ _____

_____
Approval signature of local Medical Control   Date approved

Fig. 4-7. The MPDS, v11.1 protocols. ©1978-2003 MPC.

and EMS professional organizations. It is also evident that the EMD must use a medically correct dispatch protocol system for the safe, competent, effective and non-arbitrary evaluation of, response to, and pre-arrival instructions care of citizens who access EMS systems.[43]

The topic of priority dispatching is well-documented in industry-specific literature, and is commonly a feature of international and regional EMS conferences. The Academy sponsors a comprehensive annual international summit, seminar, and conference exclusively on EMD called *Navigator.* Jurisdictions that do not provide this service (or do it poorly) are at increasing risk for failing to meet the clearly identifiable national and international standard of care.

> **The public is increasingly verbal in its expectation that dispatch life support will be provided.**

Sample of a Dispatch Life Support Protocol

To gain a sense of the flow of the pre-arrival instructions, protocol C: Arrest—Adult is detailed below. It consists of 18 panels of interrelated material. Each panel is explained along with its rationale using a male patient and female caller.

Panel 1: Patient to phone. This is the entry point. Let's say the EMD has arrived here from priority dispatch protocol 9: Cardiac (Respiratory) Arrest/Death, and also because the patient's age was determined at Case Entry to be 8 years old or above. The DLS link for a "suspected workable arrest" on protocol 9 directs the EMD to A,B,C-1. (The EMD is referred to protocol A if the patient is an infant, and B if the patient is a child age 1 through 7.) Referrals to this protocol may also come from many other situations that need cardiopulmonary resuscitation, such as when an adult patient is not breathing (or not breathing effectively) after a seizure.

The caller is advised to get the patient as close to the telephone as possible, and not to hang up. "Go do it now and tell me when it's done" ("Go *and* do it now" in the UK, Australia, and New Zealand) presses the caller into action. When the caller comes back to the telephone, the EMD asks, "Where is s/he now?" This clarifies the logistical hurdles facing callers who cannot get patients very close to the telephone. When the

1	**Patient to Phone**

Listen carefully and I'll tell you how to help her/him.

Get her/him as **close** to the **phone** as possible. Don't hang up.
Do it now and tell me when it's done.

(If I'm not here, stay on the line.)

• **Where** is s/he now?

caller returns to the telephone, the EMD might want to anticipate having to assist the caller with a "**re-freak event.**" (See Refreak Events, Chapter 5: Caller Management Techniques.) The EMD is then prompted to go to panel 2.

2	**Check Airway**

Listen carefully.

(Not breathing) **Lay** her/him **flat** on her/his **back** on the **floor** (ground) and **remove** any **pillows.**

(Breathing) **Lay** her/him **flat** on her/his **back** and **remove** any **pillows.**

Kneel next to her/him and **look** in the **mouth** for **food** or **vomit.**

• Is there **anything** in the mouth?	Yes – 13
	No – 3

Panel 2: Check Airway. The caller is instructed to open the airway according to the principles of dispatch life support. The head-tilt method, although no longer used by hands-on rescuers, provides the best "visual picture" for telephonic advice, making it the best method for dispatch life support as long as there is no reasonable concern for spinal injury (see Rule 1, protocol 30). The caller is instructed to look in the mouth to see if there is an obstruction (from vomit or another cause).

At any point when the caller is sent to the patient to check something or perform an action, even when it is not explicitly written in the script the EMD can use the universal instruction from protocol X: "Don't hang up. Go do it now and tell me when it's done." The EMD should commit this universal instruction to memory, and should be prepared to use it whenever the caller seems unsure of what she or he is doing or seems likely to hang up the phone or not return.

When the caller returns, the EMD asks whether there is anything in the mouth. In the GO TO at the bottom of the panel, the EMD has two choices based on the caller's answer. A "No" answer (always keyed in red) sends the EMD to panel 3. A "Yes" answer sends the EMD to panel 13. (Panels 13, 14, and 15 are unofficially referred to as "problem-solvers".) In this sample case, we will assume there is vomit in the mouth, so the EMD jumps to panel 13.

---

13   Clear Vomit

Turn her/his **head** to the **side** and **clean** out her/his **mouth**.

(It's okay to have a **little fluid** remaining.)

(You must **blow through** the remaining fluid.)

– 3

Panel 13: Clear Vomit. This panel prompts the caller to turn the patient's head to one side (keep in mind the possibility of a neck injury) and to clear the mouth of vomit. The EMD does not specify exactly how to do this. This is a good example of an instance where an EMD might enhance the protocol with brief advice such as "grab a towel" or "Carefully use your fingers to remove it from her/his mouth" if the caller asks how.

The two sentences in parenthesis: "(It's okay to have a little fluid remaining)" and "(You must blow through the remaining fluid)" are prompts to the EMD in preparation for the caller's inevitable concern about giving mouth-to-mouth on someone who has vomited. The EMD should provide this information

---

3   Check Breathing

Now place your **hand** on the **forehead** and your other **hand** under the **neck** and **tilt** the **head** back.

Put your **ear** next to her/his **mouth** and see if you can **feel** or **hear** any breathing, or if you can **see** the **chest rise**.

• Is s/he **breathing**?

Yes – 16
No/Uncertain/Agonal – 4

---

only if necessary. Normal-sized black font phrases in parentheses are situationally optional. Parenthetical phrases in smaller font are optional clarifiers.

Now the EMD is directed back into sequence at panel 3. Although a necessary sidetrack may be essential to solve a specific problem, the eventual sequence of

advice still leads from panel 2 to panel 3. Carefully following these pathways assure that steps are not missed.

Panel 3: Check Breathing. The first section of this panel begins with a sentence to help the caller appreciate the need for action. "I want you to see if she is breathing" is a subtle psychological boost for the caller; the task seems simple and do-able. Then the EMD tells the caller how to open the airway (remember Rule 1 from protocol 30 in the case of neck injury) and to check for breathing. The universal instruction can again be used if necessary: "Don't hang up. Go do it now and tell me when it's done." Sometimes the caller is uncertain about whether the patient is breathing, or is hesitant, or describes the patient as turning blue or making strange, peculiar, or funny noises. The EMD should, in this situation, assume that the patient is not breathing and proceed with instructions for mouth-to-mouth. There is less risk of harm in having this done to a breathing person than in hesitating or not acting in the patient's behalf. And if the answer is, "No, he's not breathing!" the EMD should be prepared for a re-freak event (see Chapter 5: Caller Management).

The EMD must pay attention to other things s/he is doing. If there is a chance during pre-arrival instructions, that the EMD might place the caller on hold while an action is being performed, the EMD should tell the caller "Don't hang up. Go do it now and tell me when it's done." and should follow this with " If I'm not here, stay on the line." Callers who find themselves on hold may hang up; those who are reassured that the EMD will come back on the line as soon as possible will be more patient.

When the caller comes back, the EMD asks another question to determine which Dispatch Life Support panel will be used next.
If the caller cannot feel or hear any breathing (or is uncertain), the EMD is referred to panel 4. If breathing is present, the EMD is then directed to panel 16. In our scenario the caller cannot detect any breathing, so the EMD goes to panel 4.

4	**Start Mouth-To-Mouth**

I'm going to tell you how to give **mouth-to-mouth.***

With the head **tilted** back, **pinch** the **nose** closed and completely **cover** her/his **mouth** with your **mouth**, then force **2 deep breaths** of air into the lungs, just like you're **blowing up** a **big** balloon.

	– 5
	*Refuses M-T-M – 8

Panel 4: Start Mouth-to-Mouth. Again, the EMD tells the caller what is going to happen next, then how to do it. Because callers must be carefully coached to do a number of steps here, this protocol continues without an operant question directly into panel 5.

5	**Check Breaths**

Watch for the **chest** to **rise** with each breath.

- Can you **feel** the air going in and out?
- Did you **see** the chest rising?

	Yes – 8
	No – 14

Panel 5: Give Breaths. Nearly everyone can relate to the sensation of blowing into a balloon, so the caller receives a clear verbal picture of what it feels like to blow into the lungs successfully. (Just as with a balloon, a good seal with the mouth is necessary to do mouth-to-mouth effectively.) If necessary, the EMD can repeat the universal instruction as well as advice to stay on the line if the caller is on hold upon her or his return.

Interestingly, when a caller is relaying this information to someone else at the scene, the EMD's instructions tend to be repeated verbatim. A tape transcription in figure 4-14, demonstrating the parts of a resuscitation attempt is a good example of the tendency to follow PAIs verbatim. The caller above has answered one of the EMD's most important verification questions, "Did you see the chest rising?" If the caller must put the phone down to go and do the tasks, the verification questions need to be asked when the caller returns.

It is rare to have two operant questions as appears in panel 5. This is called a *double question* (not to be confused with a compound question) and requires an answer to the first question *before* the second question is asked. The presence of a double question in the protocol format indicates the importance of this particular fork in the logic road. Failure to determine if the chest is rising or if the air is going into the lungs could result in an incorrect treatment and cause a delay in returning to the correct sequence. EMDs must pay special attention to this feature while in panel 5.

> The presence of a double question in the protocol format indicates the importance of this particular fork in the logic road.

A "Yes" answer means that the patient is getting air—perhaps enough to enable a successful resuscitation by the responding field personnel if all else goes well. The caller can then proceed to panel 6. However, a "No" answer means that the remaining priority is to get air into the lungs. Currently, there is no sense worrying whether the heart is beating if there is no oxygen in the blood. The EMD at this point is referred to panel 14, as follows:

14	**Change Tilt**

Tilt the **head** back more and **pinch** the **nose** closed.

Completely **cover** her/his **mouth** with your **mouth** and force **2 deep breaths** of air into the lungs, just like you are **blowing up** a **big** balloon.

	– 15

Panel 14: Change Tilt. When an airway remains blocked, first suspect whether the head is tilted enough. This panel prompts the caller to tilt the head more, and reinforces the other steps for successful mouth-to-mouth aid: pinched nostrils, and completely covering the patient's mouth with the caller's mouth. In infants, care must be taken not to hyper-extend the head (neck), which can collapse the airway like an empty hose. The EMD then moves to panel 15.

Panel 15: Airway Blocked? The most immediate priority is to get air into the patient through a patent airway. Proper coaching consists of having the caller watch for signs that air is actually entering the patient's lungs. When the caller returns to the telephone, the EMD

| **15**　**Airway Blocked?** |
| While giving each **breath**, watch very closely for the **chest** to go **up and down**. |
| Make sure the **air goes in**. |
| • Can you **feel** the air going in and out? |
| • Did you **see** the chest rising? |
| Yes – 8
No – E-7 |

asks a crucial *double* question: "Can you feel the air going in and out?" and "Did you see the chest rising?" A "No" answer refers the caller to protocol E: Choking—Adult, panel 7, in which the caller is told how to cope with a blocked airway in an unconscious person. This link demonstrates an essential cross-over capability of the protocol. Even though the original chief complaint caused the EMD to turn to the cardiac arrest protocol, the airway is still not open. This means the caller and EMD must work through an apparent airway obstruction. When a closed airway becomes open during use of the choking protocol, the EMD is referred back into protocol C: Arrest—Adult (≥ 8 years) to continue the CPR process.

In the current scenario, assume a "Yes" answer has been given to the question in panel 15. The EMD moves back to resume the sequence at panel 8 (The scripted text in panels 6 and 7, dealing with a pulse check, was removed. See the Author's Note for more information).

| **8**　**CPR Landmarks** |
| **Listen carefully** and I'll tell you how to do CPR compressions. |
| Put the **heel** of your **hand** on the **breastbone** in the **center** of her/his **chest**, right between the **nipples**. |
| Put your **other hand** on **top** of that hand. |
| – 9 |

Panel 8: CPR Landmarks. The caller is about to begin chest compressions, a primary element of CPR. Positioning is important; one should be neither too low nor too high on the breastbone (sternum). This panel begins with the words, "Listen carefully," to prompt the caller of something especially important to follow.

| **!**　**Authors' Note** |
| An official reccommendation not to check pulses in the CPR verification sequence has been approved by AHA, Canadian Heart and Stroke Foundation, European Resuscitation Council, and ILCOR. As of February 21st, 2001, the Council of Standards of the Academy's College of Fellows has officially approved this change to the protocol and is issuing new PAIs in conjunction with the April 6th version 11.1 update. Scripted text in panels 6 and 7 on the card was removed in compliance with the change, and for that reason they are not discussed here. |

| **9**　**Compressions** |
| Push down firmly **2 inches** (5 cm) with only the **heel** of your lower hand touching the chest. |
| Do it **15 times**, just like you are **pumping** her/his chest, **twice a second**. |
| – 10 |

Again, verbatim repetition of the EMD's prompts often occurs. This panel flows directly to panel 9.

Panel 9: Compressions. Here the rationale behind the separate protocols (A, B, or C) for different age groups becomes apparent. For adults, the American Heart Association, the British Heart Association, the European Resuscitation Council, the Canadian Heart and Stroke Foundation, and the Australian Resuscitation Council, all recommend pushing the chest down two inches. This could be too far for a child or infant; protocols A and B reflect the standards for these groups. The caller is prompted to do 15 compressions and then return to the telephone. The EMD enters panel 10.

Panel 10: Perform CPR. By this time, the caller is fully into the CPR protocol. Chest compressions and artificial breathing are performed at a ratio of 15 compressions to two breaths. The EMD provides encouragement, and a reminder of correct positioning and technique. The EMD continues to panel 11.

10	**Perform CPR**

With your hand **under** her/his neck, **pinch** the **nose** closed and **tilt** her/his **head back** again.

Give **2 more big breaths**, then **pump** the chest **15 more times**.

Make sure the **heel** of your **hand** is on the bone in the **center** of the **chest**, right between the **nipples**.

– 11

11	**Continue CPR**

Keep repeating this cycle of **2 breaths** then **15 pumps, 2 breaths** then **15 pumps. Keep doing it** until help can take over.

If s/he **starts** breathing, tell me **immediately**.

• (Is s/he breathing **normally** now?)

Tell me **when** the **paramedics** (EMTs) are **with** her/him.

Normal – 16

Abnormal/Uncertain – 12

End of Sequence or 18

Panel 11: Continue CPR. The EMD coaches the caller to continue until help arrives. At this point, many callers are able to continue CPR well. They are calmer because they know they are helping, and they know the EMD is right there in case they need anything. Occasionally, a patient begins breathing spontaneously. If that happens, the EMD prompts the caller to report it immediately (at which point the EMD will go to panel

16, Maintain and Monitor). The caller is also told to come back to the telephone if any questions arise.

Often, by this point in the pre-arrival sequence, the EMD is a silent, reassuring presence, waiting with the caller for on-scene help to arrive. Before the responders arrive, if the caller is still unsure and requires active intervention, the EMD is referred back to panel 10 to reiterate instructions for performing CPR. This can be repeated as often as the caller needs.

12	**Reassure Caller**

Don't give up. You've got to keep doing it.

Keep repeating this cycle of **2 breaths** then **15 pumps**. This will **keep her/him going** until the paramedics (EMTs) arrive.

– 18

Panel 12: Reassure Caller. Many lay people hold the preconceived notion that a little CPR results quickly in a miraculous (and complete) recovery. Unfortunately this is not true. (It only works on television!) The EMD reaffirms the importance of what the caller is doing. Without the caller's "bystander CPR," the patient's chances of survival are far slimmer—and in long-distant responses, downright impossible. This "problem solver" panel is present on all the CPR protocols, and the trained EMD knows to find it and use it as needed.

Example of Tendency to Follow PAIs Verbatim

EMD:	**I'm going to tell you how to give mouth-to-mouth.**	**EMD:**	**Completely cover his mouth with your mouth…**	
Caller:	Sshh, he's telling us how to do mouth-to-mouth.	Caller:	Completely cover his mouth with your mouth… *[Now on to Panel 5]*	
EMD:	**Place one hand under the neck, the other on the forehead…**	**EMD:**	**Force two deep breaths of air into the lungs just like you are blowing up a big balloon.**	
Caller:	Place one hand under the neck, the other on the forehead…	Caller:	Force two deep breaths of air into the lungs. You know, like blowing up a big balloon.	
EMD:	**… and tilt the head back.**			
Caller:	Tilt the head back.	**EMD:**	**Watch for the chest to rise.**	
EMD:	**Pinch the nose closed.**	Caller:	I can see it. The chest is rising. Okay, what now?	
Caller:	Quiet! Listen! Pinch the nose closed.			

Fig. 4-8. Example of tendency to follow pre-arrival instructions verbatim.

Call Hand-Off Example

Paramedic:	This is Mark.	Paramedic:	No problem. Was she ever unconscious?
EMD:	**Mark, she was completely obstructed. A big piece of meat came out after four thrusts. She started to breathe after about 30 seconds of mouth-to-mouth. He's pretty stressed. Make sure he's okay, too, could you?**	**EMD:**	**Yes, that was how he reported it to me.**
		Paramedic:	Okay. She's conscious now. We'll take it from here. Thanks.
		EMD:	**10-4.**

Fig. 4-9. Call hand-off example.

---

18 | Arrival Interface

When you **hear** the paramedics (EMTs) arrive, **don't** stop **CPR** (Mouth-to-Mouth) until they **take over** from you.

• (Is the door **unlocked**?)
(Send someone to **open** it now.)

Tell me **when** they're **with** her/him.

End of Sequence

Panel 18: Arrival Interface. This is an important concept in dispatch life support. When the EMD is aware that the responders are getting close (the caller can hear their sirens or says they are nearby) s/he can jump to panel 18 from anywhere else in the sequence. Panel 18 directs the EMD to tell the caller not to stop assisting the patient just because s/he can hear approaching sirens. Even when the EMD is notified by the responding units that they have arrived, it may still take several minutes for them to actually make patient contact.[5, 6] The caller must wait until the professionals can take over. (One pertinent reason to stop CPR momentarily is for solitary callers to unlock the door.) Failure to perform correct Arrival Interface is analogous to dropping the baton in a relay race, but with a penalty potentially much worse than a sporting disqualification.

This panel assists the EMD with clinical interface with field crews. Remember that until this point, no emergency responder knew more about what was happening at the scene than the EMD. When appropriate, the EMD can ask the caller to hand the telephone to one of the responders as soon as possible (see Chapter 3, Call Completion Theory). This allows the EMD to provide a 5 to 10 second patient hand-off

report, similar to what the field personnel will soon do at the emergency department. It might go something like fig. 4-9, Call hand-off example.

The DLS protocols are easy to follow after proper training and subsequent practice with each one. Comfortable familiarity with the system decreases that awful sense of inadequacy at a crucial moment. Professional EMDs should review a different portion of them daily.

Protocol Y: Tracheostomy (Stoma) Airway/Arrest

Related to the Airway/Arrest protocols is protocol Y: Tracheostomy (Stoma) Airway/Arrest. The structure of this protocol is essentially identical to protocols A, B, and C, with the important difference that the wording has been modified to assist the EMD when dealing with patients who have had tracheostomy operations. The tracheostomy operation results in a new breathing "hole" (the stoma) being created in the patient's throat. Artificial respiration must be performed using this hole rather than the patient's mouth or nose. While it is rare that the EMD will encounter this problem in providing airway/CPR instructions, protocol Y (a,b,c) insures their correct application.

---

4 | Start Mouth-To-Mouth

I'm going to tell you how to give **mouth-to-mouth.***

With the head **tilted** back, **pinch** the **nose** closed and completely **cover** her/his **mouth** with your **mouth**, then force **2 deep breaths** of air into the lungs, just like you're **blowing up** a **big** balloon.

– 5
***Refuses M-T-M – 8**

Protocol Z, the AED protocol

This protocol is an important addition to the MPDS, and will see increasing use as public access defibrillators become more widely dispersed in our communities. Protocol Z functions somewhat differently to other DLS protocols because it must be able to accommodate the timing of the "electronic protocol" stored within the AED itself; as such the Academy named it the AED Support protocol, with an emphasis on the fact that this protocol *supports* the EMD's efforts to assist a caller prepare and use an AED. As this is a novel part of the MPDS, an article discussing the AED support protocol published in the National EMD Journal and its use is reproduced reprinted at the end of this chapter in its entirety.

Protocol X, the eXit protocol

Protocol X, a new feature of the MPDS that was introduced in version 11, has some features of post-dispatch instructions and some features of Pre-Arrival Instructions. Many of the Post-Dispatch Instructions that were listed on multiple Chief Complaint protocols in previous MPDS versions have been refined and expanded on the eXit protocol. Protocol X also allows much more directed and accurate handling of potentially dangerous scenes, as well as cleaner ways to stay on the line or terminate a call.

Protocol X is a deceptively complex protocol. While the basic structure appears simple, there are several different variations that are accounted for—first vs. second party caller, alert vs. not alert patient, MEDICAL vs. TRAUMA incident, at home vs. remote scene, etc. This development leads to a columnar structure known as "free fall" rather than the more familiar matrix structure of protocols A through F. Protocol X occupies three pages in the MPDS cardset.

Pages 1 and 2 are divided into two wide side columns and a thinner middle information column. The wide column on the left has four numbered scripts for when the EMD is talking to a first-party caller (i.e., the patient). The wide column on the right has the same four numbered scripts, worded for the second-party caller.

On the first page, a narrower middle column contains **Critical EMD Information (CEI)**, and the universal instruction: "Don't hang up. Do it now and tell me when it's done." This can be used at any point in the MPDS when the caller is sent away from the phone to do something.

---

1 ☎ **1ˢᵗ Party Caller**
Help is on the way.
Don't have anything to **eat** or **drink**. It might make you **sick** or cause **problems** for the doctor.
(MEDICAL) Just **rest** in the most **comfortable position** for you.
(TRAUMA) **Don't move** around, **unless** it's absolutely **necessary**. Just **be still** and wait for **help** to arrive.
Stable – 2 Unstable or Not alert – 3

Panel 1: 1ˢᵗ Party Caller (top) and 2ⁿᵈ Party Caller (bottom), contains the basic "observe and reassure" statements. This is the default access point that is directed to by DLS links on most Chief Complaint protocols. The EMD should begin with script 1 when instructed, and move to script 2, 3, or 4 as the situation dictates. The first thing the EMD says to the caller in script 1 is "Help is on the way." Next, the EMD provides an instruction—and its justification—that is appropriate for either MEDICAL or TRAUMA patients: "Don't let her/him have anything to eat or drink. It might make you her/him sick or cause problems for the doctor." The script then gives a different instruction for the TRAUMA patient vs. the MEDICAL patient.

---

2   Routine Disconnect (⊕stable) – **2ⁿᵈ Party**
I want you to **watch** him/her very closely.
(Appropriate) If s/he becomes **less awake** and **vomits**, quickly turn her/him on her/his **side**.
(Appropriate) Please:
• Put **away** any **family pets**.
• **Gather** her/his **medications** and write down the name of her/his **doctor**.
• **Unlock** the **door**.
• **Turn on** the outside **lights**.
• Have someone **meet the paramedics**.
(Always) If s/he gets **worse** in any way, call me back **immediately** for further **instructions**.

Panel 2: Routine Disconnect, provides an elegant way for the EMD to terminate the call. The caller is given some instructions to prepare the scene for the responders (put pets away, unlock the door, etc). An associated CEI note cautions the EMD regarding asking 1ˢᵗ party callers to unduly exert themselves complying with

3 ✍ **Stay on Line** (≈ unstable) − **1ˢᵗ Party**

I'll **stay on the line** with you as long as I can.

If anything **changes,** just let me know.

(Tell me when the **paramedics** (EMTs) get there.)

End on Arrival

these instructions. This panel is used when the patient is basically stable (≈stable).

Panel 3: Stay on Line, has instructions for when the EMD intends staying on the line with the caller. Critical EMD Information in the central column recommends conditions for which it is advisable to stay on the line.

4 ☎ **Urgent Disconnect** − **1ˢᵗ Party**

I **need** to hang up now (to take **another** call).
Help is on the way.

If anything **changes,** call me back **immediately** for further **instructions.**

End

Panel 4: Urgent Disconnect. If another emergency call demands the EMD's immediate attention, panel 4 provides a script for the EMD to read the caller before disconnecting. For the first party caller, it concludes with the instruction "If anything changes, call me back immediately for further instructions." The second party caller is told "If s/he vomits or starts making funny noises, quickly turn her/him on her/his side and call me back immediately for further instructions."

5 ◊ **Control Bleeding**

Don't use a tourniquet.

I'm going to tell you how to **stop** the **bleeding.**
Listen **carefully** to make sure we **do it right.**

Get a clean, dry **cloth** or towel and place it right on the wound. Press down **firmly** and **don't lift it up to look.**

If it **keeps** bleeding, you're probably not **pressing hard** enough. Remember, keep firm, **steady pressure** on the wound.

−1
Airway − ABC-1
Amputation − 6

Panel 5: Bleeding Control, is accessed from the DLS links on several protocols and deals with bleeding control. The caller is given instructions for how to stop

bleeding. The EMD should be aware of Rule 2 on protocol 21: direct pressure should be avoided on the wound in the presence of visible bone or foreign objects.

Some useful information about when to use this rule can be found in Chapter 7 under Hemorrhage/ Lacerations and Stab/Gunshot/Penetrating Trauma. At the end of script 5, the EMD has three choices: go to protocol X, panel 1 (alert and breathing patient), go to A,B,C-1 if the airway needs attention, or go to panel 6, Amputation, if an amputation is involved. If the EMD goes to panel 6, instructions for collecting and preserving amputated parts are provided, and from there the EMD can go to A,B,C-1 or to protocol X, panel 1.

6 **Amputation**

Listen **carefully.** I want you to locate **all** amputated parts or skin and place them in a **clean plastic bag.**

Do not place the part on **ice** or in **water** as this may **damage** it.

−1
Airway − ABC-1
SERIOUS Hemorrhage − 5

Page 3 of protocol X contains one script that is very similar to panel 5—panel 13: Cooling and Flushing.

13 ◊ **Cooling and Flushing**

(Heat or Fire)
          Cool the burn for up to **10 minutes** with water.
(Chemical)
          Flush the area with a lot of **water** until help arrives.

−1
Airway − ABC-1

Here the EMD can provide instructions for cooling a heat- or fire-caused burn or for flushing a chemical burn. Similar to panels 5 and 6, the EMD can go from here to A,B,C-1 to support an airway or to X-1 to observe and reassure the patient.

The remainder of protocol X, panels 7 to 12, deal with scene safety. These are linked to from the DLS links on many protocols when specific types of dangers are identified.

Panel 7: Danger Present–Scene/HAZMAT, deals with a hazard such as chemical contamination or live electrical systems that the caller—and responder— should simply steer clear of. The caller is cautioned that it could be a very dangerous situation and told "Do not

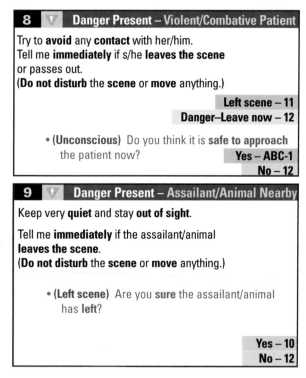

7 ▽ **Danger Present – Scene/HAZMAT**
Listen **carefully**. This could be a very **dangerous** situation.
Do not approach (or **touch**) the patient at all. Let the **paramedics** (EMTs) handle it. (If anything **changes**, call me back from a **safe place**, if possible, for further **instructions**.)
Danger–Leave now – 12
End

approach (or touch) the patient at all. Let the paramedics (EMTs) handle it."

Panel 8: Danger Present–Violent Patient, deals with a violent patient (for example following a suicide or overdose). The caller is advised to avoid contact with the patient and to tell the EMD immediately "if s/he passes out or leaves the scene."

8 ▽ **Danger Present – Violent/Combative Patient**
Try to **avoid** any **contact** with her/him. Tell me **immediately** if s/he **leaves the scene** or passes out. (**Do not disturb** the **scene** or **move** anything.)
Left scene – 11
Danger–Leave now – 12
• (**Unconscious**) Do you think it is **safe to approach** the patient now?   Yes – ABC-1
No – 12

9 ▽ **Danger Present – Assailant/Animal Nearby**
Keep very **quiet** and stay **out of sight**.
Tell me **immediately** if the assailant/animal **leaves the scene**. (**Do not disturb** the **scene** or **move** anything.)
• (**Left scene**) Are you **sure** the assailant/animal has **left**?
Yes – 10
No – 12

Panel 9: Danger Present–Assailant/Animal Nearby, deals with assailants or dangerous animals. The EMD tells the caller "Keep quiet and stay out of sight. Tell me immediately if the assailant/animal leaves the scene." The caller is further cautioned not to disturb the scene or to move anything. From script 8 and 9, the caller may tell the EMD that the violent patient, assailant, or dangerous animal has left the scene. If this happens, the EMD can go to X-10.

Panel 10: Danger Gone–Verification, warns the caller that it could still be a dangerous situation. The caller is then told that if s/he is sure the danger has gone, s/he

10 **Danger Gone – Verification**
Listen **carefully**. This could **still** be a very **dangerous** situation, but if you are **sure** the **danger has gone**, you could help the patient. (**Do not disturb** the **scene** or **move** anything.)
• Do you think it is **safe to approach** the patient now?
Yes – 1
Yes (airway) – ABC-1
No/Uncertain – 11

could try to help the patient. The responsibility for deciding on the safety of the situation is placed squarely with the caller with the question "Do you think it is safe to approach the patient now?"

If the answer is "Yes," and the patient is alert, the EMD begins with X-1. If the answer is "Yes" and the patient is not alert, the EMD begins with an airway assessment at A,B,C-1. If the answer is "No," meaning the caller is not sure it is safe to approach the patient, the EMD moves on to X-11.

11 **Danger Uncertain – Monitor Safety on Line**
I'm going to **stay on the line** to be sure you're still **safe**. If the assailant/animal **comes back**, tell me right away.
Let me **know** when the **paramedics** (EMTs) arrive.
Danger back–Leave now – 12
End on Arrival

Panel 11: Danger Gone–Monitor Safety on Line, allows the EMD to remain on line with the caller. The caller can observe the patient from a distance, and may decide it is safe to approach. The EMD must use discretion regarding the instruction links at the end of X-10 if this happens. If the assailant returns, the EMD proceeds to X-12.

12 ▽ **Danger Present – Leave Now**
(If it's too **dangerous to stay** where you are, and you think you can leave safely,) **get away** and **call me** from somewhere **safe**.

Panel 12: Danger Present–Leave Now, can be reached if an assailant or animal that was believed to have left returns to the scene, but can also be reached directly from panels 7, 8, or 9 if the EMD believes the situation is sufficiently dangerous to warrant the caller leaving immediately. Panel 12 can also be reached directly from the DLS links on protocol 7, Burns (Scalds)/Explosion; in the case of a building fire or an explosion with any

likelihood of a subsequent explosion, the EMD will be directed to X-12 and will tell the caller "If it's too dangerous to stay where you are, and you think you can leave safely, get away and call me back from somewhere safe."

Danger Awareness

As with X-12, the ultimate responsibility for assessing the danger and deciding whether to remain at the scene or to leave rests with the caller. In the MPDS cardset, this third page of the X protocol lists some important information for dealing with potentially dangerous situations. The EMD is warned that dangerous scenes, especially those involving violent people, can change rapidly, often for the worse. The EMD should reassess the situation often and should be prepared to use the link to X-12 at any point it seems prudent to advise the caller to consider leaving.

The EMD is also warned that keeping the caller on the line could place them in danger by making them more visible or by antagonizing a violent patient. Again, the scripts facilitate the process if the EMD feels it is appropriate for the caller to leave or hide.

Finally, if the caller decides to leave the scene, in many situations—especially those involving violent patients—it can be beneficial for the caller to not hang up the phone. An open phone line might allow the EMD to "listen in" on the scene gleaning information that might be useful for the responders—or crucial for their safety—can be collected.

Danger Awareness	PROTOCOL **X**
Keeping a caller on the line in some dangerous incidents could create more danger by making them visible or more accessible to a violent patient or intruder.	

Summary

The benefits of dispatch life support are significant. They include:

- **Increasing the chance a life may be saved or improved.** When a person is not breathing or has no heartbeat, brain cells die quickly. Even if a mobile response time is quoted as three minutes, that calculation is seldom truly accurate. In the first place the response times given are averages, not medians or caps. For every case that is under the average, there is another that is greater than average. Relying on averages can be very deceptive,

especially in EMS. Additionally, it is important to remember that average response times do not count the delays while the caller recognized the problem and called, while the EMD gathered information and sent field units, and while field personnel looked for the patient after arriving at the address. It is seldom possible to have help by the patient's side in less than seven to 10 minutes from the event's onset. But the EMD can create a "Zero-Minute Response" through dispatch life support.

- **A calmer environment.** People who feel helpless can be disturbed from fear, anger, frustration, and other strong emotions. They may lose self-control. People who are guided to productive, possibly life-saving actions usually become more composed. This is safer (not to mention more satisfying) for arriving field providers and allows them to concentrate on the primary emergency.

- **A sense and reassurance that something was done to help.** In many cases, the outcome is not successful. People still die. Callers tend to feel better even in the wake of a death when they know they tried to help or as they often state, "everything possible was done."

- **Fill a critical, clear public expectation of receiving pre-arrival help.** There is no longer any question that, not only can the caller perform EMD-directed instructions exactly as scripted, but the public now truly expects to receive them.

This chapter has outlined what Dispatch Life Support is, how it works, that it isn't just basic life support, and why its use is invaluable for impacting threatened lives at the earliest possible moment. It has outlined for the EMD a standard process for these challenging tasks, and why EMS systems would be remiss not to implement them. The reason for systems to provide dispatch life support should be nothing more than "it's the right thing to do."[57]

The Pre-Arrival Instruction scripts themselves require understanding, study, and frequent practice for line EMDs who may be asked to turn to them at any moment. But those who understand how helpful the scripts are, know how to use them, and who have seen them make a huge difference for terrified callers, are more than happy to make the effort.

It's okay. We can do this together.

—Jennie Greenwood, EMD
Greater Manchester, U.K.

Automated External Defibrillators (AEDs): Background, Research, and a New Protocol.

Academy-Certified EMDs to Add New Skills

Roughly a quarter of a million people die each year in the U.S. from "sudden cardiac arrest," (SCA) a common form or complication of heart disease (other causes of SCA include electrocution, drug intoxication, and drowning). Many of these "sudden cardiac arrests" result from a disturbance to the normal electrical heart rhythm called ventricular fibrillation (V-fib). In V-fib, the heart falls into a state of disordered—chaotic—electrical activity (quivering) with the result that the ventricles contract in an uncoordinated, asynchronous, and ineffective manner. In a related problem: ventricular tachycardia (V-tach), the heart beats rapidly but too shallowly for the ventricles to effectively pump blood around the body (V-tach that does not produce a pulse is treated like V-fib).

Without immediate treatment, a patient falling into V-fib or V-tach (without a pulse) will collapse and die; the only effective treatment is to restore a normal heart rhythm via an electric shock. Patients at known high risk may have equipment that can restore a normal heart rhythm implanted in their bodies: automated internal cardiac defibrillators (see MPDS protocol 19: Heart Problems/AICD). For other people, treatment at the dispatch level has, until recently, been restricted to providing CPR until trained responders reach the scene.

Waiting for responders to arrive is a very unsatisfactory situation. Each passing minute decreases the likelihood of a successful defibrillation by about 10 percent. Even allowing a (fast!) five minutes from

when the patient suffers the attack for the caller to identify the incident and call 9-1-1; for the calltaker to allocate a resource and mobilize the responders; and for the responders to drive to the scene, locate the patient, and set up their equipment, reduces the patient's chances of survival to 50:50. The proliferation of public-access defibrillation using automated external defibrillators (AEDs) can significantly reduce this time delay.

> ### AED
>
> An Automated External Defibrillator is a computerized device designed for use by minimally trained lay persons that interprets cardiac rhythms, verbally coaches the user, and then advises shock (or no shock) for electrically correctable non-perfusing rhythms. AEDs have been used for over 15 years by first responders with a high degree of accuracy and safety and are being introduced into an ever-widening variety of public-accessible locations such as airliners, airports, stadiums, large businesses, etc.

Three U.S. companies (soon to be four) manufacture and sell AEDs. About the size of a laptop computer, these machines began to appear in the homes of patients who were high-risk for V-fib but who were not appropriate candidates for having an implanted device. As they gained acceptance, AEDs

(continued on 4.25)

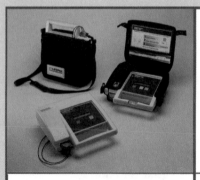

Medtronic/Physio Control
[Yellow and Black Case]

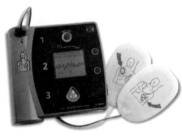

Survivalink
[Blue and Grey Case]

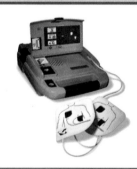

Agilent/Heartstream
[Red and Black Case]

Automated External Defibrillators (AEDs): Background, Research, and a New Protocol.

(continued from 4.24)

have been placed in progressively more locations, and can now be found in airports (and on airplanes), malls, office buildings, sports stadiums, casinos, large hotels, and even—it has been suggested—in taxi cabs!

So maybe you, the EMD, having probably never seen an AED and having almost certainly never used one, now have a call that is clearly a cardiac arrest with a caller (rescuer) reporting "I've got this shock-box thing; what do I do with it?" (Keep in mind that while defibrillator is the commonest description, regional, cultural, and age-based groups may use another name.) The new AED Support Protocol, and this article, will help.

Research Step 1: Getting started. After several requests from MPDS users for an AED protocol, the Academy organized a meeting in Salt Lake City about 18 months ago that included several Academy members and representatives from the three AED manufacturers and the American Heart Association. At that meeting it was decided that the Academy should create a supplemental pre-arrival instruction protocol that would walk the caller through the use of an AED. Formatted in the familiar style of protocol C through X, this AED card was sent out for testing at over 100 stations in 8 centers.

Research Step 2: The best laid plans. Despite what seemed to be a reasonable sample, the AED protocol was used for very few calls. And even then, we ran into problems evaluating its performance due to instructions being relayed through intermediaries. Although this suggests that AED use is currently infrequent, we believe this situation is changing, and the Academy will include the AED protocol as a standard part of version 11 of the MPDS.

Research Step 3: Refine the design. In the absence of real-case feedback, The Academy organized a second meeting for company and American Heart Association representatives and included representatives from some of the pilot centers. A day's vigorous discussion revealed several problems with the original design and suggested some improvements, although exactly how to implement those improvements remained perplexing.

The first big problem was that the machines are not entirely standardized and so must be operated in slightly different ways. For example, to turn on the Lifepak 500™ or the Heartstream ForeRunner™ unit requires the case to be opened and an "on" button to be pressed, while the FirstSave™ has no "on" button, turning itself on when the lid is opened. Similar variations appear with plugging in the pads (the pads, or electrodes, must be stuck to the patient's chest in the correct position and must be connected to the machine, some are pre-connected to the machine, others are not) and with the possible need to press an analyze button. Creating a protocol that explicitly covers all these possibilities and yet is brief and to the point is a difficult proposition.

The second big problem is that each AED is designed to give its own instructions: you turn it on and it tells you what to do. And it tells you what to do rather faster than an EMD can instruct the caller and interpret the caller's reports. This suggests the need for a protocol that simply monitors the caller's progress, preparing the EMD to jump in and help if the caller gets into difficulties of if the machine doesn't appear to be making sense. However, this "monitoring mode" approach falls over before the AED is applied (when the caller, according to currently accepted practice, must check the patient's breathing and pulse; presumably necessitating detailed instructions) and falls over again when the AED tells the caller to "Check pulse. Begin CPR!" (or some similar instruction). At this point most callers need some help, help that is both explicit and scripted into the MPDS.

The third big problem concerns this scripted help. After it is set up, the AED will generally analyze the patient's rhythm and advise giving a shock if necessary. This will be repeated for three cycles of analyze-shock. Then the AED will instruct the caller to begin CPR. Sounds easy to accommodate, until you realize that the machine will only give you one minute to begin CPR before announcing "Analyzing, do not touch patient!" Three more cycles of analyze-shock may be executed, followed by another minute of CPR, to a total of nine (or twelve) shocks. (The one-minute intervals may be discarded in favor of three-minute intervals in some countries, or there may be no limit on the total number of shocks the machine

(continued on 4.26)

Automated External Defibrillators (AEDs): Background, Research, and a New Protocol.

(continued from 4.25)

may give. The European Rescuscitation council, for example, recommends one minute of CPR after 3 consecutive shocks, and 3 minutes of CPR if no shock was advised. Check your local EMS protocols if you are unsure what is required in your area.)

So a protocol that is explicit and scripted in some places but which can step aside and let the machine take over in other places is required. And a protocol that is capable of bouncing between these two states as the AED dictates. And that can troubleshoot any stage in the procedure that goes wrong, such as when the frustrated caller reports "the pads are applied to the patient, the leads are plugged into the machine, but the machine keeps telling me to 'apply the pads' or to 'connect electrodes'."

Research Step 4: What's the secret of great comedy? The answer, of course, is timing. The same seems to hold for the secret to designing a functional AED protocol. What can you do in 60 seconds that is useful for the patient? Let's take a look at protocol C, Airway/Arrest Adult > 8. Tests here at the Academy indicate that (with a calm and cooperative caller) it is feasible to perform chest compressions (panels 8 and 9) in 35 to 40 seconds. Preceding this with a pulse check, panel 6, takes the total time to around 55 seconds. Similarly, once the caller already knows how to perform the head tilt, starting mouth-to-mouth and check breaths (panels 4 and 5) can also be performed in less than a minute. This timing gives us a handle on integrating the MPDS CPR protocol with the timing dictated by the AED.

Version 11 of the MPDS has several new features. One that is relevant to this discussion (and giving you a teaser for what you will find in version 11) is improved organization of DLS links and the addition of an eXit protocol allowing smoother handling of the final instructions in many calls. The eXit protocol has a different format from protocols A through F, comprising two wide columns (for scripted instructions) separated by a narrower column (that contains universal instructions and Additional Information). Additionally, after providing Post-Dispatch Instructions, each individual Chief Complaint protocol now has DLS links to the appropriate Dispatch Life Support protocol and panel for each major complaint handled by that protocol. DLS

links for AED-relevant situations lead the EMD to the AED Support protocol (protocol Z, for Zap!), which is formatted similar to the eXit protocol.

DLS links. Protocol 9: Cardiac or Respiratory Arrest/Death, is the primary place to BRIDGE to the AED Support protocol. From Case Entry we know the patient is unconscious and not breathing and we also know the patient's age (currently, AEDs are not supposed to be used on children younger than 8 years old). Protocol 9 Key questioning determines whether an AED is available (most municipalities are working to get all AEDs registered and many include this information in enhanced ALI information so you may already know an AED is at the caller's location). The DLS link therefore states "[if] age ≥ 8 and AED available [GO TO] protocol Z-1."

DLS	✳ Link to ☎ ABC-1 unless:		↱
Danger or Contamination		▽	X-7
Suspected **Workable Arrest**		✺	ABC-1
AED available (age ≥ 8)		⚡	Z-1
Choked first			DE-1

⚕ POST-DISPATCH INSTRUCTIONS	✪ ✪ ✪ ✪ ✪ ✪

a. I'm sending the **paramedics** (ambulance) to help you now. **Stay on the line** and I'll tell you **exactly** what to do next.

b. **(Patient medication requested)** Remind her/him to do what her/his **doctor has instructed** for these situations.

c. **(≥ 8)** If there is a **defibrillator** (AED) available, **send** someone to get it **now** in case we need it later.

On protocol 10: Chest Pain and protocol 19: Heart Problems, where there is a possibility that the patient may need an AED in the near future, a Post-Dispatch Instruction has been added: "(≥8) If a defibrillator (AED) is available, send someone to get it now and be prepared to BRIDGE to protocol Z if the patient arrests."

In cards, the AED Support protocol itself is a folded card that is stored behind the "down card" of protocol C. It is tabbed for easy retrieval. The AED protocol is designed to be used in tight conjunction with protocol C: instructions on the AED protocol often refer to panels on protocol C as we'll describe shortly. First, open the cardset to protocol C, pull the AED protocol out, unfold it, and place it alongside

(continued on 4.27)

Automated External Defibrillators (AEDs): Background, Research, and a New Protocol.

(continued from 4.26)

the open C cards in the file. (In software, links between the AED protocol and protocol C are handled for you.)

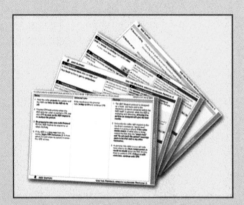

Step-by-step through the protocol. The AED Support protocol, similar to the eXit protocol, has wide left and right columns separated by a narrower central column. The left column has eight short panels for preparing the patient and setting up the AED. Current accepted practice is to confirm the patient is unresponsive, breathless, and pulseless before using an AED. Panel 2 (evaluate patient) performs this check and demonstrates the tight integration between the AED protocol and protocol C. This panel simply contains an instruction to the EMD

(not to be read to the caller) that states "Perform C1, C2, and C3 and then return to here." Protocol C is open next to the AED protocol, so the EMD goes through C-1 (patient to phone), C-2 (check airway), and C-3 (check breathing). Having completed this, the EMD returns to the AED sequence at the end of panel 2 and is directed to Z-3 and Z-4 to get the AED and place it beside the patient. If the AED is some distance away, Rule 3 directs the EMD to begin CPR with C-4 (start mouth-to-mouth) until the AED arrives.

Once the patient has been evaluated and the AED placed next to the patient, Z-5 through Z-8 deal with removing the patient's clothing, finding the AED pads (electrodes), readying the machine, and placing the pads on the patient's chest. These instructions are generic due to differences between the various AEDs. For example, Z-6 (ready machine) reads, "Open the lid if necessary and press the "on" button if there is one," and Z-7 (find pads) reads "Find the pads (electrodes) and if necessary plug them into the machine." These instructions are intentionally adaptable due to machine differences: one type of machine turns itself on when the lid is opened, others have a lid (or cover) that must be opened and an "on" button that must be pressed. Similarly, one machine requires the user to plug the pads into a socket while the other two machines should have the pads pre-plugged. (Plugs can be pulled out during set-up or the pads that are plugged into the machine may need to be replaced.)

T1 Remove Clothing

Clothing that just unzips or unbuttons can be opened and left on.

Sweaters and T-shirts may need to be completely removed or cut open.

T1 Additional Troubleshooting

Clothing can be pulled up around her/his neck while the pads are applied. It's okay if the clothing falls back over the pads when the caller performs CPR.

(continued on 4.28)

1 Get AED	T1 Remove clothing
Is there **someone there** who can **help** you? (Yes) **Send** her/him to **get** the **defibrillator**. – 2	✱ Clothing that just unzips or unbuttons can be opened and left on. ✱ Sweaters and T-shirts may need to be completely removed or cut open.
2 Evaluate Patient	T2 Machine not on
Perform C1, C2 (not breathing), and C3, then return to here when finished. **Breathing – C-16** **Not breathing – 3**	✱ Some machines begin automatically when the lid is opened. ✱ Some machines have an "on" button. It is frequently green.
3 Get AED	T3 Find/Plug in pads
(No helper) Go and **get** the **defibrillator** and **come right back** to the phone. • Is the **defibrillator** there right now? **Yes – 4** **No – Begin CPR (C-4) then – 4**	✱ The pads are usually in a flat foil or plastic package (about 6 by 8 inches / 15 by 20 cm). ✱ The pads are often already plugged into the machine.
4 Place AED	T4 Pad placement
Put the defibrillator on the **floor** next to her/his **head**, on the side **closest** to you.	✱ The pads have a picture of where they should be placed.
– 5	

Automated External Defibrillators (AEDs): Background, Research, and a New Protocol.

(continued from 4.27)

As the EMD works through these first nine panels, questions and directors ensure that everything is proceeding correctly; when a problem is encountered, the director leads the EMD to an appropriate troubleshooting section (T1, T2, T3, etc). The most common problems are listed in the middle column; more detailed information and rarer problems are listed on the back of the AED "down card."

Assisting and troubleshooting. So let's assume everything's going according to plan. The patient is bare-chested, the AED is on the floor beside him, the AED is turned on, and the cord from the pads is plugged in. Now the "fun" begins, because as soon as the pads are applied to the patient's chest the AED will and give audible, verbal (natural language) instructions to the bystander or caller (these instructions are also displayed on a small screen). The caller must now follow the instructions from the machine, and the EMD must fade into the background and try not to distract them. However, the EMD must know what's going on to allow for troubleshooting as necessary and to segue into CPR if the machine tells the caller "Check pulse. If no pulse, start CPR."

Rule 1	PROTOCOL Z
Help the caller **prepare** the patient and the AED, and **then let the AED do it's job**.	

Axiom 1	PROTOCOL Z
The AED Support protocol is designed as a front- and back-end to the electronic protocol contained within the AED itself. In general, while the AED is analyzing and shocking, **allowing it to perform as designed will give the best results**.	

In Z-9, the EMD instructs the caller, "The machine will tell you what to do. Follow its instructions. Tell me what you're doing so I'll know how it's going." (In fact, the EMD will most likely overhear the machine's instructions to the caller.)

Links are provided in Z-9 for troubleshooting analyze (T5) and shock (T6). One frustrating situation

can be that everything seems to be set up correctly but the machine continues to instruct the caller to "connect electrodes," to "apply pads," or to "plug in pads." This means that the machine cannot detect a completed circuit from pad to pad through the patient. The most likely reason for this is that the pads are not contacting the patient's skin adequately. Was the backing removed, exposing the sticky surface, from both pads? (Leaving the backing stuck to a pad would be bad.) Were the pads pressed firmly onto the skin? Are the pads placed over clothes? Does the patient have a very hairy chest? Are the pads plugged firmly into the machine? (The plugs will only go in one way round and usually they "click" in place.)

If there are problems, the EMD should try some of the common troubleshooting tips, but should not hesitate to enhance the protocol by asking the caller for help: "Can you see any problems?" If nothing seems to work, remember that you can still perform CPR as a backup (just as if there was no AED available). After making reasonable efforts, do not hesitate to follow Rule 3:

Rule 3	PROTOCOL Z
Be prepared to take over with Protocol C if the AED finishes its sequence or stops working.	

Universal Law	
If the machine or the process fails, **BRIDGE to C-4** and continue CPR.	

Also in Z-9 are some notes to the EMD concerning the likely progression of events as the AED functions. If a shockable rhythm is found here are typically three cycles of analyze-shock. (When the machine announces "stand clear" it means everyone—including the caller!) The AED may then tell the caller to "Check pulse. If no pulse, start CPR."

Follow the cycles. The end of Z-9 asks whether the AED advised CPR. If not, the EMD must attempt to discover what the machine is doing. If CPR is

(continued on 4.29)

Automated External Defibrillators (AEDs): Background, Research, and a New Protoco

(continued from 4.28)

advised, the EMD should immediately go to Z-10 where directions to perform C-8 and C-9 will be found.

---

10   Perform CPR

Perform C8 and C9. Return to here when finished or if interrupted by the machine. The machine should re-analyze and may do 3 more cycles of analyze/shock before advising more CPR.

✱ Second round of CPR advised?

Yes – 11

• **(No) What** does the machine **say?**

Rule 2   PROTOCOL **Z**

Provide CPR instructions when the AED tells the caller to perform CPR, but stop CPR **as soon as the AED begins to re-analyze the patient**.

This instructs the caller in chest compressions (although the focus group's responsibilities do not include developing medical direction, those present agreed that, with only one minute to work with, getting some blood moving was a more urgent concern than replacing the air into the patient's lungs. It is unlikely there will be any spare time between the caller finishing the 15 compressions and the AED announcing "Analyzing. Stand clear." If there does appear to be time, although it is not explicitly written in the protocol, the EMD can begin instructions for mouth-to-mouth. Regardless of how far you get with these instructions, when the AED wants the caller to stand clear of the patient, you must accept its timing and allow the caller to stand clear.

The AED will go through a second three cycles of analyze-shock. The group expressed an opinion that the first of these (the fourth shock) is often the one that is successful in converting a dysfunctional rhythm to a more normal one. After these shocks, or if a non-shockable rhythm is identified, the AED may again announce, "Check pulse. If no pulse, start CPR." At the end of Z-10 the director for "Is CPR advised?" sends the EMD to Z-11. In Z-11, rather than repeating chest compressions, the EMD

instructs the caller how to perform mouth-to-mouth (beginning with panel C-4) and continues to follow protocol C until once more interrupted by the AED. You should note here that, if the AED did convert the aberrant rhythm and a pulse is detected, the EMD will simply continue with protocol C. If the AED does not advise a shock (and the patient still lacks a pulse per AED generated request) the caller will give 2 breaths of mouth-to-mouth (having previously done compressions) and then, if time permits, do more compressions. After one minute the AED will most likely again announce "Analyzing. Stand clear."

Axiom 2   PROTOCOL **Z**

Generally the caller will respond to the machine's prompts to "stand clear" when it is giving a shock. **If the caller seems unsure** of what s/he is doing, remind her/him that the **"stand clear" and "do not touch the patient" warnings apply to her/him and to any other bystanders**.

The pattern is becoming clear. After this third round of three analyze-shock the caller has been instructed in both chest compressions and mouth-to-mouth, so should be able to perform at least one round of two breaths and 15 compressions during the one minute gaps. Most AEDs should be set up to perform nine shocks in total (some may do 12 or more). Regardless of the exact sequence, after the third (and any subsequent) rounds of analyze-shock the EMD can then proceed with C-10 and C-11.

A quick review. Once the patient has been evaluated and the AED prepared, the EMD must allow the AED to do its job. After the first three rounds of analyze-shock, or if no shock is advised and the patient is pulseless, the EMD instructs the caller to do chest compressions and then mouth-to-mouth if there is time. After the second three rounds of analyze-shock, the EMD instructs the caller to do two breaths of mouth-to-mouth and then a pulse check and chest compressions if there is time. After the third, and any subsequent rounds of analyze-shock, the EMD instructs the caller to continue with mouth-to-mouth and compressions according to C-10.

(continued on 4.30)

Automated External Defibrillators (AEDs): Background, Research, and a New Protocol.

(continued from 4.29)

The AED protocol is unusual in that it requires the EMD to alternate between highly active and highly passive roles. Note that Rules 1 and 2: "Help the caller prepare the patient and the AED and then let the AED do its job," and "Provide CPR instructions when the AED tells the caller to perform CPR, but stop CPR as soon as the AED wants to re-analyze the patient," reinforce when each role is required. And always remember that Rule 3, "Be prepared to take over with protocol C-4, if the AED finishes its sequence or stops working," allows you to intervene if things appear to be going wrong.

As time goes by, public-access AEDs will become a more routine feature of prehospital care for many cardiac arrests. Try to get access to a local AED, and work through several scenarios and drills with an AED and the AED Support protocol when you upgrade to MPDS version 11.

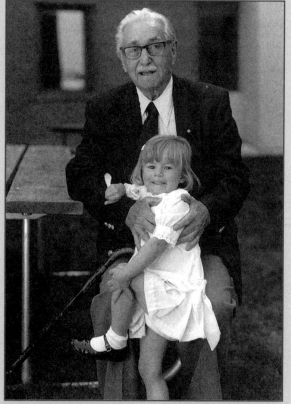

On January 13, 1986 in Salt Lake City, Mr. Robert Gilchrist, 81 y.o. cardiac arrest patient, was the first person to be saved by an AED in Mountain America. He called it "That new experiment machine." He lived an additional 7 years to age 88.

Fig. 4-10. The new AED Protocol research report by Robert Sinclair, Ph.D. Reprinted from NEMDJ.

Contents

CHAPTER 5

Caller Management Techniques

Chapter Overview

The EMD's objective is to gain control of each telephone call so the situation can be handled efficiently—while obtaining the caller's confidence and conveying a consistent impression of compassion. Of all the EMD's tasks, controlling telephone interrogation can be one of the most trying, but also at times the most rewarding. This chapter describes a series of predictable caller behaviors that can interfere with the EMD process, and innovative ways to handle them effectively.

You can only see a thing well when you know in advance what is going to happen.

— *John Tyndall*

One reason the dispatch office was the last major frontier for modernization of EMS practice was that callers were long thought to be unpredictable by nature. Most people assumed there was no way to control someone that could not even be seen. These assumptions have long been disproved, callers can indeed be worthwhile partners, even under the stress of crisis.

People enjoy being in control of their lives. They like independence. Developing the skills and judgment that lead to self-sufficiency is part of the maturation process. But when an emergency arises, control is suddenly usurped by emotion as the caller is forced to rely on a nameless, faceless person. It is easy to appreciate the feelings one might experience when forced to relinquish control under such circumstances. Many people actually revert to an earlier stage of development, which causes the caller to behave with tantrum-like behavior, just like a child.

Don't Shoot the Messenger

No one, including dispatchers, likes discomfort. Traditionally, dispatchers who received telephone calls from anxious, overly-distraught people could simply eliminate the pain by hanging up after getting essential logistical information. However, the evolution of priority dispatch has been based on the realization that many of the events surrounding an emergency are predictable and therefore more manageable. It is an error to react negatively to a caller's particular style of crying out for help, whether that be fright, anger, or obscenity. Whatever the manner of approach, the caller is, in her/his own way, expressing the same powerful need: "Please help me!" The EMD can give this help:

- Regardless of how the caller behaves.

- Regardless of whether the caller can aptly describe the problem.

- Regardless of underlying fears the caller may have

> **Sergeant Friday's First Rule of Interrogation**
> Just the facts, ma'am.

that "9-1-1 or EMS is not going to work for me." The caller's emotional (and, at times, combative) behavior may seem random and unpredictable. However, many of these behaviors actually fit a pattern common among many callers. There are certain predictable

events experienced by callers facing an emergency.[58, 59] Once the EMD knows about these events, it is easier to tolerate the discomfort and maintain an appropriate professional relationship with the caller.

Hysteria Threshold and Repetitive Persistence

Some callers are too excited to help the EMD gather appropriate information. But studies have shown that less than 4 percent are truly hysterical. Certainly, many people are very excited and are almost hysterical, but a skilled EMD knows how to control this. Therefore, the great majority of the people dialing for emergency help can, with the EMD's help, provide the information needed to make a good decision about system response and subsequent care via phone.

The concept of **hysteria** has largely frustrated humankind, but for the EMD it can also be a source of fascination. Only by studying hysteria can one hope to learn how to cope with it. Knowing how to control people who cannot control themselves is part of the artistry of dispatching.

Hysteria is a state of tension or excitement in which there is a temporary loss of control over actions and emotions. It may stem from exaggerated sensory impressions. What is more vivid and frightening to many people than a medical emergency —especially if the patient is bleeding? The key lies in questioning the common (but incorrect) assumption that hysteria is not only uncontrollable, but unchangeable as well.

> **In studying how dispatchers have helped people overcome hysteria, the most immediate observation was that the dispatcher didn't hang up the telephone.**

Perhaps the reason that hysteria has gained the reputation for being unchangeable is that it is much easier, and a much more human response, to avoid unpleasant things by terminating the event. Dealing with them head-on requires skill and energy. It is like coming across a snake in the trail. It seems easier to walk around it than to calmly entice it to move.

Indeed, hysteria and near-hysteria *can* be controlled. The challenge for the EMD is to assist the caller to regain enough self-control to bring about the most promising outcome for the patient. How is this done? In studying how dispatchers have helped people overcome hysteria, the most immediate observation was that *the dispatcher didn't hang up the telephone.* Sounds simple, but clearly it is an absolutely necessary first step. Without it, nothing can happen—no control, no assistance, nothing.

In the same way we jerk our hands from the heat of a flame or wildly swat at a struggling insect that gets caught in our hair, dispatchers have for years reflexively avoided confrontations with out-of-control callers. Such calls hurt, because people are often abusive and obnoxious in their hysteria. The dispatcher becomes the caller's target for unloading that ugly behavior. Dispatching is stressful enough as it is. Who needs to burn out because of obnoxious, hysterical callers? In an earlier dispatch era, it was an understandable and natural reaction to terminate the unpleasant experience as quickly as possible, leaving callers to fend for themselves while field personnel were responding. From this type of dispatcher sidestepping came the unflattering phrase, "putting the monkey on the back of the responder."

That approach is not valid for several good reasons. One is that controlling the hysterical caller allows the EMD to get the answers needed to make a well-informed priority response. It is also important the caller be coached in providing DLS for the patient. Finally, the self-esteem of professional EMDs inevitably improves when they can work successfully with difficult callers.

It is a myth that the caller is too upset (hysterical) to respond accurately. Ever since the Phoenix Fire Department initiated the first known successful medical self-help program in 1974, ever increasing tape-recorded documentation has been collected

> **Second, we noted that in successful re-control efforts, the dispatcher always remained calm, but firm.**

demonstrating how hysterical callers can be helped to regain control and go on to perform lifesaving acts. From studying these and other tapes, knowledge of how to help these callers has unfolded.

As mentioned, the first thing we noted was simply that the dispatcher didn't hang up! After all, once that happens, the opportunity to provide the patient with appropriate pre-arrival first aid is gone. Guiding callers "through rough waters" provides an important sense of accomplishment to EMDs; those using it have found themselves willing to *go the extra mile* with hysterical

callers to reap the emotional rewards experienced on both ends of the phone.

Second, we noted that in successful re-control efforts, the dispatcher always remained calm, but firm. It is not unusual for a caller to initially disregard the EMD's request to "calm down and listen to me." However, if the EMD repeats the request in identical phrasing over and over again, in a similar tone of voice, the caller almost always surrenders quickly. This technique is called **repetitive persistence**. The approach is very logical: if the EMD plays the role of the irresistible force, the caller must either become an immovable object or eventually yield. And, people in emotional distress will routinely yield first.

The process usually requires only one or two repetitions. Using repetitive persistence, the EMD can gain control of the call in just a few seconds. The caller gives in (or more appropriately *buys in*) and becomes a help rather than a hindrance.

The point is that most dispatchers, because of their natural dislike for hysterical behavior, have never recognized the potential for helping those faceless

> **The EMD who gets the caller on the right side of the hysteria threshold gains a worthy collaborator.**

strangers by breaking through the hysteria threshold. Hysteria renders the caller useless for performing the dispatch life support procedures that could save a patient's life. Fortunately, distraught callers have a threshold; the EMD who gets the caller on the right side of the threshold gains a worthy collaborator. By using the technique described here, that threshold is nearly always reached.

Helping the caller regain control requires the dispatcher to assume the role of "irresistible force" for a few moments, until the caller realizes two things: first, that the hysterical behavior is inappropriate, and second, that it can be changed. Once this realization is made, the caller becomes not just "okay" but begins to follow the dispatcher's instructions closely, often verbatim, as demonstrated in the following tape transcription. (We have inserted learning pointers "➜" to aid in quickly locating key events.)

This case, which occurred in 1974, resulted in the establishment of the Medical Self-Help Program in Phoenix the next year.[15] It is the first known recorded use of pre-arrival instructions (see fig. 5-4).

Phoenix Call–Baby Not Breathing (2:45 elapsed time)

Dispatcher: Fire Department.
Caller: Help me, my baby's not breathing!

Dispatcher: What's your address?
Caller: (given)

Dispatcher: All right. (address repeated)
Caller: Yes, please help me! (panic clearly present)

Dispatcher: Listen, listen to me, there is a medic on the phone, you talk to him.
Medic: Ma'am.
Caller: He's not breathing!

Medic: Hello, ma'am.
Caller: Yes.

Medic: This is a medic here in the alarm room. Now, I would like to help you. We've got a fire department truck coming there, and an ambulance. Okay?
Caller: Yes.

Medic: Now stay on the line, don't hang up, and I'll tell you what to do.
Caller: Okay, my husband is trying to give him mouth-to- mouth.

Medic: ➡ Where is the baby?
Caller: He's on my husband's lap.

Medic: ➡ Where is your husband? Is he by the phone?
Caller: He's in the living room.

Medic: Get him by the phone. Call and get him by the phone.
Caller: Okay, yes.

Husband: Look, I can't listen.

Medic: Hello, sir. Do you know how to give mouth-to-mouth?
Husband: More or less.

Medic: Okay, give the phone to your wife, and I will tell her.
Caller: Help!!

Medic: ➡ Ma'am, ma'am, now you're going to have to calm down to help your baby, okay?
Caller: My baby!

Medic: ➡ Ma'am, now you're going to have to calm down in order to help your baby.
[Note the nearly exact repetitive persistence.]
Caller: Yes.

Medic: Okay, now tell your husband what I tell you, all right?
Caller: Yes.

Medic: Okay, can you calm down?
Caller: Yes.

Medic: Okay, now tell him to give the baby a breath about every 5 seconds.
Caller: Give a breath every 5 seconds…
[Note the nearly verbatim (word-perfect) response.] (crying in the background)

Medic: Is that the baby making that noise?
Caller: No, that's my older one…

Medic: Now, he wants to give him short breaths…
Caller: He's starting to breathe a little bit.

Medic: He's starting to breathe, okay, now… (the two babies crying in the background).
Caller: They're here.

Medic: They're there, ma'am? Okay, they'll take care of your baby now.
Caller: Thank you!

Medic: You're welcome.   ⚜

Fig. 5-1. Second known recorded call where dispatch life support was performed, Phoenix, circa 1974.

For an EMD to be working closely with a complete stranger who only moments before was out of control on the telephone is a wonderful feeling and a refreshing change from the perception held by many people that the dispatcher's role is of no importance to the end result of good patient care. Not only is EMD self-esteem bolstered by this process, but the benefit to the EMS system, the caller, and most important, the patient is *clearly* evident.

Remember that hysteria is a form of regression. Although it may seem hard to believe, people who are out of control actually *want* someone in charge to tell them what to do. Crisis causes behavioral regression; a child/parent role exists when a caller looks for immediate solutions from those with the responsibility to provide care. Therefore, some people reflexively adopt a demanding, temperamental (hysterical) approach, subconsciously hoping it will work the way tantrums once did.

> **Everyone has a threshold door through their hysteria.**

The EMD, as the authority figure, must have the fortitude and patience to recognize the underlying message and bypass the frustrating method the caller may use to deliver it. It helps to mentally translate the hysterical, insistent words, "Just get an ambulance here NOW!" to mean, "Please help me cope with this awful event!" The EMD must find the self-discipline to respond *not* to the caller's *behavior*, but to the caller's *need.* Most callers care. While most callers seem unreasonable on the surface, they actually can be reasoned with during the heat of a case.

The first known, recorded case of pre-arrival instructions in Los Angeles occurred in October 1988. An untrained (in emergency medical dispatch) calltaker with less than one week on-duty experience received the frantic call, "My father is laying on the bed foaming… He's foaming at the mouth and he's not moving!" Early in his instructions occurs an excellent example of combining a calming statement with a clearly understandable reason:

Dispatcher:	Okay is he breathing now?
Caller:	No he's not.
Dispatcher:	There's no exchange of air?
Caller:	No! (screaming)
Dispatcher:	Okay, okay, if you get excited it's not going to work. 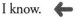
Caller:	I know.

Everyone has a threshold door through their hysteria. EMDs must sometimes challenge themselves to open it and step into the breach to recruit helpers from the ranks of out-of-control callers. This may be easy with some people and difficult with others. The question remains: If the EMD does not make the effort to find it, how can the stranger on the other end of the telephone line be helped to get across it?

The Bring the Patient to the Telephone Problem

It is amazing how many times unscripted pre-arrival instructions are begun, only to have the caller interrupt by yelling, "Bring him in here, near the phone!" When half-trained dispatchers try to ad-lib pre-arrival instructions outside of a protocol system, this problem will occur about 50 percent of the time due to the randomness of patient location. This wastes time and interrupts the train of thought and control. This is why the first panel on all the Dispatch Life Support scripts includes the command to get the patient as close to the telephone as possible. Even when just basic

---

Rules for Applying Repetitive Persistence

1. **Combine the command with a reason.** This has always been a foundation of adult learning theory. "You're going to have to calm down [the command] if we're going to help your baby [the reason]," or "We can help your baby [the reason] once you calm down [the command]."

2. **Impart the message with a positive tone.** Leaders use confidence to inspire action, not generate fear.

3. **Use the caller's name.** This is the most well-entrenched pathway into the caller's brain; he or she has heard that name since childhood.

4. **Do not alter the wording.** To do so appears to the caller's subconscious as indecision or lack of control. Repeat the described request each time in exactly the same way. Do not vary the sentence structure, tone, volume, rate, or any other vocal characteristic. Variation softens the effect of the gentle hammer the EMD is using to knock against the housing of the other person's hysteria.

5. **Never use an offensive command.** Using "Shut up," or "Just calm down" does not work. Such phrases are counterproductive and often infuriate the caller.

Fig. 5-2. Five rules for applying repetitive persistence.

The Use of Repetitive Persistence

Repetitive persistence has been shown to be the most effective method of reducing the caller's anxiety to below the hysteria threshold. Nearly all emergency medical dispatchers agree that the calls in which repetitive persistence is most necessary are often the most unpleasant to process, and they are consequently the calls where it is hardest to use the technique. Why is it then, that a significant number of EMDs find themselves struggling with the repetitive persistence technique and unable to properly use it?

Before we attempt to answer that question, let's review the proper use of repetitive persistence. Repetitive persistence is not simply repeating a request as you might with an errant child. It involves four features:

- The EMD must repeat, several times if necessary, a request for the desired action: "Sir, you must calm down..."

- The desired action must be supported by a justification that the caller will connect with: "...so we can help your daughter."

- Each iteration of the request and its justification must be said using exactly the same words.

- Each iteration of the request and its justification must be said using exactly the same volume and tone of voice.

These guidelines may sound simple enough, but very often when an EMD is asked why she or he is not using repetitive persistence correctly, the first answer is usually "I don't know." When EMDs are asked to elaborate, we often hear responses such as, "it doesn't seem natural," or, "it doesn't feel like it will work." As the evidence is to the contrary repetitive persistence does indeed work we need to examine why some of us feel this way.

The answer may lie with our prior exposure to repeated messages: when repetition is involved, messages are usually re-stated in different ways. We have been conditioned to expect this variation since a very early age. Under normal circumstances, if a message needs to be repeated it is desirable to change the way it is delivered to ensure it is properly received by the listener. For example, a mother trying to keep her child from going into the cookie jar might repeat a "stay out of the cookie jar" message in the following ways:

"Joey, you are to stay away from the cookie jar until tomorrow," then, "Joey, you cannot have any more cookies from the jar today," and finally, "Joey, the cookie jar is off limits to you for the rest of the day." This is the same message delivered in three quite different ways. Under the normal conditions of everyday life, if the sender deemed the message important enough, repetition in succession would not be uncommon but the wording of the message and the tone of its delivery would most likely be varied.

Anyone who has taken an educational methodology course will recognize that changing the wording, inflection, volume, and tone of a message is good communication technique. The repetition even if it is delivered in rapid succession is almost never presented in the same way. Repetition with variation normally helps the listener to receive the message the way it was intended. Since this is the way we are accustomed or "conditioned" to receive messages, we eventually adopt these same techniques and use them in our communications with others.

The EMD's non-visual emergency situation is, however, different from normal circumstances. To use repetitive persistence properly, EMDs are required to do the complete opposite of what they have been doing (under normal circumstances) all their lives. They are suddenly expected to ignore a lifetime's conditioning to vary repeated messages and instead use a technique that feels alien and wrong. No wonder repetitive persistence feels like it won't work. No wonder it doesn't feel natural when we try to use it.

As EMDs, we need to keep in mind that the circumstances surrounding our use of repetitive persistence are not normal: the message receiver (caller) is far from being in a normal state of mind.

(continued on 5.7)

The Use of Repetitive Persistence

(continued from 5.6)

When callers are highly stressed, overly anxious, or perhaps even hysterical, it is nearly impossible for them to be receptive to normal communication techniques. From the caller's perspective, any variation in the wording of the request or in the volume or tone of the EMD's voice implies uncertainty or indecision on the part of the EMD.

This, in turn, reinforces the caller's belief that the situation is hopeless, leads to increased hysteria and further prevents the EMD from taking control of the call, calming the caller, and offering an appropriate response.

So while life has conditioned us to vary the wording and presentation of a repeated request, in the unusual circumstances surrounding a call for emergency assistance EMDs must fight this inherent tendency. This is best accomplished by mentally preparing before each call. Along with "wiping the mental slate clean," the EMD should use this mental preparation time to focus on correctly applying repetitive persistence when the time comes. Remember, years of "conditioning" cannot be broken overnight. It takes discipline and training to learn and apply the new habit of repetitive persistence when you are calming a hysterical caller, but by understanding why repetitive persistence is a difficult technique, an accomplished EMD should be able to fully master it in a short period of time.

Repetitive persistence, to some, is an inherently difficult technique to use effectively, but another phenomenon the fact that the calls that need it most are often unpleasant and difficult to process can make it even harder.

A distraught caller, in addition to failing to respond to the EMD's requests, is also likely to be abusive towards the EMD or to use threatening language. This puts additional stress on the EMD and leaves her or him less able to repeat precisely-worded requests in a calm, controlled, and consistently-toned voice. When the caller is abusive, the EMD should use the detachment technique. This consists of detaching from the call by listening to the caller's message without hearing (or reacting to) the insults. Once the EMD has become detached from the caller's emotions, she should immediately begin repetitive persistence to take control of the call and calm the caller. In essence, the detachment technique and repetitive persistence become buffers between the caller's aggression and the EMD.

The following are important to remember when using the detachment technique:

- The caller doesn't know you, so it's not personal!

- The caller's behavior would be the same regardless of who answered the phone.

- The caller is asking for help, therefore, pay attention to the message, not to the way it is delivered.

- Remain calm and do not raise your voice, because losing your cool and raising your voice attaches you to the call.

- In your mind, picture the caller as somebody in pain, with his or her arms open, pleading for help (they are doing that). This visualization will make it much easier to empathize with an abusive caller and will also help to reduce EMD stress.

- Continue to correctly use the repetitive persistence until the caller calms down.

To correctly apply repetitive persistence, the EMD must remain calm and controlled, must be helpful but firm, and must use a constant tone and volume in his or her voice. This has been shown to have dramatic effects in calming distraught or uncooperative callers. But another important phenomenon that is relevant to repetitive persistence is that its opposite an EMD who is not calm, or who allows the caller to take control of the call, or who yells at the caller will tend to move callers towards hysteria. When the EMD behaves in this way, it leads the caller to suspect that the dispatcher is neither professional nor competent, and therefore not able to help. And when the caller concludes that the dispatcher is not able to help, increased emotion is a

(continued on 5.8)

The Use of Repetitive Persistence

(continued from 5.7)

likely outcome. Just as you can predict certain "re-freak" events, you can also expect the caller (even an initially calm caller) to be pushed towards or over the hysteria threshold whenever the EMD uses, among others, any of the following inappropriate behaviors:

- The EMD does not properly prepare the caller to receive the protocol's questions.

- The EMD implies no help will be sent until the protocol's questions are answered.

- The EMD ignores the caller's concern about help not being on the way and fails to reassure the caller.

- The EMD demeans, judges, or insults the caller.

- The EMD questions the caller's integrity.

- The EMD uses any kind of offensive or confrontational language.

An EMD should never be guilty of any of the above actions. It is of little consequence to properly apply repetitive persistence if it is the EMD's demeanor that is triggering the caller's loss of control.

The bottom line? To be well rounded and complete, every EMD must be able to appropriately utilize repetitive persistence. To conclude I will leave with you the following key characteristics of a successful repetitive persistence user:

- An EMD who fully commits, in advance of the call, to project total professionalism.

- An EMD who believes that repetitive persistence will help when dealing with a hysterical caller.

- An EMD who learns to use the detachment technique when the caller uses abusive or threatening language.

- An EMD who accepts the challenge to take control of each call and to properly use repetitive persistence whenever necessary.

- An EMD who works to remain in control so that an EMD-induced "re-freak" event cannot occur.

Variations of repetitive persistence or other repetition-type techniques have been used in psychology and psychiatry for many years. It is a widely used and enormously successful approach to solving communication problems in many situations. In EMD, the often life-or-death nature of the request for emergency assistance and the remoteness imposed by the telephone can lead to hysteria-related inhibition of effective communication. This is the perfect place to apply this time-tested technique. Commit to perfecting repetitive persistence and you'll become a better emergency medical dispatcher.   ❦

Fig. 5-3. "The Use of Repetitive Persistence," by Jose Estavenall. Reprinted from the **JNAEMD**.[60]

Post-Dispatch Instructions are being given, the EMD knows from Case Entry where the patient is which creates a clearer mental image of the scene.

Re-Freak Events

Even after effective control has been reached, the caller may cross back over the threshold when s/he is reminded of the patient's distressing state. This was given the descriptive name, "**re-freak event**." If the EMD remains calm and reassuring, regaining control tends to be easier than it was the first time. The re-freak event is triggered by three predictable points:

1. When the patient and the caller are reunited in accordance with the EMD's directive to "Get him as close to the phone as possible." The often grim sight of the patient reminds the caller again how bad the situation appears.

2. When the EMD asks for verification of the patient's vital signs (breathing and pulse). Since these are often absent, the patient is cyanotic (blue) and the caller is reminded that the situation is very real—and very critical.

3. When a friend or relative arrives and first sees the patient. At this point, the caller often vicariously

relives the initial impact and terror of when they found the patient. Their own concern and distress about the patient's condition recurs to match that of the new visitor. While the innocent inquirer is most often a friend or family member, anyone who happens upon the scene may trigger a "What happened!" event, even a responder. The caller must be coached by a calm, reassuring EMD to settle down again.

The Nothing's Working Phenomenon

This occurs when the caller has done all the right things—CPR, or the Heimlich maneuver—and sees that the patient is not improving. Most lay people (and many novice EMS providers) have the cinematic perception that things always turns out okay once life-saving techniques are done. In fact, in a typical EMS system, *saving* someone from cardiac arrest occurs actually less than 10 percent of the time—and usually only after basic life support (what the caller is doing) is followed promptly by advanced life support. During initial resuscitation, the caller often states, "Nothing's working!" in frustration, despair, and denial. The loss of control that ensues has an emotional basis similar to a re-freak event. The EMD may need to encourage the caller to "keep doing it" until EMS personnel get there.

The Relief Reaction

Paradoxically, if the patient is revived or resuscitated, the caller may tend to lose emotional ground. The combination of relief, guilt, remorse, or fear of what could have been sparks a reaction similar in effect to the re-freak event. In a sense, the caller now has the emotional latitude to vent some of the intense emotions that built up. Crying is a healthy and most common form of this relief. There are powerful internal doses of adrenaline to dissipate. While the relief event is of minor significance, the important issue here is to not let the caller lose focus and therefore not attend to the airway or miss changes in the patient's condition.

> **Don't let the caller lose focus and therefore not attend to the airway or miss changes in the patient's condition.**

The Paramedics Aren't Coming Notion

Many people do not believe that emergency services will truly work for them. The seconds between the onset of a crisis and arrival of uniformed assistance can seem like an eternity. Callers may interrupt the EMD's efforts to help with dispatch life support multiple times

---

Phoenix Call—Baby Fell in Pool (3:08 elapsed time)

Dispatcher:	Fire Department—Lifeline.	**Medic:**	Okay, what's his skin color like?
Caller:	Can you come to my house real fast? My son fell into the pool, and he's not breathing!	Caller:	Purple. It's turning purple.
Dispatcher:	All right, ma'am, give me your address.	**Medic:**	Okay, how long was he in the pool?
Caller:	(gives address)	Caller:	I don't know, maybe a minute. I don't know. I just went out to check the mail.
Dispatcher:	All right, repeat it again, please.		
Caller:	(repeats same address)	**Medic:**	Okay, now just listen to me. You're going to have to calm down now. Is someone else there with you?
Dispatcher:	Is the child still in the pool?		
Caller:	No, he's out. We're trying to give him mouth-to-mouth.	Caller:	Yes, my mother's here, and I've got my dad here.
Dispatcher:	All right, I want you to stay on the line. I have a medic that is going to give you some help while I send someone. Stay on the line.	**Medic:**	Okay, here's what I want you to do to make sure they're doing it right. How old is he?
Caller:	Okay.	Caller:	He's 2 years old.
Medic:	Ma'am, did you say you were trying to give mouth-to-mouth at this time?		*(continued on 5.10)*
Caller:	Yes		

(continued on 5.10)

Phoenix Call–Baby Fell in Pool (3:08 elapsed time)

(continued from 5.9)

Medic: Okay, I want you to tell them to put one hand underneath his neck, and the other one on his forehead. You lift his neck and push down on his forehead at the same time. All right?

Caller: ➡ Okay, hold on. (to the others) Bring him in the house. Bring him in here. Bring him in here!

Medic: ➡ Okay now, when they do that…

Caller: ➡ He's not breathing at all!

Medic: ➡ Okay, calm down ma'am listen, you're going to have to listen to me in order to help him now, Okay?

Caller: Just a minute.

Medic: Just calm down.

Caller: Okay.

Medic: All right, now, listen.

Caller: Okay.

Medic: Tell him to pinch his nose.

Caller: (to others) Pinch his nose.

Medic: And give him four quick breaths, right now.

Caller: Four real quick breaths, right now.

Medic: Four of them.

Caller: Four of them, okay.

Medic: Okay, now tell him to give him one breath about every three or four seconds, and have the other person that's there see if they have a pulse.

Caller: Okay, give him a breath every 3 or 4 seconds, and mother, you check and see if he's got a pulse. They're sending the fire department, calm down! (to medic) Are those other people on the way?

Medic: They're on their way now. They'll be there in a few minutes. I'm trying to help you until they get there.

Caller: (to others) Calm down. (to Medic) He's moaning! Is that good?

Medic: Okay, that's good! And if he starts crying, that's better.

Caller: He's opening his mouth.

Medic: He is?

Caller: Yes.

Medic: Okay, tell them to stop the mouth-to-mouth for right now.

Caller: Okay, stop the mouth-to-mouth for now.

Medic: Tell him to put his ear down close to the kid's mouth and see if he can feel any air coming in and out of him.

Caller: Okay, put your ear by his mouth and see if you can feel any air coming out. There's water coming out.

Medic: Okay, there's water coming out?

Caller: He's starting to cry.

Medic: He's starting to cry?

Caller: Well, he's moaning a little.

Medic: Okay, turn his head to the side and let the water get out.

Caller: Okay, turn his head to the side and let the water out.

Medic: You got it?

Caller: (baby starts crying) He's crying!

Medic: If he's crying, just let him cry. All right. He's going to be okay now. We'll have somebody here in a few moments. Yes, he'll be all right. If he's crying, he's breathing.

Caller: How do you know he didn't get brain damage or something from being out like that?

Medic: I beg your pardon?

Caller: Could he get brain damage or something from being out like that?

Medic: No, not if he hasn't been breathing that long. He'll be all right. Don't worry about it.

Caller: Okay, they're on their way though?

Medic: They're on their way. They'll be there to check him out in just a few moments.

Caller: Okay.

Fig. 5-4. Baby fell in pool, first known recorded call where dispatch life support was performed, Phoenix, circa 1974.

to ask, "Are the paramedics coming?" The EMD may need to confirm repeatedly that the emergency personnel are on their way. It helps to use terms a lay person understand readily. Instead of saying "en route" or "dispatched," just say, "They're on their way to help you now," or, "They've left the station already." A phrase proven useful in the U.K. and Australia is, "I'm organizing the ambulance to help you now." Avoid relaying a specific number of minutes in case the crews are unexpectedly delayed but be generally reassuring.

The Gap Theory

A new theory regarding why callers insert demands and uncooperative statements into interrogations and phone-directed advice is currently being studied by the Research & Standards Division. Called "**The Gap Theory,**" the basic hypothesis is that undisciplined dispatchers actually cause these events to happen by unnecessarily creating gaps in their interrogation and treatment sequences, in essence, relinquishing the appearance of a dispatcher-directed process to one of caller control at critical times.

These "gaps" occur (and are filled by the caller) when the dispatcher pauses:

1. To invent the next question during ad lib interrogations.

2. To mentally format full sentences out of paraphrased interrogation "questions" or treatment outlines.

3. To decide what the next question or treatment phase is in a guidelines-based process.

4. Upon losing direction when using protocols that lack an adequate graphic-user interface designed to guide uninterrupted flow through complex protocol pathways.

5. Due to lack of practice and familiarity with their own protocol.

> "Mel" always got the "bad" callers because he created them himself.

Remember that when callers are allowed to take control, then their agenda holds sway—that is, an increased frequency of insertions such as, "Don't ask all these stupid questions, just send the paramedics," or "Is the ambulance coming yet?"

An Academy master instructor relates the story of "Mel" the unfortunate EMD. According to Mel, he *always* got the bad callers. Even a superficial review of Mel's calls revealed a series of poor interrogation behaviors that encouraged the caller to take control and act out. Ironically then, Mel was right about his dilemma. He always got the "bad" callers because he *created* them himself.

Compliance to protocol minimizes control gaps and therefore problematic caller-controlled portions of call management.

Customer Service is Patient Care

Knowing that these predictable events will occur and *when* allows the EMD to prepare for them mentally, and thus react appropriately. This cause and effect understanding is as valuable to the dispatcher as a road map is to a traveller unfamiliar with the journey that lies ahead.

To successfully apply these telephone techniques, the EMD must remain firm and in charge. Do not yield to the temptation to respond to the caller's specific words. Remain in control of your own emotions. Avoid taking the hurtful things some callers say personally; there is no professional justification to end up in a shouting

> While we can't save everyone, we can help everyone.

match with an out-of-control caller. No one wins, and such acts cause totally avoidable delays in accomplishing the ultimate objective—helping the patient through emergency medical dispatch.

Remember that it is unprofessional to broadcast opinions about the caller, the caller's problem, or anything else through inappropriate words or the tone of voice. The EMD who sounds sarcastic or overburdened is prone to act on that frame-of-mind rather than on the basis of the situation at hand. The improvement of caller cooperation and the sense of satisfaction gained when one's efforts are appropriate are well worth the effort. Remember, while callers aren't usually the patients, they are customers. Treat them well. While we can't save everyone, we can *help* everyone.

Summary

It is sometimes a challenge to get quick, appropriate answers to the important questions the EMD must ask. There are time constraints. A sense of urgency can permeate every moment. But without asking the right questions, the right answers will elude even the best dispatcher and gaps in the professional sequence will continue to cause frustration for both the EMD and caller. The EMD has the opportunity to set the whole emergency response going in the right direction. A major part of the task is dealing, on the telephone, with strangers in crisis.

After millions of calls in thousands of centers around the world, the actions of most callers have been analyzed to the extent that we can accurately predict key aspects of caller behavior under various stressful situations. It is essential that each EMD understand these behaviors and, as a disciplined professional, apply the appropriate corrective techniques with strength and compassion. This is certainly not a simple task—but done well, it is an interpersonal communication art form of which EMDs rightfully deserve to feel proud.

The more details I can foresee, the more probabilities I have of saving myself.

—Italo Calvino

Contents

CHAPTER 6

Medical Conditions

Chapter Overview

This chapter guides the EMD through an assortment of ailments underlying the priority dispatch decisions that have to be made. This chapter focuses on medical conditions. It shares information about physiology (how the body functions) and pathophysiology (how the body gets sick); prehospital needs and considerations; and "the pearls" involved in providing out-of-hospital care for sick people. The specific identification of the diseases underlying many of these medical problems is difficult to do even in a fully equipped hospital.

Learning and applying the concept of priority symptoms (rather than diagnosis) and mastering the dispatch (rather than EMT, QAO, or paramedic) objectives for each Chief Complaint is a paramount goal of this chapter.

When you have eliminated the impossible, whatever remains, however improbable, must be the truth.
— *Arthur Conan Doyle*

Mastering the art of medicine takes a lifetime. To be able to function adequately as a physician takes only half a lifetime! However, there does exist a certain core of information, a group of specific *pearls of wisdom*, that form a basic understanding of medical problems and diseases. This core of information is what makes any health practitioner good at healthcare. It is the framework on which to build the remainder of what a medical person must do for each patient: operate, give care, resuscitate, cure—or dispatch.

Medical care is largely a process of setting priorities. What separates the EMD from prehospital field providers is how the information is used to set those priorities. Field personnel must regard every patient as potentially seriously ill or injured, maintaining a strong index of suspicion in each case until proven otherwise.

The EMD, on the other hand, must try to determine whose life is *more* at jeopardy given the circumstances: the responding crew, especially those using lights-and-siren; the citizens in the ambulance's path and wake; or even the patient in the situation that occurs next. Utilizing priority dispatch correctly, the EMD will prioritize resources and the mode and degree of EMS response in every case.

> **The potential to do the job right exists each time the phone rings.**

The EMD's decisions are based on the information culled from each caller. When the caller can answer Case Entry and the key questions associated with the chief complaint, the EMD can make the most informed decision about dispatch priorities. Although not every call works out as anticipated, the potential to do it correctly exists each time the telephone rings.

The EMD does not have to know a lot about the specific treatment of each medical problem to dispatch appropriately.[2] However, a basic understanding about each medical condition (and how each molds various dispatch priorities) is helpful. For one reason, it minimizes the "what if?" concerns. For example, what if a "man down" is in cardiac arrest? The traditional answer was to send the maximum response possible on every man down, just in case it was a cardiac arrest—a habit known as the *maximal response disease.*[23] Calls that are the exception to the rule (red herrings) are always possible. But the vast majority of "man down" calls turn out to be people who are breathing, and often conscious. They might have been inebriated, having

epileptic seizures, sleeping in alleyways, or something equally non-critical. With the right effort, this information can be determined by an EMD. Is there really a reason to *send in the Marines* when it is often possible to reasonably determine from telephone interrogation the absence of priority symptoms? The purpose of this chapter is to help the EMD recognize the medical basis for various patient conditions and their correct treatment. This chapter will cover the following types of medical-like conditions:

- Abdominal Pain/Problems
- Allergies (Reactions)/Envenomations (Stings, Bites)
- Back Pain (Non-Traumatic or Non-Recent Trauma)
- Chest Pain
- Convulsions/Seizures
- Diabetic Problems
- Headache
- Heart Problems/AICD
- Heat/Cold Exposure
- Overdose/Poisoning (Ingestion)
- Psychiatric/Abnormal Behavior/Suicide Attempt
- Sick Person (Specific Diagnosis)
- Stroke (CVA)
- Transfer/Interfacility/Palliative Care

Each protocol will not be fully displayed in this edition. Individual protocols may be updated during the lifetime of this text, even though the general principles remain the same. Licensed users of the Medical Priority Dispatch System™ always receive notification of Academy protocol updates, but centers not affiliated with a competent standards-based organization run the risk of becoming outdated as to the state of the art. Those receiving updates should consider them training addenda to this text. To demonstrate the complete flow of the system, protocol 30 is presented in its entirety.

The information on each protocol will be fully described and explained in this and the next two chapters. In many cases, there is repetitive information, such as certain Key Questions or Post-Dispatch Instructions. However, an understanding of how the basic body systems relate to each medical condition (and how each medical condition molds various dispatch priorities) is helpful. Also, there are certain rules, axioms, and laws that apply to more than one protocol. When this happens, a full reiteration or explanation may not occur.

In the majority of medical situations, callers are either first or second parties. Because they may be a co-worker, a spouse or child, or even a customer, callers can often provide detailed information. This allows the EMD to fully implement dispatch prioritization. The EMD can generally obtain the necessary information very quickly, because these callers are very motivated to get help rapidly for someone they know. Our job as professional EMDs is to provide the right care for all callers.

> **Professional EMDs provide the right care for all callers.**

Medical problems occur within three broad categories:

1. **Medical situations related to internal medicine.** Some part of the body has malfunctioned. The six general conditions in this group are Abdominal Pain/Problems, Chest Pain, Convulsions/Seizures, Diabetic Problems, Headache, and Stroke (CVA). They may be acute (sudden) problems, or chronic (long term, on-going) diseases.

2. **Medical-like situations related to the environment.** These are Allergies (Reactions)/Envenomations (Stings, Bites), Heat/Cold Exposure, and Overdose/Poisoning (Ingestion) problems (including Carbon Monoxide).

3. **Other medical situations.** Addressed in this chapter are Psychiatric/Abnormal Behavior/Suicide Attempt, Back Pain (Non-Traumatic or Non-Recent Trauma), and two SHUNT protocols. The SHUNT protocols are Sick Person (Specific Diagnosis), and Heart Problems/AICD. (The concepts underlying the SHUNT protocols are fully addressed in Chapter 3: Structure and Function of Priority Dispatch.)

Eight Systems of the Body. There are eight primary systems in the human body. Each of these systems has important functions that serve the body as a whole. The eight basic systems of the body are:

- Nervous
- Circulatory
- Respiratory

- Digestive
- Endocrine
- Musculoskeletal
- Genito-urinary (reproductive)
- Integument (skin)

A patient may be alerted to problems with any of these body systems when certain symptoms present. Although there are many types of symptoms, there are four *priority symptoms* of primary concern to the EMD. The MPDS attempts to identify these priority symptoms through Key Questioning. The presence or absence of priority symptoms influences both the selection of a Determinant Descriptor and the instructions provided to the caller. The four priority symptoms are as follows:

Priority Symptoms:

- Chest Pain (age ≥ 35)
- Difficulty Breathing
- Changes in Level of Consciousness
- Serious Hemorrhage

Protocol 1: Abdominal Pain/Problems

The general structure of this protocol operates from two basic Axioms.

Axiom 1	PROTOCOL **1**
True abdominal pain, except in unusual cases is **not a prehospital emergency**.	

Axiom 2	PROTOCOL **1**
Severity of **pain is not related to the seriousness** of the problem.	

These are strong but medically correct statements. But the EMD must consider this situation from a global point of view: Even cases that need surgery almost always involve a lengthy wait at the emergency center while physicians run tests, debate differential diagnoses, then prepare and staff operating suites for use. Patients may be admitted for observation periods that sometimes last days before surgical decisions are made. The unnecessary *hurry up* approach often used in the prehospital phase of patient care is considerably dangerous and of no significant value despite the sense of urgency transmitted by the caller.

People dial 9-1-1 for numerous non-emergent causes of abdominal pain, including:

- **Gastroenteritis,** more commonly known as the stomach flu (or stomach "bug" in the U.K.). It can create severe, cramp-like pain accompanied by diarrhea and vomiting. Dehydration from failure or inability to replace body fluids, especially in infants, is the biggest potential health hazard. Gastroenteritis is caused by various viruses and bacteria, has no medical cure (if viral), and is usually self-limiting in duration. The body's own defenses ultimately win this microscopic battle.

- **Appendicitis** is inflammation of the appendix, a small, worm-like section of bowel that hangs like a finger at the small bowel/large bowel junction. Appendicitis means it has become infected. Appendicitis may be characterized in later stages by specific pain in the right lower quadrant of the abdomen above the groin. The lay public traditionally fears appendicitis because of stories about "ruptured" appendixes. Before the advent of powerful antibiotics, this was a serious, and, at times fatal problem; now, the capability to rid the body of infection with antimicrobials has changed that significantly.

> **Before sending HOT, ask yourself if the time saved using lights-and-siren was significant compared to the time spent undergoing evaluation and admittance?**

Although surgery is prompt for people with a s seriously inflamed appendix, it is not hasty. The amount of time an ambulance traveling with lights-and-siren saves in terms of seconds and minutes is insignificant compared to the time spent undergoing emergency department evaluation, tests, consultations, and awaiting surgery.

- **Pelvic inflammatory disease (PID)** is an infection of the female reproductive organs. Although very uncomfortable, it is not a prehospital emergency. Complications of PID, such as toxic ovarian abscesses, require in-hospital, not prehospital care.

- **Gastritis** is an inflammation of the stomach that happens for a variety of reasons, including hangovers, dietary indiscretions, cancer, and imbalances of digestive enzymes. The pain associated with gastritis occurs in the epigastric region—at the tip of the sternum (breastbone); this can be similar in intensity and location to the sort of heart attack pain sometimes described as "severe indigestion."

- **Ectopic pregnancy** results from fertilization and fetal development outside the uterus, usually in a Fallopian tube. This tube can expand only so far as the embryo grows; eventually, it tears and bleeding ensues. Ectopic pregnancy can be life-threatening, since it is possible for a woman to bleed to death within hours without exterior evidence of bleeding. This leads to Rule 2.

> ### Rule 2   PROTOCOL **1**
>
> Abdominal pain in a female of child-bearing age (12-50) who has fainted (or nearly fainted) is **considered an ectopic pregnancy until proven otherwise**.

Frequently, symptoms of an ectopic pregnancy can present before the woman even realizes she is pregnant, hence Axiom 3.

> ### Axiom 3   PROTOCOL **1**
>
> Ectopic pregnancies often present **before the patient knows** she is pregnant.

Ectopic blood loss eventually results in the onset of shock; the first evidence of a problem may be fainting or near fainting. If a female between the (liberally defined) childbearing ages of 12 to 50 has fainted,

> **! Authors' Note**
>
> The Academy's Council of Standards has considered the issue of asking whether a woman with the Chief Complaint of abdominal pain could be pregnant and voted twice not to include it in the protocols. A patient's knowledge concerning pregnancy is not pertinent to the medical issue of "ruling out" possible ectopic pregnancy. Generally, pregnancy is not known when ectopics are discovered. The fact that a previous pregnancy test was "negative" would not alter the necessity to reconsider ectopic pregnancy if fainting or near fainting occurs in a childbearing-age female with abdominal pain.

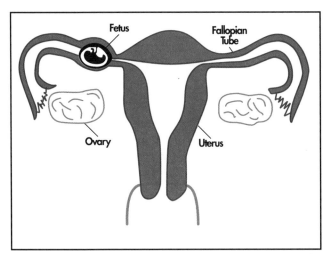

Fig. 6-1. Diagram of an ectopic pregnancy (fetus) in the patient's right fallopian tube.

the potential for ectopic pregnancy must be a concern. The actions of prehospital personnel can be life-preserving. It does no good to ask whether a woman may be pregnant, since many either do not know or will deny the possibility; age is the safest differentiating parameter for the EMD and represents the standard of care and evaluation (see Authors' Note).

- **Bowel obstruction.** Sometimes a portion of the bowel becomes blocked, causing vomiting and diarrhea. It may be due to previous surgical scar tissue or other causes, and occasionally has to be corrected surgically. Bowel obstruction is not a prehospital emergency.

- **Peptic ulcer disease.** Ulcerations (sores) in the stomach or small bowel near the stomach cause a gnawing sort of pain. These can be severe. Although unusual, ulcers can bleed and perforate without warning. Commonly, the caller does not report vague abdominal pain when confronted by the acute components of peptic ulcer disease—vomiting or passing blood from the rectum. Rather, the EMD usually hears, "He's throwing up blood!" or "Her bowel movement was nothing but dark blood!"

- **Gall bladder disease,** caused by gallstones or other obstructions of the outflow of bile into the bowel, can cause excruciating pain, usually under the right anterior rib cage extending through to the back. The pain may be mercifully brief—or may last hours.

The problem will not be fixed in the prehospital phase or aided by risking a rapid ride to the hospital using lights-and-siren.

Associated chest pain is important information that helps differentiate the minor emergency of abdominal pain from the much more serious potential of heart trouble. Sometimes, callers who initially thought the patient's pain was abdominal discover upon close questioning that the pain is actually in the chest. "Cardiac age range" is a determining factor when assigning a response to this complaint.

To avoid mistaking abdominal pain for possible cardiac pain, a higher index of suspicion is assigned to men age 35 and over and in women age 45 and over. If the answer to the key question (≥35) "Does she have chest pain also?" is positive, a GO TO prompt sends the EMD to protocol 10: Chest Pain. The universal post-dispatch instruction clearly applies to the Abdominal Pain/Problems and Chest Pain protocols, "If her condition worsens in any way, call me back immediately for further instructions."

Rule 1   PROTOCOL **1**

Epigastric pain (above navel) in cardiac age-range patients (males ≥ 35, females ≥ 45) is **considered a "heart attack" until proven otherwise**.

Sometimes, the EMD may question whether the information being reported should be handled on this protocol. This may be due to patient denial or caller confusion. In such cases, the EMD has directions in the additional information section to validate the signs and symptoms of possible heart attack.

Heart Attack Symptoms   PROTOCOL **1**

EMDs may initially receive non-specific complaints in heart attack cases. Due to patient denial or caller confusion, the following **symptoms may not be recognized as a heart attack:**

- Aching pain
- Chest pain (now gone)
- Constricting band
- Crushing discomfort
- Heaviness
- Numbness
- Pressure
- Tightness

While these symptoms are most common in the **chest,** they may also (or only) be present in the **arm(s), jaw, neck, or upper back**. These symptoms should be **handled on Protocol 10**.

Although an important goal in medical care is not to *lead* a person to say something that is not true, cardiac cases sometimes require this specific understanding to break through the atypical symptoms or denial that is so common.

Post-Dispatch Instructions. The EMD should ensure ABCs are monitored (using protocol A, B, or C) if appropriate. Treating for shock may be life-preserving. The bleeding in an ectopic pregnancy is usually entirely internal. Be clear that the patient should receive nothing to eat or drink; because, as it states on protocol X, "it might make her/him sick or cause problems for the doctor."

If the patient is nauseated or vomiting but not alert, airway control is accomplished by placing the patient on her side so vomit and other secretions can drain easily from the mouth. These instructions are available on protocols A, B, C, and X. Before hanging up, the EMD should tell the caller, "If s/he vomits or starts making funny noises, quickly turn her/him on her/his side and call me back immediately for further instructions."

Protocol 10: Chest Pain

Chest pain is a common reason people call for emergency help. It is also one of the most complicated and complex diagnostic situations, because disruption of normal function of the heart, lungs, and tissues surrounding them can occur for numerous reasons. The causes of chest pain fill entire medical texts, and are potentially (but variably) serious. Sometimes, because EMDs now probe the situation more deeply, a less than maximum EMS response may be appropriate.

Note that this protocol presumes that the patient is conscious. If not, the EMD will have initially selected protocol 31: Unconsciousness/Fainting (Near). The greatest potential for error when dealing with chest pain is to confuse it with abdominal pain or indigestion. It is true that a sensation of indigestion can be a symptom of heart attack. When in doubt, send them out!

The Age Factor in Chest Pain

The issue of prioritizing advanced life support response in chest pain patients based on age has been a mildly controversial feature of priority dispatch since its inception. The apparent low rate of heart attacks among total cases of chest pain presenting as the chief complaint at dispatch has supported the EMD's utilization of a protocol method to sort those having life-threatening events from other less lethal causes of chest pain. Twenty years ago the age for reasonably considering the likelihood of acute myocardial infarction (heart attack) was established as 35 years and older based on the then current standard of care. It remains unchanged.

Axiom 1	PROTOCOL **10**
True heart attacks are **uncommon in females < 45 and males < 35**.	

One of the largest and most respected studies of heart disease incidence began in Framingham, Massachusetts (U.S.) in 1948.[61] Some study parameters were followed for 30 years. Incidence rates of heart attacks were determined among a population of 5,127 subjects. Heart attack occurrence in men and women of various age ranges were reported as shown in fig. 6-3.

In 1995, the National Center for Vital Statistics (U.S.) reported on the 1992 death rates of 72 selected causes.[62] Of specific interest is the rate of death per a 100,000 population for acute myocardial infarction (ICD9-410). The following chart shows the percentage each age range is of all heart attack (acute MI) deaths that year.

According to Criss, the female cardiac patient will usually be in her late 50s and early 60s at the first sign of coronary artery disease and possibly in her 70s at the time of the heart attack.[63]

Statistically, chest pain in young people is rarely related to true prehospital emergencies. But once a person reaches the age range in which heart attack is more likely, the system prefers to err on the side of safety, hence, Rule 3.

Rule 3	PROTOCOL **10**
A patient ≥ 35 with chest pain is considered a **heart attack patient until proven otherwise**.	

This does *not* mean younger people cannot have heart attacks. It does mean that the dispatch standard of care is not expected to provide costly and inefficient over-response to account for these rare events. To cover this possibility, the EMD is provided some latitude of judgment.

Our review of data collected by the Centers for Disease Control and Prevention (U.S.) shows that the overall rates of acute myocardial infarction deaths (per 100,000 people) have progressively decreased during the 16-year period from 1979 to 1994. Acute myocardial infarction death rates in men have decreased from 5,153 in 1979 to 3,392 in 1994. Acute myocardial infarction death rates per 100,000 women have decreased from 3,115 in 1979 to 2,257 in 1994. Despite these dramatic decreases in the overall rate of myocardial infarction deaths, the proportions of these deaths that occur in particular age groups have remained remarkably constant throughout the 16-year period.

- Less than 0.5 percent male MI deaths occur in men under 35 years old (mean 0.41 %, standard deviation 0.02).

- Less than 0.2 percent of female MI deaths occur in women under 35 years old (mean 0.18 %, standard deviation 0.01).

- Less than 3.0 percent male MI deaths occur in men under 45 years old (mean 2.8 %, standard deviation 0.07).

- Less than 1.0 percent of female MI deaths occur in women under 45 years old (mean 0.9 %, standard deviation 0.05).

Axiom 2   PROTOCOL **10**

Medical dispatch may consider heart attack (and an ALS CHARLIE response) in certain patients < 35 when the **symptoms listed in Heart Attack Symptoms strongly suggest** the possibility.

The various types of chest pain can be confusing. For the EMD's understanding, they are separated into "Non-Critical," "Potentially Critical," and "Critical" categories in the additional information section of this protocol.

Critical Problems:

- Heart attack (clinically termed myocardial infarction)

- Dissecting thoracic aortic aneurysm

Heart Attack: In myocardial infarction (heart attack), the caller often describes the chief complaint as, "He's having a heart attack!" so the EMD may be tempted to initially select protocol 19: Heart Problems/AICD. Protocol 10: Chest Pain is the correct place to deal with a "heart attack," not protocol 19: Heart Problems/ AICD. Rather than accepting the caller's diagnosis, the EMD should evaluate the call using the questions on the Case Entry protocol, in particular question 3: "What's the problem, tell me exactly what happened?"

The same Heart Attack Symptoms information used on the abdominal pain protocol is again available to the EMD here if there is a question about certain symptoms due to patient denial or caller descriptions. This list is not intended to put words in the caller's mouth; it is intended to help clarify the sometimes-overlooked signs and symptoms of a heart attack.

A **dissecting thoracic aortic aneurysm** occurs when a weak point in the large, highly-pressurized blood vessel (the **aorta**) balloons until it either leaks slowly or bursts. An aortic aneurysm may be located either in the abdomen (with pain radiating to the back) or higher in the chest. Fortunately, it is very rare in patients under age 50. If the aorta bursts, death occurs in a matter of

---

Ten Year Incidence of Myocardial Infarction Among 2,282 Men and 2,845 Women at Risk						
Age Range	Men	(%)	Women	(%)	All Patients	(%)
30-34	5	1.1	1	0.4	6	0.8
35-44	47	10.0	8	3.3	55	7.8
45-54	133	28.4	31	13.0	164	23.2
55-64	172	36.7	105	43.9	277	39.1
65-74	97	20.7	60	25.1	157	22.2
75-84	15	3.2	34	14.2	49	6.9
30-84	469		239		708	

Fig. 6-2. Framingham (MA) Study Update Data based on 30-year follow up.[61]

Death Rates From Acute Myocardial Infarction		
Age Range	Death Rate (per 100,000)	Deaths attributable to AMI (%)
< 1	0.0	0.00
1-4	0.0	0.00
5-14	0.0	0.00
15-24	0.2	0.01
25-34	1.5	0.05
35-44	9.7	0.34
45-54	42.7	1.51
55-64	131.1	4.63
65-74	310.5	10.96
75-84	715.1	25.24
≥ 85	1622.4	57.36
all	89.9	

Fig. 6-3. 1992 Death Rate from Acute Myocardial Infarction (ICD9-410) as reported by the National Center for Vital Statistics.[62]

moments; more often, a slow leak occurs, allowing some patients to survive until surgery. Mortality for this situation is greater than 80 percent, even with surgery. The presenting symptom is usually a severe *ripping* sensation in the back. In fact the EMD may have appropriately accessed the protocol 5: Back Pain (Non-Traumatic or Non-Recent Trauma).

Potentially Critical Problems:

- Angina

- Pericarditis

- Pneumothorax

- Pulmonary Embolus

Angina. Some people have occasional chest pain that occurs when oxygen demand in the heart exceeds its supply (myocardial insufficiency). It is usually related to exertion or emotional excitement. People previously diagnosed with angina often take nitroglycerin pills or have nitroglycerin dermal patches that provide quick relief. If chest pain persists (even after being medicated), the situation could be signaling a change in the patient's cardiac capabilities for the worse.

Pericarditis. This word means "inflammation of the pericardium," which is the sac surrounding the heart. It is rarely fatal, and then, not until well into the course of the disease. It is seldom seen or recognized in the prehospital phase. One exception may be that the EMD hears about it from a caller with a specific diagnosis, if a patient recuperating from pericarditis has chest pain or other problems at home.

Pneumothorax. "Pneumo" (meaning air or lung), and "thorax" (meaning chest cavity) combines to mean *air in the chest cavity*, or air outside the normal lung passageways. Air might leak into the space between the lung and the chest cavity lining because of trauma, chronic lung disease, lung abscess, or it might occur spontaneously. Pneumothorax becomes dangerous when the capacity to exchange oxygen diminishes as the lung collapses. It can also interfere with the function of other structures in the chest, including the heart. A simple pneumothorax is usually not a dangerous problem. Much more dangerous is a *tension pneumothorax*, in which the air escaping into the thoracic cavity surrounding the lung has nowhere to go. The area blows up like a balloon, causing forced, rapid compression and collapse of the lung from the outside in, and even pushing the heart and other chest structures to the other side. This can be life-threatening.

Pulmonary embolus. is a clot in the blood supply to the lungs. Because it prevents oxygen exchange by blocking blood flow, lung tissue downstream from the clot begins to die. The affected tissue cannot rid itself of carbon dioxide or take in oxygen. Large pulmonary **emboli** are quickly fatal because life-sustaining respiration becomes impossible. Lesser emboli can cause serious breathing problems and/or sharp, specifically located pain. Pulmonary emboli tend to happen as a post-surgical complication, after childbirth, or in the wake of large-bone fractures or other situations in which the legs become immobile for long periods of time.

Non-Critical Problems:

- Esophagitis
- Hiatal Hernia (in people under 35)
- Pleurisy
- Pneumonia (except in the very young or elderly)
- Viral Illnesses
- Chest Trauma

Esophagitis. This means "inflammation of the esophagus." The esophagus is the hollow muscular tube connecting the mouth to the stomach. It can become irritated in numerous ways. The result is a severe burning sensation in the mid-line of the chest, especially when swallowing food or warm liquids.

Hiatal Hernia. This source of pain is also connected with the digestive system. A portion of the stomach protrudes into the chest through an opening in the **diaphragm**. The pain associated with hiatal hernia tends to occur after a large meal or when a patient bears down hard during a bowel movement; it causes moderate, somewhat sharp, and usually transient, pain. When stomach acid regurgitates into the esophagus due to the hernia, the pain can mimic the indigestion often associated with heart attack.

Pleurisy. This is inflammation of either or both of the membranes that cover the lungs and the chest cavity (the **pleura**). Pleurisy causes sharp pain in a specific location when the inflamed areas rub against each other during movement or respiration. There are many causes of pleurisy; the most common is viral infection. None are life-threatening by themselves.

Pneumonia. Pneumonia is an infection of the lungs. Infecting agents include bacteria, viruses, or chemical irritants. There are more than 50 causes of pneumonia and pneumionitis (inflammation of the lungs). It is most virulent, and therefore potentially compromising, in very young and very old people. Sometimes, when a person inhales his own vomit or oral secretions, a condition known as "aspiration pneumonia" develops; it can be fatal. This is why it is vital to keep the airway clear.

Viral Respiratory Illnesses. Various flu viruses can cause chest discomfort and even pleuritic (sharp) chest pain. This chest pain is often secondary to the exertion of frequent, strenuous coughing.

Chest Trauma. The EMD may receive a call that sounds medical but which is actually related to chest trauma. Someone having trouble with fractured ribs, for example, might call for help because of chest pain. Although not a prehospital emergency, people reporting these symptoms must be evaluated carefully for several reasons. Any inhibition of motion can increase the chance of infection after several days, and it hurts to take a full-sized breath with fractured ribs. Chest wall injuries may have also resulted in a slowly developing pneumothorax, bruising of other major organs in the chest (including the heart), and other problems.

Chest trauma of any duration since onset should be evaluated using protocol 30: Traumatic Injuries (Specific). In the absence of current priority symptoms, a NON-RECENT event will have a lesser classification than an acute event or one with serious symptoms complicating the problem.

The EMD's goal is not to try to diagnose chest pain. Rather, the goal is collect a constellation of signs and symptoms that help the EMD prioritize the situation appropriately. The EMD will be particularly concerned about the patient's level of consciousness and whether or not there is a sensation of "shortness of breath." SEVERE RESPIRATORY DISTRESS is defined below.

SEVERE RESPIRATORY DISTRESS

Complaints may include but are not limited to:
- Changing Color
- Difficulty speaking between breaths (only speaks words, not full sentences).

First Law of Chest Pain   PROTOCOL **10**

"Hurts to breathe" is not considered difficulty or abnormal breathing.

Second Law of Chest Pain   PROTOCOL **10**

A little chest pain may be as bad as a lot.

Patients having a heart attack sometimes experience a drenching sweat, become unusually pale (grey), or have a blue tinge around their mouths. These are considered to be signs of SEVERE RESPIRATORY STRESS.

A patient with a prior history of heart problems is more likely to have subsequent problems. And the new situation may not be the same as the old one. For example, someone with a long history of stable angina (a recurrent but transient event) may be having a full-blown heart attack. The pain in pleurisy and in some cases of pulmonary embolus is often very specific. In heart attack, it is usually generalized. Chest pain described as **substernal** (in the middle of the chest, under the breastbone) is a classic site of cardiac-related pain. Location however, is not a reliable way to differentiate the seriousness of pain at dispatch.

The use of any drugs or medications in the past 12 hours is of importance in the evaluation of chest pain, especially in the younger patient. Of particular concern is whether cocaine or any of its derivatives were ingested. Cardiac complications related to cocaine are now well-recognized.[64, 65] The severity of cardiac-related chest pain is not related to the seriousness of the underlying cause.

Post-Dispatch Instructions. If the patient is not alert and is breathing ineffectively, begin with assuring the ABCs (using protocol A, B, or C) if appropriate. If the patient is breathing normally (alert or non-alert) begin with protocol X, panel 1. The patient should rest in whatever position is most comfortable. Many people prefer to sit, or semi-recline, rather than lie flat. This is especially true when there is a sensation of shortness of breath. A patient who is not alert or who is losing consciousness should be flat on their back to facilitate blood flow to the head as well as to allow for phone-instructed airway control.

Rule 2	PROTOCOL 10

A patient having a **heart attack may worsen at any time.** Always advise to call back if condition worsens.

Depending on other needs of the EMS system, the EMD should elect to stay on the telephone with the caller on chest pain calls that appear unstable. If this is not possible (or does not seem necessary), the EMD should advise the caller, "If s/he vomits or starts making funny noises, quickly turn her/him on her/his side and call me back immediately for further instructions," and if appropriate "If s/he gets worse in any way, call me back immediately for further instructions."

Even with patients who are breathing normally or who appear alert, the EMD should be mentally prepared to move to the Airway/Arrest Pre-Arrival Instruction scripts (A, B, or C) at any time.

Protocol 19: Heart Problems/AICD

A caller describing *heart problems* can be a third-party caller, or a confused second-party caller. For example, what does it mean when someone says, "My grandmother is having a heart problem." Medically, this description is too vague. The actual problem may not even be heart related. The purpose of this protocol is to help the EMD gain more useable information. Thus, the EMD's goals are summarized in the first and second Axioms of protocol 19.

There are several similarities between this protocol and the Chest Pain protocol. Once again, the explanation of atypical heart attack symptoms is repeated within the Additional Information.

Axiom 2	PROTOCOL 19

Complaints such as cancer, leukemia, chronic illness, stroke, dehydration, infection, meningitis, etc., may incorrectly elicit an emotional response from EMDs since these diagnosis-based terms sound serious. **The caller's "diagnosis" may have nothing to do with the actual reason the patient needs help now.**

Axiom 1	PROTOCOL 19

Heart Problems are considered a specific "diagnosis." Heart problem situations range from old rheumatic fever, through benign forms of congestive heart failure, to acute angina or serious heart attack (myocardial infarction). It is occasionally reported as the Chief Complaint in cardiac arrest.

Because of denial or vague symptoms, many people do not recognize these signs and symptoms as a heart attack. A caller reporting heart problems, may report that the patient has some of these feelings. The pain is sometimes perceived as significant discomfort or pressure rather than a true pain.

Frequently, not even the hospital coronary care personnel can definitively determine if a heart attack has actually occurred for hours or days. Diagnostic proof of AMI (acute myocardial infarction, the medical term for damage and/or death of heart muscle) comes only after comparing serial electrocardiograms and blood chemistry studies (although new mobile blood chemistry strips may prove useful at-the-scene identification of acute heart attacks). A single normal electrocardiogram often cannot determine whether there was a heart attack until certain changes (or lack of them) become evident later. But any of the signs and symptoms discussed may mean heart attack. They cannot be ignored.

Often, the phrase "heart problems" is used because patients know all too well from past experience that their hearts are involved. A prior medical history may include such things as previous heart attack, takingcardiac medications (particularly nitroglycerin, **diuretics** like Lasix™, or digitalis), history of cardiac surgery in the past, and recent hospital admission for heart trouble. Patients of any age with a history of cardiac problems need to be evaluated by an advanced life support crew.

Heart Attack Symptoms   PROTOCOL **19**
EMDs may initially receive non-specific complaints in heart attack cases. Due to patient denial or caller confusion, the following **symptoms may not be recognized as a heart attack:**   • Aching pain   • Heaviness   • Chest pain (now gone)   • Numbness   • Constricting band   • Pressure   • Crushing discomfort   • Tightness   While these symptoms are most common in the **chest**, they may also (or only) be present in the **arm(s), jaw, neck, or upper back.** These symptoms should be **handled on Protocol 10.**

Some patients have **Automatic Implanted (Internal) Cardiac Defibrillators (AICDs).** AICDs are devices that help stop life-threatening heart rhythms known as tachyarrhythmia or fibrillation. During fibrillation, the heart muscle doesn't contract rhythmically, but quivers in an uncoordinated and therefore ineffective manner.

AICDs sense these life-threatening arrhythmias and administer a controlled electric shock to control them and restore a normal rhythm.

Rule 4   PROTOCOL **19**
A.I.C.D.s are becoming more common. A single firing may be normal; however, **multiple firings** or firings associated with **priority symptoms** may indicate a **prehospital emergency.** ALS evaluation for these patients is recommended.

An AICD that has fired indicated the patient has recently experienced an abnormal heart rhythm. By firing, the AICD has, in theory, restored a normal heart rhythm, but EMS examination of these patients is still indicated. An AICD that is still firing or that is firing continuously may indicate a more serious condition. Sometimes the patient will complain of heart palpitations or racing heart. A caller might report, "She says her heart won't slow down." This is one of the few times when the caller is asked to go do something with the patient during Key Question interrogation.

Rule 2   PROTOCOL **19**
The caller should be directed to **take a pulse whenever it is physically possible** (age, location, comprehension).

In the Additional Information section of this protocol, the EMD can read the "Instructions for Taking a Pulse" script to the caller. The EMD should be familiar with the technique for taking a pulse from prior CPR training.

Instructions for Taking a Pulse   PROTOCOL **19**
(Read verbatim)   **Find** the Adam's apple on her/his neck.   **Feel** on either side of it for a pulse.   **Be careful** not to push too hard.   **Count** the pulses for 15 seconds. (I'll time you.)   **How many** did you count?   • $\leq 12 = < 50$ bpm   • $\geq 33 = \geq 130$ bpm

Rule 3	Protocol 19

If the patient has a **slow** or **very rapid** heart rate (< 50 bpm or ≥ 130 bpm), **paramedics** (ALS) **should be sent.**

The generally-accepted *normal* rate for adults falls between 60 and 100 beats per minute. A fast heart rate places a powerful load on the heart. One reason heart a rate may be so fast is because of certain illicit drugs. The EMD always inquires about medication or drug use. In particular, cocaine and its derivatives can cause lethal cardiac problems. It is rare that a resting pulse rate is above 130 in an adult. This constitutes the threshold of automatic concern by the EMD.

The EMD may sometimes hear that the pulse is less than 50 beats per minute. This is also outside the normal range. Although physically fit people often have slow heart rates that are normal for them (sometimes as low as the 40s), a person complaining of heart problems should not have such a slow pulse. These patients are best evaluated by ALS personnel.

> **!** **Authors' Note**
>
> The Research Council of the Academy is sponsoring a study on the effectiveness of the EMD in obtaining an accurate pulse using this script. In addition, the Council of Standards approved a recommendation to add detection of significantly slow heart rates to this process in version 11.0.

Post-Dispatch instructions. The EMD is directed to protocol A, B, or C for the not alert patient who is breathing abnormally, and to protocol X for all other situations. Here, the EMD will allow the patient to rest in a comfortable position. The caller will be told, if it is feasible, to put away family pets, gather the patient's medications and write down the name of her/his doctor, unlock the door, turn on outside lights, and have someone meet the paramedics. These instructions can help keep the caller constructively busy if there's little else to do while awaiting help. In addition, the EMD should always advise the caller to watch the patient very closely, and can give instructions about what to do if the patient vomits or if anything else changes.

Protocol 26: Sick Person (Specific Diagnosis)

This is another, but much more commonly used, SHUNT protocol. Many consumers do not know where to begin when they call for help. Others access the emergency services simply because they are just plain sick and aren't sure what to think or do. For dispatch purposes, sick person is defined in the Additional Information section.

Sick Person	Protocol 26

A patient with a non-categorizable Chief Complaint who does **not have an identifiable priority symptom.**

For example, a basic-level EMT ambulance squad transported a man in cardiac arrest who had been described by a neighbor as having "terminal cancer." An intern at the medical center was the only one who disagreed with ending the resuscitation effort, on the basis of an incomplete medical history. As it turned out, the respiratory therapist intubating the patient noticed a deviated trachea, and a chest X-ray confirmed a large pneumothorax. Once it was relieved, the man was resuscitated. Later, it was discovered that his terminal cancer was actually prostate cancer—which is not

Axiom 1	Protocol 26

When the caller gives dispatch a previous disease or a current diagnosis, it may be because the **caller does not know what is actually causing the patient's immediate problem.**

Axiom 2	Protocol 26

A complete interrogation obtains symptoms that can be **correctly prioritized.**

Priority Symptoms	Protocol 26

The presence of:

- **Abnormal breathing**
- **Chest pain** (any)
- **Decreased level of consciousness**
- **SERIOUS hemorrhage**

necessarily "terminal" and was totally unrelated to the cause of his cardiac arrest. The cause was a spontaneous pneumothorax secondary to emphysema.

The degree of *emergency* encountered both in cases of specific diagnosis and vague multiple complaints can be variable. People with impressive-sounding illnesses can have other problems, too. Someone with incurable cancer is not necessarily terminally ill. Someone who is "just sick" may be acutely life-threatened. The EMD will not know how critical a situation is without asking all key questions. Patience and compliance to protocol is the key to getting the caller to focus on the primary, specific problem.

Rule 1   PROTOCOL 26

Find and **use** the **correct Chief Complaint** and **go to** it via the **SHUNT** pathway.

Many of the conditions and medical problems people have are tragic and painful; others are trivial. In the additional information section the NON-PRIORITY (ALPHA-level) complaints are classified as shown on the following chart. Note: Code ALPHA-1 is utilized for "No priority symptoms (complaint conditions 2-28 not identified)" and thus is not included on this chart. (fig. 6-4)

Someone with any of the listed non-priority complaints listed may be anguished. To callers, these conditions may seem terrible and unbearable. However, there is little prehospital emergency providers can do for them that warrants a HOT, or worse, a maximal response. The EMD is charged with the responsibility of utilizing the EMS system for the overall good and safety of the community. Whether the EMD uses this SHUNT protocol to access a more appropriate protocol, or remains on this one, the patient will receive appropriate care—and the EMD will have remained true to the most fundamental principle of emergency medical dispatching: practicing appropriate prioritization and therefore correct dispatch medicine.

! Authors' Note

One of the authors once drove an ambulance across the entire City of Denver running lights-and-siren for a case of hiccups.

! Author's Note

For protection of the calling public, patients, the Academy, and all dispatch agencies utilizing the MPDS, the use of any non-OMEGA codes as "no sends" or for alternative care or non-mobile evaluation is prohibited by the license agreement required to utilize this protocol. For scientific and safety reasons, there are no exceptions allowed unless under an authorized evaluative study formally approved by the Academy. A full OMEGA version can be implemented by approved Accredited agencies.

NON-PRIORITY Complaints (Alpha-level)

2. Boils
3. Bumps (non-traumatic)
4. Can't sleep
5. Can't urinate (without abdominal pain)
6. Catheter (in/out without hemorrhaging)
7. Constipation
8. Cramps/spasms (in extremities)
9. Cut-off ring request
10. Deafness
11. Defecation/diarrhea
12. Earache
13. Enema
14. Gout
15. Hemorrhoids/piles
16. Hepatitis
17. Hiccups
18. Hungry
19. Nervous
20. Object stuck (nose, ear, vagina, rectum, penis)
21. Object swallowed (without choking or difficulty breathing, can talk)
22. Penis problems/pain
23. Rash/skin disorder (without difficulty breathing or swallowing)
24. Sexually transmitted disease (STD)
25. Sore throat (without difficulty breathing or swallowing)
26. Toothache (without jaw pain)
27. Transportation only
28. Wound infected (focal or surface)

Fig. 6-4. The MPDS, v11.1 protocols. ©1978-2003 MPC.

For example, a caller who says, "My friend's real sick" may be able, with the EMD's questions, to describe that the patient is breathing normally, but is not really "with it." When asked about medical history, the caller says, "Yes, he's… I think he told me… yeah, diabetic." Now the EMD has something to go on. A jump to protocol 13: Diabetic Problems allows a prehospital response based on the diabetic-specific determinants there. Or, just because someone has metastatic cancer (an advanced form of cancer that has spread from its original site) does not mean that they are not now suffering carbon monoxide poisoning from a faulty furnace.

It is very important for the EMD to stick to the task of obtaining a report of current prioritizable symptoms one Key Question at a time. If the caller reports chest pain, the EMD will GO TO protocol 10: Chest Pain. For abnormal breathing, the EMD will GO TO protocol 6: Breathing Problems. For bleeding (or vomiting blood), to protocol 21: Hemorrhage/Lacerations.

Rule 2   PROTOCOL **26**

This Chief Complaint should be used for patients with an "unknown problem" **who are with or near the caller** (2nd party).

If the EMD gets through the Key Questions and the caller cannot describe any priority symptoms, an ALPHA-level Determinant is used. First- and second-party callers (and even third-party callers who can gain access to the needed information) who nonetheless remain vague about their problem are less likely to have a serious problem than those who are eager to report a priority symptom.

However, when third- or fourth-party callers cannot access the needed information, the existence of priority problems cannot be ruled out. Because of this uncertainty, priority dispatch provides for a higher level (in this case, more rapid) response, to assess the situation further.

Remember, standard priority dispatch always provides on-scene assessment, even in the vaguest of situations, including those who are just sick without apparent priority symptoms. It is unusual for a first- or second-party caller to have a medically serious problem and be unable to give any report of a dangerous sign or symptom—but those EMDs who do not check carefully may well regret it later.

Post-Dispatch Instructions. For the not alert patient who is breathing abnormally, ensure the ABCs (using protocol A, B, or C). For all other patients the EMD is referred to protocol X-1. The EMD should advise the caller to allow no food or drink. Some of the complaints listed on protocol 26 could eventually result in surgery; the more empty the patient's digestive system, the better. All but the most life-sustaining surgeries will be delayed if this advice is not given and followed. Encourage the second party caller, "If s/he gets worse in any way, call me back immediately for further instructions." The EMD should take care not to minimize the patient's problem, because some may be seriously ill. This is a dangerous trap that is easy to avoid by using the protocol properly.

Protocol 5: Back Pain
(NON-TRAUMATIC or NON-RECENT Trauma)
Back pain can occur for medical and traumatic reasons. This can make back pain a somewhat tricky complaint. Back pain is extremely common; it will afflict up to 80 percent of the population at some point in their lives. Fortunately, sufferers do not always summon emergency medical services. But the consequences of mishandling certain back problems can be profound. Causes of back pain can be divided into NON-TRAUMATIC and traumatic. These are listed in additional information.

NON-RECENT Traumatic Causes of Back Pain

- Bruised Spine
- Injured nerve
- Fractured ribs
- Fractured spine
- Sprained back

NON-TRAUMATIC Causes of Back Pain

- Dissecting aortic aneurysm
- Kidney stone
- Low back syndrome
- Pyelonephritis (kidney infection)
- Vertebral disc disease

Notice this protocol is titled "Back Pain (NON-TRAUMATIC or NON-RECENT Trauma)." During the key questions, the EMD will differentiate the type of back pain being reported if not evident during Case Entry Chief Complaint differentiation (Tell me exactly what happened). The EMD is referred to other, more appropriate protocols for recent trauma-related back

Axiom 1	PROTOCOL 5

Severity of **pain is not related to the seriousness** of the problem.

pain. NON-RECENT traumatic back pain is handled from this protocol. (Other GO TO prompts are included for the concurrent presence of chest pain and abnormal breathing, since these sometimes initially accompany back-related complaints until the caller has to answer the EMD's questions.)

Some people appear to be in agony, but their problem is not a medical emergency. Others will feel nothing at all, but may have the more dangerous problem. This protocol contains several elements of a SHUNT protocol as it seeks to identify incidents that could be responsible for back pain and potentially life-threatening non-obvious causes or consequences of back pain. Back pain is often caused by recent trauma or by a recent fall. If, during the key questions, it is ascertained that either of these were the case, the EMD is directed to SHUNT to protocol 17: Falls, or protocol 30: Traumatic Injuries (Specific). Back pain, when associated with difficulty breathing or with chest pain could indicate a life-threatening situation. If, during Key Questions, the presence of breathing problems or chest pain is ascertained, the EMD is directed to SHUNT to protocol 6: Breathing Problems or protocol 10: Chest Pain.

Of concern is whether anything has happened that has resulted in spinal cord injury.   Spinal injury could be suspected if the following symptoms are present (especially together):

- Abnormal Breathing
- No pain or movement below injury
- Tingling sensation or numbness in extremities

This rule has important consequences during Post-Dispatch Instructions. However, the EMD should understand that there is a reason to differentiate recent from NON-RECENT. On the Additional Information section, NON-RECENT is defined as being six hours or more since the incident or injury occurred.

Axiom 2	PROTOCOL 5

When back pain is caused by a **NON-RECENT** injury, **spinal cord injury is very unlikely.**

The second potentially critical situation related to this protocol is **dissecting abdominal aortic aneurysm**, a condition in which the abdominal aorta balloons and leaks, causing a ripping or tearing sensation in the back.

Rule 2	PROTOCOL 5

NON-TRAUMATIC back pain associated with fainting (or near fainting) in patients ≥ 50 is considered to be a **dissecting aortic aneurysm until proven otherwise**.

This is uncommon in people under age 50.[66] A key feature in slowly leaking aneurysms (besides severe back pain) is that, as blood loss accumulates, shock symptoms begin. The patient is likely to faint, or become confused and combative due to sudden loss of blood. In addition to dissecting abdominal aortic aneurysm, the other NON-TRAUMATIC causes of back pain—**kidney stones, low back syndrome, kidney infection (pyelonephritis)**, and **vertebral disc disease**—can all cause excruciating pain. First Party callers may be agitated. Kidney stones are acknowledged to be among the most painful of all health problems. Low back syndrome, kidney infections, and vertebral disc disease are not emergency situations. There is no life-saving advantage to sending crews lights-and-siren. Even though ALS personnel can administer effective pain medications, this is seldom ordered by base station physicians who must later evaluate these patients.

TRAUMATIC causes of back pain include bruised spine, fractured ribs, fractured spine, injured nerves, and sprains of the muscles and other tissues along the spinal column. For review, remember that a fracture is a broken bone. A sprain is when the ligaments, the tough fibrous connective tissues that connect bones, are stretched and torn. The pain of muscle spasms in the back cannot be appreciated by anyone who has never had the experience; still, non-emergency response is safest for prehospital crews and citizens.

> **! Authors' Note**
>
> It is said that while kidney stone pain is judged to be one of the worst pains a person can experience, it does not generate the feeling of "impending doom" that is often present with cardiac pain. This may explain why people with acute kidney stones seldom use ambulances for transportation.

Post-Dispatch Instructions. If there is no evidence of the potential for spinal cord injury, the patient can assume the most comfortable position. If there is spinal cord injury, significant movement may cause permanent spinal cord damage where none had previously occurred.

For the not alert patient who is breathing abnormally, ensure the ABCs (using protocol A, B, or C). This assures the airway and verifies breathing. In other patients, it is very important to treat for shock beginning with protocol X, panel 1, since spinal cord damage can cause loss of tone in the blood vessels, blood pools and cannot be effectively circulated. As a regular Post-Dispatch Instruction, the EMD should be sure to end the conversation with this encouragement, "If s/he gets worse in any way, call me back immediately for further instructions."

Allergies (Reactions)/Envenomations (Stings, Bites)

This protocol has two parts because callers may use similar signs, symptoms or Chief Complaints to describe either of them.

An **envenomation** is an injection of poison or other foreign substance by an animal, insect, or spider. This is analogous to a physician using a hypodermic syringe to administer a vaccination. Envenomations include all manner of events including insect bites and stings, spider bites, scorpion stings, poisonous fish spines, and bites involving snakes. Despite the fact that they are "bites," which may lead you to protocol 3: Animal Bites/Attacks, many of these venomous bites and stings may involve similar signs and symptoms to allergies– and may lead to similar consequences if left untreated. They should therefore be handled on protocol 2. (For this reason, spider and snakebites are shunted from protocol 3: Animal Bites/Attacks, to protocol 2 in MPDS v11.)

Somewhere in-between envenomations and allergies are reactions that occur from contact with certain plants (such as poison oak, poison ivy, and hogweed) and animals such as jellyfish. These incidents should also be handled on protocol 2.

An **allergy** is sensitivity to any substance to which most other people do not react. An allergic reaction may range from mild to life-threatening. The life-threatening form of allergic reaction is **anaphylactic shock**. A person reacts in minutes to the allergen (something that causes an allergic reaction). Priority symptoms include severe shortness of breath (sometimes with immediate cyanosis, or blue coloring of the skin), shallow

> **! Authors' Note**
>
> It is also reported that increased gastrointestinal tract motility is part of the anaphylaxis syndrome but this is not currently included in the standard interrogation format for EMDs.

breathing, swelling of the mouth and throat (preventing adequate breathing), and diminishing consciousness to the point of fainting, collapse, and unconsciousness (see Authors' Note). This is due to dramatic loss of blood pressure and lack of oxygen. The pulse will be weak and rapid, and the patient may be pale and profusely sweaty. Without prompt treatment, a severe reaction can be rapidly fatal.

> **Axiom 3**   PROTOCOL **2**
>
> Anaphylactic reactions (shock and collapse) **may present with a priority symptom** such as "difficulty breathing" rather than "allergic reaction" as the Chief Complaint.

In an extensive review of the medical literature, Apter and LaVallee reported that:

Anaphylaxis is a fulminant, multisystem, and sometimes fatal syndrome associated with immediate hypersensitivity. In the United States, it has been estimated to occur as frequently as once in every 3000 in-patients and may be the cause of more than 500 deaths annually. Fatalities occur in approximately 3 percent to 9 percent of the reported cases. Immediate diagnosis is imperative because the more rapid the onset, the more likely the reaction will be severe, and prompt treatment may be lifesaving. In addition, recognition is important for the prevention of further episodes. Although there are many descriptions of characteristic presentations, its unanticipated nature and the lack of specific standard clinical criteria sometimes make anaphylaxis a difficult diagnostic problem.[67]

When an anaphylactic reaction occurs, the EMD may hear, "Come quick! My mother can't breathe and is turning blue!" and turn to protocol 6: Breathing Problems. Or, "Help us, please! My son has collapsed!" In this case, the EMD may have selected protocol 31: Unconsciousness/Fainting(Near). Even if an allergic reaction presents itself in other words, priority dispatch still provides what the patient needs first: a maximal response.

Some people are plagued by allergies, which may range from being a nuisance to becoming life-threatening. Less critical symptoms of allergy may include swollen eyes, nasal congestion, sneezing, wheezing, rash, and **hives**. Hives are a very itchy rash that erupts after contact with or ingestion of an allergen. Patients occasionally experience abdominal pain and general weakness with hives.

People calling for help are often knowledgeable about their problem, since they are usually accustomed to handling it themselves.

Common **allergens** are dust, animals, pollens (hay fever), and certain foods. These rarely cause an emergency. Sulfites, a chemical preservative in some wines and foods, can cause serious allergic reactions. Some foods, including nuts, strawberries, and shelled seafood (lobster, crab, shrimp) cause life-threatening reactions in some people; so do bee, wasp, and hornet stings, and penicillin shots.

> **! Author's Note**
>
> Recorded cases of death from oral penicillin are extremely rare. The chance of a serious reaction to penicillin increases exponentially when it is given by injection. This is why prudent physicians ask patients to stay about 10 minutes in the waiting room after a penicillin shot; if a severe allergic reaction is going to happen, it is likely to start by then. This is also why prudent physicians do not often give these shots for minor illnesses anymore.

One aspect of current allergic reaction knowledge is good news to the EMD. If things are going to get bad, they usually do it quickly.

Again Apter and LaVallee, in 160 reviewed articles on **anaphylaxis**, reported that in 72 of the 80 articles in which a reaction time could be identified, the reaction occurred within 60 minutes.

> **Axiom 1**   PROTOCOL **2**
>
> Symptoms that have been present for over one hour, without increasing severely, are unlikely to get suddenly worse. **A worsening condition is a serious sign.**

> **Axiom 2**   PROTOCOL **2**
>
> A patient with a rash (including hives/itching) that is not immediately associated with breathing or swallowing problems is **unlikely to develop these symptoms.**

Occasionally, anaphylaxis may take place more than 1 hour after exposure to an allergen, usually in the setting of a depot injection or an exposure in which systemic absorption is delayed... The reaction time chosen for the criteria (Separate Criteria for Rapid Recognition of Anaphylaxis) was 1 hour... on the other hand, in 85 percent of the reviewed articles with identified reaction times, the onset of symptoms occurred withing 30 minutes.[67]

Rule 2 is the central rule to this protocol. The dispatcher's definition of severe respiratory distress includes:

> **Rule 2**   PROTOCOL **2**
>
> Determining the **presence of difficulty breathing or swallowing** (airway compromise) is a key to a proper dispatch.

> **SEVERE RESPIRATORY DISTRESS**
>
> Complaints may include but are not limited to:
>
> • Changing Color
> • Difficulty speaking between breaths (only speaks words, not full sentences).

Onset of severe allergy can be frighteningly rapid, and the patient's condition may be changing even as the caller reports the problem. Because of the relationship with airway compromise, severe cases of anaphylaxis must be noted immediately. Appropriate prehospital intervention of severe allergic reaction includes administration of **adrenaline** (**epinephrine**), which usually quickly resolves the symptoms caused by allergens; prehospital field workers can also give oxygen and, in truly critical cases, administer other advanced life support measures.

New in MPDS v11, certain bites and stings from potentially poisonous creatures such as snakes and spiders are now—more appropriately—handled on protocol 2: Allergies (Reactions)/Envenomations (Stings,

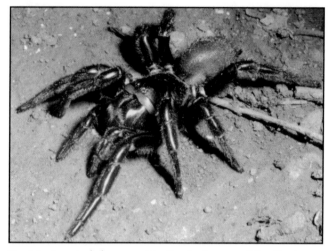

Fig. 6-5. A particularly nasty spider lives in the state of New South Wales, Australia. The funnel-web spider has a lethal history. However, there has reportedly not been a fatality from this aggressive arachnid in 15 years, largely due to the availability of an effective antivenin.

Bites). This change is consistent with the concept that protocol 3: Animal Bites/Attacks is based primarily on the mechanism of injury. A snake or spider bite is unlikely to cause significant damage from the physical bite, but it could cause potentially life-threatening problems from the poison or venom injected. Protocol 2: Allergies (Reactions)/Envenomations (Stings, Bites), handles these cases far more appropriately.

Venomous North American reptile families include rattlesnakes (of various kinds), copperheads, water moccasins, and coral snakes. This protocol was regionally modified by the Australia/NewZealand Standards Committee and approved by the College of Fellows in 1995 to reflect the considerably greater concern snake bites pose in areas of the world outside North America. The following axiom reflects this important variation.

Axiom 4   PROTOCOL **2**

Some snakebites can be lethal. While fatalities from snakebites are extremely rare in North America and Europe, they are much more likely to occur in other parts of the world.

While some snakebites can be dangerous to everyone, some people are dangerously allergic to certain animal or insect bites which cause only minor discomfort in other individuals. This should not be confused with the heightened emotions or excitement surrounding an animal attack. A severe allergy generates alarmingly rapid priority symptoms, such as difficulty breathing or unconsciousness. The caller is more likely to be focused on the priority symptom than its source. Thus the potential exists for the EMD to use protocols 6: Breathing Problems or 31: Unconsciousness/Fainting (Near) when, in fact, the underlying problem is allergic in nature. Careful consideration of the response to case entry key question 3: "What's the problem, tell

me exactly what happened?" should minimize this potential problem.

Generally, spider bites (even from the famed black widow), although uncomfortable, are not prehospital emergencies.

Rule 4   PROTOCOL **2**

Spider or insect bites (stings), unless priority symptoms are present, are **not prehospital emergencies**.

Rule 2   PROTOCOL **2**

Determining the **presence of difficulty breathing or swallowing** (airway compromise) is a key to a proper dispatch.

Although some people cannot cope rationally with spiders, there is no medical basis to support use of a lights-and-siren response to the scene.

Post-Dispatch Instructions. As snakebites are now (MPDS v11) handled on protocol 2, there is the possibility that a dangerous snake is still an imminent threat. Version11 places higher emphasis on scene safety than previous versions, so if there is a danger present at the scene, the EMD is directed to protocol X-9. Here the EMD should advise the caller to keep quiet and stay out of sight of the dangerous animal or snake and to tell the EMD immediately if the animal or snake leaves.

North American Snakebite Instructions

- Keep him/her from **moving** around.
- Keep the bitten area **below heart-level** if possible.
- **Do not** apply **ice** or a **tourniquet**.
- **Do not** give him/her **alcohol** to drink.

NAE v11.1

Australian Snakebite Instructions

- Keep him/her from **moving** around.
- (Keep the bitten limb **down**.)
- (**Bandage** the **limb** from the area of the bite to the hand/foot, then back up to the body.)
- (**Immobilize** the **limb** by splinting if possible.)
- **Tell** him/her to keep **calm**.
- **Do not move** him/her at all.
- **Wait** there for the ambulance.

AUE v11.1

Snakebite care and first aid is provided in the Post-Dispatch Instructions. There is significant variation through the world as to the proper treatment. Most of the variations seek to dispel wive's tales and old-fashioned snakebite remedies.

This protocol exhibits the uncommon situation in which medically different treatments are found and approved by different Academy Standards Committees in separate areas of the world. The Council of Standards works to always unify these issues whenever possible. Presented here is an example of an approved difference between North American and Australian protocols which is likely to undergo some consolidation in the future as experts, previously separated by oceans, meet and discuss issues and seek commonalities.

There are however, some universal recommendations. The caller should not allow the patient to move around. If possible, the bitten area should be placed below heart-level to minimize movement of the venom toward the vital areas of the body. Discourage home remedies for snakebite (particularly cut-and-suck first aid), and have the patient refrain from drinking alcohol. Ice should not be applied directly to the affected area. The use of a tourniquet is inappropriate and not advised.

Rule 5   PROTOCOL 2

If the **caller asks** whether the patient should be given their medication now, the EMD should **only give instructions included in the protocol**.

Envenomations, and particularly allergic reactions, can rapidly lead to severe breathing difficulties due to anaphylactic shock. If the patient is exhibiting extreme respiratory distress, or if the patient is not alert and having difficulty breathing, the EMD is directed to protocol A, B, or C to maintain the airway and begin CPR if necessary. Other patients, who are alert or who are not having difficulty breathing, need the supportive care provided by protocol X, starting with panel 1.

If possible, as indicated on protocol X, the EMD should stay on the line with the caller if the patient's condition seems unstable or is worsening. Dispatch life support may be needed. The EMD should be mentally prepared to start the process. If discontinuing direct contact with the caller is required or seems appropriate, the EMD should never omit cautioning the caller, "If her/his condition worsens in any way, call me back immediately for further instructions."

If a history of allergies is unknown, the EMD can have the caller look for medical alert bracelets, necklaces, or wallet cards. Many people with life-threatening allergies, such as to bee stings, rely on these devices to alert helpers as to the possible cause of a collapse. If the caller mentions that the patient has medications to treat their allergy to the substance under consideration, the Post-Dispatch Instructions on protocol 2, as well as Rule 5, clearly advise the caller or patient to administer the medications.

If the situation does not require dispatch life support intervention, the EMD can prompt the caller to gather the patient's medications, write down the name and phone number of the family doctor, and put family pets away.

We define a MEDICAL problem as being caused by an illness or other biological malady; TRAUMA is a physical injury or wound caused by an external force through accident or violence. This leads us into a conundrum with how we classify certain cards. An overdose, for example, is clearly not an illness or biological malady, and the precipitating factor the substance that the patient has overdosed on is clearly an external entity. However, no physical injury or wound is apparent.

Heat/Cold exposure is a similar situation, as is the "too much insulin" aspect of Diabetic Problems. The Overdose/Poisoning (Ingestion), Heat/Cold Exposure, and Diabetic Problems protocols are, therefore, most correctly classified as TRAUMA, but as they have repercussions that are more typical of medical events they are most easily discussed alongside the MEDICAL protocols.

Protocol 20: Heat/Cold Exposure

This priority protocol deals with two opposite but related conditions. At their worst, each can threaten life. That is, at a certain point, the body loses the ability either to reheat or cool itself without external intervention. There are three types of heat-related injury.

Heat cramps consist of cramping of large muscle masses (often the calves, thighs, or abdomen). They are most common in athletes who are training rigorously in hot conditions. A popular theory of their cause is that intracellular salt and other body chemicals become imbalanced. This condition is not an emergency and seldom generates a call for emergency help.

Heat exhaustion is also not a life-threatening or time-critical emergency. It is usually a result of overexertion on a warm, humid day and manifests with flu-like symptoms: paleness, sweating, nausea, and vomiting. Patients are very fatigued and may have a headache. Heat exhaustion is alleviated by rest in a cooler environment and increased fluid intake.

Heat stroke can be life-threatening. The body's temperature regulatory center stops functioning and the patient's temperature soars, as high as 105-108° F (40-42° C) or more. Such unnaturally high temperatures can damage the vital organs, especially the brain. Heat stroke is typically characterized by red, *dry* skin and decreased level of consciousness. It usually happens in a very hot, very humid environment where the body has little chance to evaporate sweat, radiate its own heat, or use other self-cooling mechanisms. It is likely that other *internal* factors are involved in these patients inability to regulate their core temperature. Elderly people are particularly prone to heat stroke. During heat waves, it is not uncommon in inner cities to discover patients afflicted because they cannot afford fans or air-conditioners and dare not open their windows in high-crime areas.

There are two basic cold-related injuries. **Frostbite** involves actual freezing and crystallization of body fluids at the cellular level. Frostbite generally occurs in places that receive the most cold-affected blood flow:

Rule 1	PROTOCOL **20**

Life-threatening exposure situations are **usually associated with priority symptoms**.

---

toes, fingers, ears, nose, and cheeks. It ranges in severity from temporary numbness and waxy-looking skin (referred to as **frostnip**), to completely frozen tissue that is as hard as an ice cube. Although it is not a time-critical emergency, people who have sustained significant frostbite should receive in-hospital thawing and evaluation.

Hypothermia is a more generalized response to cold, in which the body cannot maintain a normal functioning temperature. It is similar to heat stroke, except that the body temperature is sinking, not soaring. At a certain point, the mechanisms for staying warm completely fail. The surrounding air does not need to be below freezing to induce hypothermia; it can happen even at 50-60° F (10-16° C), especially in wet and windy conditions. Such environmental conditions help induce hypothermia quicker, since they readily sap body heat. Elderly people are more susceptible to hypothermia; they tend to have less body fat for insulation, and many cannot afford either to heat their homes or to eat nutritious meals. They may become hypothermic in seasons other than winter.

Axiom 4	PROTOCOL **20**

Hypothermic patients can appear dead, even to trained rescuers. A person isn't considered actually dead until they are **"warm and dead."**

Signs of hypothermia include sluggish behavior, decreased level of consciousness, pale or **cyanotic** (grey- or blue-tinged) skin, and skin that is cool or cold. The patient's level of consciousness is one of the most valuable signs. There may be a period of confusion and lack of coordination, followed by diminishing alertness as core temperature decreases. Eventually, the patient loses consciousness. Vital signs may be barely perceptible. This state of *suspended animation* has tricked more than one professional rescuer to prematurely consider the patient dead.

Survival from hypothermia depends on external sources for rewarming. Treatment begins with changing the environment. Get the patient to a dry, warm, protected shelter, remove wet clothing, and apply external sources of heat. If there are no detectable vital signs, CPR should be initiated.

Many dramatic recoveries have been documented in hypothermia cases, especially after cold-water submersion situations.

Rule 2	PROTOCOL 20

Unconscious, non-breathing, hypothermia patients should **never be considered an OBVIOUS DEATH** by dispatch or on-scene personnel and should be initially coded **9-E-1**.

For both heat and cold emergencies, the EMD should not worry about trying to "diagnose" the exact problem. This is difficult enough for the best medical clinicians once at the hospital. Stick to the search for *priority* signs and symptoms that reflect the *current* status of the patient.

Because of the connection of level of consciousness with the severity of heat- or cold-related problems, the level of consciousness and breathing status are keys to appropriate emergency response and pre-arrival care.

There is good reason to screen for other potential causes of collapse. For example, the EMD may discover that the patient also has chest pain. If this happens, the protocol directs the EMD to GO TO protocol 10: Chest Pain. Generally, heat-related emergencies generate an extra load of work for the heart, especially when there is pre-existing cardiac disease. Hot weather causes a faster than normal heart rate. If a patient suffering from a hot- or cold-related emergency also has a known cardiac history, careful cardiac monitoring will be necessary, even in someone who is otherwise alert and currently in minimal distress.

Axiom 1	PROTOCOL 20

Because a patient has a problem in a hot or cold environment does not mean the problem was caused by the environment. **Heat or cold extremes may trigger other medical problems.**

Skin color in heat stroke is often bright red, and in hypothermia is grey- or blue-tinged. The redness in heat stroke can be differentiated from sunburn by looking at parts of the body that were not exposed to the sun. Skin temperature of the patient's chest or abdomen is another clue. This is the core of the body; if its temperature is cool, hypothermia is more likely.

Post-Dispatch Instructions. Heat- and cold-related problems generally do not lead to breathing difficulties so it is unlikely the EMD will need to monitor or maintain ABCs on protocol A, B, or C. Supportive care, beginning with protocol X, panel 1, combined with appropriate warming (for cold-related problems) or cooling (for heat-related problems) is probably all that will be necessary. The EMD should keep strongly in mind that heat- and cold-related problems can rapidly lead to decreased levels of consciousness, and airway compromise is therefore a real possibility. If any question exists, the airway should be opened according to protocol A, B, or C and if necessary CPR should be started, using the appropriate Pre-Arrival Instruction scripts described in Chapter 4: Dispatch Life Support. Note that in hypothermia, the caller may have initially reported they couldn't discern a pulse in alive patients.

In heat exposure cases common sense dictates advising the caller to separate the patient from the aggravating source of heat. Air conditioning should be turned on if it is available. When the weather is the source, a cooling effect can be created by removing outer clothing, and applying cool water to the patient's body, especially in the groin, armpits, and nape of the neck. Fanning adds to the cooling effect. Any clothing not removed at the patient's request can be soaked in cool water and re-soaked intermittently. The temperature will drop readily, but helpers need to be careful not to over-cool the patient or to let the temperature rise again. Care of true heat stroke requires careful monitoring at a hospital.

Axiom 2	PROTOCOL 20

A change in skin color may be a **significant sign in exposure situations.**

In cold exposure, the patient must be protected from further cold. It is essential to remove wet clothing. Get the patient into appropriate shelter and provide external warmth by whatever means are reasonably possible. Callers should not be so overzealous that the patient suffers burns; for example, a hot water bottle to the armpit and groin should not be so hot that it causes contact burns. Be aware that a disoriented patient may not be able to complain. In some cases, rescuers might contribute their own body heat to the victim. Never allow the patient to drink alcohol, which may counter-act treatment. Light cases of frostbite (frostnip) can be rewarmed by being held against warm skin, such as under the armpits. Deep frostbite is a different matter, as Axiom 3 demonstrates.

Major cases of frostbite require carefully monitored rewarming in water of a specific and narrow tempera-ture range. This is best done in the controlled environ-ment of the emergency center. *Do not advise* rubbing affected parts, since the frozen crystals of intracellular fluid can act like knives on microscopic tissue struc-tures. The patient should also be advised not to smoke. This can seriously affect already compromised tissue.

Axiom 3	PROTOCOL 20

Gradual rewarming of the frozen part is the **single most effective measure for preserving viable tissue.**

Protocol 23: Overdose/Poisoning (Ingestion)

The dispatch definition of **overdose** is "an intentional act of taking a potentially toxic substance." The dis-patch definition of **ingestion** is the "accidental intake of a potentially toxic substance." Callers commonly describe an ingestion as "poisoning."

Axiom 1	PROTOCOL 23

Because overdose patients have a motive for their actions, they are **frequently misleading about the time, amount, or type of medication taken.**

Overdose and poisoning (ingestion) situations range from mild to life-threatening, and from sincere pleas for help (as with the panicked parent of a child) to outright and dangerous rejection of professional medical help. In some cases, especially among elderly people who have many medications and may have difficulty keep-ing them straight, an excessive dose may occur inad-vertently if the patient forgets that medication has already been self-administered (this is not called an "overdose" since the cause was not intentional). People who have attempted suicide by poisoning may or may not be cooperative with the EMD.

Axiom 2	PROTOCOL 23

Overdose is an intentional act. Even if the amount or type of substance is not dangerous, these patients **need social or psychological intervention** and occasionally protection from themselves.

Overdose patients may also pose a safety hazard for responding crews. Nonetheless, scene medical evalua-tion and intervention is a moral necessity.

Poisoning may occur through various means: injection, ingestion, inhalation, and via skin contact. The best measure of how the patient's body is coping with the toxins is level of consciousness and alertness, followed by abnormal respiration. The dispatcher is reminded in the additional information section that SEVERE RESPIRA-TORY DISTRESS should be selected if any information sug-gests ineffective breathing or severe difficulty, such as changing color or difficulty speaking between breaths.

Axiom 3	PROTOCOL 23

Tricyclic antidepressants can cause collapse and unconsciousness very quickly, even though initially the patient may appear all right. Updated name lists of currently marketed brands can be kept at dispatch for reference.

People get into a wide array of substances. There are thousands of chemicals readily available for mistaken or purposeful misuse. Of particular interest to medical per-sonnel are caustic agents, antidepressants, narcotics, aspirin or acetaminophen (such as Tylenol™), iron-con-taining vitamins, and sedatives. Acids and lye are caus-tic materials and will eat flesh and internal tissues;

Axiom 6	PROTOCOL 23

Cardiac medications can cause collapse and unconsciousness very quickly, even thought the patient may initially appear to be all right. Medications prescribed for high blood pressure, arrhythmias, and congestive heart failure are the most dangerous. They are common in many households.

causing extensive damage. (The acid described here is different from the street name for the mind-altering drug LSD.) One of the dangerous overdose substances to handle are the tricyclic antidepressants.

Certain heart medications are common in many households. These can have undesirable effects if taken in excessive doses or inappropriate situations. Axiom 6 keeps this possibility in the EMD's focus.

In general, there is increased public awareness regarding recreational drug use. In addition to the common understanding of the deleterious (long-term) effects of drug use, and the commonly understood short-term consequences of overdose, certain recreational drugs can have very specific effects. These are delineated in Axioms 4 and 5.

Axiom 4	PROTOCOL 23

The ability of **cocaine** to induce strokes and heart attacks is of serious concern. Cocaine has several **derivatives** and **street names** such as "crack" and "blow."

Street and common-usage names for these drugs are different in many cities, and even in different neighborhoods in the same city. In addition, drug-culture language can evolve rapidly. The EMD should make it his or her responsibility to keep abreast of current local drug jargon to allow effective use of protocol 23. (Similarly, understanding of current heart and antidepressant medication terminology will be a valuable asset.)

Axiom 5	PROTOCOL 23

Narcotics (heroin, morphine, Demerol™) can cause a rapid loss of consciousness and respiratory arrest. Supporting the patient's breathing is essential. The effects of narcotic overdose can be treated with a specific drug (**naloxone**) in the prehospital environment.

Of the 660,532 cases of adult exposures (age > 19 years) reported to the American Association of Poison Control Centers in 1995, 5.3 percent (35,008) were ingestions of antidepressants. 168 resulted in death (23 percent of all reported fatalities). Antidepressants were the second leading cause of death in all reported cases.[68, 69]

Small children are curious about their environment and tend to explore by putting things in their mouth. In general, a report of poisoning in a child up to the age of 11 is considered unintentional, although suicide attempts by children in the this age range do rarely occur. Of the 2,023,089 human poisoning cases reported to the American Association of Poison Control Centers in 1995, only 2 of the fatal cases were attributed to an intentional act of a child in the 6 to 12 year age range. There were no fatal cases in the less than 6 year age group.

! Authors' Note

At the inception of priority dispatch in 1978, tricyclic antidepressants were more easily identifiable by their similar sounding names—Mellaril,™ Elavil,™ Triavil,™ Tophranil,™ etc. Today such identification is more difficult and requires Medical Control involvement to routinely update a list of brand and chemical names if used in a dispatch reference book.

The introduction of regional poison control centers (PCCs) in the U.S. has provided an authoritative source of information about poisonings.[70] When the caller reports an accidental ingestion in a patient who is *conscious and alert*, the EMD can refer the case to a regional poison center. This extension of the evaluation process by an expert in these specific problems, routinely determines the safety of home care as managed by the staff at the poison center. Automatic callbacks determine the status of the patient. Any untoward changes in condition result in a mobile response. This is the only time in the standard priority dispatch system that callers may not receive an initial prehospital response. If there is a reasonable chance of intentionality, a BRAVO-level response should be selected. Calls back from a poison

Rule 3	PROTOCOL 23

If an OMEGA (Ω) referral to a Poison Control Center is not locally approved, the appropriate response is locally determined. **"Home care"** which has been used by regional Poison Control Centers with great success is an OMEGA (not an ALPHA) code because an EMS response may not be necessary.

Poison Control and the EMD

Since the beginning of the Poison Control Center (PPC) concept in 1953, the role of these expert information and treatment resources has expanded as they became better understood. Regional PCCs, began forming in the 1970's, staffed with toxicologists (experts in the pharmacology of poisons).

A process called "Home Care" for handling childhood poisonings has proven effective by these Regional Poison Centers.

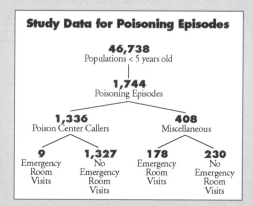

Study Data for Poisoning Episodes

46,738
Populations < 5 years old

1,744
Poisoning Episodes

1,336
Poison Center Callers

408
Miscellaneous

9
Emergency Room Visits

1,327
No Emergency Room Visits

178
Emergency Room Visits

230
No Emergency Room Visits

The Medical Priority Dispatch System currently includes one response level that does not fit into any of the standard 4-tier response categories. Ingestions (non-intentional poisonings) in children age 1 to 11 are referred by direct electronic telephone transfer to the regional PCC and no mobile response is initially sent. After evaluation by the PCC "interrogator," the patient may be referred to an ED. Rarely, response by EMTs or paramedics will be initiated by the PCC if necessary. This referral "response" by dispatch is called the OMEGA (Ω) process.

Referral of this category of callers by medical dispatchers to a Regional PCC is very safe and highly effective, both from the economical and medical standpoint. In 1983, the Journal of Pediatrics published a study by Chafee-Bahamon and Lovejoy, "Effectiveness of a Regional Poison Center in Reducing Excess Emergency Room Visits for Children's Poisonings."[71] The following excerpt may interest the emergency medical dispatcher:

Findings of this study indicated that, like reported poisonings incidents, the majority of pediatric emergency room visits for poisonings are not severe enough to warrant hospital care. Moreover, the overwhelming majority of poisoning visits are from persons who do not contact a poison center…these visits do not represent efficient use of the medical services of hospital staff. Staff rarely do more than confirm the history of the ingestion and either send the patient home without treatment or give milk or ipecac, all of which could be done at home with the assistance of a poison center. It appears, however, that regional poison centers perform patient assessments better than other sources of telephone triage.

Local poison centers, which are usually operated by emergency room staff, have been found to be significantly less proficient than regional poison centers in taking a history and making appropriate treatment recommendations. From these studies, it is likely that staff at regional poison centers, who are specially trained in taking histories of poison exposure and who have more time to spend with callers, generally make more accurate assessments than both emergency room staff and practicing pediatricians.

The majority of pediatric patients seen in the emergency room for a poisoning incident had made unnecessary visits to the hospital. By using a PCC, physicians would benefit their patients by saving time and expense without jeopardizing their patients' health.

The OMEGA response that refers pediatric ingestions to a PCC has been used in Salt Lake City for over 20 years and has long been proven medically effective. Each year in the U.S., there are 850,000 acute poison exposures in children under age 5 alone.

This study indicates that 23% (195,000) either go directly to the ED or call 9-1-1. While many parents wisely call the PCC directly, those who call 9-1-1 and report a conscious and breathing child, *without priority symptoms*, should be immediately electronically transferred to the PCC. A joint written policy with your Regional PCC outlining the mechanical procedures involved, should precede this activity and be approved by your Medical Director.

Follow-up reports from PCC to the dispatch center on patient outcome can be routinely obtained. In summary, this innovative association of PCC with medical dispatch centers is safe and without question medically appropriate. ⚜

Fig. 6-6. "Poison Control and the EMD," revision of an article by J. Clawson, originally published in JNAEMD.[72]

> **Rule 2**   PROTOCOL **23**
>
> When approved and arranged by local medical control, most asymptomatic ingestions (not including antidepressants, cocaine, narcotics, acids, or alkalis) should be referred to the regional Poison Control Center. If Poison Control's evaluation indicates the necessity of a mobile response **they will inform medical dispatch.**

control center should be coded as a CHARLIE-9: Poison Control Request for Response, unless more severe specifics warrant a DELTA-level.

Regional poison control centers are dedicated solely to poison issues and research. They are staffed by poison information specialists, pharmacists, and toxicologists and are the most likely to have the best evaluation and treatment resources available. These are different from the "poison control" service offered by individual emergency departments, which do not have the same in-depth capabilities as regionalized centers.[70]

EMS systems in the process of customizing prehospital responses need to identify their regional poison center when planning local referral policies for this protocol. Using a regional poison center makes sense in economic terms. Unnecessary transport and treatment for

> **! Authors' Note**
>
> When callers are transferred to Poison Control Centers, we advise a complete (verifiable) hand off. This means not staying on the line with the PCC call evaluator. During three-way calls, both 9-1-1 and PCC calltakers have become confused as to whether a mobile unit would be sent or not.
>
> Standard written policy should clearly direct that upon transfer of the caller, PCC should now take full control of the case and that dispatch of mobile units will not occur until a callback is made requesting a mobile response. This joint, written policy should be in place at both PCC and the dispatch center outlining the entire call transfer and re-call procedure.

poisonings is costly. In Salt Lake City, for example, data extrapolated from a study conducted in 1978 showed that appropriate use of the poison center resulted in a savings of $1.5 million a year in transport, physician, and emergency department billings. (See a complete report of a large Poison Control Center's statistical experience with EMD referral in Appendix H.)

There is a danger for field providers when trying to help overdose patients. The sad fact is that those who are serious about dying may not want emergency medical assistance. More than one suicidal patient has tried to take a few would-be helpers along. The EMD must attend carefully to the hazards that can occur in these cases. Police coverage on overdoses (intentional) is standard in many EMS systems.

> **Rule 4**   PROTOCOL **23**
>
> Consider call tracing if there are problems with location, identification, or information cooperation. **Carefully and tactfully determine the patient's exact location.**

Post-Dispatch Instructions. If the patient is violent, the EMD is directed to protocol X, panel 8 where the caller should be advised to avoid any contact with the patient and to tell the EMD if the patient loses consciousness or leaves the scene. If an overdose patient is over 8 years old, there is the possibility s/he could be violent. The EMD should keep in mind that a nonviolent patient could become violent during the interrogation or during provision of pre-arrival instructions; if this happens, the EMD should therefore be prepared to move to protocol X, panel 8. Danger awareness notes on protocol X help the EMD remain focused on the safety of the second-party caller and of the responders.

An unconscious patient, or a patient who is both not alert and ineffectively breathing, needs the airway support provided by protocols A, B, or C. In extreme cases, the EMD should be prepared to initiate dispatch life support for the patient whose breathing is in question. Other patients need supportive care provided by protocol X-1.

There are three reasons to keep a suicidal patient on the phone. First, patients in this situation are experiencing a lot of emotional pain. A kind word and a helping hand offered by a professional EMD may be just the right thing when they need it most. Second, suicidal

> **1** ☎ **1ˢᵗ Party Caller**
>
> **Help** is on the way.
> **Don't** have anything to **eat** or **drink**.
> It might make you **sick** or cause **problems** for the doctor.
>
> (MEDICAL)
> Just **rest** in the most **comfortable position** for you.
>
> (TRAUMA)
> **Don't move** around, **unless** it's absolutely **necessary**.
> Just **be still** and wait for **help** to arrive.

people are unpredictable; empathetic distraction by keeping them on the telephone may prevent them from changing their minds about wanting help while EMS crews are on the way. Finally, staying on the phone increases the safety of field providers because we know more about where the suicidal patient is and what he is doing.

Safety is the first concern. If there is significant danger, the caller should be advised to "keep very quiet and keep out of sight," (X-9). If the patient is violent, the caller should be advised to observe the patient from a distance if it is safe to do so, but to "try to avoid any contact with her/him." The EMD should advise second-party (and curious third-party) callers to beware of attack. The caller should only try to protect the patient from himself if it clearly appears safe to do so.

Protocol 25: Psychiatric/Abnormal Behavior/Suicide Attempt

Mental health emergencies vary widely. They include suicide attempts or suicidal gestures, drug/alcohol abuse or withdrawal, emotional or hysterical reactions to life's events, and normal grief. There is also a wide range of mental illness, including **depression, mania, bipolar disease (manic/depression),** and **schizophrenia.** Sometimes it is difficult to distinguish psychological

A Call to Remember

On October 2, 1991, I had a call to remember. I received the call on our non-emergency line from a gentleman wishing to commit suicide. He stated he had a loaded gun and was going to kill himself and anybody who tried to enter his house. He said he doesn't trust anybody but [our company] and called us because he likes us…He refused to give his phone number…He kept instructing me not to call the police.

After talking and listening to him for quite some time, I gained his trust. I also realized he was very drunk and depressed. Knowing we couldn't help this man until we knew where he was, I came up with a scheme. I started wriggling the phone cord so it made a crackling sound and told him that I was afraid we were going to get disconnected because of a bad phone line, and I wanted a way to call him back since we had become such good friends. He finally gave us his phone number and [a colleague] immediately called the police and the phone company to trace the address.

Meanwhile, I remained on the phone with the patient and kept him talking about his family and his troubles. I also started asking questions about his gun and talked him into unloading it and locking the ammunition in one room and the pistol in another.

Once the patient had calmed down, I had to put him on hold a couple of times to answer emergency calls. I started telling the caller that I had a good friend, who I go fishing with, at the police department that I wanted him to talk to (a police negotiator). He refused at first, but after repeatedly telling him that he could hang up and call me back if he didn't like my friend, he agreed. While the negotiator (who was outside the patient's house with a cellular phone) talked with the patient, the SWAT team surrounded the house.

The patient eventually let the police department into his house and called me back to tell me he was mad at me for calling the police. My response to him was an honest one: "I didn't call the police. My supervisor did because he thought it was in your best interest."

Before they left for the hospital, he called back and told me that he was finally going to get the help he wanted, and thanked me. I was on the phone with him for nearly two hours!

You never know who'll be on the other end of the line when it rings. ⚜

Fig. 6-7. "A Call to Remember" by Franz Malcher.[73]

Axiom 2	PROTOCOL 25

Certain serious medical problems can be confused as "just a psych problem." It would be a **serious EMD error to not respond at all**. These problems include insulin shock, severe blood loss, lack of oxygen, delirium tremens (DT's), overdose, liver or kidney failure, etc.

Axiom 4	PROTOCOL 25

Delirium tremens (DT's) is a severe metabolic derangement that has a surprisingly high in-hospital mortality rate and **should not be underestimated**.

problems from medical problems; sometimes they go hand in hand. (This complication of diabetes is discussed in the next section, protocol 13: Diabetic Problems.)

Axiom 3	PROTOCOL 25

Certain stages of insulin shock can easily be **confused with alcohol intoxication or psychiatric problems**.

People in psychological distress need sensitive, humanistic helpers. Perhaps because prehospital providers must rely more on their interpersonal capabilities than on the more high-tech medical skills available at the emergency centers, they tend to be excellent at establishing good interpersonal rapport with mentally unbalanced people. Yet psychological and behavioral emergencies often pose a significant chance for harm to emergency crews.

Suicide and psychiatric patients are often less inhibited about lashing out and assaulting others verbally and physically. This is especially true when patients begin to feel cornered or trapped by on-scene personnel.

Axiom 1	PROTOCOL 25

Behavioral emergency patients (at any level of consciousness) are considered to be a **potential risk to themselves and others**.

Because of the high risk to prehospital care personnel, many EMS system protocols require law enforcement backup on *psych* calls, particularly when violence is likely. The EMD will determine during Key Questions whether a weapon is involved, and pass this information along to responding crews.

Occasionally, a caller teases the EMD by claiming to be suicidal yet refusing to give the location of the call. A procedure for tracing calls not electronically located should be pre-established and used without delay when needed.

Axiom 5	PROTOCOL 25

It is reasonable to utilize a police only response when a person is **THREATENING SUICIDE** (no injuries have occured). This choice must be **approved by local policy** between the law enforcement and EMS-provider agencies.

Post-Dispatch Instructions. Safety is the first concern. If there is significant danger, the caller should be advised to "keep very quiet and keep out of sight," (X-9). If the patient is violent, the caller should be advised to observe the patient from a distance if it is safe to do so, but to "try to avoid any contact with her/ him." The EMD should advise second-party (and curious third-party) callers to beware of attack. The caller can try to protect the patient from himself but only if it clearly appears safe to do so.

Keeping a first-party caller distracted with conversation and reassuring words that someone cares may make a very real difference in the outcome of the call. If appropriate, the caller can encourage the patient to lie down and try to be calm.

Rule 1	PROTOCOL 25

If the actual type of suicide attempt is determined to be overdose, carbon monoxide, stab, gunshot wound, or laceration with serious bleeding, go to and **dispatch from that more specific protocol**.

The case in figure 6-9, demonstrates a near perfect pre-arrival instruction case involving a hanging situation in Derbyshire, U.K. However, the modification by the new EMD of *one* word (see arrow) in the protocol

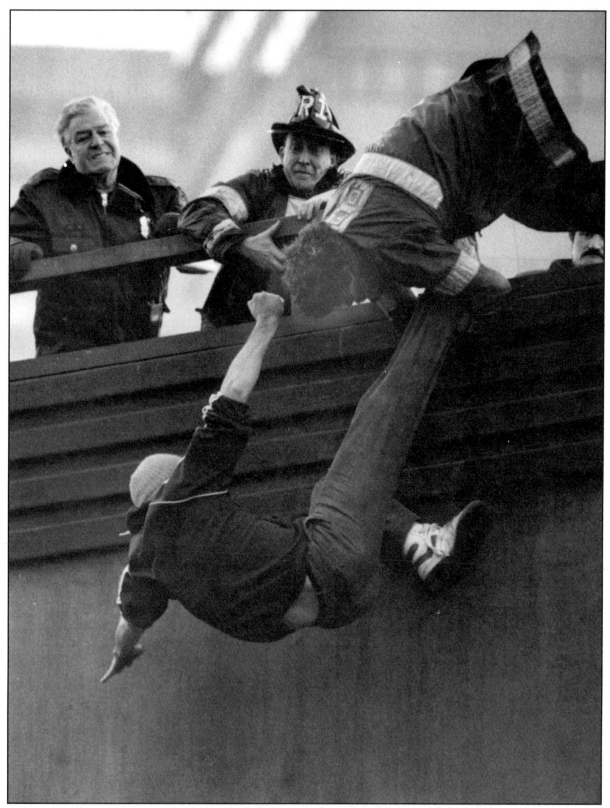

Fig. 6-8. Suicidal jumper takes rescuer with him. (Photo by Rick Sennott/Boston Herald, used with permission.) Both the firefighter and the jumper survived. The jumper was critically injured but the firefighter less so after he landed on the jumper.

Rule 2	PROTOCOL 25

1st party callers who are threatening suicide should be **kept on the line until responders arrive**.

delayed the eventually successful resuscitation by 59 seconds. This is the first known, recorded pre-arrival instruction case in the U.K.

As you can see, the protocol "knows the rules" as this brand-new EMD quickly realized when the caller could not untie the leather belt knot pulled tight under the patient's full weight.

Post-Dispatch Instructions	CASE ENTRY

(Hanging and not OBVIOUS DEATH)
Cut her/him **down** immediately, loosen the noose and see if s/he's **breathing**.

In hangings, the caller is advised on Case Entry to *cut* the patient down immediately, if possible, and begin CPR unless the patient is obviously dead. In this case the scene should not be disturbed and all evidence preserved. (Avoid cutting the knot itself as this is at times important evidence in hanging cases.) OBVIOUS death can be defined for the dispatch environment: If there is any question whether death is obvious—it is not.

If it seems safe to disconnect, the EMD should tell the caller to call back immediately for further instructions if the patient's condition worsens in any way or if the

Rule 4	PROTOCOL 25

Constricting or suffocating materials, such as rope, wire, or plastic bags, should be **removed prior to the provision of PDIs**. Care should be exercised to preserve potential crime scene evidence (i.e., the noose should be cut or loosened rather than untied).

Excerpt from a Hanging Case in the United Kingdom

EMD: Hello, can I help you?
Caller: I've got a suicide. Can you, can you come quickly?

EMD: Give... give me the address, my luv.
Caller: (given)

EMD: (repeated back) Where's that?
Caller: Quickly, he's hung himself and I can't get him down.

EMD: Is somebody else with you?
Caller: No, I'm on my own.

EMD: ➡ Can you try and get him down?
Caller: I'll... I'll try.

EMD: Try and get him down. I'm going to stay on the phone. The ambulance is on the way. (background noise from the dispatch center.)

EMD: You've got my clock in Dave? It's a hanging. A hanging.

EMD: Hello, my luv, have you got him down?
Caller: I can't and he's unconscious and everything.

EMD: Can you... can you not try and get him down? Can you not...
Caller: ➡ He's tied himself to the rail on the stairs... he's... a... with a belt and I can't undo it.

EMD: Is there any way you can get some scissors and cut him down? Get a, get a set... get a chair and cut him down with some scissors, all right? (background noise of dispatch center.)
Caller: I've got him.

EMD: You've got him down, right. How old is he?
Caller: Er... 35.

EMD: 35. Is he conscious at all?
Caller: No.

EMD: And he's not breathing?
Caller: No, he's gone blue.

Fig. 6-9. Example of how substitution of a single word in a protocol ("**get** him down" instead of "**cut** him down") delayed life-saving care 59 seconds. Amazingly, the patient made a full recovery and checked out of the hospital against medical advice.

EMD's First Rule of OBVIOUS DEATH

If there is a question whether death is
OBVIOUS— it is not.

---

patient leaves the scene. In lower-level behavioral
emegencies, or in situations where the caller has another
person there to help, they can gather the patient's
medications, write down the doctor's name and
telephone number, and put away any household pets,
unlock the door, turn on the outside lights, and meet the
responders.

Protocol 13: Diabetic Problems

Diabetes mellitus is a disease resulting from lack of
(or insufficient quantity of) a hormone called **insulin**,
which is produced by the **pancreas**, a small gland located behind the stomach. Insulin is required by each cell
in the body to regulate the uptake of blood sugar
(or **glucose**). Glucose is the first choice of most cells to
produce the energy needed to function.

Think about this analogy. The cell is a furnace, sugar is
the coal, and insulin opens the furnace door. Through
insulin's action, coal (sugar) is allowed to pass through
the furnace door (cell membrane), where it can be
burned. If enough insulin is not provided by the pancreas, excess sugar builds up in the blood (outside the
furnace door), where it cannot be used, eventually causing uncontrolled diabetic illness.

Hypoglycemia/Insulin Shock (rapid onset)

Too much insulin has depleted the body's
available blood sugar. Since the brain's most
usable fuel is sugar, it is the first organ at risk.
This is **more serious if the patient is not alert,
and is commonly confused with alcoholic
intoxication**.

Cells respond to low blood sugar by using other, less-
efficient fuels, for energy. As they get desperate for food,
they may burn fat, protein, or even muscle tissue.
The combustion by-products of these tissues are
difficult for the body to eliminate efficiently. As they
build up, they slowly become toxic (poisonous),
especially to the brain. This results in a gradual decrease
in consciousness usually occurring over many hours or
days. Lack of insulin and the resulting inability to use
sugar as cell food is known as **diabetic ketoacidosis**.

(Ketoacids are the toxic by-products of these second-
and third-choice fuels.)

Later in this gradual process, the pattern of breathing
may change. The description of a deep breathing
pattern (**Kussmaul breathing**) by the caller may be
interpreted as a "No" to the Key Question, "Is he
breathing normally?"

Low blood sugar can result in behavioral abnormalities.
Axiom 3 ensures the EMD will keep this in mind.

Axiom 3   PROTOCOL **13**

An **early sign of low blood sugar is abnormal
behavior**, which may include agitation, agres-
siveness, confusion and/or combativeness.

If the lack of insulin goes uncorrected too long, the
patient's alertness slowly deteriorates to coma—a state
of unconsciousness from which the patient cannot be
aroused. This problem is serious, but prehospital
providers' care, although supportive, can do little to
correct it. It requires careful rebalancing of insulin,
fluids, and electrolytes. This is done in-hospital and can
literally take days. Since this problem is generally slow
in onset and usually occurs in previously known
diabetics, the patient is brought to medical care long
before complete coma occurs and thus does not enter
through the 9-1-1 pathway. Only infrequently does
a patient initially discover their diabetes through an
emergency presentation.

Diabetic Ketoacidosis (gradual onset)

Pre-coma state resulting from insufficient
insulin. Unable to use sugar as fuel, the body
burns its own tissue (fat, muscle). The ketoacids
(acetones) produced are "toxic" to the patient
and cause a slowly increasing illness state.
This is **not considered a prehospital medical
emergency** but requires medical evaluation
and treatment.

Of more concern to the EMS system is the condition
known as **insulin shock**. It occurs in diabetics who take
insulin, usually by injection one or more times a day.
The diabetic has a three-part goal: to inject the right
amount of insulin (sugar regulating facilitator), to eat
the right amounts of certain foods (blood sugar), and

to exercise equivalently (burn sugar for energy). This carefully calculated balancing act can sometimes go awry. The wrong amounts of each can result in too much insulin in the blood, which has the effect of too many open furnace doors too rapidly using up available sugar fuel.

> ### Diabetic Coma (later onset)
> Unconsciousness or decreased level of consciousness occurring later in untreated diabetic ketoacidosis. Without an accurate history, this problem may be difficult to tell from insulin shock. **Airway control is the first priority in post-dispatch instructions if the patient is unconscious.**

At this point, two factors come into play. First, the process of employing secondary fuels shift into gear much too gradually to make up for the dramatic loss of sugar caused by too much insulin. Second, the brain does not use alternative fuels well and thus, its function begins to be compromised. The patient's ability to think can diminish rapidly. The decrease in consciousness is relatively rapid in insulin shock, and is the reason emergency calls for insulin shock are relatively common.

> ### Rule 4   PROTOCOL 13
> If the **caller asks** whether the patient should be given their medication now, the EMD should **only give instructions included in the protocol**.

In insulin shock, there is some controversy about the seriousness of low blood sugar regarding brain damage. While airway control in full unconsciousness is paramount, there is no need for a lights-and-siren response to conscious but not alert patients. Some patients carry medications specifically for diabetic emergency problems. The DLS instructions as well as Rule 4 remind the EMD what to do if the caller asks about these medications.

It is generally not advisable to provide telephone treatment of oral sugar, unless long response times are common. Scene blood sugar analysis (when the responders arrive) may not be reliably diagnostic of the underlying problem if phone-directed treatment has occurred between the call and a relatively short (10 to 20

> ### ! Authors' Note
> In 1995 the American Association of Poison Control Centers reported only 3 deaths in the U.S. attributed to administration of insulin. All were intentional suicides.

minute) arrival. However, if response times are expected to be very long ($\approx$1 hour or more), no harm is likely to be done by administering sugar—but due to the dangers of the patient aspirating materials into the lungs, the EMD should exercise extreme caution in allowing the caller to administer anything orally to a patient who is not fully alert.

Although the variations of the disease state itself can be confusing, the main factor on which dispatch determinants are sorted is singular and straightforward: the patient's level of consciousness.

> ### Rule 1   PROTOCOL 13
> Determining the **level of consciousness is the key** to correctly assigning the prehospital response.

Other instances of specific diagnosis are usually dispatched using protocol 26: Sick Person (Specific Diagnosis), but not this one.

> ### Axiom 1   PROTOCOL 13
> Diabetes is a "diagnosis" that **EMD's may accept at face value** because of its high degree of accuracy.

> ### ! Authors' Note
> Diabetic Problems is one of the few chief complaints not named for priority symptoms or incident types, but are diagnostic groupings. Historically, it has been demonstrated that callers do not report that a patient is diabetic unless they have an actual knowledge of the patient's condition.

Field determination of why a diabetic has lost or is losing consciousness can sometimes be difficult. Since the consequences of insulin shock are more serious, scene treatment sometimes consists of empirically giving sugar by intravenous injection. Additional sugar "incorrectly" given in diabetic ketoacidosis does not injure the patient; giving it to someone in insulin shock can be curative.

Behaviors related to insulin shock often mimic those of people who have imbibed too much alcohol: they can stagger, slur their speech, and may not follow simple commands. Unfortunately, some diabetics have been thrown in the "drunk tank" by law enforcement personnel only to be found dead a few hours later.

Axiom 2   PROTOCOL 13
A **significant potential for error** is to confuse alcohol or drug intoxication with low blood sugar from too much insulin (insulin shock).

The EMD will want to know if the patient is alert—completely awake—and behaving normally. Abnormal behavior in the diabetic patient may include abnormal speech. A diabetic going into insulin shock may be able to talk, but is likely to display slurring or halting speech. The EMD should keep in mind that answers indicating slurred or abnormal speech in response to "Is s/he behaving normally now?" is indicative of abnormal behavior.

Some diabetics are not dependent on insulin. Their bodies still make some insulin (but not enough or make it irregularly) and with careful attention to diet and/or the aid of oral medication, the situation is more easily controlled. Since these diabetics rarely become dangerously hypoglycemic, an unrelated cause of unconsciousness may have occurred prompting the call for help. The EMD is more certain of a diabetes-related situation if the caller knows the patient is insulin-dependent.

Rule 2   PROTOCOL 13
EMDs should **not advise administration of oral sugar to symptomatic diabetics**. There is no clinical evidence of improved outcome by such EMD intervention, while the potential for airway obstruction in the not alert patient is high.

Post-Dispatch Instructions. First, the caller should assure the ABCs (using protocol A, B, or C) if the patient is unconscious or is not alert and breathing ineffectively. Other patients need supportive care and observation provided beginning with protocol X-1.

One common home remedy is to try to get the not alert diabetic to take in some sugar. This could backfire causing serious problems if the sugar substance gets into the lungs because of lack of airway control.

The caller can be advised to collect the patient's medications. Diabetics usually keep their insulin in the refrigerator. The family pets can be isolated, and the caller can write down the family doctor's name and telephone number.

As indicated on protocol X, the EMD should stay on the line with potentially unstable or worsening conditions wherever possible. This is particularly important when you are dealing with a potentially unstable or worsening first party caller, because if their condition suddenly worsens they may not be able to call you back. Be aware that diabetics in insulin shock can drool (dribble in the U.K.) profusely. Profuse drooling can have the same effect as vomiting, so the EMD should pay particular attention to instructions for vomiting: "If s/he becomes less awake and vomits, quickly turn her/him on her/his side." The final post-dispatch instruction for the caller is obvious in all diabetic situations, "If s/he gets worse in any way, call me back immediately for further instructions."

Protocol 12: Convulsions/Seizures

A seizure is an abnormal firing of brain cells, usually resulting in jerking movements followed by an unconscious or semi-conscious period.[74] **Seizures** manifest in various ways and occur due to many causes. The type of seizure for which emergency units are most often summoned is a generalized, tonic-clonic seizure (formerly and still commonly called "**grand mal**"). The patient suddenly becomes, first completely stiff or tense (sometimes this initial phase is heralded by a vocal cry), with arms and legs extended (tonic phase). The patient then begins to jerk rigorously, with arms and legs contracting and then relaxing in unison (clonic phase). These two phases represent the convulsion phase.

Axiom 2   PROTOCOL 12
All actively seizing patients **appear to have** abnormal or absent breathing.

In this type of seizure, the patient *always* loses consciousness, may foam at the mouth (their sputum may be pink- or red-tinged, since tongue biting is common), and they may be **incontinent**. Witnessing a seizure can be frightening, as the patient may appear not to be breathing.

Protocol 6: Breathing Problems, is not the best place to handle a seizing patient, even though the patient may appear to be not breathing. This is because protocol 6 does not take into account the likelihood that the seizure will end quickly and the patient's breathing status may be different after the seizure. Rule 3 justified the EMD choosing protocol 12: Convulsions/Seizures for a seizing patient who is not breathing.

Rule 3	PROTOCOL **12**

When the initial **Chief Complaint appears to be seizure, go to Protocol 12** regardless of consciousness and breathing status.

Fortunately, the convulsion phase is over in about 60 seconds.

Axiom 4	PROTOCOL **12**

Tonic-clonic (grand mal) seizures generally **last about 60 seconds.**

This means that the convulsion phase in most seizures ends before the call to the EMD is concluded, (in most cases, before the EMD has even received the call). Afterward, the patient is **post-ictal**, a state of confusion, sleepiness, and occasionally combativeness. Even if the patient is turning blue, most seizures end long before brain damage would begin. The heart is still beating during the convulsion, even though breathing has effectively stopped temporarily. Afterward, if a patient is not breathing effectively (irregularly) after a quick, direct evaluation, the EMD will immediately begin dispatch life support.

Rarely, the jerking or twitching will not end, or will return without an interlude of mental clarity in between. This is a potentially life-threatening variety of seizures known as **status epilepticus** (status mean to keep going as is). The dispatch definition of a **continuous seizure**, found in Additional Information is "a seizure

CONTINUOUS Seizure	PROTOCOL **12**

A seizure **still in progress at the end of the interrogation** and after a physical verification by the caller (EMD must stay on the line to check).

MULTIPLE Seizures	PROTOCOL **12**

The occurrence of more than one seizure in a patient who **remains unconscious or not alert between episodes.**

still in progress at the end of the interrogation and after a physical verification by the caller (EMD must stay on the line to check)." Some continuous seizures actually start, stop, then start again; in other cases, the jerking motions simply continue, although they are much less violent—more like twitching. A clarifying point is that the problem must be considered continuous if the patient does not become mentally clear (awake) between seizures.

Recurrent Seizure	PROTOCOL **12**

Epileptics may have more than one seizure in a day. These are considered recurrent seizures if the patient is able to regain consciousness between episodes.

The term **epilepsy** refers to people in whom seizures are recurrent. Seventy-five percent of epileptic people have seizures due to **idiopathic**, or unknown, causes. Medication can prevent most epileptic people from suffering frequent seizures. Some epileptic patients do not take their medicine regularly (or at all) for economic or emotional reasons. Some have occasional break-through seizures despite medication, or may have recurrent seizures that are hard to control even with medication. Commonly, a caller has encountered a stranger who is having a seizure and does not know if the patient has had them before. Most medical practitioners would readily agree that Axiom 3 is correct.

Axiom 3	PROTOCOL **12**

A seizure patient with an **unknown history of seizures** has most likely had seizures before.

Types of Seizures	PROTOCOL 12

- **Generalized**
  Absence (petite mal)
  Atonic (drop attack)
  Myoclonic
  Tonic-clonic (grand mal)

- **Simple Partial**
  Focal/Local

- **Complex partial**
  Temporal lobe/Psychomotor

There are several other types of seizures. One is "absence," or staring, seizures (formerly called "petit mal"); here, the patient (usually a child) is momentarily mentally absent from whatever is going on. Although it is not the same as daydreaming, a child may be told it's like a brain "time-out." Other types of seizure include Jacksonian, focal, psychomotor, and temporal lobe seizures. These have only a general interest to the EMD since calls to EMS are almost always either for generalized or febrile seizures.

Nearly all febrile seizures occur in children who develop high fevers between the ages of 6 months and 5 years (23 months average). They affect 3 to 5 percent of all children by the age of 5 years. It is generally believed (but not proven) that feb-rile seizures occur not due to the extent of the fever, but due to how rapidly it rises. Febrile seizures may occur in the same child on more than one occasion, but this does not constitute epilepsy. The risk of death from a febrile seizure is reported in the medical literature as virtually zero.[75]

> **To not dispatch to or transport a patient who has had a febrile seizure is a grave error.**

Axiom 5	PROTOCOL 12

Reducing fever in a child after a febrile seizure **is of little value** as the precipitating factor is believed to be the rapid rise of temperature. The fever itself is of no harm and may even help the body battle the infecting microbes.

While febrile seizures are very frightening to the parents, this form of seizure is almost always limited to one event during the fever's rise. While these seizures are benign (not life-threatening) and are not prehospital emergencies (requiring only supportive care and observation enroute) they may mask a life-threatening brain infection called meningitis. To not dispatch to or transport a patient who has had a febrile seizure is a grave error, since meningitis, if not discovered in the emergency department or doctor's clinic, can be cerebrally devastating or fatal. Meningitis must *always* be ruled out in children with febrile seizures by competent physicians physically attending the patient.

One reason a report of a seizure cannot be trivialized, even though the great majority of them are due to epilepsy, is because another significant but less frequent cause of seizures is cardiac arrest.

The brain is quickly affected when it runs out of one of its prime sources of fuel—and there are mainly two: blood sugar and oxygen. Without immediate recognition and rapid resuscitation, the patient may incur irreversible brain damage, or may die.

Axiom 1	PROTOCOL 12

Seizure-like activity can be an **initial symptom of cardiac arrest**.

Rule 1	PROTOCOL 12

A seizure in a person ≥ 35 is considered a **cardiac arrest until regular breathing is physically verified** by the caller.

The potential for brain damage in cardiac arrest should be obvious. Because of the possibility of cardiac arrest, seizures are initially regarded as potentially critical prehospital complaints until normal breathing is verified as present.

Verification of breathing should ideally be done after any convulsive episode has stopped. Generalized seizures entail tremendous amounts of physical activity, and accurate assessment may not be reliable until after they stop. However, since recognition and calling, plus call processing, will take longer than approximately 60 seconds (the length of the seizure), the caller should always be directed to verify breathing (and any continuous seizure activity) at the end of the

Should Pediatric Febrile Seizures Be Treated Over the Phone?

Priority dispatch protocols automatically determine whether a seizure victim is a child or not by asking the age question on the Case Entry protocol. However, no specific use or special treatment occurs as the result of this information in response coding or post-dispatch instructions for the following reasons:

The determination of whether a seizure in a child or infant is *febrile* in nature cannot be done at dispatch or even by at-scene personnel for that matter. It is a diagnosis of exclusion accomplished only after emergency department physician evaluation and laboratory work—including (most always) a spinal tap. Poorly taught, if at all, in EMS texts is the differential diagnosis of febrile-*appearing* seizures in which the physician must "rule out" the presence of meningitis as an uncommon but potentially fatal cause of fever or seizure in little children. Once this has been done, the remaining true fever-only induced seizures have a mortality rate, as reported in the medical literature, of "virtually zero."

While there are some differing medical opinions regarding the necessity to lower fever in children, standard febrile episodes of fever of 105° F (40.5° C) or less are routinely benign. When fever is the cause of a seizure in a child (most occur under age 6) the seizure is grand mal in presentation, lasts less than 45 seconds, and leaves the child without the usual extended period of post-ictal confusion common in the adult epileptic. In addition, these seizures are uniformly solitary in occurrence.

With this in mind, *reducing the fever is of little, if any, value after the seizure has occurred* since it will not

recur (if truly only febrile in cause). The fever itself in these cases is of no particular harm to these children and may even help in the body's battle against the infecting microbes.

After a seizure, cooling procedures are to be performed only under hospital and clinic supervision since, if one should recur, the child could potentially drown or at least have a frightening event in a bath tub, sink, shower, or high up on a counter top. My personal experience with cooling little children in the ER is that it is at best an uncomfortable and frightening experience for the child and adds no discernible benefit to the prevention of secondary seizures. For these reasons, it is not warranted as an EMD-mediated post-dispatch procedure.

Regarding protocol adherence, the trained EMD should follow the protocol cards. The issue of ad hoc dispatcher actions would always be legally judged as to their correctness and, specifically, as to whether such extraneous treatments contributed to a negative outcome. This would be quite unlikely; but, in the bathtub scenario, it is possible and even predictable given the reality of all the phone calls to and from family, clergy, neighbors, and physicians that occur as the result of a "frightening" seizure. Mom or dad leaves the child for a "minute or two" to answer the phone, the door, etc. Why then chance giving extra, potentially harmful instructions?

As far as DLS treatment of seizure victims is concerned, as with all instructions in the MPDS, it is medically correct policy to follow the protocol verbatim.   ❈

Fig. 6-10. "Should Pediatric Febrile Seizures Be Treated Differently From Adult Cases?" revised and reprinted from JNAEMD.[76]

interrogation. A report at this point that the jerking or twitching is still present on direct observation is a grave sign and should be interpreted by the EMD as a continuous seizure episode. Even though the patient is breathing (maybe only shallowly) during continuous seizures episodes, respiration should be aided unless it is clearly regular.

If, after the seizure, the caller finds the patient is not brea-thing, the GO TO column directs the EMD to the age-appropriate dispatch life support protocols for assessing airway (A-1, B-1, or C-1) on the way to full resuscitative efforts.

Additional causes of seizures include trauma (new or old), brain tumors, meningitis, alcohol withdrawal, and drug abuse (especially cocaine and amphetamines). Diabetics may be prone to seizures when they go into insulin shock. Recall that insulin shock occurs when blood sugar falls below normal levels due to too much insulin.

A serious complication of pregnancy called **eclampsia** can also cause seizures. While eclampsia is not well understood, it usually occurs in the last half of a pregnancy. The gradual condition leading up to this kind of seizure is called pre-eclampsia and is marked by high blood pressure and edema (water retention) in the ankles and face. If the patient is a female between the childbearing ages of 12 and 50, the EMD should inquire if she is pregnant.

If a specific head injury preceded the seizure, the situation is acute, and medical response must be prompt and sophisticated. Certain head injuries can cause rapid swelling of or bleeding into the brain, generating a seizure. Rapid action by surgeons can relieve the situation and may

Diabetics may be prone to seizures when they go into insulin shock.

be lifesaving. Each year, according to the Epilepsy Foundation of America, 190,000 Americans sustain seizure-producing head injuries from auto accidents alone, and 50,000 of them will be recurrent and resistant to therapy.[74] Abusively shaking infants or young children violently can also rupture blood vessels in their heads, causing seizures as an early sign of an internal head injury.

Post-Dispatch Instructions. First, the EMD must stay on the line with the caller until the patient's seizure stops, and then verify breathing.

During the seizure, the caller should move dangerous objects away from the patient (or pad those that cannot be moved). No one should try to hold down the patient or suppress the jerking motions of the **clonic phase**. Another persistent old wives' tale is to put something between the teeth of a person who is seizing. This is never advisable! Tongue biting, if it's going to happen, occurs at the

Jamming a pencil or screwdriver into a seizing patient's mouth will cause nothing but expensive dental harm.

beginning of a seizure. Jamming a pencil or screwdriver into a seizing patient's mouth will cause nothing but expensive dental harm. A tongue, on the other hand, is relatively less expensive to stitch and less susceptible to long-term damage.

The EMD must clearly explain to the caller not to do these things. In fact, at least one prehospital liability lawsuit was generated in the aftermath of dental harm caused by such unnecessary aid.

Rule 2   Protocol 12

Check ABCs very carefully before initiating CPR after a seizure.

While the chest compressions of CPR should not be done while the patient is still jerking or twitching, immediate assessment of the airway and breathing status should begin as soon as interrogation and dispatch have been accomplished. Initiating the Pre-Arrival Instruction sequence is correct here if the patient is not *clearly* breathing normally although now post-ictally unconscious.

The trick here is not to be fooled by the presence of agonal (dying) respirations often associated with cardiac arrest. This type of useless irregular breathing (once the heart has already stopped) appears as a fading series of fish-like gasps for air with periods of several seconds in-between. It generally lasts only 20 to 30 seconds but can last longer in some cases. Staying on the line and reassessing *effective* breathing is paramount to correct EMD care of a seizure patient.

If the patient is breathing regularly, the EMD should proceed with supportive care and observation provided by protocol X-1. Ensuring the caller watches the patient closely (protocol X-2) is critically important, and the EMD should be mentally prepared to verify the patient's airway and to begin CPR (protocols A, B, or C) should the situation dictate it. The caller can turn the patient gently onto her side. Do not leave the patient. Observe breathing closely.

If an improving patient wants to get up, bystanders should not allow unattended wandering until functioning skills are fully normal. Seizure patients are often too confused to listen to reasoning. It is wise to create limits for their movements, such as closing the door to the room, balcony, or stairs. Time (accompanied by careful observation) should put an end to the mental confusion.

Protocol 18: Headache

Statistically, even laymen know that headaches are rarely serious problems. However, emergency calls in which the Chief Complaint is "headache" cannot be taken lightly. The sudden presentation of a severe situation usually results in (or from) other Chief Complaints such as unconsciousness or stroke. Nonetheless, even when information received from case entry key question 3, "What's the problem, tell me exactly what happened?" does not lead the EMD to protocol 31: Unconscious/Fainting (Near), or to protocol 28: Stroke (CVA) there may very well be a significant underlying cause for an isolated, sudden, severe headache.

When this is the case, many of the symptoms of the more serious underlying causes (such as stroke) are reiterated on the headache protocol, so an appropriate response should still be correctly selected.

Most headaches worthy of a call for help are painful, but some are more serious than others from the prehospital point of view. Listed in Additional Information are three types and causes of headaches: NOT SERIOUS, POSSIBLY SERIOUS, and SERIOUS.

NOT SERIOUS headaches, in terms of EMS intervention, are tension headaches, sinus headaches, migraine headaches (frequently one-sided and excruciating, but not life-threatening), and cluster headaches (similar to migraine).

Rule 1	PROTOCOL **18**
Sudden, severe onset of a headache is considered to have a **more serious underlying cause until proven otherwise**.	

Axiom 1	PROTOCOL **18**
Sudden and severe headaches, especially when associated with speech or movement problems (numbness or paralysis), **may represent the early onset of a serious condition**.	

Axiom 3	PROTOCOL **18**
Patients who call an ambulance for a headache generally have a more serious underlying cause than patients who arrive at the emergency department on their own.	

POSSIBLY SERIOUS causes of headache include hypertension (high blood pressure) and meningitis (an infection around the brain).

SERIOUS causes of headache are **subdural hematoma**, **subarachnoid hemorrhage**, and **stroke (CVA)**. Subdural hematoma is a blood clot inside the skull, a rigid structure that provides no room for swelling without forcing brain tissue into abnormal and lethal areas. The cause of bleeding may or may not be due to trauma. The blood collects under the dura mater, the toughest layer of the three brain coverings. Subarachnoid hemorrhage is bleeding into a different layer of the brain's coverings. Finally, stroke is any event—a thrombus (clot) or a hemorrhage—that disrupts the supply of blood to a part of the brain. Any of these may be lethal or permanently disabling. In the past, several of these conditions were essentially not changeable especially while the patient was in the prehospital environment.

At the time of this writing, significant research and re-evaluation of stroke as a medically treatable problem is occurring. The College of Fellows' Council of Standards closely followed relevant new information and provided medical dispatch leadership regarding the proper application of priority dispatch methods to prehospital, clot-caused stroke management. Several important modifications were introduced in v10.3, which have been carried forward to v11.

> **Axiom 2**   PROTOCOL **18**
>
> Some **younger people have STROKES** (often fatal) from a ballooned blood vessel called a berry aneurysm that expands and then breaks. This condition is present from birth (congenital). Early symptoms include sudden, severe headache.

A special type of stroke (berry aneurysm) sometimes occurs in younger patients—even teenagers and young adults. Its singular herald symptom may only be the sudden, severe headache of which the EMD is most concerned.

The EMD's goal is not to just discover whether the patient has any priority symptoms, but whether any evidence of symptoms listed in the Key Questions may suggest a more severe intracranial problem. The Key Questions include whether the patient's speech is normal, and whether there is any numbness, paralysis, or weakness in an arm or leg.

Post-Dispatch Instructions. The EMD assures the ABCs for the patient who is not alert and is breathing abnormally using protocol A, B, or C as appropriate. For other patients, the supportive care and observation provided by protocol X is required. If the EMD must disconnect the call, the last instruction to the caller should be "If s/he gets worse in any way, call me back immediately for further instructions."

Protocol 28: Stroke (CVA)

Stroke, as one of its other names (cerebrovascular accident) implies is a disruption of the cerebral (pertaining to the head) vasculature (blood vessels). Stroke is most commonly a disease of the elderly; however, it is not limited to the elderly.

Stroke is also defined for the EMD in the additional information section as a "disruption of blood flow to the brain or part of the brain due to blood clot or hemorrhage. Hemorrhage additionally causes increased pressure within the skull. Clots can be spontaneous or caused by trauma. Paralysis or weakness of one side, trouble speaking, altered level of consciousness, and respiratory changes are all common symptoms."

Blood clots travel through the blood vessels until they plug a passageway. Disrupting the downstream blood supply causes injury or death to the brain cells there.

> **Axiom 1**   PROTOCOL **28**
>
> **Cerebrovascular Accident** (CVA) and "brain attack" are commonly used terms for **STROKE**.

> **Axiom 2**   PROTOCOL **28**
>
> Just because the caller says the problem is a "stroke" **does not necessarily mean** that this diagnosis is correct.

Hemorrhage (obviously) disrupts blood flow, and, because the skull is rigid and limits swelling, it also causes increased pressure as the blood pushes into and around the brain. Stroke is a difficult call for several reasons. One is because what the caller thinks is a stroke may not be. The EMD usually needs more information.

In addition, it is important the prehospital provider not waste time at the scene.

There is a form of stroke called a transient ischemic attack (TIA; also commonly known as "little strokes"). In TIA it is believed that part of the brain is deprived of blood (and oxygen) long enough to cause symptoms, but not long enough to cause permanent damage. A patient has various signs and symptoms of a CVA, but the episode resolves completely and spontaneously within 12 hours.

> **Rule 1**   PROTOCOL **28**
>
> In order to correctly identify potential **STROKE** patients, and to correctly identify priority symptoms, **always follow the key question interrogation sequence.**

> **Axiom 3**   PROTOCOL **28**
>
> Alert **STROKE** patients should be treated as if they can hear and are aware of their surroundings. If the patient is conscious but not talking, **verbal reassurance may be helpful**.

While the use of lights-and-siren to the scene is not advised in the new treatment process of stroke,

Rule 2	PROTOCOL **28**

Some **STROKES** can now be effectively treated, but the time for successful therapy is quite short. Lights-and-siren are not recommended; however, there should be a sense of urgency. **STROKE must receive an immediate response that is not subject to delay.**

attention to the emerging stroke treatment methods should place the EMD at a higher level of alert regarding these calls. Once again, being prompt and efficient pays at dispatch.

Post-Dispatch Instructions. The caller may be excited and will need the EMD's best interpersonal talents. As with all protocols, before moving to the DLS links

read the post dispatch instruction: "I'm sending the paramedics (ambulance) to help you now. Stay on the line and I'll tell you exactly what to do next."

If the patient is not alert and is breathing abnormally, the EMD should direct the caller to verify the patient's airway using protocol A, B, or C, and to initiate CPR if necessary. Most stoke patients need the supportive care and observation provided by protocol X.

Be aware that even though many stroke patients may appear to have a decreased level of consciousness, the nature of stroke can result in a patient who does not respond as though she or he is fully conscious but who is, nevertheless, completely aware of her or his surroundings. Encouraging the caller to verbally reassure the patient can be very helpful in these situations. Stroke patients may drool excessively (dribble in the

Using EMD for Acute Stroke Identification—Official Academy Position Statement

Stroke could become one of the defining elements of the driving force behind prioritized EMD. In recent years, thrombolytic therapy with tissue plasminogen activator (t-PA) to break down blood clots that precipitate "brain attacks," has resulted in new hope for people who suffer stroke.

Clinical studies have shown that, if given during the early stages of a stroke, t-PA can indeed improve outcomes for many stroke victims. The National Institute of Neurological Disorders and Stroke (NINDS), t-PA Stroke Study Group, concluded in its 1995 paper, Tissue plasminogen activator for acute ischemic stroke, "Despite an increased incidence of symptomatic intracerebral hemorrhage, treatment with intravenous t-PA within three hours of the onset of ischemic stroke improved clinical outcome at three months."[77] Appropriate t-PA administration improves the long-term outcome in a significant number of patients. Overall, t-PA treatment is beneficial, despite the fact that it does cause serious intracranial bleeding in some patients. For 11 percent of patients, if they get to hospital rapidly, and are treated by a stroke team using thrombolytic drugs, they'll go home rather than to a long-term care facility."[78]

Earlier interventions lead to improved patient outcomes (as "time is muscle" during acute MI,

"time is brain cells" during stroke) and the goal should be a 90-minute time to treatment, rather than the latest acceptable treatment time of three hours.

This short window for effective intervention has led to the widespread realization that, as stated in USA Today, "People having strokes should be treated with the same urgency as those suffering heart attacks."

Patient groups are calling for "...a major overhaul of outmoded stroke responses nationwide, upgrading stroke to a time-dependent, urgent medical emergency."[79] This publicity has led to many agencies proposing that for all requests that report stroke-like symptoms, response be upgraded to an obligatory lights-and-siren mode both to the scene and during transport of the patient.

We believe that in most situations the small time savings of a L&S response to the scene will not alone make a significant difference in stroke outcomes and that the initial response should be the same as for chest pain in the absence of symptoms which suggest the patient is arresting.

(continued on 6.40)

Using EMD for Acute Stroke Identification—Official Academy Position Statement

(continued from 6.39)

For chest pain without these symptoms, CHARLIE (not DELTA) determinants drive responses for the cardiac age-range patient. We believe the similarities between stroke and acute MI warrant changes in protocol 28: Stroke (CVA), now that there is an intervention that significantly improves the outcome for many stroke patients if given soon enough.

In stroke, the situation is in many ways analogous to acute MI. Therefore, we believe there should be more parity between the stroke and chest pain protocols by upgrading the Stroke dispatch protocol to drive determinants that are similar to the CHARLIE determinants on the Chest Pain protocol. However, protocol 28: Stroke does not warrant the DELTA drivers we use in protocol 10 (chest pain). These DELTA determinants are driven by priority symptoms that suggest the patient is arresting and requires on-scene treatment within two or three minutes.

If a patient is arresting, effective on-scene intervention (defibrillation) by first responders can make an enormous difference, but the window of opportunity is extremely short. On-scene intervention for stroke patients is still very limited and will likely remain so until the on-scene use of neuroprotective drugs can be shown to be effective. In the meantime, the existing CHARLIE determinants do not imply that stroke (or MI without evidence of arrest) is not time-sensitive, but rather that it is reasonable to respond to stroke and acute MI without L&S and to only respond with L&S when there is evidence that the chest pain patient is deteriorating or arresting.

A stroke patient should call 9-1-1 as soon as symptoms appear, hence a need for increased public awareness and education. Pepe, et al., in their 1998 paper, Ensuring the chain of recovery for stroke in your community, point out that, "The sheer logistics of reaching and retrieving patients, even in a 'scoop and run' mode, leads to significant time lapses, a concept often unappreciated by those unfamiliar with the delivery of emergency patient care in the out-of-hospital setting."[80] They show that typical delivery of a patient to the ED will not take place for at least 30 to 50 minutes after a stroke is recognized by the patient or bystander. (This breaks down to 15 minutes from caller recognition to EMS-professional identification of the stroke at the scene; 10 to 20 minutes on-scene time; and 5 to 15 minutes transport time.) The NINDS guidelines: Rapid identification and treatment of acute stroke,[81] recommend that a physician should evaluate a stroke patient within 10 minutes of arrival at the ED, and that a stroke specialist should be available or notified within 15 minutes. In order to avoid giving thrombolytic treatment to a patient with a brain hemorrhage, a CT scan must be done. The CT scan should be started within 25 minutes, the results available within 45 minutes, and treatment (when appropriate) started within 60 minutes.

Hunt, et al.,[36] measured that a typical L&S run saves, on average, 43 seconds over a COLD run. While this saving seems surprisingly small, there are other studies that appear to confirm these results.[11] Even allowing for rural versus metropolitan differences, it seems likely that a L&S response is probably only saving one or two minutes over a COLD response time.

In a rapid (15 to 20 minute) "scoop and run" delivery to a facility where the CT turn-around is also fast, an extra couple of minutes for a COLD ambulance journey to the scene is a small, but significant, portion of the time taken before the t-PA injection-but the total time is still likely to allow treatment of patients within a 90-minute window. In a conventional ALS response and delivery (30 to 50 minutes) to a facility that does not meet the NINDS guidelines for CT scanning, the time lost by a COLD response will very likely still be less than one percent of the total time and is therefore probably not alone a major source of delay.

While these time constraints do not really suggest that the "time criticality" of thrombolytic stroke treatment warrants the extra risks of a L&S response, we do need a response mode that confers the same sense of urgency without the use of lights and sirens, i.e., one that gets the patient there quickly, but without creating unnecessary hazards for emergency personnel or civilians. Stroke is indeed a time-critical medical emergency, but it is saving hours (through public education) and minutes (through ED compliance with the NINDS time guidelines) that is important, not saving seconds that can place others at unnecessary risk.

(continued on 6.41)

Using EMD for Acute Stroke Identification—Official Academy Position Statement

(continued from 6.40)

In 1996, the Academy stated, "It is the temporary position of the Academy that, at this time, no changes are necessary within protocol 28's key questions, post dispatch instructions, or determinant codes. However, in light of changing science, we recommend the addition of a new in additional information, to state:

'The adoption of in-hospital administration of clot dissolving drug therapies may require special assignment of units equipped to evaluate patients for this therapy in areas adopting it for trial and on-going treatment. Based on the current consensus recommendation to provide this treatment within 3 hours of the occurrence of stroke symptoms, the use of lights-and-siren (HOT) responses is generally not indicated at the present time unless priority symptoms are present.'"

More recently, at the 1998 Council of Research meeting the Council recommended several additional modifications that emphasize the availability of thrombolytic treatment, but also recognized that other elements in the survival chain (such as pre-notification of stroke response teams at the receiving hospital and eliminating unnecessary ALS procedures at the scene) will have greater impact on stroke survival. Further, the Council stood by the 1996 recommendation that L&S responses are not generally indicated for stroke when priority symptoms are not present.

Since the 1998 Council of Research meeting, the Academy has continued to examine the stroke issue in great detail. For a number of reasons, the Council of Standards has now established an age-dependent triage for stroke and stroke-like symptoms. The new determinants appear as follows:

C-6 Breathing **normally** ≥ 35

C-5 **STROKE** history

C-4 **Numbness** or **tingling**

C-3 **Speech** or **movement** problems

C-2 **Abnormal** breathing

C-1 **Not** alert

B-1 **Unknown** symptoms (3rd party caller)

A-1 Breathing **normally** < 35

The version 10.3 changes have been approved by the Council of Research and then were formally ratified by the Council of Standards—effective July 20, 1998.

The 10.3 changes will improve the MPDS in several ways. Statistically, the age range given would only fail to upgrade less than three percent of all strokes, and less than one percent of all ischemic strokes, to the CHARLIE response. The recommended ALS capability of the CHARLIE response for stroke would increase the sense of urgency when compared to the BLS capability of the current ALPHA response, and might even improve the patient's reception at the ED.[82] Finally, upgrading stroke to an ALS-level response sets the scene for on-site intervention when new neuroprotective drugs gain approval.

As with all MPDS determinant-driven response modes, local medical control has the final word on who, when, and how field personnel actually respond. Due to differences in response configuration options, available facilities, and local driving conditions, this situation may be somewhat different among systems. While any delay in the stroke patient's chain of recovery is undesirable, in most circumstances the extra time taken by a COLD response to the scene is a very small portion of the total (call-to-treatment) time. Stroke is a time-sensitive medical emergency and should be responded to with a sense of urgency comparable to that used in response to chest pain suspected to be due to myocardial infarction.

Therefore in the absence of additional priority symptoms, for both Chest Pain and Stroke the Academy recommends dispatching an ALS-level response without the use of L&S (see "Response Determinant Methodology" protocol). As more data on thrombolytic treatment becomes available, the precise nature of t-PA's time criticality will become clearer. For now, it appears that the benefits of the small time savings of an L&S response may not outweigh its additional risks.

Fig. 6-11. Priority dispatch evolves to accommodate changes in treatments and accepted standards of care. Stroke management has recently undergone radical changes due to the introduction of thrombolytic therapies. This position statement presents the rationale for changes to the MPDS first released in version 10.3 (now updated to v11.1). "Using EMD for Acute Stroke Identification," by Sinclair, R. and Marler, J. Reprinted from the JNAEMD.[83]

Axiom 4	Protocol 28

The likelihood of a **patient who has a history of STROKE** having another **STROKE** is greater than the likelihood of a member of the general population having a first **STROKE**.

U.K.). Profuse drooling can have the same effect as vomiting, so the EMD should pay particular attention to instructions for vomiting: "If s/he becomes less awake and vomits, quickly turn her/him on her/his side." The final Post-Dispatch Instruction for the caller is obvious in all impaired-consciousness situations, "If s/he gets worse in any way, call me back immediately for further instructions."

Protocol 33: Transfer/Interfacility/Palliative Care

A central assumption of priority dispatch design is that the protocol must deal with obtaining necessary information from lay (non-medical) callers representing the public-at-large, who are generally reporting perceived emergencies. However, part of the reality for many systems (especially primary municipal and private ambulance dispatch centers) is that callers often are medical, nursing, or medical-clerical personnel from health care facilities requesting a variety of EMS transport and care combinations.

Calls for interfacility transfers have created a moderate dilemma for the EMD: Whether or not to interrogate the nurse or doctor per the protocol.

Several years of development and site testing has led to the addition (with v11.1 of the MPDS) of a protocol specially designed to improve handling of these calls, protocol 33: Transfer/Interfacility/Palliative Care.

Rule 2	Protocol 33

Use this protocol only when taking calls from a **medical care facility** that have been **made as the result of an evaluation by a nurse or doctor**.

Since these calls involve patients with pre-existing (and changing) conditions, traditional priority symptom-based Key Questions (completely awake and breathing normally), while present, are situationally clarified by

Rule 1	Protocol 33

This protocol is for patients being **currently cared for by medical professionals** that require additional care, diagnostics, or reevaluation at at different medical facility.

asking, "Is this a sudden or unexpected change in her/his usual condition?"

A basic tenent of the standard 32-protocol evaluation is that the caller can impart no significant diagnostic value to the process, just observational or third party relayed data. This is not the case with calls from trained and experienced medical employees. As the TV game show host used to say, "Who do you trust?"

Protocol 33 places the professional EMD in a cooperative dialogue with the medical professional currently responsible for the patient. In these situations the EMD is not the professional with the greatest knowledge of the patient's current medical or historical condition (see fig. 6-12).

The use of this protocol requires the highest level of professional demeanor, tact, and communication at the EMD's command. The EMD must realize that, unless clearly known otherwise, the requesting medical location is allowed to call the shots—especially when calling on non-emergency lines. Protocol 33 creates a standard framework for this interaction.

Due to significant regulations recently imposed by governmental health oversight groups such as HCFA

Purpose & Use of Transfer, Interfacility, and Palliative Care Protocol

To offer a **response level** based on a **joint** medical professional and EMD evaluation of the patient's medical condition and basic clinical signs. This occurs when urgent, unscheduled transport of patients is requested from medical environments such as:

* extended care facilities
* Hospice (terminal care)
* nursing facilities
* palliative home care (attended)

Fig. 6-12. Purpose and Use of Interfacility and Palliative Care Protocol. MPDS, v11.1 protocols. ©1978-2003 MPC.

(Health Care Finance Administration) in the U.S. and the NHS (National Health Service) in the U.K., earlier and more accurate data on patients in the course of their care is being required. HCFA enforces ambulance payment schedules based on both demographics and clinical data. Protocol 33 contains several "if appropriate" questions that help to determine required billing information not normally gathered in standard EMD interrogation.

Often transfer of a patient from one facility to another involves the use of special equipment or additionally trained personnel. Key Questions 6 and 7 clarify requirements that, in the absence of protocol 33, often remain undetermined until after responders have arrived.

A special feature of protocol 33 is the user-defined ACUITY levels (I, II, and III). A given ACUITY level

ACUITY Levels I, II, III

Before using the ACUITY Level (I, II, III) determinants, local Medical Control must **define** additional dispatch center **policy** and **authorize** (☒) approved **patient conditions below** (list both acuity level and title):

☐ _____   ☐ _____
☐ _____   ☐ _____
☐ _____   ☐ _____
☐ _____   ☐ _____
☐ _____   ☐ _____
☐ _____   ☐ _____
☐ _____   ☐ _____
☐ _____   ☐ _____
☐ _____   ☐ _____
☐ _____   ☐ _____
☐ _____   ☐ _____

_____   _____
Approval signature of local Medical Control   Date approved

Fig. 6-13. Acuity Levels I, II, III. The MPDS, v11.1 protocols. ©1978-2003 MPC.

Problem Suffixes

The suffix codes help to delineate the type of problem for specific response and safety purposes:

T = Transfer/Interfacility
P = Palliative Care

Fig. 6-14. Problem Suffixes, MPDS, v11.1 protocols. ©1978-2003 MPC.

! Authors' Note

This was received from one Protocol 33 Beta-test site:

I have had the opportunity to discuss the use of this card with my communication center staff. They all feel like it is a good card with the recent changes that have been made. I have also used this card myself while working in the communication center. I have taken the time to talk with some of the Nursing Homes and Clinics on the telephone. Until is it explained to them the reasoning behind the questions some of them felt it was still too much. Once I explained each question, it seemed relations improved and they could see the benefit also. The card has been utilized a total of 733 times in our center in March and April of this year (2000), of which 404 were [coded as] ALPHA, 327 were CHARLIE, and 2 were DELTA responses.

contain various non-critical patient conditions and situations that trigger a pre-assigned clinical transport capability as listed in the medically approved fill-in list (fig. 6.13). This allows for three different response types in the non-emergent ALPHA tier. These can be defined in ways useful to each particular ambulance service based on crews, equipment, and time requirements.

Several Beta-test sites helped define these ACUITY levels (see Authors' Note).

Delays in patient contact, which are often avoidable, frequently occur because of the responders' lack of information regarding the exact location of the patient in a medical complex. Rule 4 advises the EMD:

Rule 4   PROTOCOL **33**

Obtain and relay any **special directions** needed to **locate** the patient in a **medical complex.**

Axiom 1	PROTOCOL 33
A **nurse or doctor with the patient**, is likely to give an accurate assessment of the patient's condition.	

Central to the initial correct selection of protocol 33 is the fact that a doctor or nurse who is with the patient, or who has recently evaluated the patient, is likely to give an accurate assessment of the patient's condition.

As with any remote evaluation of a scene, the EMD will not always be able to differentiate any given facility's capability of providing emergency supportive care. If, on occasion, this occurs, Axiom 2 and Rule 5 may be utilized.

Rule 5	PROTOCOL 33
Do not hesitate to use Protocols 1-32 when any question exists about the patient's care environment.	

While protocol 33 represents several years of project evaluation and testing, the varied aspects of both ambulance service resources and care facility needs leave many issues of exact protocol structure and use unresolved. Development of this protocol will continue at the Academy until the design attains more universal applicability. Proposals for change forms are not only requested, but welcome.

Axiom 2	PROTOCOL 33
It is not necessary to seek permission from the nurse of doctor to **upgrade the response level**.	

The MPDS offers a unique opportunity for the private and public ambulance industry in America. A significant part of ambulance service care—the required response—can be uniformly determined throughout the US by the EMD's selection of response (determinant) codes based on compliance to a medically approved interrogation. If thousands of centers utilize exactly the same evaluation and coding system, and utilize standard QA procedures to ensure their accuracy, government and insurance payers (HCFA) can be assured of a reasonable level of standardization and impartiality in any reimbursement request made throughout America.

Summary

This chapter has presented a brief introduction to various common emergency medical problems from a practicing EMD's perspective, including several SHUNT protocols. These help the EMD access the most appropriate priority dispatch protocol when callers initially describe vague Chief Complaints. In the next chapter, the protocols for trauma are presented.

Obviously, the descriptions of the various disease processes are very brief and basic. The intent is to provide the EMD with a working baseline medical knowledge about certain emergency conditions, to explain the reasons for particular interrogation objectives, and provide the rationale of various treatments and response determinants.

While the underlying causes of many of the problems described in this chapter are difficult to specifically determine (diagnose), the EMD does well by carefully following protocol. The objectives of dispatch evaluation are not those of EMTs, ambulance officers, paramedics, and physicians—albeit similar. The EMD, like the emergency physician, is rarely the end-point of any patient's care. The First Law of Emergency Medicine clearly applies here.

First Law of Emergency Medicine
Anything can happen in emergency medicine (and usually does). You don't have to know everything, you just have to know what to do with it.

It takes time for an EMS system to shed the habit of sending a maximal response in many of these situations. It takes time to see how public safety and advanced life support availability to the overall community are enhanced without negative impact to the patient. The reality of many medical problems (or the prehospital worker's ability to influence outcome) is different from how awful they seem when described by callers.

Of all the treatments possible, the first to consider is to do nothing.

—*Gerasim Tikoff, M.D.*

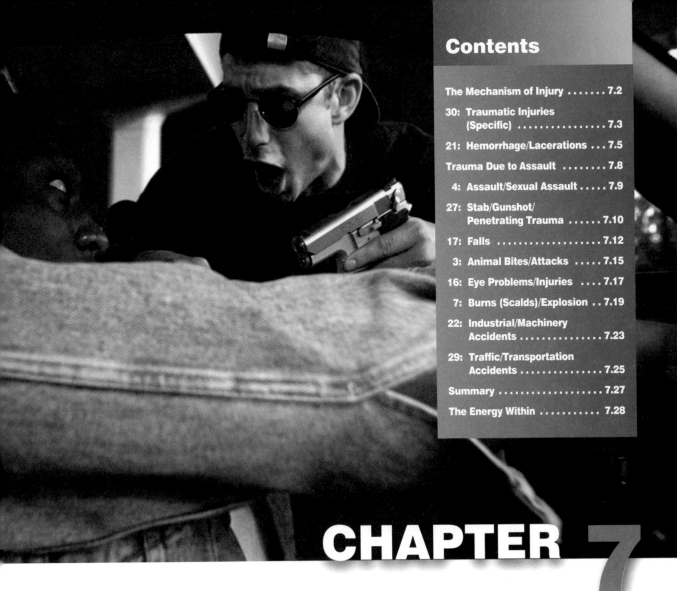

Contents

CHAPTER 7

Trauma Incidents

Chapter Overview

Many dispatchers perform their jobs without basic emergency training or practical experience with emergency medical problems. EMDs, as part of the emergency medical team, need a special familiarity with medical principles. Murder, mayhem, and a meaner society places the EMD electronically at the scene of many difficult and sad situations.

The purpose of this chapter is to introduce information related to this element of emergency care—trauma (or injury).

This chapter is valuable for EMDs who have training and experience in prehospital care; it is essential for those who do not. Information is presented from the dispatcher's perspective, not that of field personnel. There are important differences.

When you're confused, beat up and hurting, nothing feels as good as some calm, capable, credible, concerned person paying attention.
— *Alan Brunacini*

Trauma is the leading cause of death for people less than 45 years of age. Between ages 15 and 24, trauma causes 79 percent of deaths. It greatly surpasses all major disease groups as a cause of lost years of life. Each year, more than 4 million years of future work-life are lost to injury, compared to 2.1 million years to heart disease and 1.7 million years to cancer. The impact of non-fatal injury is of similar proportions.[84]

Callers seldom describe a specific set of signs or symptoms when someone sustains an injury. Instead, they tend to describe what has happened. For example, it is much less likely that the EMD will hear, "We have a person with a fractured femur on Farm Meadow Lane" than, "There's been a terrible accident on Farm Meadow Lane!" Or, "My child has puncture wounds" rather than, "My little boy was attacked by a dog!"

As a result, chief complaints for injuries are defined within priority dispatch in terms of incident types. In this chapter, the following incident types are described:

- Animal Bites/Attacks

- Assault/Sexual Assault

- Burns (Scalds)/Explosion

- Eye Problems/Injuries

- Falls

- Hemorrhage/Lacerations

- Industrial/Machinery Accidents

- Stab/Gunshot/Penetrating Trauma

- Traffic/Transportation Accidents

- Traumatic Injuries (Specific)

These are the actual titles of the Priority Dispatch Protocols that practicing EMDs use. Traumatic circumstances that are usually critical in severity are addressed in Chapter 8: Time-Life Priority Situations.

TRAUMA is usually described according to the incident type because more callers tend to be in third-party positions. They have witnessed an event—a shooting, fall, electrocution, explosion—without necessarily being personally involved. They can tell you what happened but may not know the specific injuries, or even whether or not the people involved are conscious or breathing.

The Mechanism of Injury

Some traumatic incident protocols are designed to pose certain questions that are not symptom-based (or even medical) in nature. Many are safety-related questions and questions designed to gain essential information about the mechanism of injury such as how far the patient fell.

Remember, the specific questions that are asked during an interrogation (examination) are based on the objectives that must be met for the proper handling of that Chief Complaint-based situation.

On the surface, the term "mechanism of injury" is just a fancy way of describing what happened. A prehospital emergency care provider learns to assess how significant the forces were against the patient's body in order to develop an appropriate level of concern for the potential of injuries.

> ### ! Authors' Note
>
> The unusual force of the car accident involving Diana, Princess of Wales, fueled recent debate about the conflict between apparent injuries versus the very visible mechanism involved in such crashes.

The clinician uses mechanism of injury as a guideline for choosing appropriate care. For example, a ground-level fall is a minor mechanism of injury; a fall from the third story window would be a far more significant mechanism of injury.

Sometimes, the mechanism of injury alone dictates what emergency care is provided to a patient who otherwise seems to have only minor injuries. The patient's apparent well-being is not congruent with the standard of concern. There may be slow internal bleeding or a developing head injury for which symptoms have yet to manifest.

Victims of auto-pedestrians accidents are a prime example of how the mechanism of injury outweighs the apparent seriousness of injuries described to the EMD. Mechanisms of injury such as the patient being trapped or ejected from the vehicle are keys used by the EMD in assessing the situation remotely. Mechanism of injury is discussed in more detail under Protocol 29: Traffic/Transportation injuries later this chapter, and in the article "The Energy Within" reprinted from the *National EMD Journal* at the end of this chapter.

For example, there are frequent references to protocol X, which contains nearly-universal dispatch life support instructions. Protocol X and the general concepts of the ABCs are presented in depth in Chapter 4: Dispatch Life Support. As another example, these two Key Questions are found on many protocols:

- Is s/he completely awake (alert)?
- Is s/he breathing normally?

These questions are extensions of the information gathered on the Case Entry protocol, when the mere presence of breathing and consciousness was the focal issue (primary survey). Now, the EMD wants to refine the assessment. What is the *quality* of respiration and *level* of consciousness (secondary survey)? A higher level response usually results for not alert patients or those with abnormal breathing. A frequently occurring Axiom is seen in several TRAUMA-related protocols:

Axiom 2	PROTOCOL **30**

Medical Dispatch should always try to **obtain complete information**. Even if law enforcement personnel initially request "paramedics," response should be driven by specific priority problems (see SEND Protocol).

Allied emergency agencies, such as law enforcement groups, commonly notify EMDs of TRAUMA incidents. They are known as fourth-party callers. Just as a lay caller must answer the EMD's Case Entry protocol questions, fourth-party callers must also answer certain questions for case evaluation objectives to be met. Police (and police dispatchers) calling to report an accident use the SEND card. This specialized "mini-protocol" was developed for allied public safety professionals, to remind them of the EMD's needs. (For a full explanation of the SEND protocol, see Chapter 3: Structure and Function of Priority Dispatch.)

Protocol 30: Traumatic Injuries (Specific)

Sometimes the caller doesn't follow the norm and describes a specific injury, such as, "My friend has broken his arm!" In these cases, the EMD uses protocol 30: Traumatic Injuries (Specific) after completing the Case Entry protocol.

On this protocol, the EMD has two general objectives that guide response determination. First, is the injury old or new? Second, can the injured area be classified

as not DANGEROUS, POSSIBLY DANGEROUS, or DANGEROUS? These are meant to be classifications and are not predictive in nature.

To put the answers to these questions in perspective, the EMD refers to additional information where NON-RECENT is defined:

NON-RECENT	PROTOCOL **30**

Six hours or more have passed since the incident or injury occurred.

A NON-RECENT injury in someone *without* priority symptoms is not as time-critical as other situations, regardless of what part of the body is injured. In general, a lower-priority (COLD) response can be sent.

To classify potential injury severity, the EMD refers to the classification table in the Additional Information section (see fig. 7-1).

Some callers might anxiously shout, "Come quick! She's hurt herself!" This indicates there may be a specific injury. Through the Key Questions, the EMD will determine the site of the injury (if possible), and can then make a dispatch decision based on injury severity, not heightened emotions.

In general, peripheral (extremity) injuries are considered less serious than central injuries. Injuries to DANGEROUS body areas are those to the abdomen, chest (when breathing is abnormal), head (when the patient is not alert), or neck. POSSIBLY DANGEROUS body area injuries are those to the chest (when breathing is normal), genitalia, head (when alert), upper leg (known as the femur), or pelvis. Injuries to other parts of the body are grouped as NOT DANGEROUS. There is a parallel between the EMD's severity designation and how a field provider assesses mechanism of injury and scores the severity of the injury.

When the initial complaint of a specific injury does not include mention of bleeding, the EMD is correct in selecting protocol 30: Traumatic Injuries (Specific). However, if bleeding from a single area is the initial Chief Complaint the Hemorrhage/Lacerations protocol should be selected. When the initial problem, whether an injury or bleeding from a specific area is in question, these protocols may function interchangeably.

If, during the secondary interrogation on protocol 30, the caller answers "Yes" to the question, "Is there any

DANGEROUS Body Area PROTOCOL **30**

- Chest (abnormal breathing)
- Head (not alert)
- Neck

POSSIBLY DANGEROUS Body Area

- Abdomen
- Amputation (excluding finger/toe)
- Back
- Chest (breathing normally)
- Genitalia
- Head (alert)
- Leg, upper (femur)
- Pelvis

NOT DANGEROUS Body Area

- Ankle
- Arm
- Collar bone (clavicle)
- Elbow
- Finger
- Foot
- Hand
- Hip
- Knee
- Leg, lower (tibia)
- Shoulder
- Toe
- Wrist

Fig. 7-1. The MPDS, v11.1 protocols. ©1978-2003 MPC.

serious bleeding?" it is not necessary to SHUNT protocols. Priority dispatch is designed to dispatch such cases from protocol 30 (either BRAVO-2: SERIOUS hemorrhage, or DELTA-1: DANGEROUS body area). Current response theory includes sending the fastest (usually closest) unit for both BRAVO and DELTA levels.

Axiom 1 PROTOCOL **30**

The presence of **SERIOUS hemorrhage** requires a rapid response from the **closest available emergency unit**.

If the same anxious caller reports that it's a finger which has been cut, the EMS response will be less urgent than if it's a knife to the chest.

In cases of amputation, one Key Question determines whether the amputated part has been found. Interestingly, complete amputations seldom involve severe bleeding, since the body has a fail-safe mechanism to pinch severed arteries closed. Incomplete amputations on the other hand, can produce SERIOUS bleeding especially if sharply cut.

A caller reports, "My father fell and hurt his back. Now he says he can't move his feet. Come quick!" Symptoms that can occur when the delicate spinal cord, housed inside the backbone, is bruised or torn are also listed in the additional information section. Symptoms of spinal cord injury are: no pain or movement below the injury, numbness or tingling sensations, and abnormal breathing. In a case like this, the EMD is actually referred during the Key Questions to go to a more specific protocol: 17: Falls.

Post-Dispatch Instructions. Post-Dispatch Instructions for protocol 30 depend largely on the individual case. Unless unique circumstances exist, the patient should not be moved. In minor situations, the patient may have already moved from the site of injury. In one case, a sixth grader heard a loud snapping sound while wrestling with a boy in the churchyard prior to confirmation class. She sat through an hour of the lesson, bolt upright, self-splinting her arm, until the pastor asked, "Are you all right?" She burst into tears of pain and fear. Her collarbone was broken.

If a patient has already moved, encourage the caller to have the patient rest in their current position. People with dislocated shoulders and broken collarbones, for example, prefer to sit and lean forward, self-splinting the affected arm with the other. Do not make them lie down.

The EMD should tell callers not to splint injuries. The best medicine for most fractures, whether obvious or not, is non-movement and reasonable comfort until properly trained and equipped crews arrive.

If the scene is dangerous, the EMD is referred to protocol X-7. Here, the EMD will warn the caller of the suspected danger and ensure the caller does not become a second casualty. If the scene of the incident is not dangerous, for the patient who is both breathing abnormally and not alert, the EMD should ensure the ABCs according to the instructions on protocols A, B, or C. Pre-Arrival Instructions for the alert patient (breathing normally or abnormally) who is not bleeding significantly are found on protocol X-1 and involve keeping the patient comfortable and preventing her/him from eating or drinking.

For the patient who is bleeding significantly, X-5 provides pre-arrival instructions: the caller should apply direct pressure by laying the cleanest cloth available over the site and applying pressure directly to the wound. (The caller can use a hand if the bleeding is serious and nothing else is available.) Direct pressure should be firm and uninterrupted; the caller should not look to see if the bleeding has stopped, since doing so releases the pressure and interrupts clotting. If the bleeding soaks through the cloth, another goes over it and firm pressure is continued.

Rule 2	PROTOCOL 30
Direct pressure on the wound should be **avoided** in the presence of **visible fractured bone** or **foreign objects**.	

Protocol 30 advises the EMD to avoid direct pressure on a wound that contains visible bone fragments or foreign objects. This prevents unnecessary pain for the patient and reduces the chance of further complicating a serious injury.

SERIOUS bleeding, where blood is spurting or copiously pouring from a wound should take precedence over this rule as controlling possibly lethal bleeding is more important than worrying about the patient's comfort, or non-life threatening fracture. The EMD should exercise reasonable judgment when making this type of decision.

In cases of amputation, the caller should locate the amputated parts. There can be detrimental consequences in transporting the victim to the hospital only to discover that the amputated part is still at the scene. Amputated parts should be placed in a clean plastic bag. A very large body part may require a clean garbage-sized bag. Amputations should not be soaked in fluid. The bag can be put in a cool container, but not on ice. Freezing must be avoided.

Dangerous transport speed is not necessary to ensure re-attachment. Seconds do not count here. Proper care of the patient and the amputated part is much more important. Finally, if you need to terminate the call, advise the caller, "If s/he gets worse in any way, call me back immediately for further instructions." This is an excellent universal precaution any time the EMD hangs up before field personnel arrive.

Protocol 21: Hemorrhage/Lacerations

For some reason, humans hate the sight of blood. They panic easily when the red stuff leaks. It used to be that any excited call for bleeding routinely elicited an emergency *over* response. Many ambulance crews can relate stories of responding HOT across town in rush-hour traffic on "a cutting," only to discover a pale would-be cook with a minor finger laceration. Typically, the cook had run cold water over the wound immediately after it occurred. Bleeding always looks worse when blood mixes with water, and running water thins the blood so it doesn't clot as well, either. At least the water was cold!

This protocol is titled "hemorrhage" for a good reason: The word "bleeding" sounds too much like the word "breathing," especially when the caller is excited or there is a lot of static on the radio. This has confused more than one EMD and EMS crew.

Problems associated with bleeding include difficulty controlling the hemorrhage. Loss of enough blood volume can cause hypovolemia (low blood volume), which eventually leads to circulatory collapse and profound shock. Simplistically, shock occurs because there is not enough blood to fill the circulatory system and take oxygen to the vital organs (the brain, liver, kidneys, lungs, and heart). Early symptoms of shock include dizziness, paleness, sweatiness (diaphoresis), and extreme thirst. Later in the process, a person may collapse. Serious shock is uncommon and seldom results from bleeding from minor injuries or peripheral wounds.

Axiom 2	PROTOCOL 21
In most cases, **external bleeding is not as serious as it appears**. Internal bleeding **(from rectum, vomiting, coughing up blood, or 3ʳᵈ TRIMESTER vaginal)** is more serious and **may result in hypovolemic shock**.	

Internal bleeding may be due to either a traumatic or a medical cause. It may become apparent through vomiting, coughing up blood, or bleeding from the rectum. New, undigested blood is bright red. Vomited, digested blood strongly resembles coffee grounds, or, in the case of rectal discharge, black, "tarry" stools.

Traumatic internal bleeding may stem from a blow received in contact sports, an assault, or from hitting the steering wheel in a traffic accident. Certain internal organs can bleed profusely when ruptured, particularly the liver and spleen. Internal bleeding can cause fatal hypovolemia. People in such circumstances need rapid access to a good trauma surgeon in a ready trauma center.

All cases of internal bleeding, except bleeding with urination, are considered either DANGEROUS or POSSIBLY DANGEROUS. Bleeding associated with urination but not associated with significant injury is not a prehospital emergency, although it should be evaluated promptly. However, if a patient has blood in the urine after some type of trauma, the situation is graded as POSSIBLY DANGEROUS.

Rule 1   PROTOCOL 21

EMDs should not delay transport by sending paramedics if a BLS unit at the scene can transport immediately. En route rendezvous is preferable over any transport delay in serious trauma cases.

Axiom 3   PROTOCOL 21

Bleeding is often over-treated to the exclusion of locating and treating **more serious but less obvious injuries and problems**. This often includes failure to perform simple airway maintenance.

SERIOUS Hemorrhage

Uncontrolled bleeding (spurting or pouring) from **any area** or any time a caller reports "serious" bleeding.

MINOR Hemorrhage

Controlled or insignificant external bleeding from any area.

Because IV fluid replacement is usually the realm of paramedics, they are sent when the potential for shock is high. Otherwise, basic life support crews know how to prevent shock, and can often reach the scene and transport promptly.

As every good surgeon knows, uncorrected internal bleeding always ceases—when the patient does. This ironic law helps us to appreciate the importance of undetected internal bleeding.

Second Law of Surgical Medicine   PROTOCOL 21

All bleeding always stops!

DANGEROUS Hemorrhage   PROTOCOL 21

- Armpit
- Groin
- Neck
- Rectal (serious)
- Vomiting (bright red)

POSSIBLY DANGEROUS Hemorrhage

- Abdomen
- Arm, upper
- Chest
- Coughing up
- Face
- Leg, upper
- Mouth trauma (abnormal breathing)
- Urinating (traumatic)
- Vaginal (not pregnant/post-partum)
- Vomiting (coffee grounds)

NOT DANGEROUS Hemorrhage

- Ankle
- Back
- Buttock
- Finger
- Foot
- Forearm
- Hand
- Leg, lower
- Mouth trauma (breathing normally)
- Nose
- Rectal (minor)
- Scalp
- Toe
- Urinating/Catheter (non-traumatic)
- Wrist

Fig. 7-2. The MPDS, v11.1 protocols. ©1978-2003 MPC.

The EMD differentiates bleeding by checking the area classification list in the additional information section. This process allows the EMD to determine the most appropriate, realistic emergency response.

The quality of the bleeding is also taken into account. A history of **hemophilia**—and, by extension, patients who bleed freely due to blood-thinning medicine—boosts any reports of bleeding in NOT DANGEROUS levels to BRAVO. A small cut or bruise can mushroom to a more serious problem for these people.

> ## ! Authors' Note
>
> Having previously read the Second Law of Surgical Medicine, several readers have inquired about the First Law. This law also has dispatch relevance to both stab and gunshot wounds and states, "Nothing bleeds more than the aorta," to which an occasional careless surgeon wielding a sharp scalpel can shakenly attest.

> ## Axiom 5   PROTOCOL 21
>
> It is sometimes **harder to control bleeding in people who have bleeding disorders** (such as hemophilia) or who take blood thinners (such as warfarin). In these people, **MEDICAL** bleeding warrants the upgraded BRAVO response, but **MINOR** traumatic bleeding should be evaluated on a case-by-case basis.

MPDS v11 increases the distinction between TRAUMATIC bleeding and MEDICAL bleeding. MEDICAL bleeding is most often internal bleeding, and will sometimes be discovered when the patient is bleeding through an inserted tube. It is important for the EMD to make a careful selection of bleeding *through* a tube vs. bleeding from *around* a tube at its insertion site.

> ## Axiom 4   PROTOCOL 21
>
> Bleeding from a wound **around** an inserted tube should **not** be considered "hemorrhage through tubes." Hemorrhage through tubes may indicate **internal bleeding** which may benefit from **ALS care.**

The majority of external bleeding is characterized by oozing, such as the bloody (but not serious) bleeding common to abrasions (scrapes) and minor lacerations (small cuts). Even though small cuts bleed a lot at first, by the time the EMD can evaluate and treat a bleeding patient, most bleeding has already slowed or stopped.

There are two types of serious external bleeding: arterial and venous. Arterial blood is bright red, because it has just been enriched with oxygen as it coursed through the lungs. Arteries spurt when they bleed because arterial blood is moved by the pulse associated with each heartbeat. Arterial bleeding can cause significant, rapid blood loss, and can be difficult to control. It can be *fatal.* Fortunately, this is rare. Any report of arterial bleeding raises the severity of the situation—regardless of the site of the injury—to a minimum of serious hemorrhage.

Venous bleeding is less emergent; blood passes through veins at a lower velocity and lower pressure. Venous bleeding has a steady flow and is dark red because it has been depleted of oxygen and is on its way back to the lungs for more.

Seldom does the caller simply report only bleeding when a situation is critical. The EMD is more likely to hear a report of a not alert or NOT BREATHING person, a shooting or stabbing, or some other facet of the problem that leads to a different priority dispatch protocol. Either way—whether the EMD turns to the incident-type protocol (e.g., protocol 27: Stab/Gunshot/Penetrating Trauma) or this one—the call will be handled appropriately.

If vaginal bleeding is reported, the EMD is prompted to GO TO another protocol 24: Pregnancy/Childbirth/Miscarriage. One cause of internal bleeding in females is ectopic pregnancy, where a fertilized egg implants and grows in an abnormal site outside the uterus (womb). A woman can bleed to the point of fainting with little or no external bleeding evidence.

In cases of amputation, the caller is more likely to blurt out the most vivid aspect of the call: "He's cut off his finger!" than to report "bleeding" as the chief complaint. Amputation of a finger is a specific injury, handled on protocol 30: Traumatic Injuries (Specific).

If bleeding of the mouth is complicated with abnormal breathing, the case is classified as POSSIBLY DANGEROUS. This increased classification is also necessary when bleeding with urination can be attributed directly to trauma.

Post-Dispatch Instructions. As always, the EMD is reminded to ensure the ABCs (using protocol A, B, or C) if appropriate. Recall that attention to bleeding control and treatment for shock (handled on protocol X) is an important element of dispatch life support.

About 95 percent of bleeding can be controlled with direct pressure, assuming it is done correctly. A tourniquet is almost never needed. However, it is not uncommon for emergency crews to encounter an overzealous would-be first aider trying to apply one. Improperly done, a tourniquet can result in either worsened bleeding (because the venous flow is shut off but arterial flow is not), or in tissue damage to the limb.

The caller should avoid direct pressure on a wound that contains visible bone fragments or foreign objects. This prevents unnecessary pain for the patient and reduces the chance of further complicating a serious injury.

Rule 2   PROTOCOL 21

Direct pressure on the wound should be **avoided** in the presence of **visible bone** or **foreign objects**.

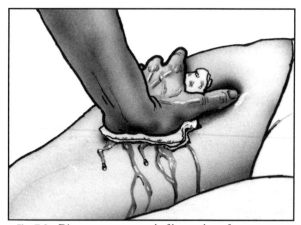

Fig. 7-3. Direct pressure control of hemorrhage from an upper leg laceration.

SERIOUS bleeding, where blood is spurting or copiously pouring from a wound should take precedence over this rule as controlling possibly lethal bleeding is more important that worrying about the patient's comfort or a non-life threatening fracture. The EMD should exercise reasonable judgment when making this type of decision. In thousands of emergency calls, most paramedics have never witnessed a case requiring a tourniquet. It is not part of EMDs' standard of care and practice. For these reasons, an explanation of how to

apply a tourniquet will not be given here. Those interested are welcome to learn about proper application of a tourniquet from a reliable source.

Control of nosebleeds is usually simple and is provided in the Post-Dispatch Instructions.

Post-Dispatch Instructions   PROTOCOL 21

(Nosebleed) Tell her/him to **tightly pinch** the entire soft part of her/his **nose**, right **under** the nasal bone.

Tell her/him to sit **forward** and don't sniff or blow. Just **pinch** her/his nose **firmly** until the emergency unit arrives.

Having the patient lean forward ensures the blood will not run to the back of the throat and into the stomach which can nauseate the patient or cause vomiting and gagging. Do not allow the patient to blow her/his nose. This disrupts clotting and can restart the bleeding.

Patients with blood loss who feel dizzy or faint should be encouraged to lie down. Maintain body temperature; if it is cold, advise helpers to protect the patient from the elements. "If s/he is cold, keep her/him warm." Finally, if you need to terminate the call, advise the caller, "If s/he gets worse in any way call me back immediately for further instructions."

Trauma Due to Assault
The next two protocols focus on trauma due to assault. Such injuries must automatically raise safety issues for emergency responders and callers in the EMD's mind. In a few unique places, EMS is provided by law enforcement officers; they have the skills and equipment to protect themselves and conduct the criminal investigation. In most places, however, the agencies are separate. The EMD must ensure that police or sheriff's officers are also asked to respond on potentially dangerous scenes (see Legend of Symbols–Police Notification fig. 3-4).

These protocols cover the most common assault situations: Assault/Sexual Assault (Rape) and Stab/Gunshot/Penetrating Trauma. The EMD should remember that the initial complaint may not always reflect the true situation. When a caller says something general, "My neighbor is bleeding," or vague, "I feel awful, and I need some help," during Case Entry, the EMD should inquire why, "Tell me exactly what happened?" This may net a reply such as, "Yeah, her father just shot her!" or that the caller has been beaten by her husband.

Assault cases often come through the police dispatcher, raising again the need to use the SEND protocol. This way, on-site police have a ready reference to remind them what initial information to relay to their dispatchers, who can then provide the EMD with specifics matching the basic priority dispatch inquiries. Achieving such cooperation is important and may require effort and patience to achieve good interagency cooperation.

Protocol 4: Assault/Sexual Assault

Assaults are a common, predictable source of emergency calls. Circumstances may include drunken brawls, fistfights, family disturbances, even unprovoked attacks by strangers. Weapons may be fists, feet, scraps of iron or lumber, bricks, or even lamps, crutches, or ladies' purses. A caller may report specifics, such as a report of uncontrollable bleeding, fractures, cuts, bruises, unconsciousness, or a sexual assault.

A difference between this Chief Complaint and protocol 30: Traumatic Injuries (Specific) is that assaultive or criminal behavior was involved. Safety issues are important in many of these cases and certain questions up front in this protocol may provide essential scene management information for responders.

The EMD needs to know what part or parts of the body are injured. The goal here is to determine whether the injury is to a NOT DANGEROUS, POSSIBLY DANGEROUS, or DANGEROUS body area. It is also important in rape situations to ask whether there are any other injuries. In the Additional Information section is the same list as protocol 30: Traumatic Injuries (Specific) (see fig. 7.4).

This information dictates, to a large extent, which dispatch determinant will be chosen. Any report of SERIOUS bleeding influences the Dispatch Determinant, as does whether the situation is recent or NON-RECENT.

> **Axiom 2**   PROTOCOL **4**
>
> Injuries to **DANGEROUS** or **POSSIBLY DANGEROUS** body areas take response precedence in sexual assault situations.

NON-RECENT injuries (defined in additional information as greater than six hours) are unlikely to get suddenly worse and are usually not life-threatening. One of the challenges in these cases is highlighted by the Axioms for this protocol:

> **Axiom 1**   PROTOCOL **4**
>
> Assault complaints are generally **3ʳᵈ party** calls and are often received by police dispatch first.

The SEND protocol is included in the Additional Information section to underscore the cooperative interagency nature of this complaint.

> **DANGEROUS Body Area**   PROTOCOL **4**
> - **Chest** (abnormal breathing)
> - **Head** (not alert)
> - **Neck**
>
> **POSSIBLY DANGEROUS Body Area**
> - **Abdomen**
> - **Amputation** (excluding finger/toe)
> - **Back**
> - **Chest** (breathing normally)
> - **Genitalia**
> - **Head** (alert)
> - **Leg, upper** (femur)
> - **Pelvis**
>
> **NOT DANGEROUS Body Area**
> - **Ankle**
> - **Arm**
> - **Collar bone** (clavicle)
> - **Elbow**
> - **Finger**
> - **Foot**
> - **Hand**
> - **Hip**
> - **Knee**
> - **Leg, lower** (tibia)
> - **Shoulder**
> - **Toe**
> - **Wrist**

Fig. 7-4. The MPDS, v11.1 protocols. ©1978-2003 MPC.

Rule 1	PROTOCOL **4**

The **preservation of evidence** in sexual assault situations may be of much greater eventual importance to the patient than initial response and treatment of physical injuries.

Rule 2	PROTOCOL **4**

Sexual assault patients often require a very **high level of compassionate care**.

Rape is a form of assault (sexual assault) with unique characteristics. It is a crime of violence and hate, not of passion. Ultimately, preservation of evidence could be of paramount importance to patient's the long-term well being.

In addition to physical injury and violation, it is also a source of immediate emotional trauma. One misconception about rape is that it is always best to send a woman to help a female victim. The gender of the responding helpers is usually less important to the raped person than is achieving a sense of security and safety. One woman, after being raped repeatedly for several hours finally escaped and called for help. The first person in a uniform to arrive was a very large male police officer. In her mind, all she wanted was to feel safe. Being comforted by this man in a nonsexual manner worked for her. At the same time, however, the EMD must recognize that rape can result in terrible physical injury. Clearly, there are multiple physical, emotional, and psychological levels of concern to be balanced.

Axiom 5	PROTOCOL **4**

Medical Dispatch should always try to **obtain complete information**. Even if law enforcement personnel initially request "paramedics," response should be driven by specific priority problems (see SEND Protocol).

The EMD will inquire during the Case Entry protocol whether more than one person was injured. With multiple victims, the chaos and safety issues that can occur increase the level of response. Another safety-related issue is whether the assailant is still nearby. If so, the EMD will advise responding crews accordingly. Field personnel should know to enter the area cautiously and when to wait for police backup to arrive.

Post-Dispatch Instructions. First, if the assailant is nearby, the EMD cautions the caller to remain safe using protocol X-9. If the assault is still in progress, the EMD advises the caller to stay out of harm's way until the police arrive. If safe to do so, the EMD can ask the caller to ensure the ABCs (using protocols A, B, or C) if appropriate, or can control bleeding (X-5) or ensure patient comfort (X-1). The scene should be left as undisturbed as possible. The caller should not move or touch any weapons.

The caller can try to find any teeth that have been knocked out. Current first aid is to wrap them in a moist, clean cloth and put them in a clean container.

!   Authors' Note

Ziploc™ plastic bags appear to be the new lay-person's container-of-choice for various dislodged or cut-off body parts (e.g., teeth and fingers).

Teeth can often be reseated at the hospital, if done without significant delay (usually within two hours). Even tooth chips can now be re-cemented into place, preventing expensive dental work.

Rape victims (either gender) must be encouraged not to change their clothes, bathe, shower, or go to the bathroom. These activities destroy valuable evidence that may lead to the conviction of the assailant. Unfortunately, legal action may not be an immediate priority to rape victims. They just want to get the filthy feeling associated with the rape off their bodies. The EMD should *tactfully* try to get them to stay as they are while providing a compassionate helping hand.

Protocol 27: Stab/Gunshot/Penetrating Trauma

The demographics of gunshot wounds vary greatly between the U.S. and other countries. More recently, U.S. surgeons and internists have claimed gunshot wounds should be declared a public health epidemic,

Rule 5	PROTOCOL **27**

Protocol 27 should **not be used for insignificant or peripheral puncture wounds** such as household pins, needles, tacks, or stepping on nails. **Use Protocol 21 or 30** as appropriate.

like AIDS.[85] Gun-related deaths reached 39,720 in 1994 and included 13,593 slayings and 20,540 suicides.

Much of the information about stabbings and gunshot wounds is similar to that of assaults. The first priority is the safety of uninjured people, including the caller. Information that there are multiple victims should be sought after carefully during the Case Entry protocol and always generates a DELTA response. Additional Information about the use of the SEND protocol is identical to that on protocol 2: Assault/Sexual Assault.

Axiom 1	PROTOCOL **27**

Immediate transport for CENTRAL wounds should always be considered vital since patients often require operative intervention and trauma center care.

Axiom 2	PROTOCOL **27**

When a problem is NON-RECENT, the presence of current priority symptoms is the issue of most concern, not the location of the injuries per se.

The SEND protocol is also included in the Additional Information section because stabbings and shootings are so often reported by other emergency agencies. Another similar concern is whether the injury can be defined as *recent*, so the definition of NON-RECENT is also included on this protocol. NON-RECENT shooting and stabbing injuries—defined as those six hours or older—are not time-critical emergencies (or the patient would probably be dead already).

One of the EMD's primary goals when confronted by a shooting or stabbing is to determine whether wounds are CENTRAL or PERIPHERAL. A report of multiple wounds, regardless of their location on the body, automatically raises the severity of the case and will generate a delta response. For single wounds, a chart is

Rule 2	PROTOCOL **27**

From a prehospital standpoint, **CENTRAL** wounds are generally much **more serious** than **PERIPHERAL** wounds.

provided to remind the dispatcher which is which. The remaining Axiom and Rules posted on this protocol support this goal.

Besides the trunk, the shoulders, buttocks, groin, and hips are also considered CENTRAL. Stabbings and shootings to the CENTRAL body are best handled by advanced life support providers because IV fluid replacement can be necessary. However, definitive care for these people rests in the surgical suite.[86]

The EMD may or may not receive reports of SERIOUS bleeding. Post-Dispatch Instructions will vary,

Rule 3	PROTOCOL **27**

PERIPHERAL wounds are considered those below the elbow or the knee. Any area that is not clearly **PERIPHERAL** is considered **CENTRAL until proven otherwise**.

CENTRAL Wounds	PROTOCOL **27**

- Abdomen
- Arm, upper (armpit)
- Back
- Buttock
- Chest
- Elbow
- Groin
- Head
- Hip
- Knee
- Leg, upper
- Neck
- Shoulder

PERIPHERAL Wounds

- Finger
- Foot
- Forearm
- Hand
- Leg, lower
- Toe
- Wrist

Fig. 7-5. The MPDS, v11.1 protocols. ©1978-2003 MPC.

depending on the caller's report. Many penetrating wounds cause little or no external bleeding. A caller may report that there is no bleeding, yet the patient may still be bleeding to death internally. However, if this is the case, the onset of the symptoms of shock will serve as a warning, such as diminishing mental alertness often characterized by fainting (or near fainting) earlier on.

The EMD will also have concerns for the safety of arriving field providers and lay persons at the scene. One question asks whether the assailant is still nearby. The answer will influence which Post-Dispatch Instructions apply.

Post-Dispatch Instructions. Shootings, stabbings, and other penetrating injuries that result from violence directed at a person represent a major challenge to the EMD's secondary mission to save lives. Rescuers sometimes take greater than normal risks to help people who have been shot or stabbed. Early advice to the caller (X-9) is, "Keep very quiet and stay out of sight," and for field responders to consider safety. Always verify law enforcement's prompt involvement.

Callers should be instructed to tell the EMD if the assailant leaves the scene and to not disturb the scene or move weapons. This preserves the crime scene. Tell callers that law enforcement officers and the emergency medical personnel are being sent, but that they may not hear them arriving, since responders in many locations do not use lights-and-siren all the way to scenes of violence.

If safe to do so, the caller can begin dispatch life support starting with the Pre-Arrival Instructions on protocol A, B, or C for the not alert patient who is breathing abnormally, protocol X-5 for serious bleeding and protocol X-1 for other situations; these include allowing the patient to rest in a comfortable position and ensuring the patient does not have anything to eat or drink. Impaling weapons, such as penetrating knives, should not be pulled out.

The EMD should also tell the caller to avoid direct pressure on a wound that contains visible bone fragments or foreign objects such as knives. This prevents

unnecessary pain for the patient and reduces the chance of further complicating a serious injury.

However, unlike bone shards or fragments of foreign objects that are found on other protocols, penetrating trauma often involves a clean wound with a well-defined penetrating object. In these cases, it might be possible to control bleeding by applying pressure around the object (without pressing on it).

If the EMD cannot remain on the telephone with the caller, the final instruction should include calling back if the patient (or assailant) leaves the scene.

Protocol 17: Falls

Many variables determine the severity of a fall, such as how far a person fell, how they hit the ground, what caused the fall, and the age of the person. While some people have miraculously survived falls from great height and others have died falling only a few feet, the EMD's rule for assessment is based on the distance they fell as defined in Additional Information.

That is, a six-foot-tall person who falls from a standing position has had a ground-level fall; a person who falls out of a second story window has fallen at least 10 feet.

LONG FALL	PROTOCOL **17**
The patient has fallen from a distance of **six feet/two meters or higher** (i.e., lowest part of the body was above 6ft/2m).	

Long falls are considered potentially critical until proven otherwise.

Rule 2	PROTOCOL **17**
In a **LONG FALL** versus ground-level fall, **distance is a key factor in determining response**.	

Many times, the caller has witnessed a jump or fall from a significant height but knows little more. Bystander first aid may be difficult or impossible when a caller is some distance from the patient and is not personally in contact with the situation.

Rule 4	PROTOCOL **27**
Direct pressure on the wound should be **avoided** in the presence of **visible fractured bone** or **foreign objects**.	

Axiom 1	PROTOCOL **17**
LONG FALLS are often 3rd party calls.	

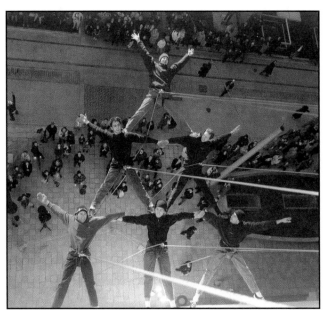

Fig. 7-6. Rapeller (young lady at top) moments before falling over 70 feet. Used with permission. Salt Lake Tribune, 1997.

Callers may have difficulty estimating the height of a fall. Ask how many stories the patient fell; each story of a building is typically 10 to 12 feet high. Try asking the caller to estimate how many times his own height the fall was. If a person is six feet tall, and the patient fell three times his height, the fall was approximately 18 feet.

EMD's First Corollary to Rule for Long Falls

Other than ground level falls, if the caller is **unsure of the distance fallen**, a LONG FALL should be selected.

Keep in mind that these are the exceptions, rather than the rules. Prevention of permanent injury—particularly to the spinal cord—are important rescue and treatment priorities. On this protocol, complaints of abnormal breathing could be related to spinal cord injury to the neck. An injury situated high enough in the spinal cord causes abdominal muscles not normally used for breathing to do the work, resulting in an abnormal, see-saw-like breathing pattern.

The Additional Information section in this protocol is packed with important material. In addition to three Axioms and four Rules, there is a table that the EMD uses to differentiate NOT DANGEROUS, POSSIBLY DANGEROUS, and DANGEROUS injuries according to the area of the body involved. Types of injuries are reviewed in a list (abrasions, amputations, contusions, dislocations,

fractures, and lacerations), as are situations in which possible spinal cord injury could be suspected.

Other key factors are:

- **The part of the body that was injured.** The reference chart in the Additional Information section shows which body areas are considered NOT DANGEROUS, POSSIBLY DANGEROUS, or DANGEROUS.

- **When the fall happened.** Injuries and incidents six hours old (or more) are considered NON-RECENT. Patients are extremely unlikely to be life-threatened as a result of NON-RECENT injuries unless priority symptoms such as altered consciousness, abnormal breathing, or SERIOUS bleeding are present.

- **Whether there is any SERIOUS bleeding.** Typically, if the bleeding is the worst part of the incident, this emerges as the chief complaint and the EMD might

DANGEROUS Body Area	PROTOCOL **17**
• **Chest** (abnormal breathing)	
• **Head** (not alert)	
• **Neck**	
POSSIBLY DANGEROUS Body Area	
• **Abdomen**	
• **Amputation** (excluding finger/toe)	
• **Back**	
• **Chest** (breathing normally)	
• **Genitalia**	
• **Head** (alert)	
• **Leg, upper** (femur)	
• **Pelvis**	
NOT DANGEROUS Body Area	
• **Ankle**	
• **Arm**	
• **Collar bone** (clavicle)	
• **Elbow**	
• **Finger**	
• **Foot**	
• **Hand**	
• **Hip**	
• **Knee**	
• **Leg, lower** (tibia)	
• **Shoulder**	
• **Toe**	
• **Wrist**	

Fig. 7-7. The MPDS, v11.1 protocols. ©1978-2003 MPC.

have initially selected protocol 21: Hemorrhage/ Lacerations. Using either protocol will result in an appropriate response. This information also assists the EMD in determining what to address during Post-Dispatch Instructions.

Age affects the type of injuries suffered in a ground-level fall. When a youthful person trips on a curb, it may generate just a few minor scrapes and bruises. However, the same fall could fracture the brittle bones and fragile soft tissue of an elderly person. In fact, elderly people often fracture hips or other bones in falls from a normal standing position.

Axiom 2   PROTOCOL **17**

Ground-level falls in elderly patients commonly result in hip fractures which are **not prehospital emergencies**.

If an elderly person has an apparent hip fracture, the injury may be painful, but it is not life-threatening. An isolated injury in an elderly person, such as a hip fracture, does not justify use of emergency travel mode. The reason the patient fell can also influence determinants.

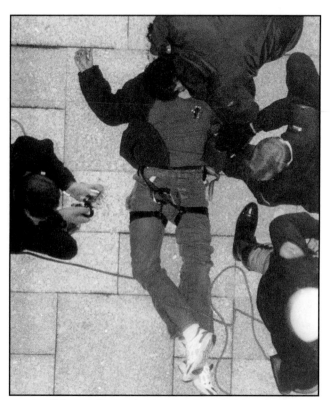

Fig. 7-8. Fallen rapeller. Used with permission. Salt Lake Tribune, 1997.

Rule 1   PROTOCOL **17**

Always consider that the patient's fall may be the **result of a medical problem** (fainting, heart arrhythmia, stroke, etc.).

Any fall associated with alteration or loss of consciousness (such as fainting) is potentially critical; it could have been caused by a transient heart arrhythmia, dehydration, abnormal blood chemistry, seizure, stroke, or other underlying causes.

At times, the cause of the fall or injury becomes more evident during interrogation, influencing selection of a more specific protocol. "She fainted!" prompts the EMD to go to protocol 31: Unconsciousness/Fainting (Near). "He had the power saw on. I think he's been electrocuted!" sends the EMD to protocol 15: Electrocution/Lightning with its special safety features.

Post-Dispatch Instructions. The EMD's instructions to the caller can prevent devastating injury.

Axiom 3   PROTOCOL **17**

Prevention of permanent nerve injury is a **major goal of rescue and treatment**.

Spinal and head injury are significant and important possible consequences of any fall. A quarter of a million Americans are living with spinal cord injuries. Cure Paralysis Now (an association for the advancement of the cure for spinal cord paralysis) reports that yearly there are 32 new spinal injuries per million population—about 8,000 new injuries each year. A further 5,000 people, who suffer severe spinal trauma, die before reaching the hospital. Most spinal cord injuries result in paralysis or loss of function. Paralysis occurs when the neural connections between the brain and the limbs are severed or damaged. Paraplegia refers to spinal damage that paralyzes just the lower limbs, while quadriplegia affects the arms and the legs; paraplegia and quadriplegia are further classified as complete (total loss of sensation and function below the injury level) and incomplete (partial loss).

Statistically, when the entire spinal injury population is examined, incomplete quadriplegia results from the largest fraction of spinal cord injuries ($\approx$31 percent), closely followed by complete paraplegia ($\approx$28 percent), incomplete paraplegia ($\approx$23 percent), and complete quadriplegia ($\approx$18 percent). These proportions change markedly in different age groups, with spinal injuries in older populations leading to proportionally more quadriplegia (65 percent in the over 60 group and almost 90 percent in the over 75 group).

Around 80 percent of people who have spinal cord injuries are male, and the highest injury rate occurs in younger people (age 16 to 30). Motor vehicle accidents are the leading cause (≈44 percent) followed by acts of violence (≈24 percent), falls (≈22 percent), and sports (≈8 percent; 66 percent of sports-related injuries are from diving, and over 90 percent of all sports-related spinal cord injuries result in quadriplegia). In older populations, falls become the most common cause of spinal cord injury (and acts of violence and sports-related injuries become less common).

People who suffer complete spinal cord lesions above the third cervical vertebra (C3) die before receiving any medical attention. Those that survive C3 cord injuries usually remain dependent on mechanical respirators. Over 80 percent of patients who survive the first 24 hours after a spinal cord injury are likely to still be alive 10 years later, but less than one percent will experience a full recovery. From an emergency medicine perspective, half of all patients who suffer spinal cord damage will present with additional injuries.

Some dazed patients have gotten up and walked around with neck fractures without recognizing significant pain or deficit after a trauma incident, but this could risk injury to the spinal cord. Symptoms of possible spinal cord injury are reviewed in the additional information section.

Spinal Injury Suspected if: PROTOCOL **17**
• Abnormal breathing • Diving accident (or jumping into water from a height) • **LONG FALL** (≥6ft/2m) has occured • Massive facial or head injury present • No pain or movement below injury • Tingling sensation or numbness in extremities • Unconsciousness at a trauma scene

In cases where spinal injury is suspected, it is important to tell the caller not to move the patient. In the unusual event of an unavoidable life-threat, such as a fire or imminent explosion, the EMD must use good judgment in recommending whether the patient be moved.

In the event of a dangerous situation the EMD is directed to protocol X-7, where instructions include warning the caller about potential dangers and recommending the caller remain at a safe distance. If the fall resulted in SERIOUS hemorrhage, the EMD begins bleeding control with protocol X-5. Patients who are not alert and breathing ineffectively require airway verification and maintenance, and possibly CPR, as directed by protocol A, B, or C.

EMD's First Rule of CPR Liability in Trauma
You can't be any deader than dead.

All other patients will benefit from the observation and supportive care from protocol X, beginning with panel 1. Instructions to the caller not to let the patient eat or drink, and to encourage the patient to "just be still and wait for help to arrive," will reduce the possibility of spinal injury and later surgical complications. Instructions for putting away family pets, collecting medications and physicians' names, and meeting the paramedics may also be appropriate.

Protocol 3: Animal Bites/Attacks

Few animal bites pose serious, even life-threatening harm, and therefore most are not prehospital medical emergencies.[87] Occasionally, however, an animal attack may be vicious. A severe incident may involve a zoo or escaped exotic animal in a location otherwise devoid of large indigenous mammals (like Australia). An EXOTIC animal for dispatch purposes is defined in the Additional Information section.

EXOTIC Animal PROTOCOL **3**
Any animal that may be **poisonous, dangerous,** or **whose risk is unknown.**

For example, one man experienced a severe reaction when his pet Gila monster—a poisonous lizard—bit his neck when he picked it up (to comfort it!) after accidentally dropping the poor reptile.

Assessment of animal bites involves using a table in the Additional Information that classifies bites as involving DANGEROUS, POSSIBLY DANGEROUS, and NOT DANGEROUS body areas. This table (which is consistent on protocols that involve traumatic injury) is only used for mammal bites or for other animals which are clearly not EXOTIC or poisonous.

As the mechanism of injury/harm is more appropriately handled by the protocol that deals with allergies, bites from snakes and spiders, and other venomous penetrations, (stings) from various creatures, are handled on protocol 2: Allergies (Reactions)/Envenomations (Stings, Bites). This axiom is helpful for gaining a rational assessment of what are often fear-producing events.

SUPERFICIAL Bites	PROTOCOL 3
Minor, usually **shallow** (non-penetrating) wounds **without priority symptoms;** even in **DANGEROUS** or **POSSIBLY DANGEROUS** body areas.	

This is because most mammal bites are superficial or isolated on an extremity—a peripheral bite. They usually do not bleed severely because mammal bites typically involve multiple puncture wounds from pointed teeth. Some bites can result in strange amputations. One poor fellow got into a fight with a biting patron at a bar, and lost both the tip of his nose and an ear! (Information related to amputation care can be found on protocol 30: Traumatic Injuries (Specific).) Interestingly, when skin has been broken by a human bite, there is very high likelihood of infection. If the skin and underlying tissues have been ripped or torn, bleeding can be serious, even on a peripheral area of the body. While lions, tigers, bears, crocodiles, and other wild or

Axiom 1	PROTOCOL 3
Most mammal bites are **not prehospital emergencies**. However, **large** animals (lions, tigers, bears, crocodiles, sharks, horses, etc.), **EXOTIC animals**, and even some dogs (pit bulls, rottweilers) are capable of inflicting serious injuries. In these rare cases, a **maximal response** is indicated.	

large animals may only live indigenously in certain habitats in the world, injuries from too close an encounter with one may occur even in urban areas. Zoos, animal parks, carnivals, and strange (even illegal) pets, may be the cause of a rare, but critical, use of this protocol as these animals can cause devastating—and sometimes fatal—injuries.

In 1997, the Centers for Disease Control (CDC) reported that:

From 1979 through 1994 attacks by dogs resulted in 279 deaths in the U.S. Such attacks have prompted widespread review of existing local and state dangerous-dog laws, including proposals for breed-specific restrictions to prevent such episodes.[88]

During 1995 and 1996 at least 25 persons died as the result of dog attacks, twenty (80%) occurred among children 5 months to 11 years of age. All the attacks by unrestrained dogs off the owner's property involved more than one dog and rottweilers were the most commonly reported breed. Most of the 55 million dogs in the U.S. never bite or kill humans.[88]

ATTACK	PROTOCOL 3
A **mauling** (or savaging) which produces **serious, multiple wounds** or **injuries,** as opposed to a single or limited number of "bites" or "stings." Also, any event **in progress.**	

DANGEROUS Body Area   PROTOCOL 3
- Armpit
- Chest (abnormal breathing)
- Groin
- Head (not alert)
- Neck

POSSIBLY DANGEROUS Body Area
- Abdomen
- Amputation (excluding finger/toe)
- Back
- Chest (breathing normally)
- Genitalia
- Head (alert)
- Leg, upper (femur)
- Pelvis

NOT DANGEROUS Body Area
- Ankle
- Arm
- Collar bone (clavicle)
- Elbow
- Finger
- Foot
- Hand
- Hip
- Knee
- Leg, lower (tibia)
- Shoulder
- Toe
- Wrist

Fig. 7-9. The MPDS, v11.1 protocols. ©1978-2003 MPC.

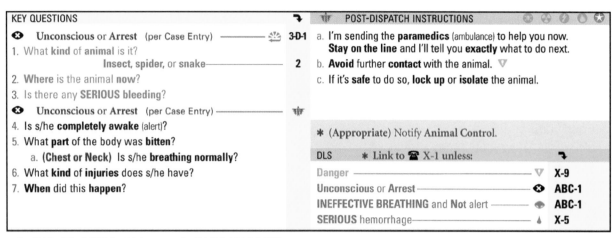

KEY QUESTIONS	↱	POST-DISPATCH INSTRUCTIONS
✪ Unconscious or Arrest (per Case Entry) —— ☸ **3-D-1**		a. I'm sending the **paramedics** (ambulance) to help you now. **Stay on the line** and I'll tell you **exactly** what to do next.
1. What **kind** of **animal** is it?		
Insect, spider, or snake———— **2**		b. **Avoid** further **contact** with the animal. ▽
2. **Where** is the animal **now**?		c. If it's **safe** to do so, **lock up** or **isolate** the animal.
3. Is there any SERIOUS bleeding?		
✪ Unconscious or Arrest (per Case Entry) ——— ⚕		✱ (Appropriate) Notify Animal Control.
4. Is s/he **completely awake** (alert)?		
5. What **part** of the body was **bitten**?		DLS ✱ Link to ☎ X-1 unless: ↱
a. **(Chest or Neck)** Is s/he **breathing normally**?		Danger ——————————— ▽ **X-9**
6. What **kind** of **injuries** does s/he have?		Unconscious or Arrest———————— ✪ **ABC-1**
7. **When** did this **happen**?		INEFFECTIVE BREATHING and Not alert ——— ☁ **ABC-1**
		SERIOUS hemorrhage——————— ⬦ **X-5**

Fig. 7-10. The MPDS, v11.1 protocols. ©1978-2002 MPC.

When an animal attack or bite is involved, the EMD should try to determine the animal's current location for the safety of responding crews, assess appropriateness of Post-Dispatch Instructions and the need to dispatch an animal control officer.

> **! Authors' Note**
>
> The historical evidence about pit bull and rottweiler attacks continues to mount in the U.S. supporting their specific addition to the protocols. One city in the U.S. recently passed an ordinance that states, in part: To keep pit bulls already licensed in the city, owners must prove they are insured or bonded against damages of up to $50,000 for injuries or deaths from pit bull attacks.[89]

Post-Dispatch Instructions. First, those at the scene should be advised to avoid further contact with the animal. Most local laws require animal bites to be reported to the police, animal control officers, or local health department authorities. Inform the caller that these personnel will be notified. Reports of animal attack are important to community health because of the possibility of rabies or other serious disease that can be transmitted by sick animals. If possible, the caller should lock up or isolate the animal for evaluation by health officials; if this cannot be done safely the EMD should go to protocol X-9, where the caller will be advised to keep quiet and out of sight. If the animal has left the scene or has been contained and the patient is unconscious and arresting (or not alert and breathing ineffectively), begin with airway verification and maintenance on protocol A, B, or C and be prepared to progress to CPR if the situation dictates. SERIOUS hemorrhage should be controlled according to the directions on protocol X-5. All other patients will benefit from the supportive care and observation provided on protocol X, beginning with panel 1.

> **! Authors' Note**
>
> This protocol exhibits the uncommon situation in which medically different treatments are found and approved by different Academy Standards Committees in separate areas of the world. The Council of Standards works to always unify these issues whenever possible.

Protocol 16: Eye Problems/Injuries

Significant eye injuries are rare, but because one of the senses is threatened, they can cause high anxiety. There are many causes of eye problems. These may range from mild (usually) to severe (rarely). A table in the Additional Information section classifies eye problems,

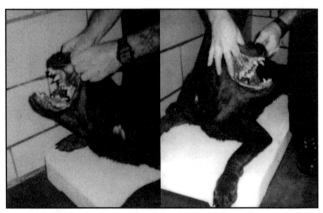

Fig. 7-11. Euthanized rottweiler following its fatal attack on a child in Kansas City, Kansas, U.S.

differenciating them as MINOR, MODERATE, or SEVERE injuries and MEDICAL eye problems. Because of the different causes of eye problems, there are several Axioms and Rules governing their prioritization.

Axiom 1	PROTOCOL **16**
Flash burns from working with or near an arc-welding device **are rarely serious** and often present with a delayed onset of pain.	

Axiom 2	PROTOCOL **16**
Abrasions or scratches from small foreign objects or contact lenses are **usually superficial** but are very painful.	

Rule 2	PROTOCOL **16**
Severe thermal burns to the eye almost always affect the face or head and should be **handled on Protocol 7.**	

MEDICAL eye problems should not be confused with injuries. Weeping or tears from allergies, infections, and other non-traumatic causes are rarely prehospital emergencies.

Abrasions, contact lenses, and small foreign objects are all listed as MINOR eye problems. Care of this type of injury is a basic-level first aid skill.

Axiom 3	PROTOCOL **16**
Chemical injuries to the eye are usually not prehospital emergencies. In general, alkalis (lyes) are worse than acids. **Immediate, continuous flushing with water is required.**	

However, chemical burns are listed as MODERATE on the classification list because of common variations in local responses. By listing this as a separate sub-determinant code 16-A-1 MODERATE eye injuries from 16-A-2 MINOR eye injuries, agencies can elect (or not) to send hazardous materials specialists in addition to the ambulance crew because of the possible nature of the chemicals involved.

An orbital fracture occurs when the bones surrounding the eye socket are broken. Major injuries can result in

Axiom 4	PROTOCOL **16**
Major injuries caused by direct blows to the eye include orbital fractures, hyphema (blood in front of the iris), and retinal detachment. **Penetrating wounds of the eyeball are considered very serious** and require careful, gentle care.	

SEVERE Eye Injuries	PROTOCOL **16**
• Direct blow	
• Eyeball cut open	
• Eyeball leaking fluid (traumatic)	
• Flying object	
• Penetrating object	

MODERATE Eye Injuries	
• Chemical burn	
• Chemical in eye	

MINOR Eye Injuries	
• Abrasion	
• Contact lens	
• Small foreign object	
• Welding (flash burn)	

MEDICAL Eye Problems	
• Allergy	
• Infection	
• Tears	

Fig. 7-12. The MPDS, v11.1 protocols. ©1978-2003 MPC.

blindness; the less eye fluid lost, the better. Another severe injury is eyeball displacement, which signals severe trauma both to facial structures and to the eyeball and optic nerve. The outcome of either situation may depend on the careful and gentle application of Post-Dispatch Instructions.

> **Rule 1**   PROTOCOL **16**
>
> For **SEVERE eye injuries**, no treatment should be given until emergency units arrive.

A direct blow or a flying object that lands against the eye or pierces it can potentially cause a severe injury. The chance of partial or complete vision loss is especially high if the injury involves leakage of either of the fluids inside the eyeball. These fluids, **vitreous humor** and **aqueous humor**, give the eyeball its shape and grapelike compressibility. They do not regenerate well if their integrity is interrupted.

In trauma situations, it may be difficult for the caller to ascertain whether the eye fluid is leaking; caution the caller not to touch the area to find out. The fluid referred to in key question 3 should never be confused with other watery discharges from non-traumatic medical conditions (such as infections) or allergies (such as hayfever).

> **! Authors' Note**
>
> The absence of a traumatic mechanism of injury was not accounted for in this protocol in the 10.2 version. This resulted in a BRAVO rather than an ALPHA response code for occasionally reported "yes" answers to Key Question 3 when medical problems were encountered. The Council of Standards rectified this by adding a trauma qualifier to the key question, "(Trauma) Is the eyeball cut open or is fluid leaking out of it?" and by adding "Medical Eye Problems" to the minor classification list in version 11.1.

One of the overriding concerns of an eye injury is whether there is associated head TRAUMA, although it is unlikely that a caller would report an isolated eye injury as the Chief Complaint if a head injury were also present. If there is any report of a change in level of consciousness, the EMD should suspect a larger problem might exist.

Very rarely, a Chief Complaint of such eye problems as sudden-onset blindness stems from NON-TRAUMATIC causes. The most familiar is retinal detachment. There is a thin membrane, known as the retina, that hugs the back surface of the inside of the eye and collects light images then transmits them via the optic nerve to the brain. It channels information to the brain for interpretation. Sometimes it spontaneously detaches from the wall of the eyeball. In extremely unusual cases, sudden onset, NON-TRAUMATIC blindness occurs for other brain-related medical causes. Prehospital treatment is gentle care and gentle transport. This is apparently a very rare emergency occurrence as the authors' have not heard of a dispatcher encountering one.

Post-Dispatch Instructions. There is no time to lose with chemical injuries; the caller must flush the patient's eye(s) immediately with copious amounts of water. Continue this until help arrives. The fluid stream should be gentle but steady, as squirting water causes unnecessary discomfort.

If there is any chance the eyeball has been cut or torn, there should be no irrigation. This could dilute or wash away the vitreous or aqueous fluid, or introduce infection. The eye should not be touched or bandaged by bystanders. Penetrating objects must not be removed. Prehospital care of this injury requires the attention of trained basic life support professionals. Since both eyes move together, they may cover both eyes with a non-compressive dressing (working around a penetrating object). This minimizes spontaneous eye movement until hospital intervention is possible.

Generally, any patient with an eye problem must be encouraged not to rub or press the eye.

Protocol 7: Burns (Scalds)/Explosion

There are many ways to be burned. The EMD may hear a report of heat injury (such as steam or an iron), fire-related injury, electrical injury, chemical burns, or injuries related to an explosion. The EMD determines whether there are multiple patients in burn and explosion incidents from the Case Entry protocol. Expect the person calling to report burns and explosions to be unusually excited—but rarely hysterical. These are frightening events. Explosions may be mass casualty events; in these cases, the EMD may also use the local disaster protocol.

There are definite safety issues related to this protocol. The EMD will need to know if the patient is away from the source of the injury and danger. Keep in mind, too, that burns are not always accidental. Burns are an unfortunately common source of child abuse; a child may be dipped into scalding water, burned with cigarettes, pressed against a heater grate, or become the victim of other cruel realities.

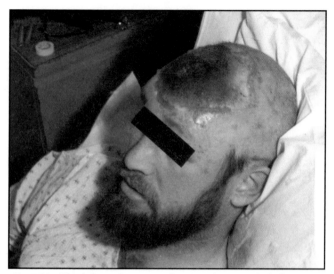

Fig. 7-13. Third-degree burn extending into the patient's skull.

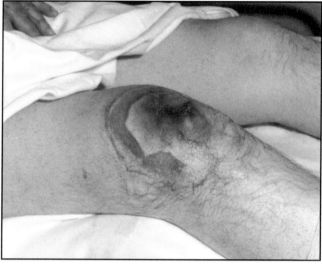

Fig. 7-14. Complete third-degree burn that required cross-leg, full-thickness flap grafts.

Malicious acts involving burn injuries are not limited to children. In a bizarre series of acts of vengeance, one U.S. city had several episodes in which hot grease or boiling water was poured onto the genitals of a sleeping, unfaithful partner. And one unsuspecting EMT, unwisely pursuing an enraged husband into the kitchen, was burned when the man threw a pot of boiling water at his face. Criminal situations sometimes underlie burn injuries. If an EMD suspects a burn injury due to interpersonal violence, responding crews should be notified and police cover sent.

> **! Authors' Note**
>
> Occasionally concerns may arise regarding the presence of burns to the face and why a higher response is not specifically afforded to it in the MPDS coding options. A burn to the face can be associated with more serious burns to the airway. The current protocol correctly handles this possibility by assessing the two most important signs and symptoms of an airway burn: difficulty breathing and/or not alertness. The medical concern with missing an airway burn has been stressed to paramedics and emergency department personnel to remember when caring for an *unconscious burn* victim. A conscious victim would be very unlikely to have a significant airway burn without concurrent priority symptoms; at minimum, some difficulty breathing.

> **Rule 4**   PROTOCOL **7**
> All electrical burns are considered to be **worse than they look externally.**

Electrical burns are potentially very serious, yet they can appear minor. Electrical current can devastate internal body tissue. It follows the path of least resistance, so if it enters at the hand, for example, it may burst out at the foot after causing a swath of injury through the body. Cardiac injury is to be suspected and can be fatal.

Electrocution patients must be treated and monitored very carefully. Usually, electrocutions, including lightning strikes, resulting in serious injuries will be called in as such; the EMD will use protocol 15: Electrocution/Lightning (Chapter 8: Time-Life Priority Situations).

Chemical burns can also be deceptive. Once a dangerous chemical contacts the skin, it can continue to burn through several layers of tissue. The best aid is to flush the area copiously and continuously with water. Many chemicals cannot simply be wiped away. Additional first-aid instructions should be sought from a regionalized poison control or burn center.

Burns can be categorized as superficial, partial, or full thickness. These terms correlate with a medically, near obsolete, but more familiar system: first, second, and third degree burns.

• **Superficial burns** (first degree) involve reddening and pain on the skin surface. A sunburn is the most common form of superficial burn.

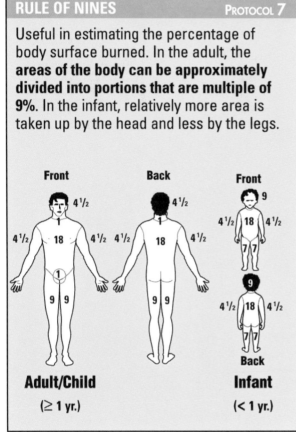

Rule 2   PROTOCOL **7**

Use the **RULE OF NINES** to determine the approximate size of the burn for response assignment purposes.

RULE OF NINES   PROTOCOL **7**

Useful in estimating the percentage of body surface burned. In the adult, the **areas of the body can be approximately divided into portions that are multiple of 9%.** In the infant, relatively more area is taken up by the head and less by the legs.

Front   **Back**   **Front**

Adult/Child   **Infant**
(≥ 1 yr.)   (< 1 yr.)

Fig. 7-15. The MPDS, v11.1 protocols. ©1978-2002 MPC.

- **Partial-thickness** (second degree) burns involve blistering of the skin, with reddening and considerable pain, since the nerve ends are exposed and injured but not deadened. Blisters may not appear rapidly. The blistering may consist of huge, fluid-filled blisters; it is not uncommon for these blisters to easily pop with movement or rough handling. It is best to leave them intact to minimize the risk of infection.

- **Full-thickness** (third degree) burns penetrate the skin and invade underlying tissues such as fat, muscles, nerves, even bone. Skin grafting will be needed. Because the nerves have been deadened, full thickness burns are not as painful—except that adjacent tissue usually has partial-thickness burns, which are painful.

Part of the EMD's task is to gain a basic idea of the extent of the burns. The RULE OF NINES is the time-honored method for determining the extent of a burn injury. However, the EMD should not to get bogged down with the mathematics of this rule, but should estimate quickly as close to the described sized as possible—*without going under*. Keep in mind that burns are often obscured by clothing or soot. The exact percentage of burns is nearly impossible to determine accurately in the field—and over the telephone. The EMD uses a general idea of the extent of burns based on the RULE OF NINES when providing the most helpful PDIs.

Diminished levels of consciousness in burn or explosion situations may occur because of smoke inhalation, oxygen deprivation, or head TRAUMA. Difficulty breathing is similarly common. Where there is smoke, there is often smoke inhalation. People can have minor burns, yet sustain life-threatening injuries from the smoke (and from carbon monoxide which is almost always present in smoke). Smoke is also heavily laden with other toxins. SEVERE RESPIRATORY DISTRESS, which can result from smoke or other inhalations, is defined in the Additional Information as changing color (often turning blue or purple) or difficulty speaking between breaths.

Rule 3   PROTOCOL **7**

Relay to responders a **simple description of burned areas**, not the **RULE OF NINES** percentage (%). A description is the more useful form of information.

The EMD should also be alert for some symptoms that are defined as INEFFECTIVE BREATHING (see the Case Entry protocol Additional Information Section).

A priority for the EMD is to ask whether anything is still burning and whether there are other environmental hazards. Although this point may seem too obvious to believe, assumptions are easy to make. If fire suppression or hazardous materials teams are not sent along with the emergency medical care providers, when needed, the results could be dreadful.

First Law of Burns   PROTOCOL **7**

If someone was burned, something might be burning.

Short by a Measure: Burn Size Assessment

Very often, personnel at community hospitals aren't so good at estimating the size of burn wounds before transferring patients to a burn center. Errors are wildest on smaller burns, with more accurate assessments observed with larger burn sizes. So say a medical team recently in the Journal of Trauma.[90]

Burn Size Assessment: The difference is not merely academic; burn size determines the allocation of resources, medical management, insurance reimbursement, and other healthcare areas. For a prospective study, the records of 132 burn patients were reviewed. In almost half of the cases, the pre-transfer computation of burn size was overestimated by 25 percent or more. Eighteen percent were overestimated by 100 percent or more.

The largest errors were seen on the smaller burns, which makes sense since a smaller discrepancy can calculate out to be a larger proportion. But more critically, the authors found that 60 percent of the referring hospitals had no "apparent formal method" for accurately measuring burn size. Even where available, illustrated charts were "poorly utilized." There are no new lessons here, except that despite the wizardry of modern technology, the value of a mnemonic such as the Rule of Nines should not be underestimated.

Fig. 7-16. Overestimation of burn size study by Hammond and Ward.[90] Reprinted by permission of JEMS, April 1988.[91]

Post-Dispatch Instructions. Advise the caller to stop any ongoing burning process. Flaming or smoldering clothes should be doused with water, smothered with blankets, or rolled against the ground. If the caller is *safely* able, the patient should be removed from any hazardous area. Impress on the caller not to go in if there is *any* question of danger. The EMD may be dealing with a caller whose physical capabilities are not up to their willingness to help.

Axiom 3   PROTOCOL 7

Most scene care for burn patients is **supportive and compassionate.**

Once the caller has extinguished any burning or smoldering clothing and has been reassured that help is on the way as outlined in the Post-Dispatch Instructions, the EMD should refer to the DLS links on protocol 7. As many situations, as minor as sunburn to as major as large explosions or fires, there are several DLS links from protocol 7 and the EMD should carefully select the correct one.

The highest priority is scene safety. In a building fire, or in an explosion situation where subsequent explosions are possible or likely, the EMD's first priority should be to ensure that the caller does not become another casualty. In these situations, the EMD turns to protocol X-12, and advises the caller "If it's too dangerous to stay where you are, and you think you can leave safely, get away and call me from somewhere safe."

If the EMD (and caller) believe the scene is safe, the next priority should be airway control if appropriate. If the patient is arresting, or if the patient is not alert and breathing ineffectively, the EMD begins with airway evaluation on protocol A, B, or C as appropriate and continues with CPR if necessary. If there is SERIOUS hemorrhage or amputation, the EMD should turn to protocol X-5, to initiate bleeding control and amputated part recovery. The choice between evaluating the airway or controlling bleeding in the patient who is not alert, breathing ineffectively, and bleeding badly is a difficult one, and must be decided on a case-by-case basis depending on the severity of bleeding, level of consciousness, and nature of breathing difficulty.

The alert patient who has been burned will benefit from cooling the burned area. Instructions for cooling and flushing burns are given on protocol X-13. A good method is running a gentle stream of water across the injury at a faucet, or even with a garden hose. If this is impossible, a clean rag can be dipped in cold water and

---

Axiom 1   PROTOCOL 7

Pediatric patients or patients with **large burns** may develop hypothermia when **exposed to prolonged cooling with water.**

Axiom 2   PROTOCOL 7

Use caution when cooling burns in cold climates or in areas with prolonged response times.

---

applied gently to the injury. Remind the caller to cool the rag with fresh water periodically, as it will quickly draw in heat from the injury.

Burns are emotionally and physically devastating. Often, once cooling has been started, compassionate care by the EMD (and caller) is the best course of action for any patient.

While burns are often extremely painful and relief from cooling is often significant, the EMD should be aware of the danger of hypothermia developing in a burn patient if cooling is too aggressive or prolonged. This is a particular issue with pediatric patients or in situations where the climate is very cold or the response times are fairly long.

Chemical burns should be generously flushed with water until prehospital crews arrive (X-13). This is best done with a garden hose, a sink hand sprayer, or in a shower. If the chemical is dry, the victim should brush away as much of it as possible before removing the clothing, and then flush with water.

The EMD should begin with protocol X-1, for patients who are not handled by the specifically-linked exit instructions; however, all burn patients, regardless of other Pre-Arrival Instructions, will additionally benefit from the reassurance and observation provided by protocol X-1.

It's an unfortunate reality that, with the exception of attending to the ABCs, the successful treatment of serious burn victims is a long-term proposition in the hospital, requiring extraordinary empathy and compassion. This level of caring can begin with the *first*, first responder.

Protocol 22: Industrial/Machinery Accidents

A study released in 1998 by the Centers for Disease Control and Prevention found that machinery accidents accounted for 13 percent (11,520) of all job-related deaths (88,622) from 1980 to 1994. Interestingly enough, homicides (13.5 percent) only surpassed machinery accidents in the job-related category beginning in 1990. Among industries, construction-related jobs showed the highest share of deaths (18.2 percent) followed by transportation (17.7 percent), and manufacturing (14 percent).[92]

Industrial and machinery accidents, although low in comparison to other 9-1-1 complaints (approximately

Axiom 1	**PROTOCOL 22**

The **number of people** involved (or hurt) should be determined during Case Entry whenever possible.

Rule 2	**PROTOCOL 22**

If **LIFE STATUS** is **QUESTIONABLE** at the end of all interrogation, a **maximal response should be sent** (DELTA-level).

Axiom 2	**PROTOCOL 22**

Even though these calls are generally 3rd party, it is important to **determine if the patient requires extrication** from machinery.

0.1 percent or less in a sample of MPDS computerized centers), are often a challenge for the EMD to accurately process due to the third and fourth party nature of these events. Significant difficulty with identification of the specific Chief Complaint is often at the core of most calls from industrial settings. The concept of the SHUNT pathway materially aids the EMD in the processing of these situations. The EMD may SHUNT to a different protocol if more specific information, regarding cause of the incident is discovered during Key Questioning.

The first thing the EMD may hear is something like: "Come quick! There's been a machinery accident at International Bumper!" Because of the tie-in to an industrial setting, the EMD begins with this protocol but may move elsewhere as the scenario unfolds. It is important for the EMD to initially determine the *medical* nature of the emergency, as Axiom 1 and Rule 2 demonstrate. Correctly asking, "What's the problem, tell me exactly what happened?" is critically essential here. Questionable life status is defined in the Additional Information as:

LIFE STATUS QUESTIONABLE

Existence of any information suggesting:

- Abnormal Breathing
- Cardiac Arrest
- Major injury
- Unconsciousness
- Uncontrollable bleeding

As the specifics emerge the EMD may find that a person has an arm stuck in a meat grinder, was involved in a tractor rollover, or had a forklift accident. The range of possibilities is endless. Unfortunately, those calling EMS to report industrial or machinery accidents are often third- or second-party callers that have had to leave the scene or area to call. If so, another rule immediately applies.

> **Rule 1**   PROTOCOL **22**
>
> If the patient is caught (trapped or pinned) in machinery, a **maximal response should be sent**, including the appropriate extrication team.

Another reason it is important to ask, "Tell me exactly what happened," is to provide the responders with information relative to the important objective expressed in Axiom 3.

> **Axiom 3**   PROTOCOL **22**
>
> It is very helpful for the **responders to know if the case is TRAUMA or MEDICAL** since different equipment must often be carried long distances to the site.

The EMD continues using this protocol when the patient is trapped or caught in the machinery. Otherwise, because this is a SHUNT protocol, the Key Questions provide several GO TO prompts. If the patient was electrocuted, the EMD selects protocol 15: Electrocution/Lightning. If the patient fell, the EMD selects protocol 17: Falls.

There may be a vague report that the patient is injured. In fact, the EMD may have heard this initially, for example, if the caller said something like, "Come quick! Joe's hand is stuck in the auger. I think it's pretty chewed up!" But there may be more information, and during the Key Questions the caller might remember other pertinent information: "Oh yeah! He fell when the damn goat butted him. He says his back is hurting, too."

There is always the possibility that the "accident" is really a MEDICAL event. If this is the case, the EMD is referred to protocol 26: Sick Person (Specific Diagnosis). If the EMD has already determined that a sick person is still trapped in machinery, the determinant response codes will be selected from the Industrial/

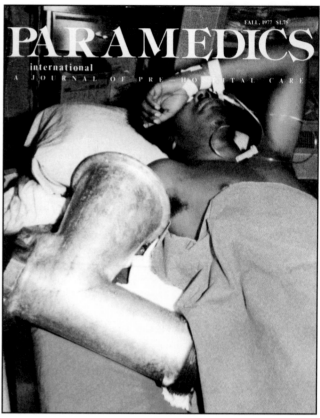

Fig. 7-17. This amazing photo graphically demonstrates a severe machinery entrapment. Used with permission, JEMS magazine, Fall 1977.

Machinery Accidents protocol. However, it will be helpful for responders to know when illness is a contributing cause to any accident.

Industrial and agricultural operations tend to be sprawling and access confusing. It may do no good for EMS to respond to the farmhouse if the injured farmer is in a field best reached through a gate off a dirt road a mile away. Also, patients are sometimes moved from the site of the accident. The caller may know the farmer is being brought to the house by tractor, so the EMD should inquire about the patient's actual location, and how to best access it.

Post-Dispatch Instructions. First, if it is safe, bystanders should be advised to turn off any running machinery. This is both for safety and for ease of communication. Handling an emergency call is hard enough without having to contend with noisy distractions.

The patient should not be moved unless he or she is in danger. In some industrial situations there could also be dangers to the responders or caller; when this is the case the caller should be advised (X-7) to, "Listen carefully.

This could be a very dangerous situation. Do not approach (or touch) the patient at all." All patients will benefit from the supportive care and observation provided by protocol X-1. Patients who are already up and walking should be encouraged to sit or lie down. This is a judgment call; in many cases, the patient was already moved (from fire or imminent danger) before the call came in.

Determine a clear, specific meeting point for the emergency unit and repeat it to the caller for verification. Because industrial and machine accidents tend to occur in hard-to-locate places, the EMD can instruct the caller to make the best access route very clear to responding crews. Many large industrial complexes have several gates and many entrances; someone should stand by each gateway or door on the way to the patient to provide direction to emergency personnel. Those personnel should also be advised to watch for successive waves of rescuers.

Assign someone to guide the first-in emergency unit all the way to the patient. This person can meet the EMS vehicle at the gate and ride in. For very difficult locations, industrial site personnel should be posted at regular intervals to direct EMS responders to the next guide. If the call is at a remote part of a ranch or farm, similar guidance measures should be established.

Protocol 29: Traffic/Transportaion Accidents

U.S. drivers traveled almost 2.5 *trillion* miles in 1995. There are approximately 200 million registered vehicles in the U.S. alone.[93] Traffic accidents are among the most common reasons people call for emergency medical help. In fact, they are usually referred to now as collisions, not accidents, since research has demonstrated that most are avoidable or preventable incidents. Traffic incidents can range from simple, one-car, non-injury events to complex, multi-patient, multi-vehicle, critical injury situations.

People may sometimes be trapped in the wreckage. According to the U.S. National Highway Traffic Safety Administration, in 1995, there were some 6.6 million motor vehicle accidents reported, with 3.3 million injuries and 41,798 fatalities. In all, about 33 percent of all accidents result in injuries of some type. Less than one percent (0.6 percent) of accidents are fatal.[93]

During the Case Entry protocol evaluation, the first three questions posed are location, callback number, and Chief Complaint. When hearing, "There's been a traffic accident!" the EMD should turn directly to protocol 29: Traffic/Transportaion Accidents (Road Traffic Accidents or RTAs in the U.K. and Australia) *after* determining the number of patients. There, the Key Questions generate the answers to the remaining Case Entry protocol questions (plus others).

While turning to protocol 29, the EMD should follow Axiom 1 and Rule 2:

Axiom 1   PROTOCOL **29**
The **nature of the accident** (such as a rollover) and **number injured** should be determined during Case Entry.

Rule 2   PROTOCOL **29**
The patient's **age does not formally need to be determined initially in traffic accidents** (and other multiple patient events). If individual patient assessment is possible, age should be determined at that time.

Sometimes patients are treated by field providers solely because the "mechanism of injury" suggests the need. That is, the traumatic forces they have apparently survived should have caused worse injuries; this is an important precaution. Throughout MPDS v11, increased emphasis has been placed on mechanism of injury concerns. The EMD uses an index of suspicion

---

3. What's the **problem**, tell me **exactly** what happened?

        Hanging ————————————————————————— 🌱 **9-E-3**

        Underwater ——————————————————————— 🌱 **9-E-6**

  a. **(Not obvious)** Are you **with** the patient **now**?

  b. **(Not obvious)** How **many** (other) people are hurt (sick)?

        Traffic/Transportation accident ——————————— **29**

        Multiple victims ——————————————————— **CC**

Fig. 7-18. The MPDS, v11.1 protocols. ©1978-2002 MPC.

HIGH MECHANISM PROTOCOL **29**

Any evidence to suggest serious injuries to any patient as a result of the mechanism of injury. Incidents may include:

a – All-terrain
b – Auto-bicycle/motorcycle
c – Auto-pedestrian
d – Ejection
e – Personal watercraft
f – Rollovers
g – Vehicle off bridge/height

---

for certain HIGH MECHANISM traffic incidents: all terrain vehicles, auto-bicycle/motorcycle, auto-pedestrian, ejection, personal watercraft, rollovers, and vehicle off bridge/height. These accidents prompt a DELTA-level response regardless of reported injuries, since the mechanism of injury makes injuries potentially critical. The EMD should understand the concept of HIGH MECHANISM before s/he has need of it during use of protocol 29.

In general, HIGH MECHANISM of injury is a consequence of the kinetic energy of the collision and is possible when there is high speed involved in an accident or when the items involved in the accident are very large or of significantly different sizes. The list of specific HIGH MECHANISM events on protocol 29 only contain those most commonly seen in the EMS system. Almost any collision, from horserider vs. tree to semi-truck vs. train, could potentially involve such injuries.

Axiom 4 PROTOCOL **29**

A traffic accident in which injury to a **NOT DANGEROUS** Body Area is **reported but not verified by a 1ˢᵗ party caller**, should be classified as Injuries (29-B-1) because of the mechanism of injury.

Axiom 3 PROTOCOL **29**

In **single vehicle** accidents (car vs. pole, car off the road) consider medical problems such as fainting, heart attack, diabetes, etc. as a **possible cause**.

Patients in traffic collisions often sustain serious head injuries. Not uncommonly, breathing is affected. SEVERE RESPIRATORY DISTRESS is defined on several other protocols (see for example protocol 6).

The EMD must determine whether there are injuries, and, if there are, whether they can be classified as NOT DANGEROUS. A list of areas of the body where injuries are statistically considered NOT DANGEROUS is supplied in Additional Information.

If there is a report that patients are trapped, the EMD must be sure the appropriate extrication crew is also dispatched. Likewise, for cases involving hazardous materials. People sitting in cars are, at times, confused with "trapped" victims. Clarification here is important to prevent over-response of specialized extrication personnel.

In single-vehicle incidents, the EMD should also try to ascertain *why* such an incident occurred. This, of course, may not be possible but again "a thing not looked for is seldom found." Underlying MEDICAL causes—including seizures, or even inadvertent carbon monoxide poisoning—occasionally precipitate accidents. This information does not change the EMD's actions, but does add to the complexity of some of the traumatic events confronting them.

MAJOR INCIDENT PROTOCOL **29**

Any evidence to suggest serious injuries to multiple patients or a need for increased resources due to the size of the event. Incidents may include:

a – Aircraft   d – Train
b – Bus   e – Watercraft
c – Subway/Metro

Axiom 2 PROTOCOL **29**

A caller who is in close proximity to a non-hazardous scene should be asked to return to the patient(s) to **check ABCs** and for **SERIOUS hemorrhage**.

Post-Dispatch Instructions. Because traffic collisions do not always occur near a telephone, the caller may be miles from the scene. Increasingly, someone with a cellular phone will call for help. The caller's involvement

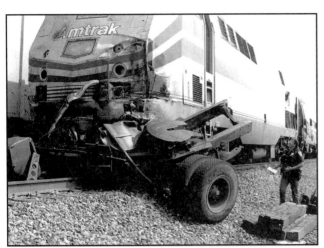

Fig. 7-19. Example of severe mechanism of injury often occurring in vehicle versus train accidents.

Rule 1   PROTOCOL **29**

The **head-tilt is the preferred method of airway control** in the dispatch environment. When a neck injury is likely, an attempt should first be made to open the airway without moving the neck. If this is unsuccessful, then advise to **gently tilt the head back**, a little at a time, until air goes in and the chest rises.

---

at the scene may be complicated by other traffic or precluded by a variety of dangers present.

Advise lay people to leave patients in the positions found, unless their airway clearly needs attention. In one situation, an unconscious patient was found trying to breathe with a closed airway in a car that was hanging off the edge of the road over a creek 20 feet below. Bystanders very carefully opened his airway, but did not attempt to remove him from the car, as the additional motion could have sent the car off the edge. If the need for airway control becomes apparent, remember Rule 1 of Protocol 29.

This is to protect the spinal cord, which should be kept as immobile as reasonably possible until X-rays are taken of the spine.

Bystanders should be advised *not* to splint any injuries and they should *not* move the patient unless he is in immediate danger. Some people are concerned about the risk of fire or explosion at a traffic accident. We know that cars do not blow up nearly as often as they do in the movies. Once the accident is over, the risk of fire in minimal, since fires are most likely to occur during or shortly after impact. The caller can minimize the hazard by simply turning off the ignition.

The caller can also be advised to keep involved parties near the scene. People who can walk after a car accident have a tendency to wander away to find a telephone and notify friends of a delay. If the accident is in an out-of-the-way place, the EMD should direct the caller to watch for the various emergency crews to arrive, and direct them to the patient(s).

Summary

Remember when your mother continuously admonished you, "Watch what you're doing, you're going to get hurt." Because none of us has completely learned yet, this necessarily lengthy chapter must introduce the EMD to a wide variety of traumatic incidents.

The priorities for determining the EMS response often allow basic life support providers to do what they do best—basic trauma care. This includes orthopedic care, spinal immobilization, and bleeding control. When a basic-level provider is allowed to manage scenes of minor to moderate trauma, advanced life support providers in multi-tiered systems are more available for types of calls clearly benefitting from their specialized skills.

There are times that trauma and the way it has occurred and therefore how it is reported generates the need to use other priority dispatch protocols. The EMD sometimes SHUNTS to a different, more relevant protocol once certain more detailed (specific) facts about the call are known. This is an important pre-designed *safety net*. Priority dispatch has the scope to be as specific or general as needed, so the patient's varied problems can be evaluated and handled with the *right* degree of emergency care and response.

> *What you see but can't see over is as good as infinite.*
>
> —*Thomas Carlyle*

The Energy Within

The Energy Within

Mechanism of injury (MOI) is the exchange of forces that results in an injury to the patient(s). In an auto accident, the mechanism of injury is the process by which forces are exchanged between the auto and what it struck, the patient and the interior, and the various tissues and organs as they collide with each other within the body. From that, we can begin to mentally reconstruct the scene or incident and determine if the mechanism was significant .

Since the EMD is remote from the incident and cannot see what happened, we must base our evaluation on the history given to us by our callers and other more subtle pieces of information known to the EMD (knowing the speed limit or traffic patterns of a street where an accident has occurred).

This article will assist the EMD in identifying those incidents where the MOI must take precedence over known injuries when formulating a response. Identifying the most appropriate chief complaint will also be discussed along with those Post-Dispatch Instructions (PDIs) that facilitate better patient safety, triage, and care.

EMD Survival Tools. When choosing the most appropriate chief complaint, EMDs must also consider the MOI. For example, a broken arm caused by a fall from a bike is significantly different than a broken arm caused by a bike versus motor vehicle accident. The arm injury is what we see, but there are more significant life-threatening injuries until proven otherwise in any HIGH MECHANISM type incident. Using this philosophy, a patient involved in an auto-pedestrian, bike, or motorcycle incident is considered to have serious injuries until proven otherwise.

When faced with an individual who fell from a rooftop and who is complaining of minor back pain, again, EMDs will consider this to be a true life-threat and dispatch a DELTA-2 response (Protocol 17, Rule 1) unless the injury is determined to be NON-RECENT (6 hours or more since injury).

Clinically speaking, the reported mechanism may indicate the injuries EMS providers can expect to find upon their arrival. A patient involved in an industrial accident where the chest was hit with a heavy object may have an impaired ability to exchange oxygen due to damaged vital organs within the chest. In these conditions, patients will often present with SEVERE RESPIRATORY DISTRESS as described by the MPDS. In addition to impaired air exchange, there can be other damage from a variety of traumatic forces or mechanisms. The aorta is attached to the body at the top of its arch by the ligamentum arteriosum. This structure holds the aorta in place and is the most common area for shear (deceleration) injuries.

Like the ligamentum arteriosum, the ligamentum teres holds the liver in place within the abdomen. In a deceleration type force, this structure can cause severe injury to the liver, resulting in significant internal bleeding. Other commonly injured organs when deceleration forces are applied to the body are the brain, kidneys, heart, and lungs. This is the reason we try and get specific types of information from our caller. Traffic/Transportation Accident, we ask if anyone was ejected, trapped, or if the incident involves a pedestrian, motorcycle, or bicycle.

According to 1996 accident statistics analyzed by the National Highway Transportation Safety Administration (NHTSA), rollover-type motor vehicle accidents constituted only 13% of light truck towed crashes but accounted for 41% of the significant injuries. It is believed this is due to ejection or entrapment injuries.

On Protocol 17: Falls, we ascertain what caused the fall, and most importantly, how far the individual fell. Once again, the EMD is evaluating and treating the MOI surrounding the traumatic event.

Platinum Ten Minutes, The "Golden Hour" is a term coined by the founder of trauma center care, Dr. R. Adams Cowley. It refers to the one-hour period following severe injuries. Studies show that patients who receive surgical intervention for their injuries in that time frame have improved outcomes. In EMS, we put this thought into everything we do.

(continued on 7.29)

The Energy Within

(continued from 7.28)

Prehospital providers work with the Platinum Ten Minutes, as that is the portion of the Golden Hour we can affect.[86] From on scene arrival of the first EMS providers to being enroute to an appropriate level care center should be no more than 10 minutes whenever possible. This is one reason for Rule 1 on Protocol 21.

If you look at Protocol 15: Electrocution/Lightning you will notice that there is no BLS-only response for someone who has been injured by electricity. The reason for this is that the energy will "go to ground" and must pass through many vital structures within the body in the process. This kind of mechanism produces injury and damage to many vital tissues, organs, and systems within the body. An effort has been made in the MPDS to better respond to those injuries that are more serious. The protocol evaluates and separates injuries by anatomical location, PERIPHERAL and CENTRAL. PERIPHERAL injuries are defined as anything below the elbows or knees, and CENTRAL injuries are above or including the elbow or knees (Protocol 27, Rule 2). This is because the structures and vessels above these anatomical lines are larger and have the propensity to bleed more severely. This severe bleeding causes a change to the patient's level of consciousness and therefore needs rapid intervention. This medical "pearl of wisdom" may also affect the EMD's decision with regards to PDIs and staying with a caller until EMS is on scene.

Law and Order (of Motion). The Law of Inertia, as described by Sir Isaac Newton, helps explain what happens during a motor vehicle accident (MVA). The first part of the law states: "A body in motion will remain in motion unless acted upon by an outside force." Let's use two motor vehicles moving at 65 miles per hour as an example. One car brakes itself to a stop while the other strikes a cement wall. Both vehicles' motion is stopped by an outside force, but with significantly dissimilar outcomes.

The Law of Conservation of Energy states: "Energy can neither be created or destroyed. It is only changed from one form to another." When a vehicle stops itself by using the braking mechanism, the energy of

motion is dissipated into heat through friction into the brakes.

In a MVA, this same energy is dissipated very quickly and changed into sound as the vehicles collide, heat is caused by twisting metal, and injuries occur to the occupants as they collide with the interior of the vehicle.

The "Tonnage Rule" Explained. Kinetic Energy is the energy of motion. It is a function of an object's mass and velocity. The formula used to measure kinetic force illustrates that it is twice as damaging to be hit by a two-pound ball as to be hit by a one-pound ball. It is three times as damaging to be hit by a three-pound ball and so on.

As speed increases, there is an even larger increase in kinetic energy. Being hit by a one-pound baseball traveling at 20 miles per hour is four times worse than being hit with the same ball traveling at 10 miles per hour.

When dealing with auto-pedestrian accidents involving children, there is a triad of events we expect to occur. Children are obviously smaller and lower to the ground than adults are, and we can describe what will happen when they are struck. This phenomenon is known as Waddell's Triad. When a child is struck, the vehicle's bumper will hit the child in the hip and upper leg area, the hood will strike the child in the chest, and the child becomes airborne. The third injury in the triad is caused when the child lands headfirst on the ground.

Kinds of Trauma. Clinically, trauma is defined as a physical injury or wound caused by external force or violence. These wounds can be either blunt (closed) or penetrating (open). A way to look at blunt trauma is the transmission of energy, rather than the object (missile), which produces damage to body tissues or systems. With penetrating trauma, the object (missile) causes the damage as it passes through the body or tissue. With penetrating trauma, energy may also be passed on to surrounding tissue if the energy or force of the object is significant.

(continued on 7.30)

The Energy Within

(continued from 7.29)

When evaluating trauma from the EMD's perspective, we will see both types of traumatic mechanism forces. Most significant injuries associated with motor vehicle accidents fall into the blunt injury pattern while the majority of injuries caused by gunshot or stab wounds fall into the penetrating type.

MOI and The Fourth Law of EMD. EMDs are taught non-discretionary compliance to the protocol. As an instructor, I am often asked why we send a "maximum" response to a patient who has been struck by a vehicle and only reports minor injuries. EMDs, like their field provider counterparts, will treat the MOI regardless of known injuries. Until an on scene assessment of those injuries has ruled out possible underlying trauma, this patient is said to be at risk. In this fashion, we observe clinical practices produced to safeguard patients against unreasonable risk. Even the sub-determinant numbers allow agencies to front-load their system where significant injuries may have been produced by a given MOI. A patient injured in an MVA involving Hazardous Materials is at greater risk for secondary injuries and contamination. The only way to protect the system and our patients is to complete a thorough interrogation of all callers reporting these incidents.

Getting it Right. Faced with a patient who has fallen and sustained a fractured extremity, EMDs must decide which Chief Complaint protocol is more appropriate, fall or traumatic injuries specific. When faced with this question, Brett Patterson of the National Academy's Curriculum Board, produced the following guiding statement:

"If the Chief Complaint includes scene safety issues, choose the protocol that best addresses those issues. When the Chief Complaint involves trauma, use the protocol that best addresses the mechanism of injury (MOI). When the Chief Complaint appears to be medical in nature, choose the protocol that best fits the patient's primary symptom, with priority symptoms taking precedence."

So for the patient who has fallen off a roof and broken a leg, Protocol 17 is best as it deals with the mechanism of the injury. For the individual who tripped on the rug and broke a leg, Protocol 30 is most appropriate. With a report of a broken nose from a bar fight, Protocol 4 deals with both the injury and the safety of everyone involved and is therefore most appropriate. In this same scenario, a caller may report that the patient has a bloody nose. From Protocol 21, the response level would be an ALPHA-level, but using the more appropriate Protocol 4, the level changes to a BRAVO response due to the mechanism of injury.

DLS and MOI. Beyond evaluating the MOI and sending those resources best fitted to deal with suspected injuries, EMDs must be able to provide callers with Post-Dispatch Instructions (PDI) that effectively deal with these scenarios.

The EMD's concern for those patients involved in significant MOI incidents revolves around several key issues.

Traumatic incidents are frequently associated with risk-laden environments. Whenever there are safety issues on PDIs, they are followed by a cautionary symbol. ▽ This denotes to EMDs that this is safety related and must be adhered to. If a caller reports that someone has been struck by a vehicle on an interstate, the caller should be told not to approach the incident unless they feel safe in doing so (Protocol 29, PDI b). When dealing with an electrocution injury, the EMD must read PDI d, which states: If safe to do so, turn off the power…

An appropriate safety guideline for EMDs can be found on Protocol 15 AI which states: "Don't take more victims to the scene."

The meaning here is clear: never put someone else in danger trying to save or help a patient who is known to be in a dangerous environment.

First, Do No Harm. The above-listed First Law of Medical Dispatch is designed to prevent further injury for everyone involved. Of prime concern to the EMD is that the individuals on scene not be allowed

(continued on 7.31)

The Energy Within

(continued from 7.30)

to do something they believe will help, but may cause exacerbation of existing injuries, or primary injury to the intended rescuer. Remember, the road to hell is paved with good intentions. The MPDS Post-Dispatch process deals with the appropriate do's and don'ts that are appropriate and/or possible for callers and the patient.

Airway Control, How and When. As I travel and teach MPDS protocols, one of the most frequently asked questions is "How do I open the airway of a trauma victim without damaging their spinal cord?" Since the only method taught by the Academy is the head-tilt neck-lift, the majority of EMDs feel confused. As remote clinicians, we work in a non-visual environment. This means we can use only those methods that can be easily described and understood by our callers. Trial studies show that untrained individuals are unable to understand other somewhat complicated airway control techniques such as the head-tilt/chin-lift or the jaw-thrust maneuver.

Recent injury studies show that cervical spine injuries are most likely compromised by flexion, rotation, or lateral-type movements. Extension of the c-spine is rarely associated with increased neurological compromise. For EMDs, it comes down to this, if a patient has an uncontrolled airway, they will die. Complications may occur from opening an airway, regardless of which method is used. But remember, if someone has a complication, they are alive, and that is our primary objective. Clearly, the EMD must assess whether any patient mandates aggressive airway control prior to instituting those interventions. This is yet another reason for a complete caller interrogation as the Key Questions are designed to look for those situations that require DLS. For a patient who has fallen and is unconscious with snorous respirations, the EMD may contemplate not getting aggressive, especially if the person is lying on their side. But if the EMD believes for any reason that the patient's ability to exchange oxygen has been compromised,

airway control measures must be taken immediately. If the EMD isn't sure if the patient needs airway control it is better to provide instructions; remember, patients without an airway aren't going to live to walk anyway!

Wow, He's Getting Worse. A trauma patient involved in an incident with significant MOI can worsen quickly and without warning. With significant MOI patterns, whenever possible, the EMD should stay online with the caller and monitor patient condition until EMS providers are on scene. If the EMD allows a caller to hang up for any reason, there needs to be clear, specific instructions regarding what to do if conditions change prior to EMS arrival.

(Protocol "X" has just such a statement located on the bottom of panel 2.) These instructions are very specific and alert the caller to our biggest concern—a change in the patient's level of consciousness. Reading the relevant PDIs from the appropriate Chief Complaint protocol and protocol X is the minimum for all trauma callers who are allowed to disconnect. For the patient who is bleeding, callers need to be reminded not to lift the bandage to look at the injury. They should be told that someone needs to keep pressure on the wound until EMS is on scene. Whenever the EMD suspects exposure is an issue, keeping the patient warm is desirable.

Summary. The EMD is the only clinical provider asked to make decisions about the MOI and appropriate patient care without actually seeing the scene or their patient. Protocol compliance, coupled with the EMD's professional knowledge and skill, has been shown to be a powerful tool for appropriate resource allocation and patient treatment in a remote environment. I would encourage all EMDs to scan the trauma-related protocols and look for those tools and safety valves the MPDS utilizes to better treat mechanism of injury. Your understanding of these processes will make you more confident in your ability to accurately deal with trauma-related scenarios in a fashion that is safe, effective, and reproducible.

Fig. 7-20. "The Energy Within," by Brian Dale. Reprinted from NEMDJ, Summer 1999.

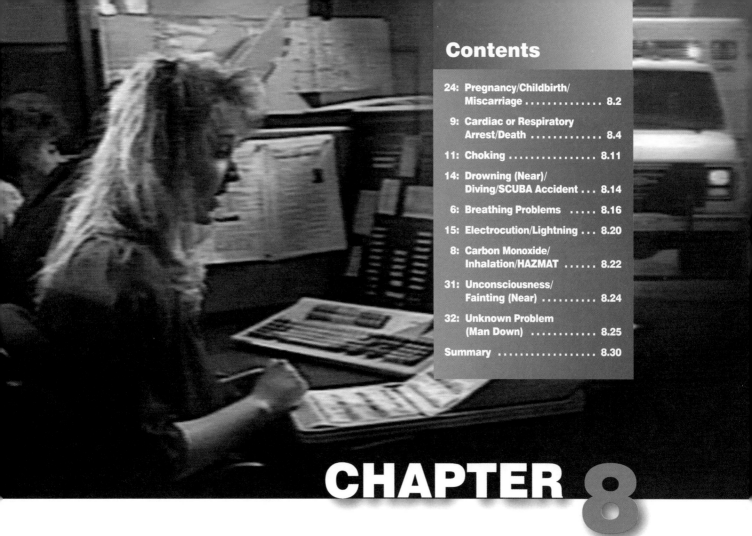

Contents

CHAPTER 8

Time-Life Priority Situations

Chapter Overview

Critical priorities are estimated by outcome to be about 5 to 10 percent of the emergencies that are telephoned into EMS systems. That adds up to a large number of people worldwide needing time-critical or lifesaving assistance every year. The Medical Priority Dispatch System™ identifies nine situations in which a problem poses an immediate time critical or life risk possibility to the patient. Some are medical in nature, others are due to trauma.

Time- or life-critical calls represent some of the closest emotional ties the EMD will have with callers. This can generate a lot of pride—but sensations of frustration as well. Clearly, priority dispatch (especially dispatch life support) has an impact on patient survival. The EMD can make a difference! However, there are losses. In cardiac arrest of all types, the average save rate is less than 1 in 10. To win is to beat the odds! The EMD should not expect to save every life. Priority dispatch provides the potential to save lives, but does not guarantee success every time. EMS is a best-efforts ball game; the won/loss score must not be allowed to define the quality of those efforts.

Listen to the newborn infant's cry at birth—see the death struggles in the final hour—and then declare whether what begins and ends in this way can be intended to be enjoyment.

—Søren Kierkegaard

Time-life priority situations occupy a significant proportion of the EMD's likely call volume. These calls are often difficult as callers are frequently involved with emotionally charged and highly stressful situations. Time-life calls are also difficult because the sense of urgency can lead to calltakers rushing their interrogations and making serious mistakes. The very real possibility of hazardous environments for some of these calls only adds a further level of complexity. In this chapter we will cover the following Chief Complaints:

- Breathing Problems

- Carbon Monoxide/Inhalation/HAZMAT

- Cardiac or Respiratory Arrest/Death

- Choking

- Drowning (Near)/Diving/SCUBA Accident

- Electrocution/Lightning

- Pregnancy/Childbirth/Miscarriage

- Unconscious/Fainting (Near)

- Unknown Problem (Man Down)

Three of the protocols detailed in this chapter—Pregnancy/Childbirth/Miscarriage, Choking, and Cardiac (Respiratory) Arrest/Death—are known as BRIDGE protocols. Recall that this means the protocol itself serves an intermediate role between the Case Entry protocol and the Pre-Arrival Instructions. Through the answers to the Chief Complaint Key Questions, the EMD verifies where to begin in the sequence of Pre-Arrival Instructions before turning to the Dispatch Life Support protocols.

Protocol 24: Pregnancy/Childbirth/Miscarriage

This protocol is a BRIDGE protocol. Numerous unpredictable things can happen to a pregnancy over the course of nine months. One point of differential concern is whether a woman is engaged in full-term childbirth or whether the problem is a complication of pregnancy, such as miscarriage.

Pregnancy is separated into three trimesters, each consisting of three months. The first trimester is from 0 to 3 months (0 to 12 weeks); the second trimester is from 4 to 6 months (13 to 24 weeks); and the third trimester is from 7 to 9 months (25 to 40 weeks). Normal gestation ranges from 37 to 41 weeks; *quickening*, or the first noticeable movement of the fetus, usually occurs in the 18th to 20th weeks.

> **! Authors' Note**
>
> In Australia and New Zealand the number of weeks defining each trimester is slightly different.
>
> | | |
> |---|---|
> | 1st trimester: | 0 to 13 weeks |
> | 2nd trimester: | 14 to 27 weeks |
> | 3rd trimester: | 28 to 40 weeks |
>
> This represents an approved cultural variation in standards.

Miscarriage is the term for loss of pregnancy at a stage when the fetus is not capable of living outside the uterus. This is generally prior to the 26th week, although modern technology is rapidly redefining the definition of neonatal viability. The dispatch definition of miscarriage is when the fetus or products of conception are delivered in the first trimester or in the second trimester up to 20 weeks (5 months).

Other complications of pregnancy include **placenta previa** and **placenta abruptio**. The **placenta** is the highly vascular filtering organ of pregnancy that is attached to the uterine wall and through which the fetus derives nourishment and casts off waste products. In placenta previa, the placenta lies either partially or fully between the fetus and the uterine opening into the birth canal. A sign of this potentially life-threatening condition is *painless* bleeding in the last trimester. Placenta abruptio is sudden, premature, tearing of the placenta away from the uterine wall, usually in the last trimester. It is very painful. Either complication can cause life-threatening bleeding.

> **BRIDGE protocols function as an intermediate step between Case Entry and the delivery of pre-arrival instructions.**

The birth process (**labor**) goes more slowly for **primigravida** women (those having their first baby) than for

> **Axiom 1**   PROTOCOL **24**
>
> In general, first full primigravida patients **progress through labor more slowly** than second plus, full multigravida patients.

multigravida women (those who have delivered more than one child). Labor occurs in three stages.

Stage 1: Dilation of the cervix in preparation for passage of the infant through the birth canal. This part of labor can take many hours, especially for primigravida women.

Stage 2: The period from completion of cervical dilation through expulsion of the child. At this point, labor pains tend to be severe and frequent. For dispatch purposes, delivery is considered imminent in a first-pregnancy when labor pains are two minutes apart (or less). Delivery is considered imminent in multigravida women when labor pains are five minutes apart or less. Rupture of the amniotic sac of fluid may produce a gush of fluid.

A normally positioned infant descends head-first through the vagina, so the top of the head finally begins to show during contractions; this part of the process is called **crowning**. Birth is imminent and the EMD must prepare immediately for another patient.

Rule 1	PROTOCOL **24**

When crowning (top of baby's head is visible) **and/or pushing is present, turn to PAI Childbirth–Delivery sequence "Check Crowning"** (F-5) since **birth is IMMINENT**.

Rule 2	PROTOCOL **24**

Presentation of the cord, hands, feet or buttocks first **(BREECH) is a dire prehospital emergency**. Often the only chance for survival of the baby is at the hospital. (See also PAI Childbirth–Delivery sequence "**BREECH** or **CORD**" F-15.)

Once the baby is delivered, the EMD and the caller must be concerned with the well-being of two people. Each needs careful attention. In particular, the baby must be dried and kept warm, since mild hypothermia occurs easily in newborns.

Stage 3: Delivery of the placenta, also known as the afterbirth. Callers must carefully preserve the afterbirth in a clean plastic bag or basin for inspection. This way, the physician can determine whether the placenta was normal and completely delivered. Partial delivery of the placenta can result in severe bleeding, and retained portions of the placenta can cause serious infection.

The determinants depend in several cases upon whether the pregnancy is first, second, or third trimester. A premature baby is prone to more complications. Sometimes, a mother laboring with a premature baby or those faced with an unexpected out-of-hospital arrival will try to delay birth. This should never be done.

Axiom 2	PROTOCOL **24**

Any attempt to prevent or delay birth can **cause serious brain damage to the baby and even death**.

Once the birthing sequence has begun, there is little that anyone can to do to safely stop it. However, the EMD should understand that, since premature labor and miscarriages may require the same labor as a full-term baby, there is often a pall of disappointment or grief. The EMD can help responding crews prepare for a potentially less-than-happy event.

Third trimester bleeding may be severe, even life-threatening. (The EMD must also remember that a woman can bleed significantly into the abdomen and not bleed externally at all.) Light spotting is not unusual in the first trimester and tends to not to be a time-critical problem. Sometimes, a caller reports an injury to the abdomen of a pregnant woman. Everyone fears injury to the fetus. Fortunately, nature has made it quite difficult to injure a fetus in blunt trauma. In this case, the EMD will select protocol 30: Traumatic Injuries (Specific). There, an abdominal injury is categorized as DANGEROUS. If stabbing or gunshot wound to the abdomen is reported, however, the situation may be much more serious.

It is not uncommon that the caller may report a seizure in a pregnant woman. There is much concern about **eclampsia**, a rare but serious late complication of pregnancy. Its more common precursor, **pre-ecamplsia** involves a triad of symptoms: hypertension (or elevated blood pressure, which is hard on the developing fetus), water retention, and a predisposition to seizures. If a pregnant woman is already having seizures (eclampsia), the EMD will use protocol 12: Convulsions/ Seizures.

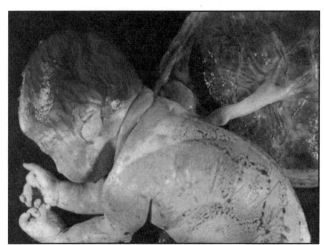

Fig. 8-1. Another possible birthing abnormality is a "nuchal cord" in which one or more loops of umbilical cord are wrapped around the baby's neck. The Childbirth—Delivery PAI advises the EMD how to deal with this problem.

Post-Dispatch Instructions. In a first- or second-party caller situation, the EMD should plan to stay on the phone until help arrives. Tell the caller *not* to try to prevent birth. Some uninformed people will do practically anything, like crossing the woman's legs, to try to prevent birth outside the hospital. Once childbirth is active, it is extremely dangerous to try to stop it.

Once the baby enters the birth canal, the woman often has the sensation, due to rectal stimulation, of needing to have a bowel movement. The EMD should tell the caller not to let the woman sit on the toilet. Some babies have been born into the toilet—a hard start for anyone! Instead, the woman should be encouraged to lie down and take deep breaths in between the labor pains. This will conserve her energy for pushing later.

If birth is imminent, occurring, or has happened, the EMD should assure the caller that help is on the way and go directly to the appropriate pre-arrival instruction panel in protocol F. The EMD will begin with F-1 if birth is imminent, F-5 if delivery is occurring, F-8 if the baby has been born and is breathing, or F-17 if the baby has been born but is not breathing.

Other general principles surrounding childbirth are also found on these protocols. For example, if the baby has been delivered, the caller must dry the baby and keep it warm. A good technique is to lay it on the mother's chest and cover them both carefully, being sure that the child's airway can still be monitored closely. There is no hurry to cut the umbilical cord; this can be done by the paramedics. If ambulance response time is lengthy, the EMD can also warn people at the scene to expect delivery of the placenta within about 20 minutes of the baby's birth.

One final precaution: Childbirth is one of the few usually happy events for EMS providers. It is easy to assume that the parents are excited, too, but this may not always be true. Some people want their babies more than others. Initial parenthood can be frightening. The EMD should be cautious about always assuming this is a happy event until the caller's demeanor indicates the prevailing sentiments at the scene. Then, congratulations are in order!

Protocol 9: Cardiac or Respiratory Arrest/Death

This BRIDGE protocol serves as a buffer between the Case Entry protocol and Pre-Arrival Instructions. Cardiac and respiratory arrest are clearly time-critical events. The following rules embodies one of the most important concepts in prehospital care.

Rule 3   PROTOCOL **9**
An unconscious person in whom breathing cannot be verified by a 2nd party caller (with the patient) is considered to be **in cardiac arrest until proven otherwise**.

The EMD knows during Case Entry interrogation that the chief complaint is critical when the answers to, "Is he breathing?" and, "Is s/he conscious?" are a panicky, terror-stricken, "No!" When the EMD asks what the main problem is, answers will range from, "I think s/he's dead!" to, "I can't get her/him to wake up!" Even before turning to protocol 9, the EMD sends a maximal response because breathing and consciousness are absent. In other situations, the call may come in as, "S/he's breathing funny."

Axiom 1   PROTOCOL **9**
"Funny noises" reported by the caller generally means the patient is unconscious with an uncontrolled airway and often represent agonal (dying) respirations at the **beginning of a cardiac arrest**.

Agonal respirations are the curse of our ability to straightforwardly identify cardiac arrest over the phone.[94] What appears to the caller to be some form of breathing in these unconscious patients is actually ineffective "last-gasp" respiratory attempts as the breathing center in the brain stem eats up the last bit of oxygen left in its breathing pacemaker. These gasps are not effective breathing in any way and seldom last longer than a few seconds, however, in some cases can last over a minute. The abnormal nature and appearance of these gasps cannot be overemphasized. In any patient reported as unconscious, if the caller provides the least suggestion that breathing is irregular, funny, peculiar, strange, or gasping, assume agonal respirations and select protocol 9: Cardiac or Respiratory Arrest/Death. If later pre-arrival instruction verifications reveal that the patient is actually still breathing, the re-coding of the event should be done.

Respiratory arrest that occurs by itself is unusual. It is much more prevalent in infants than any other age group. When someone stops breathing, the heart also soon stops as blood oxygen levels decrease and can no longer sustain the heart. Certain situations, such as choking (when quickly reversed) or drug overdoses (if patients are maintained with mouth-to-mouth breathing) will not necessarily deteriorate into full cardiac arrest. Drowning, severe respiratory insufficiency from long-standing lung disease, and rapid, excessive alcohol intake are other causes of cardiopulmonary arrest that often begin with respiratory failure.

Outright cardiac arrest is most often associated with heart attack. Of some 650,000 sudden deaths from heart attack per year, 350,000 occur *before* the patient gets to the hospital. That means that every minute and a half in the U.S., someone goes into cardiac arrest from a heart attack alone. There are other causes: heart disease, specific diseases in other organ systems, poisoning, anaphylactic shock, severe bleeding (more internal than external), and electrocution.

The EMD must be sensitive to the emotions involved in all sudden prehospital cardiac arrest situations, particularly those involving children. In previously healthy infants who are less than one year old (average age: 6 months) found in cardiac arrest, Sudden Infant Death Syndrome (SIDS) may be the culprit. These particularly tragic situations generate extreme guilt and hysteria in a family. New advice about placing infants ready for sleep on their backs, rather than prone, has significantly reduced deaths due to Sudden Infant Death Syndrome (SIDS) worldwide.

Rule 2	PROTOCOL 9

A healthy child (or young adult) found in cardiac arrest is considered to have a **foreign body airway obstruction until proven otherwise**.

The first Key Question on this protocol again asks, "Did you see what happened?" This is obviously repetitive to the central question posed on Case Entry. It is asked again on purpose because of the great importance of identifying the correct Chief Complaint in an apparent arrest situation. As Bernard Malmud stated, "If your train's on the wrong track, every station you come to is the wrong station." The correct treatment depends on identifying the correct Chief Complaint. The issue of choking always being considered in previously healthy children and young adults is central to this question. If the arrest was witnessed, it is very reasonable to inquire whether the patient choked on anything first as the type of treatment provided after this fork in the evaluation road for a choking patient would be completely different and ineffective. Again, the protocol "knows the rules."

Many people think a person who stops breathing will turn blue. This is not necessarily true. While a report of a person turning blue is good evidence that an oxygenation problem exists, a patient must have a certain amount of blood volume to become cyanotic. If a ruptured aortic aneurysm, ectopic pregnancy, or other bleeding has caused significant loss of blood volume, the patient may be deathly pale (grey), not blue. If a caller reports that the patient is blue, the EMD can confirm this as a potentially critical problem.

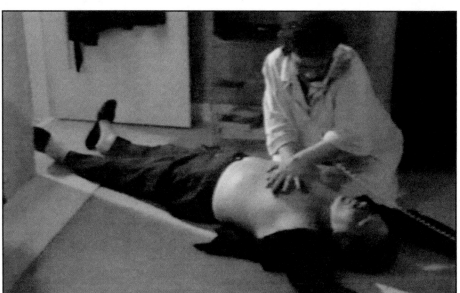

Fig. 8-2. After dragging her motionless, non-breathing husband nearer the phone, a terrified wife is calmed and begins CPR. From *Anonymous Hero*, ©1987 Pyramid Film & Video, Santa Monica, California. Used with permission.

Whenever a caller *volunteers* that the patient is turning grey or *blue*, an override of the the determinant response level is in order.

EMDs who face the task of teaching dispatch life support measures on the telephone to strangers in crisis must be basic life support trained themselves. That gives the EMD a sense for what the caller is being asked to do. Basic life support training includes airway obstruction clearance techniques, mouth-to-mouth breathing, and CPR for adults, children, and infants. All are tasks an EMD might reasonably expect to help a caller do using pre-arrival instructions. Regardless of field experience, delivering telephone instructions in critical cases is difficult and very different from being at the scene. The EMD is forewarned to stick to the script.

The EMD should ask the caller if they saw what happened. Unwanted surprises will be avoided this way. For example, if the caller has not yet mentioned that the patient was electrocuted, that fact could come to light with this question. If the arrest was witnessed, the EMD should inquire whether the patient choked on anything first. If so, the EMD will turn to protocol 11: Choking. If the caller suspects the patient is dead, the EMD should tactfully ask why.

In some cases, it is clear that death is obvious. Wild dogs have half-eaten a frozen body, which has just been found by the river in winter. A decapitation has occurred. The stench of decomposition and a horde of flies surrounds a body found after several hot summer days. A person uncovers the hot tub on Monday for the first time since Saturday's bash and finds a floating body. In cases in which there is *no question* about the situation, an EMS system may elect, when user-defining its dispatch priorities, to send less than a maximal response to confirm the suspicion of irretrievable death. Some situations of obvious death are listed (see figure). The use of the OBVIOUS DEATH categorization is growing.

> As coroner, I must aver, I thoroughly examined her. And she's not only merely dead, she's really most sincerely dead!
>
> —E.Y. Harburg
> Motion picture lyricist
> "The Wizard of Oz"

In February, 1998, USA Today reported that:

> *One of every 10 people nationwide spends the last year of life bedridden by illness, and half suffer physical or mental ills that restrict their ability to function, says a study out today. The study, by the National Center for Health Statistics, is the first in more than a decade to examine how Americans die, says lead author Jim Spitler. Researchers examined more than 2.2 million death certificates and interviewed scores of survivors for more details. Among other findings: 56 percent of people die in hospitals or other medical settings; 19 percent die in nursing homes; and 21 percent die at home.*[95]

It is essential that the EMD carefully follow the complete listed questioning sequence to determine that what initially appears to be "obvious" is indeed *unquestionably* obvious. The term "unquestionable" was initially defined verbally for an inquisitive EMD in Salt Lake. The answer he was given can be used again here. "Unquestionable, Frank, means that you are willing to bet your job on it." He replied, "That's good enough for me, Doc." In essence, if you're not completely sure, do not select a 9-BRAVO-1. It's that simple.

> But we've got to verify it legally to see if she is morally, ethically, spiritually, physically, positively, absolutely, undeniably, and reliably—Dead!
>
> E.Y. Harburg
> Motion-picture lyricist
> "The Wizard of Oz"

OBVIOUS DEATH   PROTOCOL **9**

Local Medical Control must define and authorize (☒) any of the patient conditions below before this determinant can be used. Situations should be unquestionable and may include:

☐ Cold and stiff in a warm environment
☐ Decapitation
☐ Decomposition
☐ Explosive gunshot wound to the head
☐ Incineration
☐ **NON-RECENT** death
☐ Severe injuries obviously incompatible with life
☐ Submersion (> 6hrs)
☐ _____
☐ _____

Approval signature of local Medical Control   Date approved

Fig. 8-3a. The MPDS, v11.1 protocols. ©1978-2003 MPC.

EXPECTED DEATH	PROTOCOL **9**
Local Medical Control must define and authorize (☒) any of the patient conditions below before this determinant can be used. Situations should be unquestionable and may include:	
☐ Terminal illness	
☐ **DNR (Do Not Resuscitate) Order**	
☐ _____	
_____	
Approval signature of local Medical Control Date approved	

Fig. 8-3b. The MPDS, v11.1 protocols. ©1978-2003 MPC.

In addition, v11 introduced the third standard protocol OMEGA for classifying EXPECTED DEATH. Many systems have well-defined policies that allow for terminal patients to pass away in dignity without the useless chaos of a resuscitation attempt. The direct dispatch referral of authority to law enforcement, the coroner, Hospice, or mortuary personnel is locally defined and approved by Medical Control and the public safety administration in keeping with current policy and the law. As with the determination of OBVIOUS DEATH, EXPECTED DEATH situations must be unquestionable. The confirmed presence of a **DNR** order is often required.

DNR (Do Not Resuscitate) Order PROTOCOL **9**
A physician's order directing medical personnel to not attempt to revive a patient using CPR or other extraordinary means.

Rule 1 PROTOCOL **9**
Often, when faced with a dying **DNR** patient, **callers just want reassurance that they are doing the right thing.** However, if the caller believes the **DNR** should be ignored or is uncertain if the **DNR** is valid or in place, an appropriate response and resuscitation attempt should be made.

Post-Dispatch and Pre-Arrival Instructions. First, assure the caller that help is on the way. Specific words of reassurance are provided in the Post-Dispatch

Instructions section of this protocol, "I'm sending the paramedics (ambulance) to help you now. Stay on the line and I'll tell you exactly what to do next."

Callers are especially prone to panic in critical cases. The EMD should use repetitive persistence and other calming techniques. For example repeat, "You must calm down and do exactly as I say to help your father," verbatim until the caller becomes more composed.

Version 11 of the MPDS places increased emphasis on caller and responder safety than previous versions. One consequence of this is the flexibility to instruct callers to leave the scene or to not begin Dispatch Life Support if the scene appears to be dangerous. Protocol 9, like many other version 11 protocols, directs the EMD to X–7 if there is any danger present. If the patient choked before arresting, the EMD is directed to Pre-Arrival Instructions for unblocking the patient's airway. If the scene is safe, and the patient did not choke first, the EMD turns to protocol A, B, or C to begin CPR.

If someone is doing CPR already, so much the better! The EMD, however, is not saved from the task of relaying telephone instructions. The EMD should attempt to coach the lay rescuers to be sure the care is delivered as correctly as possible. This is often welcomed by those at the scene. More importantly, statistics from many studies show that a major component of successful resuscitation rests with immediate bystander CPR.[96] If CPR is not being done, the EMD should turn to the appropriate Pre-Arrival Instructions. The appropriate starting points are listed on the Post-Dispatch Instructions section (protocol A-1 for infants, B-1 for children, C-1 for adults, and Y-1 for adults with stomas).

Axiom 2 PROTOCOL **9**
Agonal respirations can be confused with "still breathing" before they fade away during an arrest.

The major area for potential errors in cardiac or respiratory arrest is in misidentification by the caller, either in *not* realizing that it has occurred, or in thinking that it has occurred when it has not. When the EMD asks, "Is s/he breathing?" during the Case Entry protocol, the caller might confuse agonal breathing for respiration consistent with life.[94] CPR is sometimes begun inappropriately on post-ictal seizure patients. The worse scenario of the two is failure to identify a cardiac or respiratory arrest because of inaccurate patient assessment. Whenever breathing appears at all uncertain to a second-party caller, arrest should be suspected until further evaluation proves otherwise.

With EMD coaching, the caller is more likely to perform CPR correctly. The scripts ask certain questions to confirm accurate assessment: Can respiration be seen? Is the chest rising? Does the caller feel air movement on her cheek as she bends over the patient's face? Is the person turning blue? In the end, the EMD's axiom must be, "When in doubt, send them out," meaning, always err in the direction of patient safety if any doubt exists.

Two examples of actual situations requiring telephone-instructed CPR are given here. In one case, the EMD was heard talking to her colleague while the caller was away from the phone, saying that she couldn't believe there was really time to do so much instruction, and that it probably would be to no avail (see arrow). Yet the patient was resuscitated! This case, in figure 8-5, "I think My Wife Has Died" is an example of CPR treatment over the phone from a period prior to the formal use of scripted pre-arrival instructions, and should be judged in that context for its learning value of both what to do—and what not to do.

The case "Making a difference in Wales," fig. 8-6 is the first known of its kind in which a patient with an implanted pacemaker that had suddenly failed was

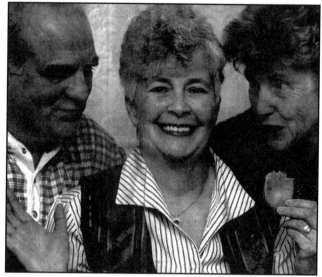

Fig. 8-4. Carol Simmonds holding her faulty pacemaker, flanked by her thankful husband Harold and amazed neighbor Dorothy Chick.

successfully resuscitated solely through the advice of an EMD. Robert Bevan recalls the event and the interesting way he became stationed in the Control center.

One of Mrs. Simmonds pacemaker wires fractured where it exits the device. Apparently the pre-arrival CPR instructions resulted in a reconnection of the wire thereby reactivating her heart beat via the pacemaker. Local medical officials credited the pre-arrival resumption of her heart activity with preventing likely brain damage.

I Think My Wife Has Died

EMD:	Fire Department	Caller:	Pardon?
Caller:	Paramedics I think. I think that my wife has died.	**EMD:**	**May I have the telephone number your calling from?**
EMD:	**What's your address, sir?**	Caller:	467-4585.
Caller:	1738…	**EMD:**	**How long has she been down do you know?**
EMD:	**1738?**		
Caller:	Logan Avenue.	Caller:	Pardon?
EMD:	**How old is your wife?**	**EMD:**	**How long has she been down?**
Caller:	69, she's a stroke victim and she has heart trouble.	Caller:	She was just sitting in a chair.
EMD:	**Is she breathing?**	**EMD:**	**Do you know how to do CPR?**
Caller:	No, not that I can tell. I can't find a pulse either.	Caller:	Know what?
EMD:	**Can I have the telephone number your calling from?**		

(continued on 8.9)

I Think My Wife Has Died

(continued from 8.8)

EMD:	**Do you know how to do CPR?**
Caller:	CPR means what?
EMD:	**That's about the chest compressions, to get her heart going. Do you want me to try to tell you how to do it?**
Caller:	What's the point in that? Why don't the paramedics come?
EMD:	**They're on the way, sir. The other dispatcher has dispatched them but...**
Caller:	Go ahead.
EMD:	**Okay, are you close by her now? Okay, can you get her onto the floor?**
Caller:	All right.
EMD:	**Okay, lay her on the floor on her back. Okay, are you close by her now?**
Caller:	I am.
EMD:	**Okay, tilt her head back. Put your one hand behind...**
Caller:	I don't have her on the floor.
EMD:	**You don't have her on the floor?**
Caller:	No, just a minute. (pause) Okay, I've got her on her back.
EMD:	**Okay, go back to her and put one hand behind her neck and the other on her forehead and tilt her head back, that'll open her airway, and then bend down and see if you can feel if she's breathing. Okay, if she's not breathing take one hand and pinch her nostrils closed, cover her mouth with your mouth and breath four deep breaths into her and watch to see if her chest rises, okay, then come back to the phone.** (pause—radio traffic)
Caller:	Okay.
EMD:	**Okay, did she breathe?**
Caller:	No.
EMD:	**Okay, did her chest rise?**
Caller:	No, not noticeably...I'm not sure.

EMD:	**Okay, I'm going to tell you what to do now until they get here, okay? Go back to her and feel on each side of her Adam's apple on her neck, and feel if there's any pulse, okay, if there's not a pulse you're going to give her two more quick breaths, and then you place your hands on her sternum—do you know where that is, in the middle of her chest—okay? Then you press, 15 times, once a second, and then stop and give her two more breaths and watch for her chest to rise, then go back and press again 15 times. With both your hands use the weight, your body weight, to do that, okay. I'm going to stay on the phone. You go do that now. If she starts to breathe or she gets a pulse you come back and tell me, okay?**
Caller:	I can't feel any pulse now.
EMD:	**Okay. If you do that, that'll make her heart beat and that'll circulate the blood to her brain. So go and do that for her now.**
Caller:	That's on her sternum?
EMD:	**Yes. Take your fingers and follow up her rib cage to the center of her chest and put the heel of one hand there and put the other hand on top of it, and then press down about 2 inches on to her chest and do that once a second, 15 times, and then give her two breaths and then start it again.**
EMD: →	**(to the dispatcher) I can't believe I'm doing this! I know she's dead. I can't believe they're not there yet. I'd never think there'd be time for anybody to be doing this!** (pause—radio traffic)
Caller:	Paramedics are apparently here now.
EMD:	**Okay, ... (unintelligible)... (caller hung up).**

Fig. 8-5. "I think my wife has died," Salt Lake City, Utah, 1984. This patient survived but not long term.

Making a Difference in Wales

I started my career in South Glamorgan Ambulance Service working in the busiest station in the Trust at Blackweir. When South Glamorgan and Gwent and Powys Ambulance Services merged, I took the opportunity for promotion and transferred to another busy station at Bassaleg as a Leading Ambulanceman. While at Bassaleg it was suggested to me that I take an MPDS course being run at Ty-Bronna in Cardiff. After four days of sitting on the most uncomfortable chairs known to mankind, I left Ty-Bronna having qualified in MPDS as the second highest on my course, but what to do with it now?

A few short months later I was approached and asked would I like to be seconded to Caerleon Control? The thought of no more aching back or knees, no more drunken yobs on Saturday night shifts, coupled with the knowledge that I had recently written off £50,000 worth of motor car I had collided with when answering a 999 call, finally swayed my mind. So off to Caerleon I went.

During this secondment on a typical wet and cold January evening in 1996 I was working an afternoon shift along with my colleagues Malcolm Cook and the MPDS coordinator Graham Davies, the 999 line rang. Being the Control Assistant, I immediately answered, listening to the dulcet tones of the operator announce, "This is B. T. (British Telecom) Bangor connecting you to 01495–271203." Hello, I thought, it's in my home town!

Flipping open the cardset in front of me, I launched into Case Entry, "What's the exact location of the incident please?"

"Quick, my mother-in-law has stopped breathing." Using the skills taught on the course I then asked the question again to which I was told "12 Risca Road, Crosskeys"—only seven doors from my house.

"What's the problem there please," I asked, knowing full well what the answer would be, I flipped the cards to the well-thumbed protocol 9: Cardiac/Respiratory Arrest. Feeling despondent now because I had realized who actually lived at the address, I continued with the Key Questions to be told, "She's turned blue and isn't breathing." Another deft flick of the wrist ensured that I was now on the resuscitation protocol.

"I'm going to tell you how to do mouth-to-mouth now," I told the caller who by now was understandably frantic with worry.

"We are already doing it," she replied.

"Okay," I said but I'm going to tell you how to do it properly, listen carefully." By now my worst fears were realised. The patient was not breathing and had no pulse. During the lifetime that was the call, Malcolm mobilized an ambulance from my old station of Bassaleg, which is only six miles away, but at the time, might as well have been 60. It was a comfort to know the crew of the ambulance were old colleagues who would give the patient every chance that there was.

After several cycles of CPR came the heart-stopping moment when the caller joyfully announced, "She's breathing again."

What to do now? I couldn't find anywhere on the cardset that covered this one—instant panic. So reverting to my previous life as an operational ambulanceman, I gave some enhancements to the script that I hoped might help (and hopefully wouldn't land me in it if the case was reviewed either).

In the eight minutes it took the ambulance crew to arrive the patient had gone from full-blown cardiac arrest to breathing on her own with a good pulse, and therefore had every chance of survival. And, as you can see here today, did! It later transpired that Carol had a pacemaker in situ that had malfunctioned and the act of CPR had managed to restart it. I hasten to add she has a new one now which appears to be working fine.

As an operational ambulanceman I was lucky enough to have resuscitated several people successfully "hands-on" so to speak. But when faced with doing it through a bundle of wires, it's a totally different thing as you are never sure the person on the other end is doing everything correctly. But thankfully, on the day in question, they were.

Nothing could or can compare with the feeling of sheer delight knowing that I had made a difference in somebody's life.

And, no, I never did get into trouble for my enhancements of the script as the case wasn't reviewed! 🔱

Fig. 8-6. "Making a Difference in Wales," from an address given by Robert Bevan at the Academy Accreditation Ceremony of the South East Region of the Welsh Ambulance Service, U.K., 1998.

Malcolm Woollard and Graham Jones of the South East Region of the Welsh Ambulance Service lent this fascinating insight into the effect of pre-arrival instructions in their system:

I also wanted to confirm the bystander CPR data that we discussed. Clinical audit profiles, taken from paramedic run sheets, show that prior to the introduction of MPDS only three percent of cardiac arrest victims received bystander CPR. Since MPDS implementation this now averages forty percent (as witnessed by paramedics on arrival of the ambulance). We can't think of anything else to blame this on other than PAIs (no new citizen CPR scheme has been introduced in this time, etc.).

Protocol 11: Choking

Choking is a critical pre-hospital emergency. Without a pathway for air, a person will die unless the situation is rapidly reversed. Time is of the essence. Most people feel the effects of hypoxia within moments, especially when they panic. Unconsciousness probably occurs 3-5 minutes into fully obstructed choking, with decreased level of consciousness preceding it by a minute or two. As Dr. Henry Heimlich first taught:

1. The patient **cannot breathe.**

2. The patient **cannot talk.**

3. The patient **collapses.**

If a patient is found unconscious, the rescuer's first clue that the problem is due to choking might occur when efforts to open the airway fail, and the chest refuses to inflate during artificial respiration. People can choke on

Rule 1	Protocol 11

A healthy child (or young adult) found in cardiac arrest is considered to have a **foreign body airway obstruction until proven otherwise.**

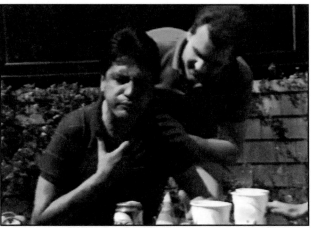

Fig. 8-7. Choking victim, who cannot talk, first clutches his neck, gaining the attention of an onlooker. From *Anonymous Hero,* ©1987 Pyramid Film & Video, Santa Monica, California. Used with permission.

just about anything. A common culprit is meat, especially at parties, where an abundance of alcohol, laughter, and a too-large bite of the roast lethally combine. In children, who experiment endlessly with taste, any item might become lodged in the airway, especially hot dogs (which are usually cut into choke-sized pieces).

There are two types of choking. One involves a complete obstruction of the airway, in which no air can pass in or out of the lungs. Speaking with a complete obstruction is impossible, since the vocal cords vibrate due to the passage of air. One should always ask a victim of suspected choking, "Are you choking?" If, with a terrified expression, the person in distress indicates a nonverbal "Yes," or grabs their throat in the universal choking sign, the Chief Complaint is quickly confirmed (see fig. 8-8).

The other type of choking is partial obstruction of the airway. In these cases, people can inhale and exhale enough to gag, cough, and make noise. There may be anything from normal coughing, to coughing with distinct wheezing sounds between coughs, to a high-pitched whistle in near-complete obstruction.

The final type of choking is not actually choking. More appropriately dubbed "gagging," the patient has a near choking episode, or more commonly, inhales some liquid substance which produces violent gagging or coughing. While very frightening, gagging, by definition, is not life-threatening. Communication centers using ProQA™ consistently report that about 25 percent of all patients initially reported as choking are actually an 11-A-1 determinant when evaluated correctly.

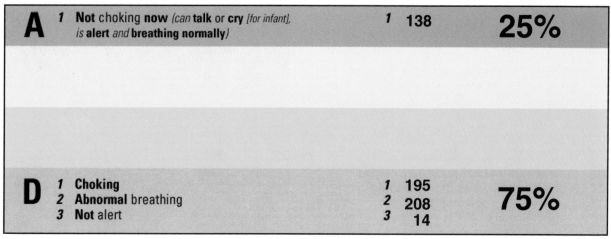

A	*1*	**Not** choking **now** *(can **talk** or **cry** [for infant], is **alert** and **breathing normally**)*	*1*	138	**25%**
D	*1* *2* *3*	**Choking** **Abnormal** breathing **Not** alert	*1* *2* *3*	195 208 14	**75%**

Fig. 8-8.   MPDS, v10.3 protocols. ©1978-98 MPC. Included are percentage breakdowns from ProQA™ of 555 specific determinant codes dispatched from protocol 11: Choking, which occurred in Cleveland, Ohio in 1995.

First aid for complete airway obstruction is the Heimlich maneuver. (Some still incorrectly refer to it as the abdominal thrust.) This technique is taught in the basic life support (CPR) class required of all EMDs. The best approach for partial airway obstruction is to let the affected person try to clear the airway alone. This can be frustrating because there is nothing to do except be encouraging, watch and wait. Because there is a small risk of internal injury with the Heimlich maneuver, it is better if the patient can inhale enough air to cough; a cough generates expulsive forces many times greater than the best force that a helper could generate. Only if the victim of a partial obstruction begins to pass out should the EMD instruct the caller to try an obstructed airway maneuver, since the patient can no longer make efforts to clear his own airway.

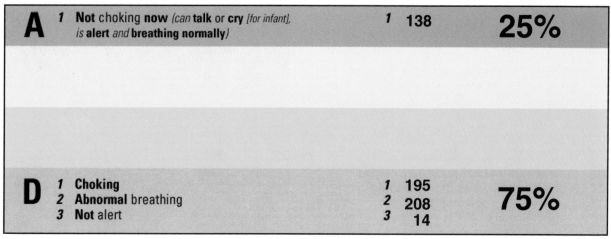

Fig. 8-9.   Nearly unconscious choking victim, receives first of several sitting Heimlich maneuvers by the caller who has just put down the phone. From *Anonymous Hero*, ©1987 Pyramid Film & Video, Santa Monica, California. Used with permission.

Choking is often resolved rapidly by on-scene helpers, before prehospital providers can arrive, and sometimes even before the call to 9-1-1 is complete. Although the choking episode has ended and the emergency is past, people at the scene often remain emotionally charged, so the EMD should understand the caller's residual excitement. Field personnel should evaluate people who have had a choking episode to be sure all portions of the obstructing object are gone. Foreign objects that lodge in the lungs may cause infection and other side effects.

The EMD will need to know if, after choking, the patient is now breathing normally. Wheezing or funny noises may indicate a still-partially obstructed airway. Swelling or other soft tissue trauma may also cause this. The EMD needs to know if the patient is completely awake and what the patient choked on, if known. Different substances can present unusual challenges for rescuers. The variety of things that can choke a person to death is astonishing and includes a marshmallow, a piece of meat, a slippery marble, or an errant denture plate.

Post-Dispatch Instructions. When complete airway obstruction occurs, assure the caller that, "I'm sending the paramedics (ambulance) to help you now. Stay on the line and I'll tell you exactly what to do next." If the caller is panicked, the EMD should use repetitive persistence (detailed in Chapter 5: Caller Management Techniques) to help calm the caller. To review, repeat the phrase verbatim and with a steady tone of voice.

Rule 3	**Protocol 11**
Before ALPHA-response selection the caller needs to **verify that the patient is not choking now** (can talk or cry, is alert and breathing normally).	

Choking on a Marshmallow

EMD:	**Fire Department.**
Caller:	(gives address).
EMD:	**(repeats address).**
Caller:	Yeah.
EMD:	**What's the problem?**
Caller:	What?
EMD:	**What's the problem?**
Caller:	She's choking on something! (someone hollering in background that she's suffocating) She's suffocating! She's not breathing. She's suffocating!
EMD:	**Okay, who is she?**
Caller:	Um, (gives name). You have to get over here fast!
EMD:	**How old is she?**
Caller 2:	(yelling) Hey, get somebody over here right away, she's almost dead!
EMD:	**What's... how old is she, sir?**
Caller 2:	She, okay, I mean, 76 years old, or 78.
EMD:	**What's she choking on?**
Caller 2:	Marshmallow in her throat.
EMD:	**Is she getting any air at all?**
Caller 2:	No! That's why I need an ambulance here, and somebody here fast.
EMD:	**Okay, what's the phone number that you are calling from?**
Caller 2:	(gives phone number).
EMD:	**Do you think you can calm down enough to maybe do the Heimlich if I tell you how?**
Caller 2:	Well, start... (unintelligible)...and I'll see what I can do for you.
EMD:	**Do you know how to do it?**
Caller 2:	No, I don't, ma'am.
EMD:	**Is she...**
Caller 2:	She's almost dead now.
EMD:	**Is she sitting up? Or is she...**
Caller 2:	No, she's laying on the floor now.

EMD:	**Okay, does she have any pillows underneath her?**
Caller 2:	No, none.
EMD:	**Okay, she's laying flat on the floor?**
Caller 2:	Yes she is, ma'am, on her side.
EMD:	**On her side?**
Caller 2:	Yes.
EMD:	**Okay, roll her over on her back.**
Caller 2:	(to someone at the scene) Help me roll her over on her back. She's suffocating from a marshmallow that went down her throat.
EMD:	**Okay, and she's not getting any air at all, right?**
Caller 2:	No!
EMD:	**Okay, now straddle her hips with your legs.**
Caller 2:	Yeah, what do I do now?
EMD:	**Okay, now put the palm of your hand right under her rib cage, in the middle.**
Caller 2:	Okay, I've got that.
EMD:	**Just put the other hand on top of it...**
Caller 2:	Yes.
EMD:	**...and push. (pause) Did anything happen?**
Caller 2:	No.
EMD:	**Okay, try it again. Do you see how it's trying to force it out of her throat?**
Caller 2:	Yeah, but I don't think she's going to respond, ma'am. I'm being honest.
EMD:	**Okay, there is nothing coming... You can't get it to pop out?**
Caller 2:	No, I can't.
EMD:	**Okay, why don't you keep doing that, and they're right around the corner. They'll be right there.**

Fig. 8-10. "Choking on a Marshmallow," Salt Lake City, Utah, 1983. The patient survived after the caller tried one more time. This early call demonstrates pre-scripted dispatch life support sistuations. Note the premature termination of the call on "radio" arrival of the responders.

A good choice of words is, "Listen to me carefully so we're sure to do it right." When possible, use the caller's name to help penetrate the strong interfering emotions. Repeat more than once if necessary.

The EMD then turns directly to the pre-arrival instructions. Protocol D-1 is the start point for choking infants and children; protocol E-1 is the start point for choking adults.

The Council of Standards, based on a strong recommendation of the Research Council, first approved the use of chest thrusts in the treatment of choking infants for version 10.3. This has been continued in version 11.0. Back slaps and back blows are not approved under DLS standards.

In situations of partial airway obstruction, the EMD should tell bystanders not to interfere with the victim's attempts to expel the foreign body. They should not give back blows, since that could cause the object to lodge further (and more completely) into the airway. Bystanders must lend support and encourage the victim to remain calm. Panic tightens the muscles in the throat precisely when it is most important for them to relax and open. Bystanders should not interfere with coughing. The EMD can reassure the caller that if the patient can talk or cough, the airway is open and enough oxygen should get to the brain.

Occasionally, a partial airway is so close to being fully obstructed that the patient's efforts to clear the airway become increasingly feeble. If the patient loses consciousness, the EMD may need to instruct the caller in obstructed airway maneuvers. A choking person must never be left alone. Some people who realize they are choking excuse themselves from the table before anyone knows there is a problem; they are later found, dead, in the bathroom or kitchen.

Figure 8-10 is a fascinating transcription of an EMD giving Pre-Arrival Instructions in 1983 to a caller confronted by a choking incident. This case occurred before scripted protocols were in full use in this center. Though successful, several "errors" by today's standards are identifiable, especially at the end of the case.

Protocol 14: Drowning (Near)/Diving/ SCUBA Accident

Technically, a **drowning** is when a person dies from suffocating in a liquid environment. A near-drowning is when a person begins to drown but is rescued and revived. Drowning can occur in a variety of situations, such as bathtubs, seizures occurring near water, overdose, inebriation, or falls. Sometimes a mother is distracted from giving a young child a bath and returns to find the child unconscious in the water. A swimmer might be hit by a passing motorboat, or a diver left unconscious after misjudging his rise from a depth. Cars sometimes go off the road and into lakes and rivers.

Rule 1	PROTOCOL **14**

The current location of a drowning patient (in water, underwater, out of water) **should be determined on Case Entry** during "What's the problem, tell me exactly what happened?" This insures proper use of **ECHO** coding for patients underwater or not breathing.

A *diving accident* to most people is an injury that occurs as a result of entering the water haphazardly. Hitting the bottom of a pool or a submerged object is very hard on the head and neck. Body surfers may be slammed head-first by a large wave against the ocean floor. Such incidents demonstrate a clear mechanism of injury for possible spinal injury. In fact, some callers may report, "My buddy broke his neck!" leading the EMD initially to the "Traumatic Injuries (Specific)" priority protocol. Either way, the patient will get the appropriate prehospital response once the evidence of possible neck injury becomes apparent.

To people who enjoy the sport of SCUBA diving, a "diving accident" may pose an entirely different scenario. Diving injuries related to SCUBA can be life-threatening. Problems usually occur as a result of a too rapid change in pressure caused by poorly controlled ascent from depth. The most dangerous are air emboli (when nitrogen bubbles expand and wreak havoc at the intravascular level), and **decompression sickness** (also known as the bends). Treatment requires care in a **hyperbaric oxygen chamber**, where the victim can be recompressed through specialized therapy and mechanically "brought to the surface" properly.

People in cold-water, near-drowning incidents have a better chance of survival than those in warm or hot water. The water does not necessarily need to be freezing! Temperatures even as relatively warm as 70° F (20° C) can cause hypothermia.

Axiom 1   PROTOCOL 14

Victims of cold water drowning **can remain underwater for long periods of time before death or brain damage occurs**. An automatic body reflex is triggered in cold water, called the "diving reflex." Inhaled cold water may also lower blood and body temperature. The heart usually remains beating for a few minutes after submersion.

The "diving reflex" allows air-breathing aquatic mammals to remain underwater for extended periods of time. Cold water reduces the body's need for oxygen and causes the heartbeat to slow. This limits the amount of blood going to the periphery, re-directing the increasingly limited amounts of oxygen available to go to the vital organs.

Even if no heartbeat or respiration can be detected, begin CPR immediately; the protective effect of the diving reflex ceases when the body is removed from cold water.

Axiom 2   PROTOCOL 14

The **"diving reflex" is more pronounced in children under four years of age**, possibly because of a similar reflex experienced during childbirth enabling the fetus to survive on limited oxygen.

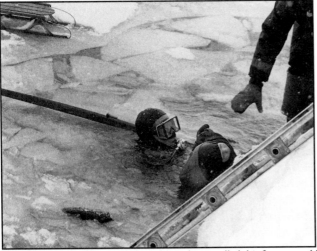

Fig. 8-11. After 20 minutes of searching, divers pulled this four-year-old child from icy Lake Michigan in cardiac arrest. Appropriate emergency care led to a full recovery. (Photo by Chicago Tribune, ©1985, Chicago Tribune Company, all rights reserved, used with permission.)

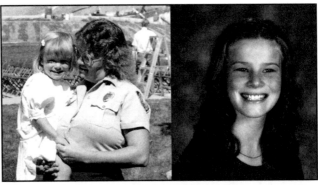

Fig. 8-12. The little girl on the left (Michelle Funk) is a near-drowning survivor who was underwater for over 63 minutes. Holding her is the EMD who handled the call for help. The young woman to the right is Michelle in 1997.

Rule 2   PROTOCOL 14

A submerged patient, regardless of time underwater (≤ 6 hours), is considered **resuscitatable by definition until proven otherwise**, especially in a cold-water situation.

EMD's First Rule of Hypothermia

They're not dead until they're warm and dead.

In one remarkable case, an 18 year-old student was trapped in a submerged car in a frozen pond for 38 minutes. Although pronounced dead at the scene, he gasped while being loaded into the transport vehicle. Resuscitation led to a complete recovery, and he returned to college two weeks later. Another case involved a 42 year-old physician who was underwater for 10 minutes. He suffered no physical damage, and later resumed his medical practice. Other cases are illustrated in figs. 8-11 and 8-12.

Axiom 3   PROTOCOL 14

For drowning victims **not responding to mouth-to-mouth ventilation**, the Heimlich maneuver may be recommended in the course of providing CPR when the rescuer responds that the airway is blocked. (See PAI ABC-15.)

In near-drowning, fluid may pass into the patient's lungs, although the actual incidence of this is debated. The chance of infection and other physical reactions from getting foreign material in the lungs can generate serious problems within a few hours. "Approximately 15 percent of near-drowning victims who are conscious at the time of admission die of delayed 'drowning' from pulmonary and cerebral causes."[5] Near-drowning victims should be encouraged to be evaluated at a medical center.

Even if a near-drowning victim is alert and breathing normally, and has no apparent injuries, the caller should be warned that breathing problems may be delayed and can develop relatively quickly. An advanced life support crew may be better equipped to handle some of the consequences of near-drowning or diving accidents when the patient is demonstrating any effects or symptoms.

> ### Rule 4   PROTOCOL 14
>
> In diving accidents where there is any suspicion of neck injury, **tilting the head or moving the patient should be avoided** if at all possible.

On-scene helpers may sometimes remove the patient from the water and into a shelter. This information affects the EMD's Post-Dispatch Instructions if spinal trauma is suspected. If the patient is in the water, or lost in the water, the EMD needs to summon a specialized dive or rescue team.

Post-Dispatch Instructions. The caller's first instinct may be to attempt a rescue; which may not be wise.

> ### Rule 3   PROTOCOL 14
>
> Each year potential rescuers drown themselves attempting to save drowning people. The caller should be advised to **attempt a rescue only if it is safe to do so.**

If the patient is not breathing and out of the water, the EMD should have selected protocol 9 to begin airway assessment and CPR. If the patient is breathing then proper, direct use of protocol 14 occurs. In either case, the safety advice in the Post-Dispatch Instructions on protocol 14 should be given when appropriate. For example, in an adult, if, upon initiating mouth-to-mouth ventilation, the airway is blocked and the chest does not rise (C-5) the protocol will retry, recheck, and direct the EMD (C-14) to attempt change the tilt angle

and if that doesn't work, will continue (C-15) to the Heimlich maneuver on the patient per current AHA guidelines.

> ### Rule 5   PROTOCOL 14
>
> The **head-tilt is the preferred method of airway control** in the dispatch environment. When a neck injury is likely, an attempt should first be made to open the airway without moving the neck. If this is unsuccessful, then advise to **gently tilt the head back**, a little at a time, until air goes in and the chest rises.

With the special precautions about neck injury in mind, the EMD should ensure the ABCs if appropriate. If the patient is still in the water, the EMD should instruct the caller to keep the patient floating on the surface; this is less likely to disturb the integrity of the spinal cord. It is possible to do mouth-to-mouth breathing in the water, supporting the neck in a neutral position. It is best for would-be helpers to wait for trained rescuers to extricate and treat the patient properly.

Near-drowning often involves great gulping of water into the stomach. If large amounts of fluid begin to drain from the mouth or the patient begins to vomit, the caller should position the patient so the fluid can drain away from the lungs.

Hyperbaric (decompression) chambers are an important resource for EMS providers for several reasons. In cases of SCUBA accidents, the EMD should know the location of the closest one. A good resource is the **Dive Alert Network** (DAN), which knows the pertinent telephone numbers. EMDs who do not live near the ocean should not presume that there is no local SCUBA activity. Enthusiasts can be found anywhere. One of the largest SCUBA diving clubs in the U.S. is in Michigan.

Protocol 6: Breathing Problems

Breathing can be affected for medical, mental, chemical, physical, and traumatic reasons. Breathing problems are among the most common of chief complaints. They are often serious, because human survival depends on adequate supplies of oxygen. In severe cases, the EMD may hear a panicky report of a patient who is *turning blue, fighting for air*, or *making funny or peculiar noises*. This overview of breathing problems is intended to endow the EMD with a sense of the complexity of the issue. It will not make anyone an expert in discerning which breathing problems are serious and which are not.

In reality, many causes of breathing trouble are not very serious. However, these are impossible for an EMD to separate from the potentially dangerous or lethal causes over the telephone. For this reason no ALPHA or BRAVO response categories are found on this protocol. Several dispatch concepts help define and clarify the seriousness of certain breathing problems generally.

Difficulty breathing can be divided into three basic categories: primary—the problem is within the lungs; secondary—the problem is in the upper airway; and tertiary—where the problem is not in the lungs or airway. The degree of distress of any of these problems can range from mild to life-threatening.

Rule 1   PROTOCOL **6**

INEFFECTIVE BREATHING discovered during key questioning should be coded as **SEVERE RESPIRATORY DISTRESS** (DELTA).

Rule 2   PROTOCOL **6**

Breathing broblems are **potentially life-threatening** until proven otherwise.

Primary causes of breathing problems. In these cases, the problem is within the lungs.

- **Acute pulmonary edema.** "Edema" is fluid retention in a body space—in this case, the lungs. Fluid build-up occurs for a variety of reasons (altitude sickness or acute heart failure). Caused by the sudden failure of the left side of the heart to pump efficiently, the resulting **acute pulmonary edema** can be both sudden and rapid.

- **Asthma, emphysema, or chronic bronchitis.** These illnesses as a group are known as **chronic obstructive pulmonary disease** (COPD) or COAD for airway disease in the U.K. and Australia. Through different mechanisms, **asthma**, **emphysema**, or **chronic bronchitis** obstruct air flow in the small passages of the lungs, or cause breakdown of those passages so oxygen exchange is impaired.

- **Pulmonary embolus.** A clot of blood, fat, or even thicker amniotic fluid (in delivering mothers) lodges in a lung, preventing downstream blood flow. This causes lung tissue to starve and eventually die, and can be very painful. (Pulmonary embolus was discussed Chest Pain, Chapter 6: Medical Conditions.)

- **Heart failure.** In heart failure, the heart fails to pump well, which causes fluid to back up into the lungs. The blood comes in faster than it is pumped out. In a sense, the patient is drowning in his or her own fluid. This may be a chronic (congestive) or sudden (acute) condition. It can cause profound shortness of breath, especially in acute cases.

- **Pneumonia.** Infections of the respiratory system often persist in the lungs and create excesses of fluid and phlegm that decreases or blocks respiration for a segment or larger area within a lung or lungs bilaterally. These conditions usually respond well to proper antibiotic treatment (if bacterial, not viral, in cause).

Secondary causes of breathing problems. In these cases, the problem is in the upper airway.

- **Croup and epiglottitis. Croup** is a viral infection, most common in children (the equivalent in adults is laryngitis). Its most distinguishing characteristic is a cough that sounds like a barking seal. It usually manifests at night, a few hours after a child has gone to bed and lain flat a few hours, resulting in benign swelling. **Epiglottitis** is a serious bacterial infection that can be life-threatening. It involves the sudden onset of inflammation of the epiglottis, which is the flap of tissue that covers the windpipe when swallowing. Critical cases of epiglottitis occur primarily in children, since their airways are smaller than adult airways. A child with epiglottitis is usually very quiet and still, sitting upright or leaning forward. Drooling (dribbling in the U.K.) is common because the swollen epiglottis makes breathing and swallowing difficult. The danger is that the infected epiglottis can swell so much that it completely obstructs the airway (like a sticky marshmallow). Gentle handling and prompt hospitalization are important.

- **Tracheitis.** Inflammation of the trachea usually caused by an infection.

- **Choking.** Both full and partial foreign-body obstruction were discussed in protocol 11.

- **Allergic reactions.** These were discussed in protocol 2. The primary problem is soft tissue swelling of the throat, causing a mechanical obstruction that may not be alleviated by positioning of the head. One reason advanced life support is so important for breathing problems is the provision of anti-allergic medications and the skill of endotracheal intubation, in which a tube can be used to bypass such problems.

Rule 4	PROTOCOL **6**

If the **caller asks** whether the patient should be given their medication now, the EMD should **only give instructions included in the protocol.**

Tertiary causes of breathing problems. In these cases, the underlying problem is not in the lung or airway, although this may not be apparent on evaluation.

- **Hyperventilation syndrome.** While hyperventilation means "fast breathing" (hyper = fast, and ventilation = breathing), **hyperventilation** syndrome is different from other forms of rapid breathing. A syndrome is group of signs and symptoms representing a distinct medical problem.

  While *true* hyperventilation syndrome is not a critical situation, other causes of **tachypnea** (rapid breathing) may signal serious underlying conditions, such as heart disease or a pulmonary embolus (lung clot).

  The EMD must be careful *never to presume to be able to diagnose hyperventilation syndrome via telephone.* It is never to be "no-sent" or sent a lower "underride" response in violation of protocol. Several dispatch lawsuits have involved a failed dispatch diagnosis of hyperventilation (see Archie Case and Lam Case in Chapter 11: Legal Aspects of EMD).

  Hyperventilation syndrome, usually due to a benign cause such as anxiety or emotional upset, includes a group of classic symptoms. In addition to rate and depth of respiration, an early sign is numbness or tingling in both hands and sometimes around the mouth or earlobes. If hyperventilation persists unchecked, the hands (and sometimes the feet) spasm in a painful way that draws the fingers (and toes) together and upwards (carpal-pedal spasm). Extreme hyperventilation can also cause chest pain.

These symptoms can generate increased anxiety, making the syndrome a self-perpetuating cycle. All of the signs and symptoms occur because of a too-rapid loss of carbon dioxide from the blood; the cure is time. Breathing must slow down and blood gases balanced. Heart attacks often present in a similar way, especially as described by lay people.

Axiom 1	PROTOCOL **6**

While true **hyperventilation** is a benign (not serious) condition, EMDs should **never assume it exists**. Advising breathing into a paper bag is considered to be **EMD malpractice.**

- **Heart attack.** The cause of breathing problems related to heart attack is similar to heart failure. Basically, the pump malfunctions and cannot keep up with the body's needs, causing fluid to back up in the lungs. Mild heart attacks can result in congestive (chronic) heart failure while severe attacks can cause immediate pump failure if enough heart muscle is damaged.

- **Stroke** (cerebrovascular accident or CVA). A stroke patient may appear to have breathing problems as he or she struggles to maintain normalcy; in particularly severe strokes, breathing compromise may necessitate artificial respiration. Some stroke patients may snore or make crowing sounds because they cannot control their head position, and therefore, their airway.

- **Diabetic ketoacidosis.** Diabetic ketoacidosis is a complication of diabetes that manifests with

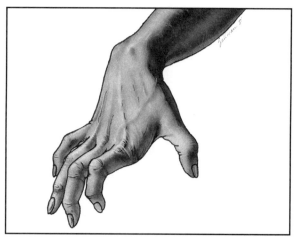

Fig. 8-13. Carpal-pedal spasm is a late, but frightening sign of prolonged hyperventilation syndrome.

diminished consciousness or coma, and relentless, rapid, deep breathing. This pattern of air hunger is called Kussmaul breathing. It resembles a rhythmic gasping. The underlying physiological process is that the body has become acidic, and rapid, deep breathing is one way to rebalance itself. Diabetes was discussed in protocol 13.

• **Seizures.** Seizures are sometimes reported as "breathing problems" due to sudden unconsciousness and lack of airway control. Cyanosis is not common during the clonic (jerking) phase but may ensue as the actual seizure stops and the postictal phase lingers. This is not a primary breathing problem for the patient, but rather a predictable aspect of a seizure. Seizures were discussed in protocol 12.

• **Drug overdose and substance abuse.** Some drugs—both prescription and recreational—cause respiratory insufficiency or arrest if used to excess. Drugs such as heroin, morphine, and others act on the breathing centers of the brain and inhibit (or stop) breathing. Some overdoses can be reversed with certain medications available to field responders; for others, a respirator will breathe for the patient in the hospital until the body eliminates the drugs naturally. In either case, the caller may need to provide mouth-to-mouth resuscitation, with the EMD's help, until emergency personnel arrive.

• **Cardiac arrest.** As a person enters cardiac arrest, unusual breathing efforts—called agonal respirations—may cause confusion among bystanders.[94] Literally, these are dying breaths. These occasional, irregular attempts to breathe—after the heart has stopped—may range from gasping to near-normal but irregular deep breaths, and may include vocal sounds. A caller distracted by this terminal abnormal breathing might not notice cardiac arrest until the EMD asks the key questions. A caller who reports that the patient is making funny noises is often describing agonal respiration or at least an unconscious person with an uncontrolled airway.

Alertness is an excellent, but late, indicator of the seriousness of a breathing problem, since a diminished level of consciousness signals severely reduced oxygenation of the brain. One pitfall to avoid is the failure to be sure the patient is choking. If this is the case, the EMD is prompted to GO TO protocol 11: Choking. Another somewhat unreliable indicator that the situation is serious is a change in skin color. If the patient has a history of heart problems, this may suggest an underlying cardiac event, since there is an essential link between the heart and lungs. Symptoms of SEVERE RESPIRATORY DISTRESS are listed here.

SEVERE RESPIRATORY DISTRESS

Complaints may include but are not limited to:
• Changing Color
• Difficulty speaking between breaths
(only speaks words, not full sentences)

Post-Dispatch Instructions. The EMD will initially work with the caller to ensure the patient's ABCs (using protocol) if appropriate. Airway management is obviously the primary focus. If the patient is a child who is sitting forward and drooling (indicating possible epiglottitis), airway management includes remaining calm and resisting the temptation to look in the mouth. Even applying a tongue depressor in epiglottitis can cause the airway to seal off. If the patient is conscious, airway maintenance usually includes letting the patient take the position of comfort. People in respiratory distress almost invariably prefer to sit up. Several lawsuits have been brought in cases in which dispatchers made a *dispatch diagnosis* of hyperventilation and recommended breathing into a paper bag while failing to send a field crew. Don't do it.

Someone who is having trouble breathing may collapse suddenly. The caller should be instructed, "If s/he becomes less awake or vomits, quickly turn him/her on his/her side," or, "If s/he gets worse in any way,

---

Rule 3   PROTOCOL **6**

A patient having **breathing problems may worsen at any time**. Always advise to call back if condition worsens.

---

call me back immediately for further instructions." In some cases, especially those coded with DELTA-level responses, the EMD may elect—wisely—to stay on the line with the caller. Prepare to instruct the caller in CPR.

Axiom 2   PROTOCOL **6**

In **conscious patients**, breathing may be helped by **sitting up**.

Protocol 15: Electrocution/Lightning

Electrocution is a high-level prehospital medical emergency. Electric shock, whether encountered by a curious child chewing on a lamp cord, by an unlucky hiker struck by lightning in a thunderstorm, or by a home-repair enthusiast, varies in its effect. Factors include voltage, type of current (AC or DC), length of contact, degree of insulation and grounding, and location of entry and exit pathways to the patient's body. Significant injury is less likely when the electrical source is 110 volts (U.S. standard) versus 240 volts standardly used in Europe and Australasia as this lower voltage generally causes just surface burns. One exception to this is "immersion electrocution," which can cause cardiac arrest. (Immersion electrocution occurs when someone in a bathtub drops an electrical appliance, such as a blow-dryer, into the water.)

One reason that the effects of electricity are so unpredictable is that the extent of injury depends on which parts of the body are transversed by the current. There is an entrance and an exit that occurs as the electrical current chooses its path.

Axiom 1	PROTOCOL 15

Hidden exit wounds and internal injuries may **complicate the patient's status**.

On entry to the body, electricity may cause a trivial-appearing surface wound. As it travels through the body, it seeks the line of least resistance as it makes a pathway to the ground. Nerves, blood vessels, and other fibers make good routes. Pathways through other internal areas can also result in serious internal damage. If the heart is involved, it requires only a small amount of electricity to cause **fibrillation**, a lethal arrythmia that can be reversed only with a quick prehospital intervention called defibrillation (see AED: Chapter 4). CPR is not defibrillation. However, it buys time until a defibrillation-capable team arrives.

High-voltage shocks can cause gruesome trauma as the charge exits the body. The force of exiting current can be explosive. There is potential for other trauma, too. In one case, a 20 year-old was electrocuted at work; his

Axiom 2	PROTOCOL 15

Electrocutions and lightning strikes occurring above the ground may result in significant falls causing **injuries that may be more serious than those incurred from the electrocution or lightning**. Answering all key questions should ensure this is not overlooked.

friends pulled him out of the light rain into a construction shack, and started CPR. When paramedics arrived, they initiated standard advanced life support procedures (including defibrillation), without effect, and transported the victim about 25 minutes after arrival. He was pronounced DOA (dead on arrival) at the hospital. Later, it was discovered that the young man, a lineman for the power company, had fallen 25 feet to the ground from a pole, and had ruptured his spleen. No one had discovered this detail on the scene; bystanders didn't think to mention the fall while rescuers assumed that the situation was a straightforward electrocution. The patient bled to death.

As Bernard Malamud once stated, "If your train's on the wrong track, every station you come to is the wrong station." Remember that some victims may have been moved. They may have fallen.

A report of a long fall (more than 6 feet) in conjunction with an electrocution helps cue field personnel that there is potential for additional trauma. Responding field crews need to know if the patient has been moved so someone can assess the site for its mechanism of injury. Routinely using

The Salt Lake Tribune	Monday, October 24, 1994

Man Rushes to Aid of Brother, Dies By Electrocution

A Salt Lake-area man was electrocuted while trying to save his brother in an industrial accident Saturday afternoon at the Moroni turkey processing plant.

Clair Kendall, the surviving brother, was hooking up an electrical-service line to a piece of equipment at the west end of the plant when an electrical charge coursed through the truck he was in, the Sanpete County Sheriff's Office reported.

He collapsed and lost consciousness. His brother, Neil, ran to the truck and tried to pull Clair from danger, but he received a lethal dose of electricity.

Medics took the two men to Sanpete Valley Hospital, where Neil was pronounced dead. Clair was flown to University Medical Center and listed in critical condition Sunday night.

Fig. 8-14. "Man Rushes to Aid of Brother, Dies By Electrocution," Salt Lake Tribune, 1994.

the Case Entry query, "Tell me exactly what happened" is a valuable tool in understanding these often complex situations.

Electrocution poses significant safety hazards for rescuers and bystanders, as demonstrated by abundant Axioms and Rules.

Axiom 3	PROTOCOL 15

Each year many potential rescuers are injured attempting to help. The caller should be advised to **attempt a rescue only if it is safe to do so**.

A written policy—established locally—should be in place for the EMD to appropriately handle electrical situations. If electrical wires have fallen or there are other power sources that on-scene personnel cannot deaden, the EMD must know how to notify the emergency contact from the power company quickly.

First Law of Responders	PROTOCOL 15

Don't take more victims to the scene.

In some cases, the patient may not even yet be disconnected from the power source. Certain currents of electricity cause muscles to contract; if the patient's hands are grasping the power source (such as a bare wire), this could cause them to contract more tightly around the wire itself. If disconnection has not occurred and the power has not been turned off, significant safety issues remain.

Axiom 4	PROTOCOL 15

A bystander can be electrocuted just getting close to the patient, without even touching her/him, when high voltage is involved or the ground is wet.

The EMD will need to know whether the patient is completely awake (alert) and whether breathing is normal. The answers to these questions help the EMD determine the priority response.

Post-Dispatch Instructions. If the situation was initially reported as a possible cardiac arrest, the EMD

Second Law of Responders	PROTOCOL 15

Don't get it on you or even touch it.

may appropriately use protocol 15: Electrocution/Lightning. Once the safety issues in the first three key questions are covered, the post-dispatch instructions will assure that the necessary treatments can be safely provided.

The experienced EMD—once the cause was described as electrocution—would probably prefer to use this priority protocol to gain more exact information. The EMD will always stay on the telephone until breathing can be *safely* verified.

Rule 2	PROTOCOL 15

Advise caller to **beware of electrical risks and electrified water**. Do not advise any treatment unless it is safe to do so.

Moisture facilitates the conduction of electricity. Helpers walking through a puddle to help the victim may end up creating more victims. Even damp ground can increase the danger zone. One of the most important messages the EMD can provide is for the caller to limit the situation to one victim, despite the sometimes heart-rending nature of helplessly watching someone in distress. The temptation to react dramatically or heroically is great. The EMD must encourage extreme caution and self-restraint.

Third Law of Responders	PROTOCOL 15

If there is more than one unconscious patient on-scene, there may be scene safety implications.

If it is safely possible, the caller should turn off the power. This may mean flipping the switches in the circuit box, or simply unplugging a malfunctioning appliance from its power source. If downed electrical wires are the problem, the caller must try to keep curious onlookers at a safe distance and point out the dangers the wires may pose.

Once it is certain that the hazards are controlled, the EMD can begin working with the caller to check and assure the ABCs (using protocol). If the patient is in cardiac arrest, the process will lead to the appropriate Pre-Arrival Instructions.

Protocol 8: Carbon Monoxide/ Inhalation/HAZMAT

Hazardous materials are one of the largest-growing industrial realities of this generation. *Four billion tons of hazardous materials* (called HAZMAT) are carried by air, surface, rail, and water annually.[97] Proper manufacture, transport, and disposal of hazardous materials are difficult. The chemical names are often polysyllabic tongue-twisters (pun intended), and trying to organize the information so appropriate medical intervention can be provided is daunting.

A HAZMAT incident may involve a solitary patient with carbon monoxide poisoning or entire communities, such as when a tank car full of toxic herbicide and pesticide crashed into the Upper Sacramento River in northern California in 1991. (That incident affected the water supply of millions of people and wiped out wildlife in and around the world-class trout river for 40 miles.)

> **HAZMAT** ☢
>
> An incident involving a gas, liquid, or other material that, in any quantitym **poses a threat to life, health, or property**.

One of the most common inhalation poisons is carbon monoxide (abbreviated CO). It is a clear, odorless gas. Carbon monoxide binds to a receptor site in the hemoglobin molecule in blood, 200 times more powerfully than the life-sustaining element oxygen—preventing oxygen exchange in the lungs. This effectively "suffocates" the patient at the sub-cellular level.

Carbon monoxide poisoning is often used in suicide via a motor vehicle running in an enclosed space to generate a concentration of fumes. Carbon monoxide poisoning also occurs inadvertently. For example, when a faulty furnace is turned on in the autumn, the whole household can be affected, sometimes lethally. An exhaust leak in the family car can lead to carbon monoxide poisoning if there is no fresh air ventilation.

Entire families of recently arrived immigrants have died after using charcoal barbeques indoors. Carbon monoxide is also a major component of any fire, so people who have suffered smoke inhalation (including firefighters unprotected by appropriate gear) are

inevitably affected. Fumes, gases, and vapors accounted for 48 deaths among cases reported to the American Association of Poison Control Centers in 1995. Interestingly, *all* 48 cases were attributable to carbon monoxide of which 19 were ruled intentional.[68]

> **Axiom 1**   PROTOCOL **8**
>
> **Patients who have inhaled** smoke, carbon monoxide, or other chemicals may be **found in any stage of intoxication**. Carbon monoxide binds very tightly to hemoglobin and can lead to an **urgent situation**.

> **Axiom 2**   PROTOCOL **8**
>
> **Unconsciousness** in a patient who has inhaled carbon monoxide is a **bad sign**. Hyperbaric oxygen treatment may be necessary to prevent death or brain damage.

This priority protocol also deals with other inhalation poisonings. These may occur in a number of ways, such as when toxic or noxious gases escape their containers, or when a person inadvertently mixes two household products that together form a toxic chemical gas. For example, mixing Clorox™ and Comet™ cleanser creates chlorine—a noxious gas. Many chemicals can cause lung damage, while others negatively affect oxygen transport and other elements within the human system. In many places, money and resources have now been dedicated to specially trained HAZMAT teams. Their mission is to know how to cope with situations involving strange and toxic materials.

> **Rule 1**   PROTOCOL **8**
>
> All hazardous exposures and inhalations are considered **high-level emergencies until proven otherwise**.

An EMS system is smart to prepare for a HAZMAT situation before one happens. Special HAZMAT protocols are just as important as special disaster protocols. It is beyond the scope of priority dispatch to appropriately orchestrate a HAZMAT incident. If a HAZMAT problem occurs, the EMD should be prepared to exit the priority dispatch system and use the local HAZMAT or

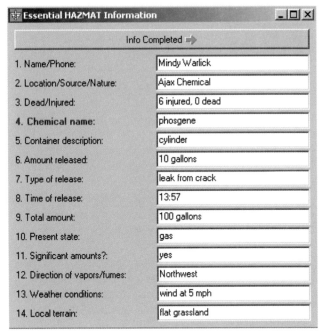

Essential HAZMAT Information	
Info Completed ⇒	
1. Name/Phone:	Mindy Warlick
2. Location/Source/Nature:	Ajax Chemical
3. Dead/Injured:	6 injured, 0 dead
4. Chemical name:	phosgene
5. Container description:	cylinder
6. Amount released:	10 gallons
7. Type of release:	leak from crack
8. Time of release:	13:57
9. Total amount:	100 gallons
10. Present state:	gas
11. Significant amounts?:	yes
12. Direction of vapors/fumes:	Northwest
13. Weather conditions:	wind at 5 mph
14. Local terrain:	flat grassland

Special log window in ProQA™ for the capture of Essential HAZMAT Information as listed on Protocol 8—Additional Information.

disaster protocol. As a starting point, however, the EMD can use the checklist for reporting a HAZMAT emergency.

Second Law of Responders   PROTOCOL 8

Don't get it on you or even touch it.

The EMD will determine the number of people involved during Case Entry and whether they are safe and out of danger. The EMD must prevent anyone—well-meaning bystanders and emergency responders alike—from going into the same toxic trap as the patient. In some instances the field personnel face one of the toughest tasks possible: having to stay outside the danger zone until the environmental hazard is contained or controlled.

Toxic exposure may also cause burns if the circumstances are explosive. If the situation includes burn injury, the EMD should GO TO protocol 7: Burns (Scalds)/Explosion. As always, level of consciousness and difficulty breathing are primary concerns. Airway tissue may swell or burn when irritated by toxic fumes, creating a time-critical emergency. The airway may become so swollen that it swells shut.

If the caller knows the nature of the fumes or other hazardous-material emergencies, the HAZMAT team will

be able prepare more specifically, and perhaps even make recommendations regarding on-scene persons before arriving. For example, if it is known that a chemical is particularly dangerous, evacuation orders for the surrounding downwind area may be issued immediately.

> **If the EMD knows the color and code number on that placard, it may be possible to have an answer for responding crews before they arrive at the scene.**

Certain loads of hazardous materials are placarded, using one of two universally acknowledged identification systems. If the caller does not know the nature of the toxins, perhaps he can describe the placard on a container or overturned truck. If the EMD knows the color and code number on that placard, the nationwide hazardous-material identification system[98] or regional poison control center may be able to help. It may be possible to have an answer for responding crews before they arrive at the scene. When the right information is available, the EMD can advise the caller (who may not know how dangerous the situation is!), responding prehospital field personnel, and anyone else—such as the media—converging on the site of potential hazards.

Post-Dispatch Instructions. Safety first! A primary goal in emergency medical services is to prevent further harm. If the caller is inside or near a hazardous place, protocol 8 directs the EMD to X-7. Here, the caller is advised that the situation could be dangerous.

Rule 2   PROTOCOL 8

Callers should be **advised not to re-enter** a hazardous or dangerous environment.

Protocol X-7 allows for two scenarios. If it is safe to do so the caller can remain where they are, but will be advised to not approach or to not touch the patient if this is appropriate. If the situation seems immediately threatening to the caller, the EMD proceeds to X-12 where the caller will be instructed to leave immediately. If appropriate, the caller could open the garage door on the way out to begin fume ventilation. Once clear of the danger zone, the caller can call again.

The EMD should advise the caller not to touch a contaminated patient. A proper HAZMAT team is the best source for safe decontamination.

Protocol 31: Unconsciousness/Fainting (Near)

When an EMD uses this protocol, the implication is that the EMD determined during Case Entry that some degree of effective breathing exists. Where problems are encountered with either verification of breathing or determining whether breathing is agonal, protocol 9: Cardiac or Respiratory Arrest/Death, would be used instead.

Rule 2   PROTOCOL **31**
An unconscious person in whom breathing cannot be verified by a 2ⁿᵈ party caller (with the patient) is considered to be in **cardiac arrest until proven otherwise**.

The difference between *unconsciousness* and *fainting* is that the first is persistent and the latter is transient (fleeting). The medical term for fainting is **syncope** (pronounced SIN-ko-pee). The EMD needs to differentiate between fainting and unconsciousness, and, when making a dispatch determination, will also use the patient's age to predict the seriousness of the situation. A single fainting episode (especially in a person under age 35) is likely to be relatively benign. In someone 35 years of age or older, fainting could, more likely, involve the heart, which elevates the potential seriousness of the situation. A patient who remains unconscious or is even "not alert" by the time the EMD finishes the Key Questions will receive a maximal response.

Axiom 1   PROTOCOL **31**
Fainting implies a state of unconsciousness from which the patient has "come to." While this is generally less serious than prolonged unconsciousness, it **does not imply a benign condition and should be medically evaluated**.

If a person has regained consciousness, the EMD must then determine that person's level of consciousness.

Axiom 3   PROTOCOL **31**
If the **caller doesn't seem to understand "Is s/he completely awake,"** ask "alert," "able to talk normally," "with it," "making sense," or a more descriptive phrase to determine any decrease in level of consciousness.

Axiom 3 reflects the importance of a responsible dispatcher to be able to enhance (not replace) the system of gaining useable information from the caller.

Causes of sudden unconsciousness range from serious to not-so-serious. Time-life critical causes include cardiac arrest and major respiratory insufficiency, severe head injury, diabetes (particularly insulin shock), hypovolemic shock, and drug overdose. Depending on the presence of priority symptoms, poisoning, stroke, heart attack, or irregular heart rhythms may be time-life critical. Typically, benign causes include seizures (especially in known epileptics), alcohol intoxication, fainting from the heat, fright, or standing up too fast.

Many people with epilepsy control their seizures well with medication; others are unable to achieve full control. Many epileptics have at least occasional "breakthrough" seizures. When callers recognize seizures and report this as the Chief Complaint during Case Entry; the EMD should always select protocol 12: Convulsions/Seizures. But some callers do not know what a seizure looks like and may initially describe a person who has "fallen out" or some other vague term. If seizure isn't initially evident then protocol 31: Unconscious/Fainting (Near) is used.

Collapse may be the first noticeable evidence of a serious medical problem, such as hypovolemic shock due to internal bleeding. Someone with a history of cardiac problems is more likely to have a critical reason for the unconsciousness or fainting. It does not matter if the exact cause is known, as long as the EMD can elicit a report of whether priority symptoms are occurring.

If a patient who is now awake has fainted more than once, the situation could be very serious. One possible explanation is undetected internal bleeding. Common causes are leaking abdominal aortic aneurysms and ectopic pregnancies. If the patient is a female in her childbearing years, the EMD will ask whether she has had any abdominal pain that might correlate with an ectopic pregnancy. The range of childbearing years has a liberal dispatch definition—ages 12 to 50.

Axiom 2   PROTOCOL **31**
The Chief Complaint and the main associated symptoms (such as fainting) are sometimes reversed by the caller in **ectopic pregnancy and aneurysm cases**.

Other respiratory problems may also have preceded the collapse. SEVERE RESPIRATORY DISTRESS is defined by reports that a patient is "changing color," or having "difficulty speaking between breaths." These are grave signs.

Axiom 4	PROTOCOL 31

"Funny noises" reported by the caller generally means the patient is unconscious with an uncontrolled airway and often represents agonal (dying) respirations at the **beginning of a cardiac arrest**.

Sometimes situations of unconsciousness involve alcohol. An unconscious person, whether because of alcohol or not, is potentially critically ill—without exception! It is vital to not judge regular clients who are often found *unconscious* on the sidewalks or in alleys. These may be transient, unkempt, sometimes unpleasant people who prefer a Skid Row existence, but no greater medical-legal liability rears its head than when someone is treated casually because of social misfortune. Alcoholics have legitimate health emergencies, often more frequently than the average population. If the caller says, "Ralph's down again, at 16th and

EMD's Third Rule of Judgment

Judging the integrity of the patient may be more foolhardy than judging the integrity of the caller.

Market," it is essential to ask the Key Questions before making a dispatch decision. The EMD should not try to second-guess the caller or the situation. It is dangerous to think, "Oh, it's just Ralph, he's probably fine." When in doubt, send them out.

Post-Dispatch Instructions. The EMD ensures the ABCs using protocol A, B, or C as appropriate. If the situation has deteriorated to cardiac or respiratory arrest, the age-appropriate dispatch life support protocol will track the EMD through the appropriate progression of instructions.

Well-meaning helpers often try to comfort patients by putting pillows under their heads. It is amazing how often an airway-occluding pillow is found when the EMD recommends removing any pillows. The caller should also have the patient lie flat. This aids oxygenated blood in getting to the vital organs, especially the brain.

EMDs First Law of Scene Helpers

Always assume there is a pillow or other object behind the patient's head unless you know otherwise.

Some awake patients may express thirst after a fainting episode, particularly if they are in hypovolemic shock from an undetected internal bleed. No food or fluids should be given, in case the patient needs surgery.

Stay on the line if the patient's condition seems unstable or is worsening. If appropriate, the EMD can hang up, but only after encouraging the caller, "If s/he gets worse in any way, call

> **No greater liability rears its head than when a caller is treated casually because of social misfortune. Alcoholics have legitimate health emergencies.**

me back immediately for further instructions." Remember, unconsciousness is not a normal state nor does a patient normally remain in that state. Be vigilant.

Rule 3	PROTOCOL 31

Stay on the line with the caller when the patient is still unconscious to ensure ABCs until responders arrive.

Protocol 32: Unknown Problem (Man Down)

Sometimes, a caller reports, vaguely, that, "There's a man down at Speer and Humboldt," or, "There's something terribly wrong in Pioneer Park, send an ambulance here right away!" Such calls may be on behalf of people in public who have been assaulted, have had a medical mishap (perhaps a seizure or diabetic emergency), or have simply decided that it's time for a nap. The general emergency level is totally variable. Without call prioritization, however, the man down category tends to be a disproportionate catch-all category.

Rule 2	PROTOCOL 32

If the actual type of problem (Chief Complaint) becomes apparent during interrogation, go to and **dispatch from that more specific protocol**.

Axiom 1	PROTOCOL **32**
Often, unknown problem calls are 3rd party. Obtaining specific symptoms may be difficult; however, a **problem isn't "unknown" until all required questioning has been completed**.	

Although the man down may end up having nothing seriously wrong with him, the EMD must not be lulled into complacency, but must remember Frenza's Law.

Frenza's Law	PROTOCOL **32**
A thing not looked for is seldom found.	

The EMD's index of suspicion must remain high in spite of the fact that this is a frequent (and often minor) situation. Man down calls are notorious for backfiring when anyone in the chain of care fails to honestly explore the various possibilities before deciding how to react.

First Law of Medical Dispatch
First, do no harm.

This law means that with proper training, sound protocols, high protocol compliance, quality assurance feedback, and continuing dispatch education, we should be making the right decision based on sound data the vast majority of the time and not have to so often "be in doubt." Certainly, there are circumstances when, because the answers to questions are vague or "gray," or the information requested is just not known, the EMD must rely on the Second Law. Signs that life status is questionable may be difficult to gather in certain situations. Existence of any evidence suggesting a threat to life—unconsciousness, abnormal breathing, or cardiac arrest—must, in the absence of more precise information, receive a maximal response. The EMD must work with the caller to see what, if any, information is available.

An interesting failure to invoke the Second Law took place July 6, 1986, at a large public safety dispatch center in the Southeastern U.S. Obviously, the Hendon case (fig. 8-15) involves a first-party caller who only produced grunting noises throughout the entirety of the

Second Law of Medical Dispatch
When in doubt, send them out. (Always err in the direction of patient safety.)

call. The calltaker apparently did not recognize that the caller had a major problem and on several occasions threatened the caller (judgment danger zone).

The Hendon case, an amazing 55 minutes long, had an equally amazing ending. Upon successfully tracing the call through Bell South, the fateful decision to only send a police unit was made. According to case depositions, on arrival, the police team found a car in the driveway, but could see no evidence of anyone in the locked house after a careful walk around the outside. The older, more experienced officer mentioned during the response in that he had had responded to this location in the past and that the occupant was an alcoholic. He then recommended leaving. The rookie officer, however, insisted that more be done, even suggesting they break in. The older officer then called dispatch and asked, "Do you still have the RP [reporting party] on the line?" Fatefully, the dispatcher replied, "Yes, but he's refusing to come to the phone." Upon hearing the dispatcher's misinterpretation of the facts, the officers drove away. Nearly a day later, the patient's son found him, lying in the house, critically ill from a massive stroke. Upon regaining some ability to speak, the caller recounted how he had actually called 9-1-1 several hours before the call transcribed here, but was hung up on. The patient apparently was not currently a drinker nor a derelict, but was a recently retired superior court judge for the region.

The Second Law of Medical Dispatch is an essential part of the application of the Medical Priority Dispatch protocols. Other ways of saying this are "when in doubt, err in the direction of patient care and safety" or, in the sense of coding selection, "come the closest without going under." Unfortunately, the application of this concept is sometimes overused as an excuse for noncompliant behavior by EMDs. We have consistently found that when protocol is followed in a careful, nondiscretionary manner, the necessity to "over-send" is minimal. Data collected from sites using the computerized version of the protocols show that overriding occurs on less than 1 percent of calls (0.6 percent in Cleveland; 473 of 79,652 calls in 1995). All overrides should be reviewed by qualified quality assurance personnel to verify that such action was medically justified.

Hendon Case (55:00 elapsed time)

Dispatcher: _____ Police, may I help you?

Caller: (grunting)

Dispatcher: _____ Police, may I help you?

Caller: (grunting)

Dispatcher: This is _____ Police, may I help you?

Caller: (grunting)

Dispatcher: This is _____ Police, may I help you?

Caller: (grunting)

Dispatcher: Hello, do... hello?

Caller: (grunting)

Dispatcher: Sir, do you need a police out?

Caller: (grunting)

Dispatcher: Hello? Sir, you need to stop mumbling... and tell me what's wrong.

Caller: (grunting)

Dispatcher: Sir, do you need a police out? What's your address?

Caller: (grunting)

Dispatcher: Hello?

Caller: (grunting)

Dispatcher: Sir, do you need a police?

Caller: (grunting)

Dispatcher: What's your address?

Caller: (grunting)

Dispatcher: What's your address, sir?

Caller: (grunting)

Dispatcher: What's your address, sir?

Caller: (grunting)

Dispatcher: Hello? This is _____ Police, may I help you?

Caller: (grunting)

1:22

Dispatcher: Sir, you need to tell me your address, or I'm going to hang up. You need to stop mumbling in my ear and tell me what's wrong.

[From this point, only key sections of the case transcript are included. The caller's grunting noises are omitted even though they occur after virtually every dispatcher query.]

Caller: (trying to articulate words)

Dispatcher: Hello? If you... Hello?

Dispatcher: What's your address?

Dispatcher: Sir, listen to me. Hello?

Caller: (grunting louder)

Dispatcher: What's your address?

Dispatcher: Do you need a police out?

Dispatcher: Hello? Do you need a police out or an ambulance?

Dispatcher: Hello? Can you tell me your address?

Dispatcher: Hello? What's your address?

Dispatcher: Hello? What's your address?

4:03

Dispatcher: Do you need a police out? Cause if you're playing on the ph... if you're playing on the phone, officer's gonna come and take you to jail.

[Time passes as the dispatcher continues to ask caller for information.]

Dispatcher: Do you need an ambulance out?

Dispatcher: Hello?

Dispatcher: Hello? Do you need a...

Dispatcher: Hello?

Dispatcher: Do you need a police out?

4:39

Dispatcher: Hello? I'm gonna hang up if you don't tell me what's the problem.

[Time passes as the dispatcher continues to ask caller for information.]

Dispatcher: Hello?

Dispatcher: Hello?

Caller: (crying and grunting)

(continued on 8.28)

Hendon Case (55:00 elapsed time)

(continued from 8.27)

Dispatcher: Do you need an ambulance out?
Dispatcher: Hello?

Dispatcher: Ma'am, do you need a police or an ambulance out?

[Time passes as the dispatcher continues to ask caller for information.]

Dispatcher: Hello?
Dispatcher: Hello?
Caller: (crying and grunting)

Dispatcher: Do you need an ambulance out?
Dispatcher: Hello?
Dispatcher: Ma'am, do you need a police or an ambulance out?

7:17
Supervisor: Ma'am, they can't help you if you don't give them an address.

[Time passes as the dispatcher continues to ask caller for information.]

Dispatcher: Ma'am, can you give me your telephone number you're calling from?

8:52
Supervisor: (in background) I've got a lady on my 9-1-1... who obviously has some kind of extreme (unintelligible). And a... can't get her... to get any information from her. (unintelligible)

Dispatcher: Ma'am, just stay on the line with me, going to try to find out where you are, okay?
Supervisor: I have a lady on my 9-1-1 who obviously has some difficulty breathing... (unintelligible)
Dispatcher: Ma'am, can you give me your address? Do you know your address?
Dispatcher: Ma'am do you know your address?

9:50
Supervisor: (in background speaking to the telephone company) We're going to try to control the phone for as long as we can... (unintelligible)
Dispatcher: Can you give me your address so I can get you some help?
Dispatcher: Hello?
Dispatcher: Ma'am, do you know your telephone number your calling from?
Dispatcher: Hello?
Dispatcher: Ma'am, can you calm down an give me your address?
Dispatcher: Ma'am, can you give me your address?
Dispatcher: Hello?
Dispatcher: Hello?
Dispatcher: Ma'am, can you give me your address so I can send you some help?
Caller: (moans) Oh, no.
Dispatcher: You don't know your address?
Dispatcher: Do you know what's the name of the street you stay on, ma'am?
Dispatcher: Hello?

11:13
Dispatcher: Ma'am, if you can give me your address and your telephone number, I can send an officer out there or send you a paramedic. But I can't send you no help if I don't know where you are.
Dispatcher: Do you know the name of your street? Hello?

[Note: entire call lasts for 55 minutes.]

Fig. 8-15. The Hendon Case.

A direct extension of the the Second Law is the Third Law of Medical Dispatch, which clarifies the need to "be in doubt."

Third Law of Medical Dispatch

Don't be in doubt so much. (With proper training, protocol, and time to do the job right, guesswork will be minimized.)

Signs that life status is questionable may be difficult to gather in certain situations. Existence of any evidence suggesting a threat to life—unconsciousness, abnormal breathing, major injury, uncontrollable bleeding, or cardiac arrest—must, in the absence of more precise information, receive a maximal response. The EMD must work with the caller to see what, if any, information is available.

Axiom 3   PROTOCOL 32

Standing patients are less likely to be in cardiac arrest than sitting patients, who are, in turn, less likely to be in cardiac arrest than patients lying motionless.

Axiom 2   PROTOCOL 32

Even though callers may be some distance from the patient, they **might have seen the patient moving,** heard them talking, or observed or been told the patient's position (standing, sitting, lying).

People sitting up sometimes go into cardiac arrest—but they are generally not moving! (A brief anoxic seizure or agonal breath may be a transient exception, of course.)

On this protocol, in particular, it's vital to stick with the system as De Luca's Law states. The purpose of this law is to protect the EMD from inadvertently creating harm.

De Luca's Law   PROTOCOL 32

EMDs will follow all protocols per se, avoiding freelance questioning or information unless it enhances, not replaces, the written protocol questions and scripts.

Sometimes, a caller later reports that the patient is wearing a bracelet or necklace that describes a chronic problem, such as diabetes or epilepsy. This information could be useful but may not be the cause of the patient's problem.

It can be helpful to responding field personnel to know where the patient is. For example, a dispatch message of "Six-fifty-two East Fourth South on a man down" creates an entirely different picture and pre-arrival plan than would "652 East 4th South, Bratten's Seafood Restaurant." Knowing the type of location in this instance might raise the possibility of choking or an anaphylactic reaction to seafood in responders' minds. A *man down* in a garage may be the result of carbon monoxide or electrocution. A business establishment may be the site of a seizure or cardiac arrest. At the park on the Fourth of July, the cause may be choking. On or near a street, the situation may be an auto-pedestrian collision, seizure, or cardiac arrest. These examples are not rules and are used only to illustrate the concept underlying Rule 1.

Rule 1   PROTOCOL 32

Relay the type of location (if known) to responding units, not just the address.

Post-Dispatch Instructions. If there appears to be any danger at the scene, the EMD is directed to protocol X-7, where the danger can be more carefully considered and the caller advised of any hazards and asked to leave the scene if appropriate. If the situation seems safe and the caller is able, the EMD can ask the caller to return to the patient and see if he is conscious, and breathing, or moving at all, and to provide a report. Together, the EMD and caller can ensure the patient's ABCs (using protocol A, B, C, or Y) as appropriate.

The caller can also help direct emergency responders to the patient. This is especially helpful in parks or other wide-open areas. One crew responding to a large park on a hanging, was sent to the "southwest corner" of the park. The crew might have spent a long time searching for the victim in the grove of trees there had not the callers waved them in. The patient was 25 feet high in a tree.

Percentage of DELTA Codes in Unknown Problem Cases					
Location (data interval)	**DELTA-Level** (% of Unk. Probs.)		**Unknown Problem** (% of all cases)		**All Cases**
Colorado Springs, U.S. (1/1/98 to 2/24/98)	22	(12.9)	170	(5.9)	2,856
Cleveland, U.S. (1/1/96 to 12/31/96)	367	(6.8)	5,385	(6.0)	89,231
Derbyshire, U.K. (1/21/95 to 10/31/95)	134	(4.4)	3,041	(8.6)	35,090
Salt Lake City, U.S. (1/1/99 to 12/31/99)	219	(6.8)	3,198	(14.4)	22,175
Melbourne, Australia (4/1/98 to 8/16/99)	902	(7.5)	12,111	(5.1)	237,443
Montreal, Canada (1/1/95 to 12/31/95)	1,072	(12.9)	8,572	(5.2)	165,418

Fig. 8-16. Percentage of DELTA (Life Status Questionable) codes in protocol 32: Unknown Problem (Man Down) cases.

Summary

This chapter, along with Chapter 6: Medical Conditions and Chapter 7: Trauma Incidents, have embodied the meat of the priority dispatch concept. Through use of priority dispatch protocols, the EMD can prioritize callers' needs without jeopardizing the quality of response. Each protocol includes a section of Additional Information to remind the EMD about various details surrounding each incident type or medical problem. The SHUNT protocols help the EMD identify priority symptoms and provide a funnel to the appropriate working protocol. What are often initially confusing complaints evolve into categorizable and useful information.

These three chapters have encapsulated for the EMD the basis of emergency medical care from a dispatch life support perspective. Many of the diseases and injuries are complex, and there was no intention to make them seem less severe and debilitating than they are for patients. However, for dispatch prioritization, there are easy and reliable methods for deciding which emergency personnel are needed and how fast. For example, body temperature in heat and cold injuries may seem important to the uninitiated, but the patient's level of consciousness has much more to do with the level of emergency response needed.

Remember that all callers with true time-priority items should get an initial emergency response of less than five minutes when this is physically possible. Callers with significant problems should have response of less than 10 minutes—which means first responders in most cases. EMS system design plays a big role in assuring these are all possible more often than not. In rural areas, distance may replace true medical need as an indicator for lights-and-siren response. And the system provides a valuable service in updating responding crews with specifics about what is going on at the scene during the often-lengthy gap between initial call receipt and arrival of responders.

With a basic understanding of the medicine underlying the priority decisions, an EMD not only knows what to do, but why certain things are true, too. In the end the ultimate goal is that every patient receives the best chance for survival and recovery.

If you can look into the seeds of time,
And say which grain will grow and which will not,
Speak then to me...

—*William Shakespeare*
MacBeth

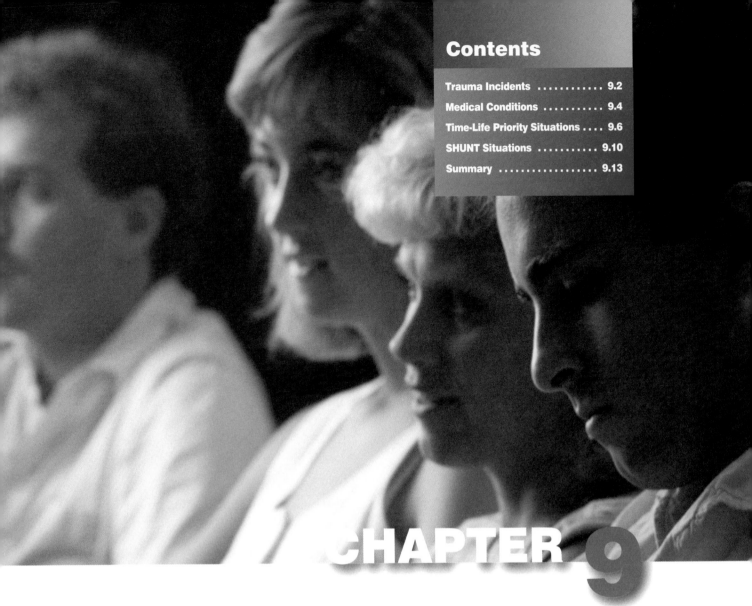

CHAPTER 9

Scenarios

Chapter Overview

In this chapter, each of the various types of priority protocols is demonstrated in full, from Case Entry (initial assessment), key questions (on-going assessment), through dispatch of resources and, where applicable, dispatch life support to case completion. The protocols chosen for demonstration are:

1. The **Trauma** protocol, 7: Burns/Explosion.

2. The **Medical** protocol, 23: Overdose/Poisoning (Ingestion).

3. The **Time-Life** protocol, 31: Unconscious/Fainting (Non-Traumatic).

4. The **SHUNT** protocol, 22: Industrial/Machinery Accident

Practice what you know and it will help to make clear what now you do not know.

— Rembrandt

In this chapter, four scenarios are played out, transcript-style, to demonstrate the process of priority dispatch using the Medical Priority Dispatch System.™ Interspersed in the transcripts are explanations or clarifications in brackets and italics. The intention is to show the progression the EMD makes from the initial call until telephone interaction ends. This means the EMD first uses the Case Entry protocol, then chooses one of the priority protocols, asks the Key Questions, applies the knowledge gained to the dispatch determinants, and sends the appropriate EMS response. After that, the EMD returns to the caller and provides the appropriate PDIs and evaluates the CEIs. In one scenario, this leads into PAIs, so the reader can understand how to use these scripts.

> **Talent is useless without training, thank God.**
> **—Mark Twain**

Trauma Incidents

In the following scenario, an EMD is shown using the priority dispatch system to address trauma incidents. These calls are for illustration purposes only, not intended as actual case material.

EMD: *[Using the Case Entry protocol]*
       EMS, what's the address of the emergency?

Caller: My little girl! She's burned! Help me! Help me!

EMD: *[Repeating, using the same phrase]* **What's the address of the emergency?**

Caller: Just send help! Hurry!

EMD: **What's the address of the emergency?**

       [The repetitive persistence now pays off.]

Caller: 1022 Masonic! Hurry!

EMD: **Please repeat your address, ma'am, for verification.**

Caller: Ten-twenty-two Masonic.

EMD: **What's the phone number you're calling from?**

Caller: 285-6163.

EMD: **Okay, please repeat the phone number for verification.**

Caller: 285-6163. Hurry!

EMD: **What's the problem, tell me exactly what happened?**

Caller: My 3 year-old is badly burned! She was on fire! Please help! *[Note that the EMD now knows the chief complaint—burns—and the child's age.]*

EMD: **How many other people are hurt?**

Caller: Nobody else, just my daughter..

EMD: **Is she conscious?**

Caller: Yes! Can't you hear her crying?! *[This obviously answers the next question, "Is she breathing?" so the EMD passes that question.]*

The little girl has been burned, but is conscious and breathing, so the EMD selects protocol 7: Burns (Scalds)/Explosion, and continues the key questioning phase.

EMD: **Is this a building fire?** *[Key question 1 is asked as it is not obvious.]*

Caller: No.

EMD: **Is anything still burning or smoldering?**

Caller: No. The fire is out.

EMD: **Is everyone safe and out of danger?** *[Key question 3.]*

Caller: Yes. Hurry! She's in so much pain!

EMD: **How was she burned?** *[Key question 4.]*

Caller: I was doing laundry and came upstairs and found her in flames in the bedroom. I think she was playing with my husband's lighter! I can't believe he…

EMD: **Is she completely awake (able to talk)?** *[Key question 5.]*

Caller: I think so, listen to her cry! *[The EMD can hear the crying child saying, "Mama! Waaah!! Mama!"]*

EMD: **Is she having any difficulty breathing?** *[Key question 6.]*

Caller: No, but she's crying so hard. *[To child:]* Oh, sweetie, it's okay…

EMD: **What parts of her body were burned?** *[Key question 7.]*

Caller: Oh look! Oh… it's all over her belly and chest, and on her right arm. It's blistering… Oh help us! My baby! *[A re-freak event occurs during the mother's assessment of the actual damage—a predictably common occurrence.]*

EMD: **Ma'am, I'm sending the paramedics to help you now. Stay on the line and I'll tell you exactly what to do next.**

Caller: Okay, okay, okay… I'm okay now.

[To her child:] Honey, I'm calling for some help.

[To EMD:] What can I do for her? Is anyone coming?

EMD: **Yes ma'am, I'm sending the paramedics–the ambulance–to help you now.**

Caller: Okay.

The EMD consults the Rule of Nines in the Additional Information section to determine the extent of burns: a child's chest and abdomen equals 18 percent, plus an arm equals 4.5 percent, totalling 22.5 percent burns. Thus, according to the dispatch determinant list, this incident is rated a 7-C-3: Burns ≥ 18% body area.

EMD: **EMS, Medic 40.**

Medic: Medic 40.

EMD: **Code Three to 1022 Masonic. A 3 year-old girl with blistering thermal burns to the chest, abdomen and right arm. Conscious, alert, breathing normally. Mother reports the fire is out. Dispatch code 7-CHARLIE-3.**

Medic: 1022 Masonic, Code 3, clear.

EMD: **Ma'am, are you still on the line?**

Caller: Yes! Are they coming? She's in so much pain! Maybe I should just drive her…

EMD: **Oh no, ma'am, that might be very dangerous. The paramedics are on their way. If you'll work with me, I can help you help her while you're waiting, okay?**

Caller: Please!

EMD: **Are you sure the fire is out?** *[confirming a lack of need for PDI-b.]*

Caller: yes.

There is no apparent danger, the child is not unconscious or arresting, the child is not exhibiting signs of INEFFECTIVE breathing, and there is no SERIOUS hemorrhage or amputation, so the EMD refers to the DLS link for cooling and flushing and proceeds to protocol X-13.

EMD: **Okay, we want to cool the burns without making her too cold. We can use the kitchen sink, if you think she'll fit. Can she sit on the counter and lean over the sink?**

Caller: I think so.

EMD: **Sit her there, and use the hand sprayer. Run a very, very gentle stream of water that feels cool over her burns. Be very careful that the water isn't really cold! That should feel good to her. Will that work?**

Caller: Let me try.

EMD: *[After a minute, hearing the child settle down.]* **How's it going now?**

Caller: Much better! She's calming down now.

EMD: **Good! You can continue cooling her for about 10 minutes, but the ambulance should be there soon.** *[The EMD now feels that it would be appropriate to terminate the call, so a transition is made to X-1 as indicated]*

EMD: **Tell her the ambulance will be there to help her soon.**

Caller: Okay.

EMD: **Don't let her have anything to eat or drink. It might make her sick or cause problems for the doctor. Just let her rest in the most comfortable position and wait for help to arrive. Do you feel comfortable handling things if I hang up now?** *[The EMD can read X-1 (TRAUMA) instructions vs. X-1 (MEDICAL) here.]*

Caller: Yes. We can manage.

EMD: *[The EMD now moves to X-2]* **I want you to watch her very closely. If you can, I'd like you to put away any family pets, gather the patient's medications, unlock the door, turn on the outside lights, and if there is some one else there have them meet the paramedics. Alright?**

Caller: Yes. We're okay now.

EMD: **If she gets worse in any way, call me back immediately for further instructions, Okay?**

Caller: Okay. I'll do that.

EMD: **Okay. Good luck. Bye.**

Caller: Thank you. Bye. ⚕

Medical Conditions

In the following scenarios, an EMD is shown using the priority dispatch system to address medical incidents. These calls are for illustration purposes only, not intended as actual case material.

EMD: **Eastedge EMS. What's the address of the emergency?**

Caller: 436 Sixty-fifth Street, in Albany.

EMD: **Would you please repeat that address for verification?**

Caller: Yes sir, that's 436 Sixty-fifth Street.

The caller, a boy, is completely calm which is not unusual when a child calls. The EMD should not judge the severity of the incident upon the caller's level of excitement—especially when the caller is a child.

EMD: **Thanks. Is that a house or an apartment?**

Caller: Apartment 6-D, it's the third townhouse down from the street.

EMD: **What's the phone number you're calling from?**

Caller: Yeah, that's 524-0880.

EMD: **Can you tell me that number again, for verification?**

Caller: 524-0880.

EMD: **What's the problem, tell me exactly what happened?**

Caller: Well, I came home from school, and my aunt—I live with her and her boyfriend—she's in bed, see, and I can't get her to make sense. She's acting drunk or something. *[The EMD does not yet have a Chief Complaint, so a clarifying question is needed.]*

EMD: **Tell me exactly why she is acting this way?**

Caller: Well, I found a couple of empty pill bottles in her hand, and she's been real depressed, see, she got fired from her job yesterday. *[Before turning to protocol 23: Overdose/Poisoning (Ingestion), the EMD will complete the Case Entry protocol.]*

EMD: **How many other people are hurt?**

Caller: Just her. She looks pretty bad.

EMD: **How old is your aunt?**

Caller: Oh, she's old—about 35.

EMD: **Is she conscious?**

Caller: Conscious, what? *[The EMD recognizes that the child does not understand "conscious," so the question is clarified using an appropriate protocol enhancement.]*

EMD: **Is she awake?**

Caller: Yeah, I think so. She's acting weird in bed, like she's drunk.

EMD: **Is she breathing?**

Caller: Yeah, sure.

The EMD does not need to ask the final question—patient's sex—since it's obvious and so selects protocol 23: Overdose/Poisoning (Ingestion). Why not protocol 25: Psychiatric/Abnormal Behavior/Suicide Attempt? The form of suicide attempt in this particular case—overdose—has its own protocol. Protocol 23 is the best match for this situation. The EMD now begins key questioning.

EMD: **Was this accidental or intentional?** *[Key Question 1.]*

Caller: From what I saw, I think she did it on purpose.

EMD: **Is she violent?** *[Key Question 2.]*

Caller: I don't think so. She's too out of it. She can get pretty mad though, sometimes.

EMD: **Is she completely awake (alert)?** *[Key Question 3.]*

Caller: What?

EMD: **Is she able to talk?** *[Key Question 2, enhanced in a way that might make sense to a child.]*

Caller: Yeah, she's talking, but she's just mumbling. Like I said, she's acting drunk.

With so many references to drunken behavior, it might be easy to be drawn into thinking this patient is, in fact, "just drunk." Whether or not that proves to be the case is completely irrelevant here, and it would be a grave dispatching error to focus on this. The EMD must progress through the protocol and provide the indicated response.

EMD: Is she breathing normally? *[Key Question 4.]*

Caller: Oh yeah, she's moaning, she's breathing. It's okay.

EMD: What did she take? *[Key Question 5.]*

Caller: You mean the pills?

EMD: **Can you tell me the names of the pills? The name is usually written on the pill bottle.** *[EMD is correctly clarifying the question.]*

Caller: The one is, um, E-lav-il.™ The other is Val-i-um.™ *[The EMD looks in the center's reference list, and sees that Elavil™ is a tricyclic antidepressant called amitriptyline generically. Per Axiom 3 in the Additional Information section, "Tricyclic antidepressants can cause collapse and unconsciousness very quickly, even though initially the patient may appear all right..."]*

EMD: **When did she take it?** *[Key Question 6, the last.]*

Caller: I don't know. I asked her, and she told me just to leave her alone. She doesn't know I'm calling, but she needs help.

EMD: **Okay, you did the right thing, and you're doing a good job helping me. I'm sending the ambulance to help you now. I'm going to put you on hold, but I'll come back as soon as I can. Stay on the line and I'll tell you exactly what to do next to help her. Okay?** *[The EMD waits for verification from the boy.]*

Caller: Okay.

The EMD puts the caller on hold, remembering that she has 15-20 seconds before the boy is likely to become anxious about being on hold too long. Using the information gathered, the EMD scans the Dispatch determinants, and sees that this best fits the 23-C-4 Determinant. That is, on protocol 23, this caller has reported a CHARLIE-level, determinant four "Antidepressants (tricyclic)" situation. She proceeds to dispatch the appropriate prehospital response.

> It's what you learn after you know it all that counts.
> —John Wooden

EMD: **Eastedge EMS, Medic Seven.**

Medic: Medic Seven.

EMD: **Code Three, 436 Sixty-fifth Street, in Albany, apartment 6-D. It'll be the third townhouse down from the street. On a 55 year-old female, conscious, breathing, tricyclic antidepressant overdose. She's not alert but is breathing normally. Dispatch code 23-C-4.**

Medic: Four-thirty-six Sixty-fifth Street, Albany, on an overdose, go ahead.

EMD: **Caller is a 12 year-old nephew, reports he found two empty bottles, one Valium,™ the other Elavil,™ in her hand. They were full last night. Time of ingestion unknown. Patient does not currently know that her nephew has called for help. He reports she is not violent. Police responding.**

This last bit of information is extremely helpful to responding crews, since suicidal patients can be hostile, especially when they have not asked for help. Per this agency's policy the EMD is reminded to notify the police by the highlighted notification symbol in the protocol.

Medic: Medic Seven, clear. *[Now, after notifying the police, the EMD turns her attention back to the caller to provide Post-Dispatch Instructions.]*

EMD: **Are you still there?**

Caller: Uh huh. She's still acting crazy.

The EMD checks the DLS links and determines that there is no immediate danger, the patient is not unconscious, and there is no evidence of INEFFECTIVE BREATHING; the default link to X-1 is therefore selected.

EMD: You'll need to go back to her to reassure her that help is on the way. Don't let her have anything to eat or drink. It might make her sick or cause problems for the doctor. Just let her rest in the most comfortable position and wait for help to arrive. Don't hang up. Go do it now and come right back to the phone to tell me when it's done. Okay?

Caller: Okay. I'll go tell her.

EMD: Are you back?

Caller: Yeah, I'm here. She's still acting weird.

EMD: That's okay. Help is on the way. I'll stay on the line with you as long as I can. Go back to her now and watch her closely and look for any changes. If she becomes less awake or starts getting worse, tell me immediately. Tell me when the ambulance arrives. Don't hang up. Go do it now and come right back to the phone to tell me when it's done. Okay?

Caller: Okay. *[After a long pause]* She seems to be much the same.

As there is time and the patient appears to be stable, the EMD decides to cover some of the things that might be useful for the paramedics from Panel 2.

EMD: Please put away any pets, unlock the door, and turn on the outside lights. If there's someone else there, ask them to meet the paramedics. If you know the name of her doctor, please write it down. Okay? Don't hang up. Go do it now and come right back to the phone to tell me when it's done.

Caller: We don't have any pets.

EMD: That's okay, just do the other things.

Caller: *[After a pause]* Okay, I'm back again.

EMD: *[Continues monitoring the patient in panel 3.]* The ambulance should be there real soon. Go back to her again and watch her closely and look for any changes. If she becomes less awake or starts getting worse, tell me immediately. Don't hang up. Go do it now and come right back to the phone to tell me when it's done. Okay?

Caller: I hear the ambulance. Should I go meet them?

EMD: Sure. You did a great job.

Caller: Thanks. Bye.   ⚕

Now let's go back, and say, for the purposes of the exercise, that a new EMD turned initially to protocol 25: Psychiatric/Abnormal Behavior/Suicide Attempt at the end of the Case Entry protocol. This occasionally happens before new EMDs are fully familiar with the Chief Complaints selection process, since the caller was reporting an attempted suicide.

EMD: **Is she violent?** *[Key Question 1.]*

Caller: Oh, sometimes. She's just lying in bed, acting weird. I don't think she would get violent right now.

EMD: **Does she have a weapon?** *[Key Question 2.]*

Caller: No, I don't think so. My uncle has a gun, but he always keeps it with him.

EMD: **Is this a suicide attempt?** *[Key Question 3.]*

Caller: I… I don't know, but she did this before and these bottles, well, they're empty and they were full this morning, so maybe...   ⚕

The fifth of the sub-questions to Key Question 3 is overdose. Now the EMD knows that the nature of this particular suicide attempt is overdose. By simply following the protocol, the EMD sees a go to prompt next to overdose. The prompt sends the EMD to protocol 23: Overdose/Poisoning (Ingestion). So, even with just a slight detour, the EMD still lands ultimately on the most appropriate protocol for this patient.

Time-Life Priority Situations

This particular EMD has had a very quiet shift, and is caught in the lethargy of a warm, breezy, springtime mid-afternoon.

He works alone for a small communication center, and nothing has happened in hours to jolt him into alertness. A conscientious professional, he had realized that the underload trap had been eroding his mental clarity. Just before this call, he got out of his chair and spent 10 minutes doing invigorating stretches. Good thing!

EMD: **Southern Springs EMS. How can I help you?**

Caller: Bob Hepburn here. Listen, my wife seems to have had a little spell. Can you send someone out to help? *[The EMD can tell by the man's demeanor and voice that he is elderly and a bit shaken, but under control.]*

EMD: **Yes, sir, we'll be glad to. Where is she?**

Caller: Now son, she's on the carpet in the living room. *[This demonstrates the need for precision in questioning.]*

EMD: **I meant, what's the address of the emergency?**

The EMD could have avoided several questions and an awkward moment if he had begun the call with this question right after "Southern Springs…"

Caller: Okay, that's…uh…silly, we've lived here for ever… yes! That's 324 Oakwood, Southeast. *[It's not unusual for people in crisis to forget even everyday information. The EMD must be patient.]*

EMD: **Could you repeat that address for verification?**

Caller: 324 Oakwood, Southeast.

EMD: **What's the phone number you're calling from?**

Caller: 272-9464.

EMD: **Please repeat your phone number for verification, sir.**

Caller: 272-9464.

EMD: **What's the problem, tell me exactly what happened?**

Caller: Well, it was just like she was fine one minute, and fainted the next. No reason that I could tell. She just fainted! She's in on the floor in there.

EMD: **How old is your wife?**

Caller: She'll be 69 next month.

EMD: **Is she conscious?**

Caller: Well, sort of. I think so, now. But she wasn't there for awhile.

EMD: **Is she breathing?**

Caller: Yep, she's breathing, but she's not herself. Say, when will those ambulance people get here?

EMD: **They'll be there shortly. We can do what's best for her if you'll just answer a few more quick questions, okay?**

Caller: Sure thing.

The EMD obviously knows the sex of the patient already, so he skips that question in the Case Entry protocol. The EMD selects protocol 31: Unconsciousness/Fainting (Near) as the most appropriate protocol in this situation.

EMD: **Is she breathing normally?** *[Key Question 1.]*

Caller: Well, it's a little labored.

EMD: **Does she have a history of heart problems?** *[Key Question 2.]*

Caller: Nope. She's always had her health. Now me… I'm different! I'm the one with all the heart trouble.

EMD: **Is she still unconscious? You go check and tell me what you find.** *[Key Question 3.]*

Caller: Well, she's not herself, but she's awake, I think. I think so, yes. *[As the patient is conscious, the EMD should ask Key Question 3a: (Conscious).]*

EMD: **Is s/he completely awake (alert)?**

Caller: Well, like I said, she's not herself. She's awake but she's none too with it if you know what I mean.

The EMD should interpret this as a conscious but not alert patient. Key Question 3-a(i) "Has she fainted more than once today?" has the prompt, "(Alert)." As the patient is not alert, the EMD does not ask this question. Key Question 3a(ii) has the qualifier (Female 12-50). As this patient is almost 70 the EMD also skips this question. The EMD scans the Dispatch Determinants. The ALPHA-level response is inappropriate because of the patient's age.

The CHARLIE determinants do not apply, either. This situation is definitely a DELTA code, but for dispatch information for responding crews and for data collection, it matters which determinant descriptor the EMD selects. There are three that apply to this patient:

D-1 **Unconscious** (at end of interrogation)

D-2 SEVERE RESPIRATORY DISTRESS

D-3 **Not Alert**

The EMD correctly chooses determinant 31-D-3 and dispatches.

EMD: Southern Springs EMS, Ambulance 38.

Amb: Ambulance 38, at Naranja and River Road.

EMD: DELTA response, 324 Oakwood, Southeast.

Amb: 324 Oakwood, Southeast, go ahead.

EMD: On a 68 year-old female, conscious, not alert, breathing abnormally. Husband reports she fainted. Code 31-D-3.

Amb: Okay.

[It isn't appropriate to include the caller's name in the responder script. Why?]

EMD: *[Switching back to speak with the caller]* Are you there, Mr. Hepburn?

Caller: Yes sir. *[anxiously]* She's really not well. Are they coming? When will they get here?

EMD: I'm sending the ambulance to help you now. Stay on the line and I'll tell you exactly what to do next.

Remember, do not give specific times. This protects the caller from unrealistic expectations, since no one can predict when the responding ambulance will arrive; trains, collisions and break-downs do happen. The EMD refers to the DLS links and determines that "Unconscious" and "INEFFECTIVE BREATHING" are both inappropriate for this patient. Therefore the EMD selects the default exit link, X-1 and continues.

> **Training is everything. The peach was once a bitter almond; cauliflower is nothing but a cabbage with a college education.**
> **—Mark Twain**

EMD: You'll need to go back to her to reassure her that help is on the way. Don't let her have anything to eat or drink. It might make her sick or cause problems for the doctor. Just let her rest in the most comfortable position and wait for help to arrive. Don't hang up. Go do it now and tell me when it's done. Okay?

Caller: Okay, I'll go tell her.

EMD: Are you back? *[The EMD proceeds to X-3 to "stay on the line with a potentially unstable patient."]*

Caller: Yeah, I'm here. She's still kind of out of it.

EMD: That's okay. Help is on the way. I'll stay on the line with you as long as I can. Go back to her now and watch her closely and look for any changes. If she becomes less awake or starts getting worse, tell me immediately. Tell me when the ambulance EMTs are right with her. Don't hang up. Go do it now and come right back to the phone to tell me when it's done. Okay?

Caller.   Okay. *[Sounding a little panicky after a pause]* I don't think she's breathing anymore. She seems to be turning blue. Where the heck's that ambulance?

At this point, the incident has worsened into a possible respiratory and/or cardiac arrest. First the EMD notifies the responding crew. He also dispatches appropriate additional EMS units if appropriate. Then, the EMD transitions from X-3 to C-1.

EMD: They're on their way, Mr. Hepburn. Listen carefully and I'll tell you how to help her. Get her as close to the phone as possible. Don't hang up. Do it now and tell me when it's done. [C-1]

Caller: I'll have to drag her from the living room. That okay?

EMD: Yes. Quick as you can but be gentle.

Caller: Okay, she's right here in the hall.

The EMD doesn't need to ask the X-1 question "Where is s/he now?" since the caller has already provided the information, so moves directly to C-2.

EMD: Listen carefully. Lay her flat on her back on the floor and remove any pillows.

Caller: Okay.

EMD: Kneel next to her and look in the mouth for food or vomit. Is there anything in the mouth?

Caller: No. I don't think so. *[EMD can proceed to C-3.]*

EMD: Okay. Now place your hand on the forehead and your other hand under the neck and tilt the head back.

Caller: My hand on her forehead and under her neck. Okay.

EMD: Put your ear next to her/his mouth and see if you can feel or hear any breathing, or if you can see the chest rise. Can you feel or hear any breathing?

The EMD proceeds to C-4 and enhances the protocol with a reassuring answer to the caller's question.

Caller: No, I don't think so. She's dead isn't she?

EMD: No sir, she's not dead. We can keep her going until the ambulance gets there. I'm going to tell you how to give mouth-to-mouth.

With the head tilted back, pinch the nose closed and completely cover her mouth with your mouth, then force 2 deep breaths of air into the lungs, just like you're blowing up a big balloon.

Caller: What then? *[It appears he hasn't figured out to give the breaths now.]*

The EMD continues in C-5 because it answers the caller's question, but the EMD takes a second opportunity to make sure the caller is giving breaths.

EMD: Watch for the chest to rise with each breath. Give your wife two breaths of air now Mr. Hepburn... Can you feel the air going in and out?

Caller: Not really.

EMD: Did you see her chest rising?

Caller: No!

EMD: *[C-14]* Mr. Hepburn, stay with me now, we need to get the air in. Tilt her head back more and pinch the nose closed. Completely cover her mouth with your mouth and force 2 deep breaths of air into the lungs, just like you are blowing up a big balloon.

[C-15] While giving each breath, watch her very closely for the chest to go up and down. Make sure the air goes in.

Caller: Okay.

EMD: *[C-8]* You're doing well Mr. Hepburn. Listen carefully and I'll tell you how to do CPR compressions. Put the heel of your hand on the breastbone in the center of her chest, right between the nipples. Put your other hand on top of that hand. Okay?

Caller: Okay. I can do that.

EMD: *[C-9]* Now push down firmly 2 inches (5cm) with only the heel of your lower hand touching the chest. Do it 15 times, just like you are pumping her chest twice a second.

Caller: Twice a second?

EMD: Yes. Twice a second for a total of 15 pumps. Okay.

Caller: Okay *[In the background the EMD can hear the caller counting and grunting as he pushes.]* Okay, I've done that.

EMD: *[C-10]* Pinch the nose closed and tilt her head back again. Give 2 more big breaths, then pump the chest 15 more times. Make sure the heel of your hand is on the bone in the center of the chest, right between the nipples.

Caller: Okay, I can do that.

EMD: *[C-11]* Keep repeating this cycle of 2 breaths then 15 pumps, 2 breaths then 15 pumps. Keep doing it until help can take over. If she starts breathing, tell me immediately.

Caller: Alright, I'll do that. Okay, I think I can hear a siren.

The EMD hears the caller counting the CPR cycles and hears him breathing between giving his wife mouth-to-mouth inflations.]

EMD: *[C-12]* Don't give up. You've got to keep doing it. Keep repeating this cycle of 2 breaths then 15 pumps. This will keep her going until the EMTs arrive."

Caller: I think they're outside.

EMD: Okay, do not stop CPR until they take over for you. Hand the phone to one of the paramedics as soon as you can. Is the door unlocked?

Caller: No.

EMD: Okay, go do that when you hear them ring the doorbell, then start CPR again until they're positioned to take over for you, Mr. Hepburn, okay?

Caller: Okay. Thanks! ⚜

The EMD hears the bell ring. Mr. Hepburn rushes to the door and lets them in. Soon, one of the paramedics is on the line.

The EMD at times provides a brief hand-off report, making sure to give the approximate time the patient has been in arrest. Finally, he asks the medic to tell Mr. Hepburn he did a good job, and lets the paramedics get to work.

This scenario shows how the EMD follows the protocol as closely as possible. Occasionally, the EMD puts in additional words such as "Okay?" when he wants the caller to confirm that he understands and will do as instructed. In some places the EMD is forced to answer the caller's questions, and rather than breaking the flow of the protocol, the EMD finds a way to answer the caller's question while still moving right along with the sequence.

If at any point the patient had vomited, the EMD would have immediately broken out from wherever he was in the protocol and gone directly to C-13. Here he would instruct the caller to: "Turn her head to the side and clean out her mouth. (It's okay to have a little fluid remaining)." If the caller expresses concern about remaining fluid, the EMD reassures him that a little is okay, "You must blow through any remaining fluid." Once the mouth has been cleared, the EMD returns to the sequence.

Similarly, if the caller reported that the patient was breathing, the EMD would go to C-16 as indicated to maintain and monitor.

SHUNT Situations

EMD: **North Slope EMS, what's the address of the emergency?**

Caller: 2600 Highland Drive. I don't know how…

EMD: **Ma'am, would you please repeat that address for verification?**

Caller: Twenty-six hundred Highland Drive.

EMD: **What is the phone number you're calling from?**

Caller: I'm at 682-9899.

EMD: **Would you say that once more, please, for verification.**

Caller: Six-eight-two, ninety-eight, ninety-nine.

EMD: **Thanks. Now, what's the problem, tell me exactly what happened?**

Caller: Well, I work with my husband at our manufacturing plant out by the airport. I was in the office, and suddenly I heard him yell that the tool he was using stopped running. Then he yelled to call 9-1-1.

EMD: **Are you with the patient now?**

Caller: No, he's down in the shop alone.

EMD: **Is he hurt?** *[The EMD still has no Chief Complaint so he enhances the question further.]*

Caller: Gosh, I can't really tell from here My office has a window overlooking the workshop floor. I…

EMD: **How old is your husband?**

Caller: He's 37.

EMD: **Can you see if he is conscious?**

Caller: Yes, he's sitting up, and shouting at me. *[To the patient:]* I'm coming honey! I'm calling 9-1-1. Be right there. *[This is enough to tell the EMD that the patient is breathing, so the EMD is done with Case Entry.]*

EMD: **Go check him. Is there a telephone that's nearer to him? Go pick it up so we can get some better information. Don't hang up. Maybe we can help him while help's on the way, okay?**

Caller: Okay, it'll take me a minute to get to the shop, okay?

EMD: **Okay. I'll get help started. Get back on with me right away, okay?**

The EMD has made a leader's decision to send the caller for better information, since the patient is conscious, breathing, and calling her. The unit has been alerted to respond. In the absence of enough useable information, the EMD turns to protocol 22: Industrial/Machinery Accidents. This is a SHUNT protocol, and may assist the EMD in determining a more appropriate protocol if the patient's wife can provide more information.

> Just as important as having ideas is getting rid of them.
> —Francis Crick

Caller: Okay, I'm on the cordless phone in the shop.

EMD: **Okay. I'm here. Is the immediate area dangerous or hazardous?** *[Key Question 1.]*

Caller: No. I don't think so.

EMD: **Where exactly is he?** *[Key Question 2.]*

Caller: He's still down in the shop.

EMD: **What happened to him?** *[Key Question 3.]*

Caller: It looks like he's hurt bad!

The EMD wants to further clarify the nature of the problem. Since the caller has already made a trip back to check on the patient, the EMD uses sub-categories listed under Key Question 2 to get more information.

EMD: **Is he caught or trapped in any machinery?**

Caller: No! He's hurt bad! It's his leg. He's bleeding. I think he got cut.

EMD: **Are you sure it doesn't involve electrocution?**

Caller: I don't think so...

   [To husband:] Jim, did you get shocked?

   [To EMD:] No.

EMD: **Did he fall?**

Caller: No, he was on the shop floor.

Finally, the EMD has the best, most useable information. The SHUNT protocol directs the EMD to go to protocol 30: Traumatic Injuries (Specific).

Key Question 1, "Is he completely awake?" could be omitted as obvious because the caller has been asking the patient questions and the patient has been answering and yelling, but the EMD decides to confirm that the patient is indeed fully conscious.

EMD: **Is he completely awake?**

Caller: Yes, but he's in a lot of pain.

EMD: **Is he breathing normally?** *[Key Question 2.]*

Caller: Yeah, but there's a lot of blood!

EMD: **What part of his leg is injured?**

Key question 3. The EMD has enhanced the question: since he already knows it's the leg, he is asking which part of the leg is hurt. This will matter when the EMD determines whether the injury is NOT DANGEROUS or POSSIBLY DANGEROUS.

Caller: It's his thigh, about halfway to his knee.

EMD: **Okay, is there any serious bleeding?** *[Key Question 4.]*

Caller: It looks pretty serious. He's got a bunch of blood on his pants.

This ends the questioning phase, since the fifth Key Question, "(If amputation) Have the parts been found?" does not apply to this situation. And the last Key Question "When did this happen?" was answered during case entry when the caller said she heard him yell and then called 9-1-1.

EMD: **I'm sending the paramedics to help you now. I'll need to put you on hold while I give them your information. Stay on the line and I'll tell you exactly what to do next.**

Caller: Okay, thanks.

Now, the EMD consults the Additional Information section, where the patient's injury—an upper leg injury—is classified as a POSSIBLY DANGEROUS body area. This is needed in order to select the appropriate Dispatch Determinant. It is not an ALPHA-level problem, since the injury is worse than NOT DANGEROUS and is not NON-RECENT. It is not a DELTA-level problem, which applies to DANGEROUS body areas, cases involving SEVERE RESPIRATORY DISTRESS (as defined in the Additional Information section), and patients

> **Utility is proven in pudding of practice.**
> —Steven J. Gould

who are not alert. Since there are no CHARLIE-level determinants, this is clearly a BRAVO-level situation. This patient has both POSSIBLY DANGEROUS body area and some SERIOUS hemorrhage. Therefore he selects 30-B-2 as this better describes the immediate problem, and then relays information about hemorrhage and area injured to the responders.

EMD: **North Slope EMD, EMS-2.**

Unit: EMS-2, North Slope.

EMD: **Respond, 2600 Highland Drive, at CCM Productions, on an industrial accident.**

37 year-old male, cut thigh with report of SERIOUS bleeding, conscious and alert, breathing normally. Wife attending. Dispatch code 30-B-2.

Unit: 2600 Highland Drive, thanks.

EMD: *[To wife:]* The EMTs are on their way. Is there a particular entrance they should use to gain access quickly?

Caller: Tell them to come in the gate at the corner of Humboldt and Nelson. My red Chevy is parked by the shop door. We'll be right there when they come in.

EMD: Okay.

[To responding unit:] EMS-2, caller advises to enter through the gate at the corner of Humboldt and Nelson, and to go into the shop door next to the red Chevy.

Unit: EMS-2, clear.

EMD: *[To caller:]* Now, listen carefully so we can help your husband while they are on the way. *[The EMD first reads PDI-b and c to the caller.]* Do not move him at all *[The EMD already knows the patient is not in danger.]*

Caller: Should I splint his leg?

EMD: No, don't splint his leg. The EMTs should be there shortly, and they need to assess the injury. Is he still breathing normally?

Caller: Yes.

Referring to the DLS links, the EMD decides from the callers answers that the patient will benefit more from bleeding control provided by X-5 than from the supportive care provided by X-1. Therefore, Pre-Arrival Instructions begin with X-6.

EMD: Good. Don't use a tourniquet. I'm going to tell you how to stop the bleeding. Listen carefully so we're sure to do it right.

Caller: Okay, no tourniquet.

EMD: Get a clean, dry cloth or towel and place it right on the wound.

Caller: Just a minute. *[Gets towel.]* Okay.

EMD: Press down firmly…

Caller: Press down firmly… okay.

EMD: … and don't let up.

Caller: … don't lift it up to look.. Okay.

EMD: If it keeps bleeding, you're probably not pressing hard enough. Remember, keep firm, steady pressure on the wound.

Caller: Okay, it seems to be helping.

The EMD knows there is no amputation, and also knows there is no airway issue with this patient. From here the EMD transitions to X-1 as indicated to provide supportive care until the ambulance arrives.

EMD: Reassure him that help is on the way.

Caller: Okay.

EMD: Don't let him have anything to eat or drink. It might make him sick or cause problems for the doctor. Don't move him. Just tell him to be still and wait for help to arrive. Don't hang up.

Caller: Okay. There's blood coming out from under the towel.

The EMD suspects this is because the caller is not pressing hard enough—this is usually the reason for unsuccessful bleeding control—so the EMD returns to X-5.

EMD: If it keeps bleeding, you're probably not pressing hard enough. Remember, keep firm, steady pressure on the wound.
[The EMD enhances this statement with:] You can push quite hard so long as it doesn't cause your husband extreme pain.

Caller: Okay.

EMD: Is that helping?

Wanting to be sure the bleeding is being controlled, the EMD asks a question that isn't in the protocol: "Is that helping?" This type of additional questioning is acceptable when the EMD needs to enhance the protocol as in this example.

Caller: Yes. It seems to have stopped it again.

EMD: *[The EMD reinforces the idea that the pressure must be maintained before returning to where he left off in X-1:]* Remember, keep firm, steady pressure on the bleeding site.

Caller: Okay.

The EMD is finished with X-1 and makes the decision that the patient is stable and that the caller is completely able to cope with the situation. The EMD therefore moves to X-2.

From the situation, the EMD can determine that the list of things to do in X-2 are inappropriate in this situation. It is unlikely there are any pets in the workshop, and any medications will be back in the house. The EMD has already given instructions to the crew regarding how to get into the shop, so turning on lights and meeting the paramedics is unnecessary. Also, as the caller is occupied with keeping pressure on the wound to control the bleeding, the EMD doesn't want her to get up and run around doing other things. Exactly what instructions are appropriate for any given case must be determined by the EMD. The EMD chooses to reinforce the steady pressure concept one more time before disconnecting.

EMD: **Do you feel comfortable handling things from here?**

Caller: Yes. They'll be here soon, right?

EMD: **They'll be there soon. Remember, keep firm, steady pressure on the bleeding site and call me back he becomes less awake or starts getting worse in any way.**

Caller: Okay.

EMD: **You've done a great job. Good bye.** ⚜

In the scenario just presented, had the caller been unable to gather specific information, the EMD would have stayed on the SHUNT protocol at the conclusion of the Key Questions. From the Dispatch Determinants on that protocol, the best possible answer would be "Unknown illness or injuries (not caught in machinery)"—again, a BRAVO response.

Summary

Priority dispatch is composed of many discrete parts. These scenarios are intended to provide a learning forum for "putting it all together." The pathway that each case takes is always unique; there were innumerable moments when each scenario could have taken a different turn, based on many "what if?" possibilities. Real-life experience with the system, when understood and mastered, should be even more fun and rewarding. The professional EMD nevers stops practicing.

Laziness is nothing more than the habit of resting before you get tired.

—Jules Renard

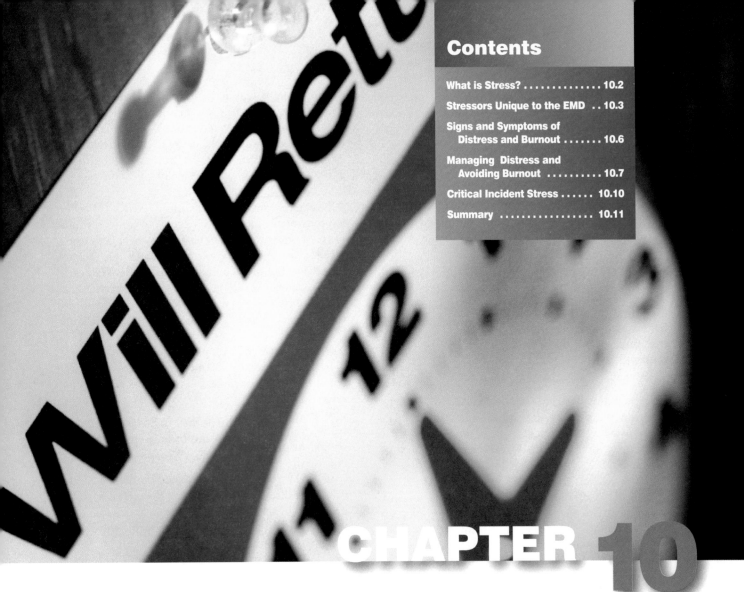

Contents

CHAPTER 10

Stress Management *in* Dispatch

Chapter Overview

Dispatching is very stressful work. Anyone who has done it knows vividly how the hot seat feels. Shifts that begin with a bang and never slow down can leave the EMD feeling drained and slightly bruised, if not totally battered. On the other hand, in slow times, waiting hours for a call can be hard in its own insideous way.

This chapter addresses stress and its negative effects. It focuses on the stressors unique to the dispatch office and offers the EMD an understanding of the way stress can build to unhealthy levels.

It also describes various strategies to recognize and cope with stress. Half the battle is learning to admit that over-accumulations of stress exist. The other half is learning to manage stress appropriately.

Dispatchers' First Rule of Randomness: Emergency calls will randomly come in all at once.

—Unknown

The EMD plays a pivotal role in emergency services. Everything that happens in the system funnels through the dispatch office. The EMD must continually make certain, rapid decisions in the *unseen presence* of strangers in crisis, relying almost solely on auditory stimuli. In relaying the call to field personnel, the EMD must be sure that the right crews get the right calls. Staying on top of the entire system at all times is another part of the complex set of challenges faced daily by EMDs.

The EMD is inevitably affected when, shift after shift, invisible callers express powerful emotions. Caller emotions may include sadness, grief, anger, anxiety, fear, or even, hysteria. Similarly, the EMD is the sedentary partner when field personnel relay emotionally laden messages by radio. When an ambulance crew is being shot at, everyone in range of that radio report, including the EMD, experiences high levels of adrenaline.

> **Stress is the nonspecific response of the body to any demand.**

The EMD's job is to direct, coordinate and communicate a constant stream of activity while remaining seated at a radio console in a protected building. Chronically high adrenaline levels are harmful, particularly to people whose jobs are fixed to chairs and consoles. The pressure to keep up with the action in a passive way can generate stresses difficult to imagine for people who have not done it.

What is Stress?

Stress is constant. It is not a disease or affliction. The classic definition of stress, coined by stress expert Hans Selye, is "the nonspecific response of the body to any demand." (Those demands are known as stressors, which are the causative agents of stress.) At the same time, a certain amount of stress is necessary for human survival. Living creatures all react to their stressors. The demands of the environment as well as the individual's reactions to them may be physical, psychological, social, or environmental. Physically, the demands of hunger, thirst, of being too warm or too cold, fatigue, and a full bladder are stressors. They force

> **Stress serves as a signal from our perceptual system to our emotional and cognitive centers that something is not right.   —D.J. Williams**

a response to biological needs: seeking food and fluids, shelter, rest, and bathroom facilities. Other stressors may include family obligations, financial strain, occupational load, and the desire to be successful. Any of these examples are forces that motivate people to seek a more comfortable and personally satisfying life.

When stress reaches overwhelming levels, the positive benefits begin to fade. Too much stress is a leading cause of or contributor to heart disease, hypertension, ulcers, lowered immunity to disease, arthritis, diabetes, cancer, alcoholism, depression, and suicide. The cost of stress is enormous. Conservative sources estimate stress costs *$20 billion per year* to the American economy; some sources extend that figure to up to $100 billion.[99]

The Greek term for bad, painful, or difficult is "dys." Dys-stress, written for the modern reader, is *distress*. In common usage, the phrase, "I'm stressed out" actually refers to distress. Distress can range from mild to severe. At the far end of the spectrum, it has earned a vivid name: **burnout**. It is also called cumulative stress reaction.[100] Burnout is what can happen to people when they invest great personal effort in a pursuit without effectively managing the accompanying stressors. In the extreme, end-stage burnout is like the way a lantern flickers out when it runs out of fuel. Stress, and to some extent, distress, are inevitable in modern daily life. But burnout is not. Those attentive to personal well-being, who learn to recognize and manage stress, need never burn out.

> **Burnout is not inevitable if stressors are properly handled.**

An important principle is that what one person regards as distressful may be precisely what another regards as fun or a worthy challenge. This relates both to the volume of stress and to the specific stressors encountered. Everyone is different. One person may love the wild rides at the fair, and the noise and the crowds; this setting may be stressful, though, to someone who favors quiet, all-alone days in a cabin in the woods. And vice versa!

> **Stress is only detrimental when we fail to recognize its signals early.**

People interested in the emergency services tend to thrive on a higher level of stimulation than most people. That is, most people are content to handle routine matters in traditional settings. They work and live in relatively tranquil places. Their lives are predictable.

They enjoy having a regular routine. EMDs have chosen an unusual lifestyle indeed! Knowing how to recognize stress and diffuse inappropriate buildup is a necessary EMD skill. Stress is only detrimental when we fail to recognize its signals early.

In addition to type and volume, stressors also vary in other ways.

- **Duration.** Some people can cope for only moments when confronting a medical emergency. Others enjoy entire careers handling those same situations.

- **Quantity.** The number of stressors in a person's life at one time.

- **Quality.** How threatening those stressors seem.

Stressors Unique to the EMD

Distress and burnout have specific (and often disastrous) effects on humans. Research has demonstrated a relationship between distress and disease. This is particularly relevant to the EMD, since dispatching is a notoriously stressful occupation. There are a variety of stressors—and considerable volume as well! Some of the stressors unique to the communication center are listed below.

> Gaining a sense of teamwork can be especially challenging in places where the EMDs work for a different agency than the people they dispatch.

Shift work. The majority of the lay public enjoys a nice, steady 9-5, Monday through Friday workweek. But emergencies don't schedule themselves conveniently; they happen at all hours of the day and night. Thus, one thing that sets EMDs apart is the hours they keep—sharing the *honor* of a 24-hour pursuit, of course, with field and hospital personnel. But EMDs are set apart even from those people because the EMD must be awake to answer the phone and set off the alert tones, pagers, and beepers. Field personnel are at least allowed to sleep—until the EMD wakes them up. Small wonder the two groups have not traditionally shared a strong sense of camaraderie!

Other team members. Dispatch center personnel are outnumbered. For each EMD, there may be many field personnel—and the EMD holds considerable power over their activities. This can result in an "us vs. them" perception. Another factor that can be divisive is that EMDs work in environmentally protected places, while those they dispatch must brave the elements. The resulting resentment is especially true during times of extreme weather conditions.

Gaining a sense of teamwork can be especially challenging in places where the EMDs work for a different agency than the people they dispatch. The resulting identity issues can also contribute to dispatcher stress. Field prehospital providers, by necessity, are typically strong, assertive, decisive, and independent. Sometimes it feels to the EMD that cooperation is lacking. Prehospital personnel like to be in control. It is an essential trait in the prehospital environment. This group dislikes being bossed around. The EMD who understands the group dynamics involved, learns quickly how to generate an air of cooperation through skillful verbal communication.

Excess audio stimulation. Having multiple ringing telephone lines to answer is stressful. EMDs do it all the time. In many places, EMDs also handle concurrent radio traffic. When one can keep up with the demand, there is a sense of exhilaration and pride. But it can sometimes be taxing to try to respond to so much with only two ears and two hands.

When the caller is a poor communicator, the task is more difficult. Some people, such as mentally challenged, drug-impaired, or elderly people, may be unable to process the EMD's questions quickly, especially when confronting an adrenaline-producing crisis. Children require extra effort, as do people who speak only a foreign language. Distraught callers must be calmed down. Sometimes, a more human response would be to end unpleasant encounters by hanging up as quickly as possible. The professional EMD should know why that is a maladaptive response, and what to do to avoid it.

> And all this is done from a chair, while listening to people on the telephone or radio, hearing their tone, fright, and need, but never seeing their faces.

Overload/underload. It seems that activity in the communication center is either feast or famine. An EMD may sit for hours and do almost nothing. Being geared up enough to handle whatever happens without being too keyed up is difficult to balance. One may need to transition from underload to overload instantly. The next call may be the first in an overwhelming series of emergencies. When several things happen at once, it is a challenge to keep everything straight! Caller anxiety, decisions about system response, needs of field personnel (such as additional units, or special services), hospital notifications occur differently for each call. It is easy to feel frazzled.

The EMD must be able to constantly shift patterns of activity. And all this is done from a chair, while listening to people on the telephone or radio, hearing their tone, fright, and need, but never seeing their faces.

Emotional involvement. The EMD can get drawn into the emotions generated by some calls despite the physical detachment from the scene. The EMD shares the tragedies and other emotional tugs of emergency medical care, especially in small communities when the EMD may know everyone involved.

With the advent of dispatch life support, the emotional investment of helping callers pays off well when things go right. And when they do not, the payoff can be painful. One EMD stayed after a continuing dispatch education session to tell her medical adviser about a recent case that illustrates this point. She recounted the exhilaration and pride of giving effective pre-arrival instructions for a choking child, only to find out later that the child had become the victim of a fatal abuse situation. The EMD was crushed by this tragic turn of events.

> **Critical decision-making requires that EMDs are in command of their emotions, not the other way around.**

Advanced prehospital care has increased the survival rate of people who go into cardiac arrest, and this is good. But EMDs must understand clearly that overall success percentages from CPR are well below 50 percent—usually more like 10 percent. Children in cardiac arrest (unless they have an airway problem that is quickly reversed) survive even less often. Despite the best efforts of the EMS system, people still die. An understandable sense of futility can arise in EMDs. A sense of responsibility for those events can arise despite the miles

that separate the scene from the dispatch office. So finding a healthy perspective toward resuscitation is important.[101] *Each loss is not a failure.* It just is.

Prolonged efforts. Some situations last for hours. Prolonged efforts generate unusual levels of stress, even if they turn out well. Whether a mass casualty incident, a trapped worker, a hostage situation, a child lost underwater, or something else, such experiences are likely to remain in the EMD's imagination forever.

Media attention. Routine situations do not draw unusual levels of media attention. The presence of newspaper reporters and broadcast media indicates that the EMS system is handling a *big* call. Performance expectations often change in a subtle way at such times. In addition to the mechanics of the call itself (plus others that come in), the EMD may have to handle information calls from the media. Although most EMS agencies have media relations policies, the fact that the media smells a story can generate an unusual sense of importance about the situation.

In 1981 EMS legal expert James George made the following prophetic statement about distress and the media:

> *EMS dispatchers bear a heavy responsibility. When a dispatcher errs in screening a call and a patient is seriously harmed or fails to survive, the dispatcher inevitably suffers great distress. Often, the event becomes a newsworthy item. The attendant bad publicity may cause an erosion of public confidence in the EMS system itself.*[18]

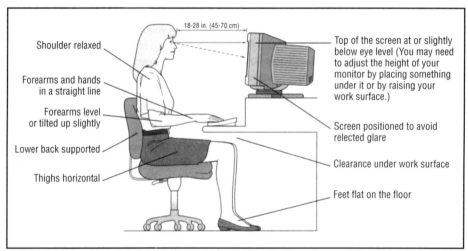

18-28 in. (45-70 cm)

Shoulder relaxed

Forearms and hands in a straight line

Forearms level or tilted up slightly

Lower back supported

Thighs horizontal

Top of the screen at or slightly below eye level (You may need to adjust the height of your monitor by placing something under it or by raising your work surface.)

Screen positioned to avoid relected glare

Clearance under work surface

Feet flat on the floor

Fig. 10-1. Work-space ergonomics and posture for reducing stress.

Personal stressors. Some calls, for some reason, evoke uncomfortable or painful personal memories. Perhaps the caller is a child saying, "Daddy is beating Mommy," and the EMD comes from a home of abuse. Perhaps a caller reports a carload of young people in a bad crash during graduation season, and the EMD lost several friends the day before their high school graduation several years ago. Situations that strike a personally difficult note must be acknowledged in order to be successfully managed. Otherwise, one might come to wonder why the job of being an EMD hurts so much "for no reason."

Ergonomics. Job setting is one *fixable* stressor. Ergonomics has to do with the environment in which the EMD works. Factors such as lighting, temperature, ventilation, airiness, furniture (especially the console and chair), visual and audio distractions, movement, and even smells can affect the EMD's ability to work efficiently.

Although some administrators regard attention to ergonomics as coddling, attention to it does make a difference. In one small dispatch setting, the all-purpose dispatcher not only answered all the phones and radio traffic, but took care of the problems people brought to the walk-in counter as well. Trying to concentrate on a fast-breaking situation *out there* was a challenge when the dispatcher had a line of people waiting (often impatiently) to pay parking tickets and register their dogs. The obvious answer was to delegate window services to someone besides the EMD.

> To be effective you must perform stress maintenance on a regular basis, with occasional "extra" treatments during more stressful periods.

Pay special attention to the chairs used by dispatchers. An EMD who feels like a pretzel because of a poorly designed chair can make life miserable for everyone (inadvertently or not). Then the field personnel might get cranky, or the EMD might even treat callers and other citizens insensitively. The entire EMS system can suffer for want of a comfortable work setting, or

---

Four Hallmarks of Distress

1. **Persistent feelings of fatigue.** This is a common signal of chronic distress. Nothing generates a refreshed, clear-headed viewpoint on life. (Some people in trouble have described sleeping 10 to 14 hours a day without achieving a sense of vitality.) This persistent fatigue may manifest itself in two ways. There is physical fatigue in which even small motions require effort. And there is emotional fatigue, in which it becomes nearly impossible to muster any emotional interest in the needs of others. The EMD's own needs consume every ounce of emotional energy. The willingness to work hard and well is dampened.

2. **Loss of motivation for the job.** People in EMS often have high ideals and unrealistic expectations for their work. They devote so much of themselves to the job initially that they must learn either to balance their efforts with outside pursuits or become disillusioned. Balancing one's view of EMS to a more realistic viewpoint can stem the tide of distress. Those who deny the distress may progress to full-blown burnout.

3. **Negativity.** People who are negative by nature become more so; those who are not tend to surprise co-workers with increasingly negative remarks. Obviously, a negative, ill-tempered EMD may not generate the best first impression for an agency in terms of public relations, especially calming distraught callers.

4. **Persistent cynicism.** This last hallmark of distress is like negativity. Usually cynical people get worse, and normally even-tempered, positive people start making inappropriately cynical remarks. A cynic is someone who "doubts the goodness of human motives." The dispatch office is a dangerous place for a cynic, where caller reports must be prioritized appropriately despite disruptive caller traits such as drunkenness, abusive language, or hysteria. Judging a caller's integrity at dispatch can be a dangerous proposition. In some ways, this is part of what caused the problem in the Dallas call-screening incident in 1984 (see Chapter 11: Legal Aspects of EMD).

Fig. 10-2. Four hallmarks of distress.[102]

simply for want of a chair that fits. Anyone who is expected to be anchored in one place for hours at a time deserves to sit in relative comfort.

Signs and Symptoms of Distress and Burnout

There are many signs and symptoms of distress that can occur in different combinations. There are emotional, behavioral, cognitive, and physical responses to stress, and they occur along a spectrum. Being in the dispatch office can be invigorating and enjoyable—if one knows how to blow off steam when necessary. That is, a person who is fine one day does not suddenly burn out the next day. An analogy would be what happens when a family moves from an address after many years. Perhaps the young couple didn't have much when moving in, but moving out is a different story! Stuff comes into a house little by little. The accumulation is only noticeable when one tries to move it out all at once. The distress associated with burnout is similar; stressors accumulate little by little, and they can become a big problem almost imperceptibly. To avoid discovering a big stress-related load, one must monitor oneself continually and do something about stress build-up.

Four Hallmarks. Most people overdosed on stress share four hallmark signs and symptoms. These may range in severity from mild and transient (for low-level distress) to severe and unyielding (see fig. 10-2).

Other signs and symptoms. The signs and symptoms of stress may occur in any combination in different people. One person may react mostly physically to a set of stressors by developing headaches, backaches, or other physical symptoms. Someone else might react mostly emotionally by becoming depressed. Another individual might have emotional, physical, *and* cognitive signs and symptoms. Most people experience a blend of emotional, physical, cognitive, and behavioral signs and symptoms.

> One trap of the downward spiral of distress is that fatigue becomes a potent obstacle to physical conditioning.

The most common physical reactions are:

* Sleep disorders

* Gastrointestinal problems

* Headache or backache

However, a variety of physical complaints may occur. In a business in which both sleep and eating habits are notoriously poor, it may be hard to say which contributes to the other, but it is well known that rotating sleep schedules and eating food of questionable volume and nutritional value are not conducive to good health! The sedentary nature of dispatching—*even without significant stress*—makes the problem of weight control difficult at best.

One trap of the downward spiral of distress is that fatigue becomes a potent obstacle to physical conditioning. Underactivity quickly becomes the norm, just when one of the best stress management techniques—physical exercise—would be most helpful.

The most common emotional reactions to distress are:

* Crying unexpectedly and for no apparent reason

* Easy irritability

* Flashes of anger

* Generalized persistent frustration

An EMD with these symptoms might become impatient with callers or try to pin the blame for frequently dissatisfying interactions on everyone else. Some people find themselves laughing inappropriately. Others claim to feel nothing, to be *numb to it all.*

Cognitive reactions to too much stress include:

* Memory loss

* Confusion

* Difficulty making decisions

* Difficulty concentrating

* Inability to solve problems

These reactions are especially hazardous to the EMD, who is in a position of great responsibility. There is little room for error when dispatching emergency crews to people in crisis.

There may be an overwhelming sense of feeling overburdened. The EMD can become increasingly hostile toward calls for help or field transmissions that make even the slightest *demand*. Administrative requests for paperwork might feel nearly insurmountable. In keeping with the common behavioral responses to such demands, distressed EMDs can certainly have a few choice words to say about them!

Diagnostic Criteria for Major Depressive Episode

There are two sets of criteria for diagnosing a major depressive episode. First, a person develops symptoms which can be characterized as "the blues" or "down in the dumps." There is a prominent loss of interest or pleasure in most or all normal activities and interests. Second, at least four of the following symptoms will have been present every day, or nearly every day, for at least two weeks:

1. Changed appetite or weight, either eating too much, or, more commonly, too little.

2. Sleeping too much or too little.

3. Psychomotor agitation or retardation.

4. Loss of interest or pleasure in usual activities.

5. Fatigue and loss of energy.

6. Feelings of worthlessness, self-reproach, or excessive or inappropriate guilt (either may be delusional).

7. Diminished ability to concentrate and think; slowed thinking and indecisiveness.

8. Thoughts of death or suicide that are recurrent.

Fig. 10-3. Clinical depression means more than simply, "having the blues." This chart lists common symptoms of true depression. [From Diagnostic and Statistical Manual of Mental Disorders, 3rd ed. (Washington, DC: American Psychiatric Association, 1980).]

Another behavioral pattern that emerges when someone feels he or she has given it all is to sit back to let others do the work for a change. Worse is when a person nearing burnout actively blocks procedural changes. The distressed EMD not only resists doing new tasks personally (such as PDIs) but also tries to rally others to block the change as well. As if this grim scenario isn't bad enough, it is also true that burnout can be both contagious and pernicious. Colleagues cannot listen to complaints and frequent threats of quitting without being affected. This is especially true if the person involved has earned a measure of co-worker respect.

> **Stress management is the responsibility of the individual first, and co-workers, supervisor, friends and loved ones second.**

High absenteeism is another predictable response to stress. This is because going to work is painful. The EMD can regain the perspective to carry on with the job happily only when the cause of the hurtful stressors are acknowledged and managed.

There are certain behaviors that signal serious distress. Addictive behaviors might begin or worsen, such as needing those after-work drinks, unusually heavy tobacco use, or compulsive eating. As someone becomes more burned out, increasingly worrisome signs and symptoms may arise. Clinical depression, defined as having four or more of the eight classic symptoms

(shown above) for two or more consecutive weeks, may occur. Additional signs of pathological burnout also include increasing suspicion or paranoia. Burned-out people accuse others of avoiding them or pressuring *(nagging)* them to get help. Such a person may emit a "leave me alone" message, behaviorally, then wonder why no one will ever go for a drink after work. Concerned co-workers, loved ones, and friends might feel confused by the mixed messages sent by the affected person.

Managing Distress and Avoiding Burnout

Stress management begins as the responsibility of the individual. The first goal is to develop ways to effectively and honestly monitor stress buildup. That way, stressors can be appropriately managed while they are still relatively minor. Stress management is much more difficult once major problems arise.

One person suffering most of the major signs and symptoms of burnout said that he knew what was happening to him, "but they don't have any programs for us to fix it." His company was not providing help, so he felt no obligation to deal with it himself. Even so, people owe it to themselves to seek help. It makes sense for stress management to be a gift that one gives oneself!

There are innumerable methods for coping with stress. Some are healthy and helpful; others are maladaptive and destructive. Collectively, the American public has much to learn about stress management; Americans consume more than 20 tons of aspirin per day, and doctors prescribe muscle-relaxers and tranquilizers and sedatives to American patients more than 90 million times a year.[99] Although there is a place for these medicines, their use does nothing to eliminate the stress likely to be causing many of the medical complaints. They only ease the pain temporarily—until it is time for the next *quick fix*.

Stress is not limited to EMS. It is a cop-out to blame a bad mood on work when at home, and on home life when at work. An honest appraisal of the various stressors present in one's life can help the EMD see them for what they are. For example, someone who is heavily in debt and thus *forced* to work massive amounts of overtime could eliminate some of the debt and do without a few extras to gain breathing room—and find some time to enjoy the pleasures that remain.

> **Any time a troubled worker can be properly counseled and rehabilitated, everyone benefits.**

A person with relatively more life experience tends to cope better with various stressors than someone with relatively little life experience. Some people just fall apart as soon as unpredictable things begin to happen, regardless of their life experience. People with access to strong resources, such as a caring family, to help them cope with a problem have an advantage over those for whom such external resources are unavailable or not helpful.

Nowadays, savvy administrators recognize the stressful nature of dispatching and genuinely try to provide an environment as reduced in stressors as possible. Education about stress and stress management is a start. Another helpful tool is having a good employee assistance program. These programs provide assistance to employees for both personal and professional problems.

Any time a troubled worker can be properly counseled and rehabilitated, everyone benefits. In addition to being a wise financial investment for the EMS or public safety agency, an emergency assistance program is also an important humanitarian gesture. The International Association of Fire Fighters figures that:

> *Approximately 18 percent of any workforce is losing 25 percent of its productivity as a result of the costs of impaired performance due to alcoholism, drug addiction, and emotional problems… Studies have shown that for every $1 invested in an emergency assistant program, the employer will save $5 to $16. These savings can be seen in a decreased use of medical and insurance benefits, savings in worker's compensation claims, fewer grievances and arbitrations, less absenteeism, less use of management time with troubled employees, less employee turnover, and less personnel replacement costs required of training a new employee. Benefits of the employee assistance program are also expressed through the improved morale of the workforce and the rehabilitation of a valuable trained employee and experienced worker. The U.S. Department of Labor estimates the average annual cost of an employee assistance program to the employer ranges from $12 to $20 per employee.[103]*

Maladaptive solutions. Some ways of trying to manage stress are suboptimal. Substance abuse is a widely-recognized maladaptive response to stress. Drowning your sorrows is never a good approach, because those feelings will re-emerge eventually, perhaps inconveniently. *Substance abuse* includes anything consumed in compulsive or addictive patterns such as alcohol and other drugs, nicotine, salt, sugar, and fatty foods. Even watching too much television puts off—but does not deal with—stress buildup.

Leaving oneself in a rut is another insidious maladaptive solution. A rut can be comfortable, since it is familiar and unchanging. But when the sides of t h e rut begin to close in and become smothering, it is time for a change.

> **An employee assistance program can provide beneficial counseling and support for employees experiencing stress.**

Yet some people claim that there's, "Nothing I can do about my stress." Look again. This may be the onset of a maladaptive stress-management technique called *learned helplessness*.

Another maladaptive response to stress is to express negative emotions (such as frustration, anger, or apprehension) inappropriately. This might include fighting (verbally or physically) with others—including children, co-workers, supervisors, spouses, even callers. These actions may provide momentary relief, but they are usually painful in the end. Some people constantly threaten to quit the job. This may feel better temporarily, because when there is an end in sight for a painful experience, it becomes more bearable. A person with a

> **Time "away from it all" is a positive way to overcome stress overload.**

toothache has worse pain while wondering whether the dentist is available than once an appointment is set. But an EMD who constantly threatens to quit has a negative attitude toward the job. It is also demoralizing to others.

Positive stress management techniques. Learning to work well with stress—since some always exists—usually involves multiple approaches. There are many good stress management techniques. Each person has to choose those which suit him or her best. And don't just pick one or two; to repeatedly follow a rigid stress management regimen plunges one into another rigid pattern. Such an approach to stress *management* may be as stress inducing as it is stress releasing! Sometimes it may feel right to jog; on other days, it might be better to relax on the couch reading a fun book. Tastes change. Moods change. Flexibility and honesty are the best tools for deciding, day to day, the best way to unload the stress of the day.

The suggestions in this stress primer are but a starting point for a pursuit which results in a sense of well-being for those who take it to heart.

- **Take time off.** Everyone needs some time off. This is what coffee breaks, lunch breaks, weekends, evenings, and vacations are for. Most people have to work for a living. But rest and recreation are vital for making living fun. People who

> **Stress in humans is a biological signal to re-evaluate our priorities.**

routinely work through the lunch hour are probably less efficient and more irritable by mid-afternoon than those who take advantage of a mid-shift break. An engine cannot last long if constantly revved up; likewise, humans cannot sustain unrelenting work pressures without being allowed to idle occasionally. One of the most difficult things for emergency providers to accept is that the EMS agency can—and will—survive without their constant presence. This is as true of volunteers as is it of paid personnel. One great stress-management technique is to learn to say the word **no**!

- **Take a vacation.** Getting away from it all is unbeatable psychic salve. Some people insist they never need a vacation, but in the end, many of these end up with forced vacations due to

stress-related illness. One person laid up for six weeks admitted (after the fact) that the time away had given him unanticipated and enjoyable perspective on his life. In the extreme, some people have found that only by quitting their jobs can they rebalance their attitudes after accumulating too much chronic stress.

- **Take time for yourself.** Another great strategy for managing stress is to stop giving so much. Daily "me time" makes for a healthier, happier caregiver and coworker. Yet taking time for oneself is typically a difficult task for a caregiver. It feels selfish, but try it! Days have a way of evaporating without getting around to it. It is hard to add "me time" to the demands of work, family, and other interests. Some people incorporate it with a specific solitary activity, such as exercise or meditation. Even 10 minutes alone in the bathroom can help.

- **Meditation is another good release.** It is a straightforward, relaxing process of taking a quick, mental vacation. This provides momentary relief from daily concerns. Some people equate meditation with the feelings of well-being they get from prayer. There are many forms of meditation. Classes are not hard to find in most places. If one type of meditation feels unsuitable, try another. Deep relaxation techniques are also very effective, and can be learned relatively rapidly and with good results.[104, 105] Instruction might be available through local wellness centers or cardiac rehab programs.

- **Increase exercise.** One of the finest day-to-day stress management techniques is increased exercise. Research has shown that depressed people respond better to therapy done in conjunction with an exercise program; similarly, stress can be minimized when there is a physical outlet.

> **Pressed for time? Try exercise. It combines physical maintenance with stress relief, an efficient way to maintain yourself at peak condition.**

Some people are horrified at the thought of jogging, bodybuilding, or other unappealing activities. They just don't like to get sweaty. That's fine. Instead, walk around the block and get some fresh air. Other sporting activities that have been reported to manage stress include fishing, darts, and other quieter forms of exercise.

- **Develop outside friends and interests.** Diffuse the concentration of stressors generated by work by developing a group of friends or interests not associated with dispatch or even public safety. Often, when people try something new (such as dispatching), they throw themselves so whole-heartedly into it that they forget about other pleasurable activities in life. Resurrect old hobbies that have gone by the wayside. Or start an activity or hobby that has always been intriguing. Get to know the neighbors better, or find some other amenable, but non-public safety, social group. Resuming a lost church habit or volunteering (and the social interaction with other people that goes with it) may work.

- **Apply self-reprogramming and rebalancing.** One last broad category of stress management has to do with deciding whether there are some personal traits that contribute to one's distress. Self-directed behavior modification in search of a more balanced approach to life may be the key to survival as an EMD. This might include a res-olution to be friendlier to and more tolerant of others, such as being more patient with hysterical callers. Try a positive viewpoint of the world and get rid of the old negative one.

Self-observation is the way to recognize unwanted personal traits. This requires unrelenting self-honesty and objectivity. It means developing a way of self-obser-vation that continues even when one doesn't realize it. For example, when calls come in thick and fast, an impatient tone may creep into an EMD's voice. It takes practice to notice which situations stimulate inappro-priate flares of temper. It also helps to observe others and decide what is effective and appealing about their style. Perhaps those qualities could be incorporated into one's personal style. This is an interesting side-effect of case review participation.

There's no rule book that says that who we are now is who we must always be. Each individual has the freedom to strive for self-improve-ment. Become a constructive self-critic and devote some energy to self-growth. Pay attention to personal behavior and internal thoughts. An internal dialogue like, "Now, what does this dirtball want?" may not be something anyone would utter out loud. But internal dialogue can reinforce negativity. Each person has the option to resolve not to call people derogatory names anymore, even internally. Practicing not judging for an hour each shift can start the process of stress management.

> **If you keep doing what you've always done, you'll keep getting what you've always gotten.**

Critical Incident Stress

Some situations in emergency services go beyond what even public safety personnel regard as normal. These situations cause extensive, acute stress reactions. Such events may range from having an entire town disappear in a natural disaster, or having someone on a response team die, to a personally tragic event.

When a critical incident occurs, previously otherwise healthy, well-balanced people encounter stressors of a magnitude that generate various acute reactions. These may be physical, emotional, behavioral, or cognitive. The most vital concept to remember is that they are *normal* responses by *normal* people in response to *abnormal* events.

The Seven Most Stressful Calls

1. Death or injury to a member of the EMS team.

2. Death or injury to a child, especially when abuse is a factor.

3. Prolonged efforts, especially those that end with tragedy.

4. Receiving an emergency call from a loved one or friend while on duty.

5. Scenes with heavy media exposure.

6. Mass casualty incidents, particularly when there is no one alive.

7. Symbolic events, such as the assassination of U.S. President John F. Kennedy in 1963, the explosion of the Space Shuttle *Challenger* in 1986, or the death of Diana, Princess of Wales, in 1997. ❧

Fig. 10-4. The seven most stressful types of calls for EMDs to handle.[106]

Many of the signs and symptoms are similar to those of chronic stress: fatigue, health problems (such as headaches, backaches, etc.), changed appetites, emotional numbing, oversensitivity, and depression. Other reactions might include insomnia, nightmares, fear, guilt, flashes of temper, and general irritability, and whole or partial amnesia for the event. The difference is that they are brought on acutely by a particular event. (These reactions can begin immediately or within a couple of days.)

Fortunately, there are several effective methods for helping people with critical incident stress. The most well-known is a system of intervention known as **critical incident stress management** (CISM), a process originally developed by Jeffrey Mitchell. The most well-known intervention, critical incident debriefing, allows people to discuss their experience in a safe, supportive, non-judgmental setting. They learn that what they are encountering is normal, and what signs and symptoms might occur. A debriefing is done, optimally, within 24 to 72 hours post-event. This process helps most people feel better within six to eight weeks and minimizes long-term problems. (Some people are affected enough that they have long-term problems or require professional assistance, but at least a debriefing helps identify these people early.) Critical incident stress debriefing is a proven, healthy way to overcome what can otherwise be a debilitating response to a powerful emotional event.

> **It is normal to react to traumatic events through stress. The trick is to recognize and deal with the reaction.**

Debriefing teams are available regionally to people in the emergency services. The most effective teams are composed of both communication and field personnel plus trained mental health workers who have received specialized training.

Summary

The job of an EMD varies widely from place to place. Some EMDs handle relatively few calls, and tasks are relatively low pressure. However, these EMDs often have the stress of knowing the people involved. Other EMDs are extremely pressured and constantly receive and process what seems to be the worst and most bizarre events society can generate. Stress and distress are inevitable in modern daily life. However, the far end of the distress spectrum, burnout, is completely preventable—*if* one is honest with self-appraisal and in managing personal stressors.

Not everyone is suited to be an EMD. For some, it is just too stressful. The addition of providing compassionate dispatch life support may be a difficult adjustment for long-time dispatchers to make. Those not suited to be competent, modern EMDs should realize this unhappy fact and move on to do something they enjoy. This is for the sake of self, the agency, field colleagues, and the public. People without enough experience to know whether dispatching is right for them must realize from the outset that they face a unique set of stressors. Stress management is essential. Even former field personnel, who know about emergencies and their peculiarities first hand, must acquire a new viewpoint when they operate a radio console.

EMD, at its best, is an invigorating challenge. It requires steady nerves, the ability to concentrate on multiple diverse tasks, and the patience and empathy to blend the impersonality of technology with highly personal events. Each person has the choice to manage stress well so that being an EMD can be a rewarding experience, not only to the caller, but to the EMD as well.

Every life has a measure of sorrow. Sometimes it is this that awakens us.

—Buddhist proverb

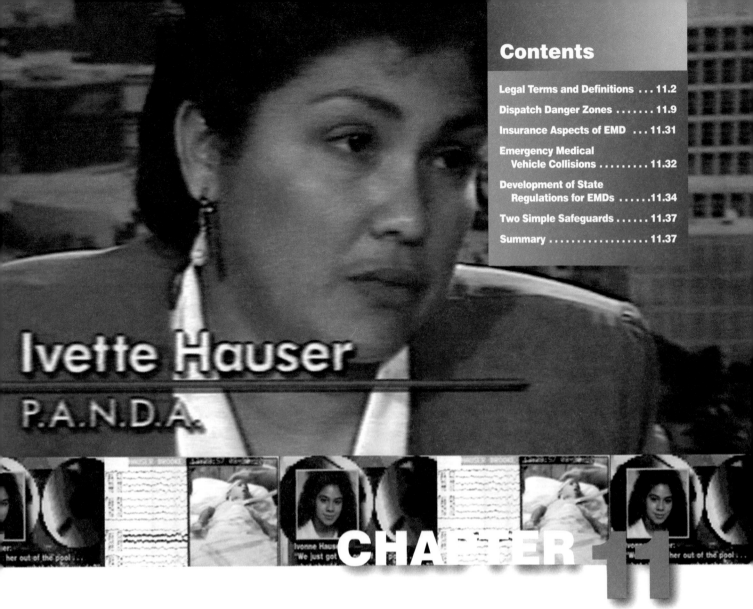

Ivette Hauser
P.A.N.D.A.

CHAPTER 11

Legal Aspects *of* EMD

Chapter Overview

This chapter summarizes legal issues surrounding EMD and the Medical Priority Dispatch System™. First, a common framework is provided through the presentation and definition of relevant legal terms and principles. Certain areas of medical dispatching which have tended to attract legal attention—"dispatch danger zones"—are presented in full, along with recommendations for minimizing vulnerability to lawsuits. Several hallmark legal case call transcripts are presented and evaluated.

Since the inception of priority dispatch, many states have generated regulations, certifications, and immunity statutes in support of the concepts that have evolved into the standards of priority dispatch and dispatch life support.

The point is, while your dispatching personnel express anxiety over the possibility
of liability for providing such a service, we may well see the day when a
municipality faces allegations of negligence for not providing such a service.

—James O. Page
September 28, 1981

The legal framework of any new development tends to be tested and defined in the contemporary courts system. The Medical Priority Dispatch and EMD concepts may also face such challenges. When the Aurora (Colorado) Fire Department, was first considering using priority dispatch and pre-arrival instructions in 1981, there was concern about the legal implications and liability for trying a new approach to an old task. Officials of the department turned to lawyer and EMS expert James O. Page, who wrote a landmark seven-page response that has since been widely quoted to diminish legal anxieties about priority dispatch. (This letter is presented in its entirety in Appendix C.)

Since the first edition of this book, concepts of priority dispatch have been embraced and implemented throughout the U.S., as well as internationally. This has resulted in an element of safety in numbers. As more EMS agencies make the transition from dispatch as it used to be to *priority* dispatch, controversies about call prioritization and pre-arrival first-aid assistance have quieted.

Since Salt Lake City implemented priority dispatch in conjunction with pre-arrival instructions in 1979, no lawsuits have been brought against any of the thousands of EMS systems using the Medical Priority Dispatch System™. Medical dispatch-related legal cases have universally reflected failure to use the concepts of priority dispatch as it is described in this book.

! Authors' Note

The legal definitions, terms, and situations discussed here refer to the U.S. legal system and may differ from the legal realities in other countries throughout the world. The authors' suggest consulting with a competent lawyer for legal advice on laws, regulations, and policies in effect for a given geopolitical area.

Adhering to a *system* of medical priority dispatch is vital. Implementing and using priority dispatch properly implies that all components of the system are in place. A legally sound priority dispatch program means personnel are well-trained and use a medically approved and scientifically-based system that includes appropriate medical control and ongoing operational supervision in a total quality management environment. Together, these elements protect against the sort of disastrous consequences that are demonstrated in the variety of illustrative cases used throughout this chapter.[107]

Although priority dispatch is relatively easy to understand intellectually, many people maintain a powerful "knee-jerk" response to the impassioned pleas of callers for help. Dispatchers still want to send too many responders on every call that *might* be bad. Statistically, and by the refinement borne by years of experience, priority dispatch has proven repeatedly that this is a hazardous attitude. Bigger is not always better. It is more appropriate to send the *right* response rather than the *biggest* one. A number of dispatch negligence lawsuits have been filed against agencies that fail to provide such a readily available system. These support, rather than undermine the priority dispatch concept. A major roadblock to the transition from traditional dispatching to priority dispatch has been to convince skeptics that every call doesn't generate a surprise.

First Law of Medical Diagnosis

When you hear hoofbeats, look for horses, not zebras, and you will be right most of the time.

Constituents of communities where dispatching procedures are not up-to-date are correct in demanding to know why telephone pre-arrival instruction assistance wasn't available to them when Uncle Harry collapsed. They are right to question whether collisions with EMS vehicles running HOT could have been avoided. Could the call have been prioritized and the correct crews sent non-emergency? The liability tide has long-since turned against dispatch policies and procedures of yesteryear.

Legal Terms and Definitions

Some familiarity with dispatch-relevant legal terminology is necessary to place into perspective what is safe and what is risky in a communication center. The following is a brief review of essential legal principles related to priority dispatching.

Duty. Duty imposes an obligation to provide a certain level of care when the general public has developed an expectation that it should be available. In broader terms it also means taking reasonable actions and protecting against taking unreasonable actions. Thus, part of providing improved care (even remotely by telephone) is that the system assumes *responsibility* to provide that level of care. The issue of duty in relation to EMD is characterized by the following expert legal opinion:

Changing social conditions constantly lead to the recognition of new duties. No better general statement can be made than that the courts will find a duty where, in general, reasonable men would recognize it and agree that it exists.[108]

Priority dispatching, including Pre-Arrival and Post-Dispatch Instructions, is now clearly the national standard in the U.S. Old-fashioned radio dispatch methods are no longer adequate or reasonable. As Page stated in his letter to Aurora:

The point is, while your dispatching personnel express anxiety over the possibility of liability for providing such a service, we may well see the day when a municipality faces allegations of negligence for not providing such a service. In view of the fact that implementation of this new level of service does not constitute a major expenditure to the municipality—and thus is an organizational/management/training issue, rather than a funding/taxation issue—I feel the case for a legal obligation (duty) to provide it becomes stronger.[109]

> One would argue there is a duty for an emergency system to take reasonable steps to avoid emergency vehicle collisions. Since prioritization of response leads to fewer of these collisions, prioritization of dispatch is a reasonable step to take to execute the duty to avoid emergency vehicle collisions.
> —Gary Horewitz

Priority dispatch also includes the important element of prioritizing response. Paramedic and attorney Gary Horewitz warns that, EMS systems involved in litigation have typically *not implemented a proper dispatch process.* As EMD has become the U.S. national standard, many states have authorized regulation of EMDs through certification and recertification procedures. Similar trends are occurring internationally.

Negligence. Once a new duty is established, the potential for accusations of **negligence** also arises. Negligence is the failure to provide the degree of care (as defined by a community or national standard) normally associated with a set of circumstances requiring that care. It may also be considered negligent not to cease, desist, or refrain from actions which come to be generally regarded as unreasonable or improper, such as continuing to employ obsolete practices and procedures. To prove negligence, four essential elements must be present:

First: The defendant must have a duty to act.

Second: That duty must be breached in some way, by acts either of commission or omission.

Third: Injury (also called damage) of some kind must have resulted directly from the breach of duty. (Damages [plural] is defined as the monetary retribution awarded in such cases.)

Fourth: There must be reasonable causation, meaning that the cause-and-effect relationship of the agency's failure to meet its duty was clearly related to the injury sustained (in contrast with the coincidence of such a breach with an injury that would have occurred in any event).

The burden of proving these four elements—duty, **breach of duty**, injury or damage, and causation—is the responsibility of the **plaintiff**, or the party alleging negligence. The party being accused of wrongdoing is the **defendant**.

Liability refers to the legal responsibility, obligation, or duty of an individual or organization to do, or refrain from doing, something.[168] If found legally responsible for damages associated with an incident in **litigation**, that individual or agency is considered liable.

The best "insurance" an EMD center has against becoming a defendant is to preclude accusations of negligence. This may be accomplished by implementing a proven EMD system, together with a quality management system that maintains a high level of compliance with protocol standards—and by protecting EMDs from undue pressures that might cause them to lose tolerance with and patience for the job (i.e., burnout). It is well understood that people who project at least the illusion of caring, through a kind tone of voice and a helpful demeanor, are less likely to be sued than those who do not. Much of this starts each time an EMD says, "Hello," and means it.

First Law of Medical Empathy

Good doctors and bad doctors both get sued. Nice doctors don't.

Some people have speculated whether there might be more potential for accusations of negligence in the area of pre-arrival instructions. What if CPR is done incorrectly by the caller despite the EMD's instructions?

Assuming EMDs follow the scripted text for post-dispatch instructions properly, they should be covered. EMDs are required to document that they have had CPR/choking treatment training prior to taking EMD training, so they have personal experience with the technique. That way, they can appreciate the subtleties of what they are asking faceless strangers to do. One study showed that the incidence of complications (such as broken ribs, lacerated internal organs and pneumothorax) was not significantly higher among people who received dispatch-assisted CPR than among people receiving either bystander or fire-department CPR.[110]

Reasonable Man. Some people are afraid that EMDs will not be able to perform the entire list of tasks every time, now that they have more to do. It takes only one burst of calls in a short period to appreciate how very busy one person sitting in a chair pushing buttons can become! Does an EMD have to deliver the same degree of assistance in every instance? Of course not.

Approximately 30 percent of callers are third party and often do not know the answers to the Four Commandment questions. In addition, there are times when the EMD is simply overwhelmed. The law recognizes that such times will occur and that it is simply not possible to give every available bit of assistance. Here, the concept of a "reasonable man" enters the equation. Under the standard definition of negligence, one of the components has to do with what a reasonable man might be expected to do under the same or similar conditions. That is, what if another call comes in while the EMD is tied up talking a caller through appropriate first aid? This fear was expressed to Page by the Aurora Fire Department:

> I cannot believe any jury in this land would ever hang a liability on a community or on a dispatcher who said, "I'm going to do the best job I can, with the information I've been trained to give, and I'm going to give it."
>
> —Arthur Miller

If a dispatcher successfully gives CPR instruction, or any Tother aid, over the telephone to one individual, but is unable to give the same to another person who calls in because of a rash of alarms at the time of the call or other circumstances beyond his/her control, can the dispatcher be held liable?

His reply:
I feel we need only to refer to one of the standard definitions of negligence. That is, failure in a particular situation to perform as a "reasonable man" would under the same or similar circumstances. What

would a "reasonable man" do under the circumstances described in your question? Obviously, the dispatcher would continue to instruct or aid the first caller to a reasonable conclusion. The alternative would be to "abandon" a patient who is known to be in a life-threatening circumstance…[109]

The possibility of conflict between taking the time to give telephone-instructed care and having another phone line light up exists, although the chances appear to be much less common than skeptics have feared. In the first seven years of priority dispatch in Salt Lake City, Utah, for example, only once was it reported that two of the three EMDs were tied up giving phone CPR instructions at the same time.

> If the worst-case scenario happens, the EMD must use the judgment that reasonably applies to the moment.

This may not be such a critical point for those agencies that have more than one dispatcher. The chance to impact, even help save, a life is worth the effort. Even EMDs who work alone might have a second call come in. If there are 600 calls per year, isn't it more appropriate to worry about the call that already exists, instead of being concerned that another might happen while the EMD is busy with Post-Dispatch or Pre-Arrival Instructions? If the worst-case scenario happens, the EMD must use the judgment that reasonably applies to the moment. Tell the initial caller not to hang up, that the other emergency line is ringing. Quickly answer it and determine its relative urgency. Depending on the second caller's response, juggle the needs of each caller the best way possible. EMDs are trained to prioritize. No more can be expected of a reasonable EMD.

The Emergency Rule. If there is only one call and the caller can provide the information related to the incident type or medical condition, the EMD can make an informed decision about care and response. If the caller refuses to provide phone-assisted dispatch life support to the patient, there is nothing more the EMD can do, and no liability for dispatch negligence is incurred. It is certainly best to try several times to convince a caller to help before giving up.

> The EMD can only be expected to respond in a reasonable manner to the various tasks at hand.

If, on the other hand, the same call comes in while there are too many other things happening at once—say, a working fire, a rash of medical calls, or a chase in progress involving a stolen vehicle—the EMD is functioning under different circumstances. The EMD can only be expected to respond in a reasonable manner to the various tasks at hand. The basis for this lies in the long-established emergency rule, which states:

> *The courts have been compelled to recognize that [a person] who is confronted with an emergency is not to be held to the standard of conduct normally applied to one who is in no such situation.*[108]

First Law of Mixed-Up Prioritties

If you're always waiting for the big one, you will miss lots of little ones.

Even public safety professionals, who are trained to handle emergencies, can encounter a demanding mix of situations that, together, are beyond their reasonable capabilities to perform. The ability to cope may vary justifiably from moment to moment in the course of a day's work in emergency services. The skeptic might then ask whether it is negligent not to have sufficient numbers of EMDs to cover every possible contingency. The answer is, no. The legal community recognizes that reasonably practical efforts to provide for normal, average, predictable levels of emergency activity, are fully adequate. When extraordinary emergency situations arise, disaster protocols are called for. Even an agency that expects to handle emergencies can be overwhelmed, creating an emergency "overload." The legal system takes this possibility into account via the emergency rule.

Foreseeability. Concerns voiced frequently about priority dispatch are: What if the caller lies? Or what if she doesn't provide essential information that the EMD would have no other way of knowing or obtaining?

Remember that EMDs are people with all the advantages and limitations of the human mind. As such, they cannot be expected to be predictors or prognosticators. No one is always 100 percent correct. If this were so, the only safely certifiable EMD would have lived long ago in King Arthur's court and would have had a long white beard and a pointed hat! Merlin excepted, EMDs must follow accepted medical protocols based on statistical probabilities that reflect a reasonable degree of patient safety. If training is adequate and procedure is

followed, errors that occasionally occur will most likely be due to incomplete or untruthful information—not lack of it.

According to the law, **foreseeability** requires only that we draw *reasonable* conclusions from the data given by the caller. That is, the EMD is not required to predict that a certain set of circumstances will result in findings reported at the scene that are not reasonably similar to the data given. A case in point: In one city, an EMD received a call from a third-party complainant that, "A man has fallen down the stairs." No further details were known. According to their user-defined responses within the Priority Dispatch System, the closest basic life support team was dispatched HOT and found not a man, but a woman. She was not on the stairs, but in her apartment. And she was not suffering from a fall injury, but had instead been stabbed in the chest with a 10-inch Bowie knife.

> **If the caller's information is incorrect, the EMD cannot be faulted, assuming that the EMD followed protocol and made reasonable efforts to obtain the appropriate information.**

Did the EMD do anything wrong? No. Legal protection for the EMD lies with the concept of foreseeability. It is reasonable to assign dispatch priority based on what the caller says. If the caller's information is incorrect, the EMD cannot be faulted, assuming that the EMD followed protocol and made reasonable efforts to obtain the appropriate information. In this case, there seemed to be a clear picture about the circumstances at hand; the call was classified according to the information available to the EMD. Many callers, especially third party, do not have accurate or complete information. In the absence of a clear picture, the best just-in-case response of the EMD is sometimes the higher response.

In fact, what had happened was that the caller witnessed the assailant running (and falling) down the stairs while escaping the scene. Had the assailant successfully evaded detection, the victim might not have been found for a very long time. A maximal EMS response would have been sent had the correct facts been known—but when the call was made, neither the EMD nor the well-intentioned caller could *foresee* the complete set of facts involved in this case.

A traditional, automatic maximal response would have ensured, of course, that the EMS personnel needed would have arrived at that scene initially. They could

The Maximal Response Disease

In the beginning the world was without light—not to mention lights-and-sirens. From the EMS standpoint such a time seems hard to imagine because today it couldn't be less true. Literally millions of "emergency" responses occur every year in the U.S. alone. Almost every one of them, in the years B.C. (before call prioritization), were run lights-and-siren, not only to the scene but often to the hospital. Ninety percent of the time however, there is no medical justification for this practice.

Closer examination of this philosophy suggests a Mt. Everest syndrome logic: "Why do we always use them? Because they're there!" From a medical standpoint, we could consider this aberrant thinking process the "Maximal Response Disease." It's a combination of always responding lights-and-siren or sending multiple vehicles. And short of the common cold, it infects more EMS response system people than any other malady.

Dispatch Misconceptions

The "disease" takes root from three traditional notions. First, it's an emergency, we've got to hurry! Years ago when hurrying was maybe all that was done for the victim, from beginning of call to end, the "hurrying" had some value—it got the victim to the treatment. Second, many systems have coupled EMS response logic to that of fire response. Unfortunately it is an apple vs. orange-type comparison. A fire gets worse by seconds and minutes, therefore, why not a prehospital medical problem? But a single cardiac arrest in a football stadium does not spread in the manner of a fire so that after a minute there are two arrests, then four, eight, sixteen, until shortly the entire stadium is in cardiac arrest. Medical problems do change, but the vast majority involve a single patient in less than a life-threatening crisis.

Then, last and unfortunately least palatable of all, running lights-and-siren in and of itself is fun and seems important—at least to some people, including a once 22 year-old EMT who will remain nameless. After one fire department first discussed the idea of sending first response EMT/engines non-lights-and-siren, a paramedic captain remarked, "What are you guys going to do, take away the last thing on this job that's any fun?"

Fortunately the maximal response disease is the dinosaur of today's progressive EMS systems. Medical priority dispatching is the method of its extinction.

The "Marine Corps" response has been touted as the method of ensuring that those in dire straits get all the help they need—and fast. So will everyone else without medically appropriate guidelines for the dispatcher to follow. In the past, EMS leaders pointed out that, in order to avoid any errors in judgment, the maximum response was always sent.

This conclusion itself, however, has become an error in judgment. Today, with significantly greater numbers of EMS-knowledgeable lawyers on the plaintiff's side of the table, we may be unable to defend against the myriads of potential cases resulting from significant delays in arriving at a critical emergency because an ALS team was tied up responding on a fractured extremity or a similar BLS call. Systems with the capability of tiered response that don't use their first-response personnel or their BLS ambulance crews (often private) and still send a "one-of-each" response, are not functioning at today's required level of medical responsibility.

Many telecommunications people believe that of the three basic areas of public safety dispatching (police, fire, and EMS), fire and EMS are more alike than either is to police dispatching. In reality, EMS and police dispatching are more alike structurally since the majority (over 90 percent) of their incidents do not involve escalating emergencies. In contrast, fire usually involves incidents that are considered escalating until proven otherwise with a few limited exceptions. There is also another very basic difference between fire and EMS that is often overlooked due to their common co-location that has contributed to maximal response thinking.

(continued on 11.7)

The Maximal Response Disease

(continued from 11.6)

Changing Dispatch Role:

Since the combination of fire and medical dispatching is very common, a clear understanding of this difference is essential knowledge to students of dispatching in general. The changing role during the unfolding of an incident can be thought of graphically as the variable width of a wedge. A report of fire begins at the point of the wedge. That is to say, the initial role of the dispatcher is simple and straightforward—get the locations and what is burning, then send the right assignment based on these two factors.

Varied interrogation sequences are not necessary. Once the first arriving unit visualizes an active scene, the process often escalates—the wedge expands as scene command relays specifics of the fire (exact location and its extent) and makes requests for additional responses.

The dispatcher gets busier with information relay as multiple command sectors are established and additional units staged.

Moveups and mutual aid are often necessary and other agencies such as police and EMS are notified as needed. The small point at the beginning of the fire dispatch wedge is based on the absolute necessity to get suppression units on the road quickly. A fire is assumed to be spreading. The extent of it can rarely be seen initially. It gets worse each second. Seconds do count here. But this set of facts for fires cannot be simply extrapolated to medical dispatching.

Caller Interrogation

By far the greatest responsibility of the EMD is up front, at the beginning of each call. The wedge is therefore reversed in EMS calls. Like the fire dispatcher, the EMD initially starts at the same place in the interrogation process. The location and callback number is, of course, identically essential. At this point the medical equivalent to the "What is burning?" question is asked, "What is the problem?" This query should elicit a Chief Complaint if one is not readily apparent at the moment the phone is answered.

The EMD must understand an important point here. At times the caller will offer the EMD information such as "He's dying!" or "Send the paramedics quick!" While these are complaints, they aren't Chief Complaints with categorizable medical information such as signs, symptoms, or Incident Types.

As you can see, "He's dying!" doesn't help you select a protocol. But then by asking "Why do you think he's dying?" you may elicit a response of "Because he's got a really bad pain in his chest and he's just pouring sweat." Age (approximate if not exact) is also determined, as well as the two most important medical questions we ask: Is he conscious? Is he breathing? You are looking for only yes or no answers at this point. Of course the answer may also be "I don't know" or "I'm not sure."

Herein lies one of the most significant concepts to understand about priority dispatching. In situations where, through this initial questions sequence, the victim is determined to be not breathing, or is unconscious but breathing cannot be verified, cardiac arrest is assumed and a maximum response is sent immediately before ever reaching a protocol! The priority dispatch concept does not waste valuable time asking more specific questions prior to response when the answers to these two important Four Commandment questions suggest an ultimate time-life threat from the start. Obtaining this entry material is an absolute baseline requirement in initiating any medical call for help.

Dispatch Protocol

Much has been said over the years about who is in charge. It ranges from who controls response through who controls the scene to who controls the patient. We know now that this role changes as we obtain more precise information from in-person visual assessment of the situation.

(continued on 11.8)

The Maximal Response Disease

(continued from 11.7)

However, from the time the call is received to vicinity arrival, the dispatcher "calls the shots." No, the EMD does not outrank the battalion chief or a seasoned paramedic. Hardly. The dispatcher is only doing what we (medical control or fire/EMS administration) have determined prior to the incident to be the correct level of response for any particular type of emergency. The dispatcher is only carrying out that protocol. But until someone arrives at the scene, no one can know more about the nature of that incident than the dispatcher.

As an analogy, compare response selection to golf. The dispatcher selects the club and the responder then drives, putts, or chips to the green. A maximal response to every emergency is the equivalent of driving a #1 wood to the hole from 20 yards out. It's just not appropriate for that situation. In the hospital, this would be the equivalent of the emergency doctor dropping everything she's doing and sprinting to the front desk to check the next patient just because she can't trust the triage nurse—also hardly appropriate. Priority dispatching has proved to be an effective, safe way to determine the nature of the emergency at the time the call is received, thus eliminating the need for maximal responding in many cases.

As may now be better understood, this outdated maximal response philosophy did not eliminate dispatch errors. It just made the real errors less apparent (ALS units tied up on BLS calls, first responders who were not needed, and emergency vehicle accidents). To professional EMDs, this potentially wasteful and even dangerous practice of maximal response should be reserved for the highest level of actual or potential crisis. Often, sending the Marines as a knee-jerk reaction has created the only real crisis present. ⚜

Fig. 11-1. "The Maximal Response Disease," revision of an article by J. Clawson, originally published in the JEMS.[23] Reprinted with permission.

have provided optimal care for that particular victim. However, to routinely take a just-in-case approach to such rare "red herrings" would mean innumerable hazardous maximal responses to minor falls and minor trauma. When the caller is willing and able to answer the EMD's questions, the EMD is right to trust those answers and prioritize the call accordingly.

Abandonment. Abandonment is the unilateral termination of a patient-caregiver relationship by the caregiver where an adequate replacement for that caregiver has not been provided, *and* when this action results in some preventable harm. The most common form of abandonment in EMS today is what plaintiff's attorneys now call dispatcher abandonment—the failure to provide pre-arrival instructions when possible and appropriate. The standard of care in the U.S. and in some other countries clearly requires intervention with telephone instructions to the caller. Omitting help is no longer acceptable.

Special Relationship. Once an EMS system performs certain acts or extends certain promises, it develops a new special relationship with its community. If there is originally no obligation to provide certain services, then a system evolves to another level, inherent promises have been made to provide a certain treatment or service. Consider the contrast between ambulance services of yesteryear with today's standard. 9-1-1 callers would find completely unacceptable the dispatch of a low-top Cadillac ambulance staffed by a single driver with questionable medical credentials. The general public holds modern EMS to a different, and higher standard. This is entirely applicable to EMD as well.

> **Whenever injury results from a dispatcher's error, the threat of costly litigation and bad publicity cast a dark shadow over EMS personnel.**[18]
> **—James George**

Legally, a special relationship can be interpreted as a right. One case, *Archie vs. The City of Racine*, Wisconsin (see no-send situation examples later in this chapter), was litigated alleging a violation of the patient's civil rights due to the specific nature of the failures involved.

Detrimental Reliance. This term came into English law several centuries ago. It describes situations in which a would-be rescuer fails to complete the act of helping, and others (who would have helped, except that they saw someone was already doing so) lost the timely chance to do so. As a result, the victim suffers. The original case involved a man who was drowning in a lake. People picnicking on shore saw him. One fellow stood forward saying, "I'll save him!" and started to swim out. Along the way, however, the would-be rescuer changed his mind and aborted the effort. The man drowned. His widow successfully sued the would-be rescuer. The law of detrimental reliance is a special way to identify a duty when there might have originally been no duty.

If the dispatcher promises to send help but doesn't, and if the caller, based on that promise, decides to not take the patient to the hospital in their own car, then the caller has relied on the dispatcher, to the caller's detriment. When, based upon the promise of another party, someone relies on that promise to their detriment, a contract may be formed—even if the first person made no promise in return. In this example, if the party making the promise fails to keep it, anyone relying on that promise may have grounds for a lawsuit for breach of promise/contract. Giving specific (eventually unreliable) timeframes for response or arrival may create this type of "implied warranty."

Tort of Outrage. A tort is a wrongful act (not including a breach of contract or trust) that results in injury. A tort of extreme or outrageous conduct could exist if a reasonable man would find that the particular conduct in question was so outrageous as to create a liability. It is sometimes found in civil litigation. A case in point occurred in Texas. Hospital-based EMTs slept at the hospital. The dispatcher called out the ambulance for a critical case, but the EMTs didn't respond. They were called again, but for some reason the dispatcher never checked to determine why they did not go on the call. It turned out that the EMT had answered the telephone, but had then fallen back to sleep. Any time a case elicits the response, "I can't believe they did that!" a tort of outrage might apply (in those jurisdictions where it is recognized).

Dispatch Danger Zones
The purpose of presenting the preceding terms and their meaning has been to provide an idea of some of the legal rules that govern the priority dispatch playing field. With these in mind, consider the body of legal action that has occurred (or has been threatened), out

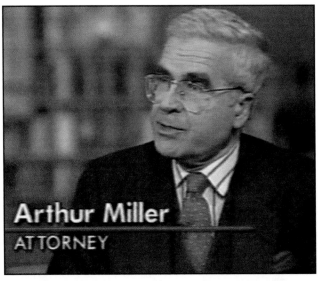

Fig. 11-2. Prominent legal expert discusses EMD legal issues on national television, Good Morning America, stating, "Litigation psychosis—people petrified because they are afraid of being sued—typically prevents human beings, like that dispatcher, from doing the right thing."

of which a body of recurrent errors and omissions now known as the "Dispatch Danger Zones" have emerged.[111]

Many dispatch negligence lawsuits are dropped or settled out of court. A common reason to settle a case out of court is that defense attorneys recognize a reasonable chance of losing. Unfortunately, without arguing a case in trial and on appeal, the issues raised cannot influence the body of dispatch-related case law. Historically, such lawsuits that we are aware of (whether dropped or settled) *never involved properly implemented and managed* priority dispatch systems. A proper system includes doing everything possible to avoid the Dispatch Danger Zones through:

- Implementation of a proven system of medical protocols

- Professional training of on-line personnel

- Having strong medical control

- Proper record-keeping

- Proper supervision of on-line personnel

- Team building

- Properly established risk management and quality assurance and improvement programs.

Conversely, lawsuits that have been filed against communication centers have usually involved one of the dispatch danger zones. The results of these lawsuits have

---

DeLong vs. County of Erie, Findings

A jury finding that defendant county, which operated a "911" emergency telephone system, and defendant city, which provided facilities and assistance for said operations, are equally liable for the personal injuries and wrongful death of plaintiff's decedent is affirmed, where the decedent, who died of stab wounds inflicted by an intruder in her home, called the "9-1-1" number to report a burglary and was told that the police would come "right away," but the call receiver failed to follow established procedures in taking down and verifying the information given by the caller and transmitted the incorrect address to a dispatcher, who radioed the call to police cars and, when the officers reported no such address existed, took no further action. Defendants assumed a special duty to provide emergency police assistance to decedent and they were negligent in carrying out that undertaking; additionally, circumstantial evidence supports a conclusion that the decedent relied on the assurance of police assistance. ❧

Fig. 11-3. Excerpt from *DeLong vs. County of Erie* (89 Ad2d 376) summary findings.

---

been less favorable for the EMS system being sued. The dispatch danger zones are listed below. Details with pertinent case histories and transcripts follow.

- Failure to verify basic information, such as the address

- No-send policies in which a caller does not receive an EMS field response

- Dispatch diagnosis

- Delayed response

- Situations in which more than one call for help had to be made

- No protocols for the EMD to follow

- Failure to follow protocol

- Requesting the caller's permission before giving Pre-Arrival Instructions

- Omission of Pre-Arrival or Post-Dispatch Instructions

- Asking to talk to the patient

- Attitude problems

- Pre-conceived notions and imposed, personal, negative impressions

- Mistranslation or misinterpretation of the caller's complaint

- Problems at shift change

- 1st Party gone-on-arrival situations

Failure to verify. Basic to the process of emergency care is knowing how to find the patient. Failure to verify addresses and telephone call-back numbers can be disastrous. In October 1976, Amelia DeLong called 9-1-1 to report that a burglar was breaking into her house. She lived at 319 Victoria Blvd., in

> **Confirmation of the caller's address and phone number is crucial. This is particularly so where the caller is a minor, or an individual whose native language is not the same as that of the dispatcher.**[18]
> **—James George**

the village of Kenmore, New York (near Buffalo). The calltaker reassured her that help would be sent right away, and recorded her address as 219 Victoria. He did not check whether her street was Victoria Boulevard (in the City of Kenmore) or Victoria Avenue (in the City of Buffalo), and then assumed it was Victoria Avenue. Buffalo police reported there was no such address as 219 Victoria Avenue and canceled the call.

Thirteen minutes after calling, DeLong ran, naked and bleeding, from her house. She had been fatally stabbed seven times. Had proper dispatch occurred, Kenmore Village police would have arrived within one minute of the original call. Her heirs were awarded substantial damages. The defendants unsuccessfully appealed to the New York State Supreme Court.[112]

The EMD must properly verify both the incident address and the caller's callback number. There are particular strategies for doing so outlined in Chapter 2: Basic Telecommunication Techniques. In the case of a failure to appropriately verify an address or phone number that turns out to be incorrect, if someone were to

---

Archie Case—First Call

Dispatcher:	**Fire Department.**
Caller:	Hi, say, this is Les Hiles and we have a lady that's really ah, I don't know, I'm not a doctor, hyperventilating. She can't hardly breathe, and I said, well let's go down to the emergency ward. Says, "I can't walk." Ah, so I say, well, I thought I could call rescue squad to get her, okay, 818 College Ave.
Dispatcher:	**What's the address?**
Caller:	818 College Avenue. I'll meet you out in front.
Dispatcher:	**What's the problem with her?**
Caller:	She just don't—just breathing like, you know, she just can't get her breath or nothing.
Dispatcher:	**How old is she?**
Caller:	Ah, excuse me. Rena, how old are you? Forty-three.
Dispatcher:	**Let me talk to her please.**
Caller:	Okay. Come here, come here. Wants to talk to you. She ain't big enough. Four hours… don't people—(makes sound of a person breathing very hard). See, I'm, I'm Les Hiles you know and I could be the best act in the world, but…
Dispatcher:	**Let me talk to her. Put her on the phone.**
Caller:	She's coming. She ever gets here. I know what's wrong with her.

Patient:	Hello.
Dispatcher:	**Hi. What's, what's, what's the problem?**
Patient:	Hyperthermia.
Dispatcher:	**Hyper what?**
Patient:	Thermia. Having a hard time breathing.
Dispatcher:	**Have you ever had this trouble before?**
Patient:	Once, once.
Dispatcher:	**Why don't you slow down a little bit and just relax?**
Patient:	And stay in my apartment?
Dispatcher:	**Just relax and don't breathe like you're breathing.**
Patient:	Okay.
Dispatcher:	**Do me a favor.**
Patient:	Yes?
Dispatcher:	**Get, get a little paper bag.**
Patient:	A little what?
Dispatcher:	**A paper bag.**
Patient:	Paper bag.
Dispatcher:	**And put it over your mouth and breathe into that. That will slow your breathing down.**
Patient:	Okay, thank you.
Dispatcher:	**Okay, bye.**
Patient:	Bye.

Fig. 11-4a. *Archie vs. The City of Racine* (627 F. Supp 766 [E.D. Wis 1986] and on appeal 826 F.2d 480 [7th Cir. 1987]).

be harmed or die, this would clearly be a breach of the standard of practice for EMDs in particular, and for telecommunicators in general.

No-Send situations. EMS legal expert James George stated in 1981:

Telephone evaluation or screening procedures are necessary to weed out non-emergency calls from true emergencies and to reduce the inappropriate and wasteful use of EMS personnel and equipment.[18]

Fundamental to priority dispatch is that every caller receives help or assistance. The Archie case, transcribed in figure 11-4, involves a situation that could not

happen in a system properly using Priority Dispatch. Note how the dispatcher's failure to follow procedures and protocols designed to reduce the risk of error can lead to tragic results, especially when accompanied by a decision not to send help. In this case, at 7:19 a.m. on May 27, 1984, in Wisconsin, caller Les Hiles reported a situation to dispatcher George Giese (*Archie vs. The City of Racine*).[113]

Almost eight hours later, Hiles called again, and Giese answered. Hiles wanted to know if his friend's "hyperventilation" should still be present after breathing so long into the paper bag. Again, an ambulance was not sent. She was found dead the following morning; the

Archie Case—Second Call

Dispatcher:	**Fire Department.**	**Caller:**	Listen to me now. Is there anything to do with the heart?
Caller:	Hi, this is Les Hiles.		
		Dispatcher:	**No.**
Dispatcher:	**Yes.**	Caller:	It isn't going to beat the heart out?
Caller:	Listen, this, this lady, ah, my little black girlfriend, I, I called before and tried the paper bag. She's still hyper-how do say that word—hyperventilating?	**Dispatcher:**	**No.**
		Caller:	Cause I know…like my chest when…I'm talking. You know who I am. Les Hiles.
Dispatcher:	**M'hm.**	**Dispatcher:**	**M'hm.**
Caller:	But she lay here for six hours. I mean, did, and I asked, "Did you ever do this before?" She said, (slurred words) "Only once in a while. But it scares me, you know, me.	Caller:	The swimmer? Okay, what I thought, my God, man, maybe it'll wear her heart out.
		Dispatcher:	**No.**
Dispatcher:	**Well, if she's hyperventilating, just, just have her do what I told you to do. She's going to have to breathe into that bag.**	Caller:	No? Okay. Say, what's your first name?
		Dispatcher:	**George.**
		Caller:	Okay, thanks a lot.
Caller:	Yeah, but.	**Dispatcher:**	**Okay.**
Dispatcher:	**Over her nose and her mouth and then slow her breathing down.**	Caller:	Thank you very much.
		Dispatcher:	**Yeah.**
		Caller:	Bye.

Fig. 11-4b. *Archie vs. The City of Racine* (627 F. Supp 766 [E.D. Wis 1986] and on appeal 826 F.2d 480 [7th Cir. 1987]).

official cause of death was pulmonary emphysema with superimposed bronchopneumonia.

Dispatch diagnosis. Failure to send help in the previous case stemmed from "dispatch diagnosis." These situations are particularly catastrophic because the consequences can be fatal to the patient, and the public's trust in the system can be utterly shaken. Consider the case that occurred December 26, 1987, involving a 42 year-old California woman, Ziporah Lam, whose family called when she suddenly experienced tingling in her arms and pain in her stomach and back. It subsequently aired on the TV news magazine "60 minutes" (see fig. 11-5).

A few minutes later, after Mrs. Lam had dutifully breathed in and out of the paper bag, her husband called again. His call was fielded by a different calltaker who took a different, but equally errant, diagnostic path.

On the recommendation of the dispatcher, Sidney Lam and his son, David, walked Ziporah Lam to their car, which was in the driveway. Their intent was to transport her on their own to a medical center. As she was placed in the passenger front seat of the car, she immediately seized. Sidney Lam attempted to provide CPR while David Lam ran back into the house and—for the third time—called 9-1-1. The calltaker of their first call answered.

The dispatcher concludes the call by hanging up the telephone. No pre-arrival instructions were provided for the victim or her family while the paramedics responded. The time lag between the Lam's third call and time of dispatch was estimated at approximately 30 minutes.

Delayed Response. The public's expectation is that when a real emergency occurs, the public safety system will react swiftly. Responses that are delayed for unacceptable reasons are fraught with risk and danger. If a delayed response contributes to a patient's escalating injury or death—decisions, actions, and inactions leading to the event will be scrutinized. Response may be negligently delayed because of a wrong address (as in the DeLong case), because of dispatcher failure to recognize the real problem or need (as in the Archie and

---

Lam Case—First Call (3:27 elapsed time)

Dispatcher David:	Fire Department. I need a paramedic, please.	Dispatcher:	Sounds like she might be hyperventilating.
Dispatcher: David:	**What's the problem there, sir?** Ah, my mom is experiencing pain in her back and her stomach and her hands are tingling.	David:	Does that require a paramedic? Ah, are you going to call a paramedic?
Dispatcher: David:	**What happened… What was she doing right before this happened?** What were you doing right before this happened, mom?	**Dispatcher:** David:	**No, not really.** Mom, it sounds like your hyperventilating.
Dispatcher: David:	**Is she anxious about something?** Ah, she was just lying in bed.	**Dispatcher:** David:	**Sir, does she have any medical history?** She had, uh, pneumonia about 4 or 5 months ago.
Dispatcher: David:	**She was just lying in bed?** Are you anxious about anything, Mom? No.	**Dispatcher:** David:	**And that's all, sir?** She thinks she is having a chest problem too.

(continued on 11.14)

Lam cases), or for other reasons listed in the remaining dispatch danger zones. It is one thing when such a situation can be explained reasonably; it is quite another when they cannot. In any event of negligence or preventative error, someone will be held accountable.

Significant delays in known lawsuits usually involve response times between 45 and 90 minutes. It is fact that there has never been a lawsuit claiming negligence for *not* responding lights-and-siren. These issues (and times) are very different.

More than one call for help. Another clear danger sign is when a caller has to make more than one call for help. This element was present in both the Archie and Lam cases. In each case, the same dispatcher handled more than one call for help from the same situation. (In the Lam case, there was a second dispatcher who took the second call; then the original dispatcher took the third call for help.)

If a different calltaker handles a repeat call and is unfamiliar with the findings of a previous interrogation, that call now becomes his call and a full primary and secondary survey is required. Even in the brief interim between calls, the patient's condition may not have been static, which could invalidate previously known details of an earlier call.

A case involving more than one call for help occurred in Chicago, Illinois in 1993. This case, since settled, might have set the record for the most repeat calls to 9-1-1 for a medical event. On the afternoon of September 15, 1993, the Reverend Eric Dale suddenly collapsed while doing repair work at home. Reportedly, at least 10 calls to 9-1-1 went unanswered before his granddaughter got through. Subsequently, five calls were eventually answered at the police 9-1-1 primary answering point and three were routed to the fire communication center at the secondary center (see figs. 11-6, 11-7, 11-8, 11-9, 11-10).

While the danger zone of "more than one call for help" is evident by the transcript, several additional danger zones are also evident. This agency claimed to use a form of dispatch protocol, however, no medical protocol compliance or any PAIs are evident in the three calls that got through to the medical dispatch calltaker.

No protocols to follow. Dispatch-related errors and lawsuits are much more likely for municipalities that have medical dispatchers working without a medically-proven dispatch protocol system. This is not a predictive warning; it is a statement of fact. It is too easy to make errors either during resource allocation or during telephone first aid instructions. Freelance decision-making is less possible within a quality managed approach to medical dispatching because of its protocol-based framework and its built-in accountability to medical control.

Lam Case—First Call (3:27 elapsed time)

(continued from 11.13)

Dispatcher: Yeah, that's the way it feels. Is she hyperventilating? Do you know what hyperventilating is? She's breathing real hard.

David: She has pain all over.

Dispatcher: Right. You get that tingling feeling all over.

David: She is getting a tingling feeling all over. She is coughing, and she looks faint now.

Dispatcher: Um, let me talk to her.

Sidney: Look, can you get a paramedic over here. My wife just isn't feeling well.

Dispatcher: Sir, we don't come out for people that aren't feeling well.

Sidney: Oh, Okay.

Dispatcher: Okay?

Sidney: She's not feeling well—it could be serious. She has vibrations in her chest... vibrations...

Dispatcher: (interrupting) Sir?

Sidney: Pardon me?

Dispatcher: Sir, did you hear when I talked to the other person?

Sidney: Pardon me?

Dispatcher: You didn't hear me talking to the other person?

Sidney No, I didn't.

Dispatcher: Okay. Sounds to me like she is experiencing hyperventilation. Now I need to talk to her to verify that.

Sidney: Okay, do you want to talk to her?

Dispatcher: Please, sir.

Sidney: Hold on.

Dispatcher: Thank you.

Ziporah: (moaning) Ohhh... I can't talk. What?

Dispatcher: Ma'am...

Ziporah: What?

Dispatcher: What's wrong with you? Why are you breathing so rapidly?

Ziporah: I'm not breathing rapidly, I am having pains.

Dispatcher: I can hear. You're breathing rapidly.

Ziporah: I'm having pains in my stomach and in my back, and my arms are all tingling.

Dispatcher: Yes, you're hyperventilating, ma'am.

Ziporah: Oh, I am having some terrible pains all over.

Dispatcher: Are your fingers numb?

Ziporah: My hands are tingling.

Dispatcher: Okay, let me talk to the young boy that was there.

Ziporah: Okay, hold on.

David: Hello?

Dispatcher: Hello.

David: Yeah?

Dispatcher: Okay, what's happening to her is, she is hyperventilating.

David: Okay.

Dispatcher: Okay, there isn't anything the paramedics can do for her. There isn't anything a hospital can do for her. The thing she needs is to control her breathing.

David: Okay.

Dispatcher: Okay, the problem is, she's taking in too much air and what you experience is your fingers start to tingle, and your arms start to tingle.

David: She has to slow down her breathing. And your head, and your chest and everything else, it hurts?

Dispatcher: Yes, it hurts because your body is not getting the proper air exchange.

David: Okay, she has to slow down her breathing...

(continued on 11.15)

Lam Case—First Call (3:27 elapsed time)

(continued from 11.14)

Dispatcher:	**Right, she has to breathe in and out into a paper sack.**
David:	All right, make her breathe out of the bag, Dad.
Dispatcher:	**Cover her nose and mouth…**
David:	Cover her nose and mouth…
Dispatcher:	**… with the bag, and have her close her eyes and relax, okay?**
David:	Okay.
Dispatcher:	**Have her do that, she has to do that for 15 minutes.**
David	You're positive that's what it is though?
Dispatcher:	**That's what it is.**
David:	It's not anything like a heart attack or anything?

Dispatcher:	**No.**
David:	Okay.
Dispatcher:	**And if in 15 minutes…**
David:	Yeah?
Dispatcher:	**You know, you got to do this for 15 minutes and if at that time she still experiences, the uh, the tingling and all that…**
David:	Yeah.
Dispatcher:	**You can take her over to the local hospital.**
David:	Okay.
Dispatcher:	**Okay?**
David:	All right.
Dispatcher:	**Thank you, sir.**
David:	Thank you.

Fig. 11-5a. *Lam vs. The City of Los Angeles,* (LASC NVC 01788).

Lam Case—Second Call (1:46 elapsed time)

Dispatcher:	**Fire Deparment 26**
Sidney:	Yeah, my son just phoned a few moments ago to describe my wife's symptoms, and they said it was, like hyperventilation.
Dispatcher:	**Yes, sir.**
Sidney:	Hello?
Dispatcher:	**Yes, sir, go ahead.**
Sidney:	And now she is throwing up. Is that part of hyperventilation?
Dispatcher:	**Okay, has her breathing slowed down now?**
Sidney:	Her breathing has slowed down a little bit.
Dispatcher:	**What…what she is suffering from sir…Does she uh, have the flu?**
Sidney:	It started as severe pain in the stomach, got up into the upper back, tingling of the hands, vibrations in the chest, throat and ears, and throwing up.
Dispatcher:	**Is she still throwing up?**
Sidney:	No.

Dispatcher:	**And if in 15 minutes…**
Sidney:	Yeah?
Dispatcher:	**Is she feeling better? Or is she feeling the same?**
Sidney:	(Asking his wife) Are you feeling any better, or are you feeling the same? (Too the dispatcher) The pain in her back is still there in the middle of her back.
Dispatcher:	**I see. Ok, but her breathing has stablized, is that correct?**
Sidney:	(Asking his wife) Hes your breathing stabilized? Yes, somewhat. She seems to be breathing a little bit easier, but uh, still fairly rapidly..
Dispatcher:	**Uh, I'd just take her to see, uh, see her doctor or take her to the emergency room and let her be seen by a doctor. Is she…has she been seen by a doctor?**

(continued on 11.16)

Lam Case—Second Call (1:46 elapsed time)

(continued from 11.15)

Sidney:	No, this just happened about 5 minutes ago.
Dispatcher:	**Might be a touch of food poisoning.**
Sidney:	Okay, so we should take her to a doctor?
Dispatcher:	**Yeah, I would just put her into the car and, you know, let her bee seen by a doctor.**

Sidney:	okay.
Dispatcher:	**Because that's a" the paramedics would do.**
Sidney:	Really?
Dispatcher:	**Yeah, you could just save yourself the money.**
Sidney:	Okay, fine.
Dispatcher:	**Okay, bye-bye.**

Fig. 11-5b. *Lam vs. The City of Los Angeles,* (LASC NVC 01788).

Lam Case—Third Call (0:32 elapsed time)

Dispatcher:	**Fire Department.**
David:	I have a heart attack victim.
Dispatcher:	**Your address?**
David:	(given)
Dispatcher:	**Telephone number?**
David:	(given)

Dispatcher:	**Okay sir, what are you doing for the patient right now?**
David:	She's… she's foaming in the mouth and choking now.
Dispatcher:	**Sir, we're on our way.**
David:	Thank you.

Fig. 11-5c. *Lam vs. The City of Los Angeles,* (LASC NVC 01788).

According to EMS legal expert James George:

An "upfront" clearly articulated written policy in support of telephone screening of emergency calls, coupled with sound guidelines and protocols for use by dispatchers would provide a ray of legal light in an otherwise murky area of heavy potential liability. A reasonable system of call screening can provide a good legal defense for both the EMS dispatcher and his employer should a charge of negligent handling of emergency calls be raised by a plaintiff.[18]

Failure to follow protocol. An individual EMD who acts beyond the boundaries of protocol loses whatever shield may be provided by the system. In a perfect world, the quality assurance system identifies these people on calls in which there are no negative consequences. It then provides immediate positive feedback and, if necessary, remedial training. As urged

> EMS dispatchers must always avoid the appearance of responding to or categorizing emergency calls in a haphazard or arbitrary manner.[18]
>
> —James George

in the Medical-Legal section of the Standard Practice for EMD (ASTM F-1258-95):

X2.1 *The agency and the EMD should understand the importance of EMD performance evaluation.*

- *Inappropriate performance or procedures, or both, can cause injury or death, or both, to field personnel or civilians.*

- *Poor work habits can lead to lawsuits against the EMD and the parent department or agency.*

- *It is important that the EMD remain informed on the correct procedures and protocols and follow them explicitly.*

- *If procedures appear faulty, the EMD should inform a supervisor for appropriate review.*

X2.2 *Civil liability for the EMD or his organization can result from the following:*

- *Caused action or omission by the EMD.*

- *Failure to supervise on the part of EMD supervisor.*

Dale Case—First Call (received 14:49:27)

Police:	**Chicago Emergency.**
Caller:	Hello, I need the ambulance
Police:	**All right, hold on, I'll connect you, hold on.**
Fire:	**Fire Department.**
Caller:	Oh, I need please, I need the ambulance.
Fire:	**What happened?**
Caller:	Please, at (given). Please hurry up.
Fire:	**Why do you need the ambulance?**
Caller:	I need the ambulance.
Fire:	**You haven't told me why.**
Caller:	Because my grandfather is having a heart attack, and he's dying.
Fire:	**Your grandfather, well, calm down, and give me the information. How old is he?**
Caller:	Huh?
Fire:	**What's his name?**

Caller:	His name is Eric Dale, please.
Fire:	**How old is he.**
Caller:	I don't know, sixty something.
Fire:	**Sixty something? What is the address, all right, what is the address?**
Caller:	(Given.)
Fire:	**What floor? What floor? Is that a house?**
Caller:	Huh?
Fire:	**Is that a house?**
Caller:	Yeah, please hurry over.
Fire:	**What is the telephone number there?**
Caller:	568...
(Fire 2):	**They are on their way, ma'am.**
Caller:	Oh, please.
(Fire 2):	**They're on their way, they are coming.**

Fig. 11-6. *Dale vs. The City of Chicago*—the first of 5 calls received at 9-1-1.

Dale Case—Second Call (received 14:49:38)

Police:	**Chicago Emergency, Mathis.**
Caller:	My, my grandfather had a heart attack, I need some help.
Police:	**Stay on the line, stay on the line, I'll put you through to the Fire Department.**
Fire:	**Fire Department.**
Police:	**Go ahead and talk to them.**
Caller:	Hello, my grandfather had a heart attack.
Fire:	**Where is this at, sir?**
Caller:	Thirty-eight West 108th Place, hurry up, he don't got no pulse or nothing.
Fire:	**All right, hon, is this a house or an apartment?**

Caller:	A house.
Fire:	**All right, they'll be there. Watch for the ambulance, okay?**
Caller:	(address given) Hurry up.
Fire:	**All right, we'll get somebody over there, okay. Bye bye.**
Caller:	He ain't moving.
Fire:	**All right, we'll be there shortly. Go watch for them.**
Caller:	Hurry up, man.
Fire:	**The ambulance is on the way, sir. Go watch for them okay?**
Caller:	I'm telling you ma'am, hurry up.
Fire:	**All right, they're on the way. Bye bye.**

Fig. 11-7. *Dale vs. The City of Chicago*—the second of 5 calls received at 9-1-1.

Dale Case—Third Call (received 14:52:25)

Police:	**Chicago Emergency, Mathis.**	Caller:	Right.
Caller:	Yes, we need the ambulance at (given)	**Police:**	**They're on their way.**
Police:	**They're on their way, they're on the way for that man that had a heart attack.**		

Fig. 11-8. *Dale vs. The City of Chicago*—the third of 5 calls received at 9-1-1.

Dale Case—Fourth Call (received 14:52:49)

Police:	**Chicago Emergency, Mathis.**	**Police:**	**Yes ma'am, for the grandfather that had the heart attack, they are rolling, they are on their way.**
Caller:	Yes, I just tried to call you, I need, the Fire Department is sending me an ambulance, 38 West...	Caller:	Okay, thanks.
		Police:	**All right, ma'am.**

Fig. 11-9. *Dale vs. The City of Chicago*—the fourth of 5 calls received at 9-1-1.

Dale Case—Fifth Call (received 14:53:54)

Police:	**Chicago Emergency.**	**Fire:**	**Where's this at ma'am?**
Caller:	Hello.	Caller:	Huh?
Police:	**Hello.**	**Fire:**	**Where at?**
Caller:	Can you please send an ambulance? My father just had a heart attack?	Caller:	One-hundred-eighth Place.
Police:	**Stay on the line. I am connecting you with the paramedics.**	**Fire:**	**They'll be there shortly, they're on the way.**
		Caller:	Please, please hurry up.
Fire:	**Fire Department, Nick.**	**Fire:**	**All right, they're on the way ma'am, okay, go watch for the ambulance.**
Caller:	My father just had a heart attack, he's dying, he's not moving.		

Fig. 11-10. *Dale vs. The City of Chicago*—the fifth of 5 calls received at 9-1-1.

- *Failure to observe recognized agency standards by the EMD or the parent organization, and*

- *Failure to observe recognized community or national standard practices.*[54]

There is basically only one degree of deviation from protocol that is sanctioned in priority dispatch. When a reasonable doubt exists regarding the right thing to do, act in the direction that insures patient safety. Dispatchers often have opinions about callers who seem frivolous, drunken, "stupid," or just plain upset.

Second Law of Medical Dispatch

When in doubt, send them out. (Always err in the direction of patient safety.)

EMDs not working within the framework of a protocol system sometimes make bad decisions based on an emotional response, sometimes even failing to send the requested resources. Perhaps it feels empowering to exert control over the callers. Or maybe a dispatcher

Follow the Protocol and Avoid Liability

The EMS coordinator of a fire department in the Midwest implementing a two-tiered response system using priority dispatch, expressed concerns that arose about response coding. First, if Dispatch codes a call COLD and the officer in charge of the fire apparatus decides to run HOT anyway, what is the potential liability exposure of the city and of the officer involved? Second, if Dispatch codes a call COLD and the officer runs COLD, but upon arrival finds a medical situation, not like what they were told, what potential liability exposure might arise? These are good questions I've been asked before in varying ways.

In answer to the first question, in my opinion, there is absolutely no reason for responding-station officers or crews to determine response mode and configuration where priority dispatch is in place and functioning. If department policy states which response mode (HOT vs. COLD) is to be determined by the EMD, a station officer's decision to do otherwise would be a direct violation of policy and procedure.

In support of the EMD as this decision-maker, no one can know more than the EMD prior to arrival, since the EMD is the only person who has talked with and interrogated the caller. The EMD's selection of a determinant code-based response is clearly the correct process since these responses are pre-planned by the department's management in conjunction with sound medical oversight input.

Should an officer change any response for his own reasons, in violation of procedure, it would be very likely that any liability incurred would rest on that officer. However, if it could be shown, perhaps a pattern in the department's failure to take corrective action in similar situations, then the department as "captain of the ship" might incur liability.

In this case, having a medically-approved protocol, training the EMDs, and also having a policy and procedure in place clearly stating who has the responsibility for response configuration and mode determination, would establish a rational and non-arbitrary process that would be legally defensible as well as correct.

The second question is an interesting converse to the first. It is apparent that the crew would have no liability for following policies and procedures and responding COLD as directed. What is important is that the EMD complies with the protocol in asking the listed evaluative questions and then codifying the data obtained. It is apparent that the EMD cannot be a prognosticator or clairvoyant in regards to scene findings. The dispatcher is only required to make a reasonable determination of the patient's problem based on the available information.

If the EMD followed the Key Questioning and picked the closest of the listed determinant codes (without going "under"), then the EMD would have met his/her duty to perform based on their training and procedure (the protocol). While in some instances, scene findings may be different than initially reported by the EMD, that does not mean that the EMD made a "negligent" mistake.

Field crews should be inserviced to understand that once the EMD has evaluated the patient and scene, three things can happen in the ensuing time of mobilization, response, and initial patient in-person evaluation — the patient can get better, get worse, or stay the same. Curing such failure of crews to appreciate this obvious, but not well-understood fact, could make life easier for everyone and prevent inappropriate criticism of dispatch from the field.

It should be pointed out that there has *never* been a case that has ever claimed negligence for not responding HOT. Furthermore, no study in the medical or public safety literature proves, or even states, that lights-and-siren saves significant time. The careful use of lights-and-siren as warning devices now more than ever requires their measured medically-correct use to prevent the terrible consequences of the predictable occurrence of emergency-vehicle collisions.

Fig. 11-11. "Follow the Protocol and Avoid Liability," revision of an article by J. Clawson, originally published in the JNAEMD.[114]

wants to avoid the wrath of field crews, who may also dislike coping with such situations. But dispatchers must balance the needs of the entire system—including those of the caller.

An interesting application of the Second Law of EMD occurred the week after EMD was first implemented in Salt Lake City, Utah in 1979, a call was fielded from an elderly woman who reported that her husband had just suffered a seizure. The interrogating dispatcher (not yet an EMD) turned to the radio dispatcher and requested an ambulance-only response. The radio dispatcher, a newly trained EMD was surprised, having just been taught that a seizure in a person over age 35 was to be considered a cardiac arrest until proven otherwise. He asked the patient's age.

"Seventy-six," said the interrogator. "Why?"

"We're supposed to send closest EMTs and paramedics on seizures in people over 35," he said.

The interrogator said, pointedly, "It says right here on these new protocols to send 'ambulance only'. "

"I think that's wrong," said the EMD. "Let's not take a chance until we can check. We'll send a maximum response this time." He did, and he was right; it was a cardiac arrest.

In fact, a typist preparing the first on-line set of protocols had inadvertently omitted the "over age 35" dispatch determinant from the protocols given to the dispatch office (obviously quality assurance was nonexistent at this time). Within hours of being trained, the new EMD made this decision based on a very important patient care-based priority. The typographical error was corrected immediately. The ASTM document also addresses this exceptional need to question established standards:

> **You can build a boat because there is a river, or because you almost drowned.**
> **—A. Seaton**

If procedures appear faulty, the EMD should inform a supervisor for appropriate review.[54]

Freelance dispatching is far different, and much less defensible than a proper clarifying enhancement of protocol.
The Third Law of Medical Dispatch helps to place the Second Law into clearer perspective.

Hauert's Ode to Freelancing

Well, I thought I knew what he said he smelled, so I sent what I heard that he felt he needed. (Quoted from a confused dispatcher.)

While this appears to some to be overly strict, time has proven it is not. In fact, there is an associated dispatch

Third Law of Medical Dispatch

Don't be in doubt so much. (With proper training, protocol, and time to do the job right, guesswork will be minimized.)

law within the protocols that clarifies that EMDs occasionally need to carefully extend the protocols to obtain the information they need to satisfy all interrogation-based objectives (see De Luca's Law).
De Luca's Law describes how to interpret what the "spirit" of the Fourth Law is and how the science of

De Luca's Law

EMDs will follow all protocols per se, avoiding freelance questioning or information unless it enhances, not replaces, the written protocol questions and scripts.

priority dispatch functionally requires nondiscretionary compliance to protocol. EMDs must comply with protocol. This does not mean they are meant to be robots. Enhancing and clarifying the protocol are appropriate and sometimes even necessary. Replacing or inventing it ad lib are not. EMD requires intelligence, training, attention to detail, flexibility of thought, and the ability to remain focused on following the protocol. EMD is not for dispatchers who want to sit back and let the system operate with no one in control. Defensible dispatching requires that an EMD gain an accurate, reproducible evaluation of the situation while avoiding arbitrary decision-making.

Fourth Law of Medical Dispatch

The science of medical dispatching requires non-discretionary compliance to protocol.

Caller "Refusal to Provide Dispatch Life Support" Example

Dispatcher:	**Hello, the City of _____ Fire & Rescue.**
Caller:	Hello, listen this guy he's sitting on the porch and he ain't breathing, he ain't breathing. (gives address)
Dispatcher:	**What's the address?**
Caller:	(gives again)
Dispatcher:	**(repeats address)**
Caller:	Big apartments, some brown, big apartments. I felt his chest—he ain't breathing, man.
Dispatcher:	**Okay. (repeats address)**
Caller:	Yeah.
Dispatcher:	**Okay, we have fire and rescue on the way. You want to give... ah... he's not breathing at all? Are you sure?**
Caller:	He ain't breathing at all. He's been smoking that shit!
Dispatcher:	**Ah... okay, we have fire and rescue on the way. You want to give him... you want to give him...**
Caller:	Okay, he's right here.
Dispatcher:	**Listen, you want to give him some help before the rescue gets there?**
Caller:	Man, that m---------- might got AIDS, man!
Dispatcher:	**We have rescue on the way, you want to help the guy?**
Caller:	I don't know. I can't help him. Shit. He ain't breathing.
Dispatcher:	**Okay, you want to give him mouth-to-mouth respiration?**
Caller:	I ain't giving him shit. I just called y'all. Please, man, y'all just get, 'cause I ain't puttin' my mouth to no shit.
Dispatcher:	**Okay, we have Fire & Rescue on the way.**

Fig. 11-12. Caller "Refusal to Provide Dispatch Life Support" example.

Consider field providers. They follow a set process in gaining their information. First they check the ABCs (and, if absent, then they follow a strict protocol, so as not to miss a step). The questions and examinations of their ongoing assessment are then based on the Chief Complaint and the objectives of the care process.

Compare the legally sound EMD system to the protocols followed by field providers.[29] Both are concerned with the ABCs. If the ABCs are compromised, both the field provider and the legally sound EMD follow a carefully prepared protocol that:

1. Minimizes the chance of missing a step.

2. Efficiently addresses the most life-threatening issues first.

The ongoing assessment of the field provider and the well-prepared EMD are both concerned with follow-up assessment and care, based on the Chief Complaint. While the field provider follows a set protocol for care, the EMD follows a set protocol for case entry. Each protocol has a set of questions and cues to clarify the condition of the patient and to ensure that the proper protocol is followed. Any additional questions asked by the EMD should enhance the protocol, not replace it, by utilizing clarifying questions and information to ensure that the proper protocol is being followed.

A standardized system of protocols is not only the most legally defensible dispatch system, but it also makes it possible to have a standard for the thorough review of calls. Quality assurance and review are very important components of a legally defensible dispatch program. They also provide evidence that reasonable steps are being taken to implement a sound (constantly improving) dispatch system. Review of a call is possible, in part, because a standardized system allows objective identification of any deviation from the standard dispatch framework.

> **The mental picture of a minimally-trained or untrained dispatcher "winging it" through telephone-instructed CPR has frightened more than a few city attorneys.**

Please Don't Ask Permission

Obtaining permission is a necessary part of responsible life—"Can I borrow the car?," "Would you like to go to the prom?," "Will you marry me?" It is implied that a rational adult has a right to say yes or no—in essence, exercise self-determination. However, the world of emergency medical dispatch is different. Everyone we deal with is not rational, healthy, or calm.

In 1975, the first documented pre-arrival instructions were given, establishing the prototype for a branch of medical dispatching science that would evolve over the next 15 years into Dispatch Life Support.

As an offshoot of pre-arrival instructions, some EMDs and dispatch centers require the caller to consent to receive and perform pre-arrival instructions for the benefit of the patient. One U.S. system in the Pacific Northwest qualifies the provision of pre-arrival instructions with the permissive questions "Do you want to do CPR?" and "Do you want to help?"

What medical or legal basis exists for asking the caller's permission prior to helping the victim? This notion probably emanated from the medical process of obtaining formal consent prior to treating or operating on a patient. Here the similarity ends. In the medical world, the *patient* is asked for a personal, verbal permission to proceed with recommended treatments based on a calm, informed description of the pros and cons of those treatments.

Several things are wrong with a permission- based pre-arrival instruction system. First, since when do we ask a bystander, even a interested or committed one, whether or not they want to "help" the patient? Didn't they just call and ask for help? We don't let the caller dictate by request what the specific mobile response will or won't be. Likewise, we shouldn't ask for their opinion on the appropriateness or lack of treatment for the person who we have just determined needs it.

Second, regarding legal consent, who has the right to deny emergency care to a critical unconscious or dying person? Not a relative, child, or even a spouse. Ask Page, Lazar, Ayres, Horewitz, or Wolfberg. If they agree that it is inappropriate, then why ask a perfect stranger?

Third, the "permission camp" incorrectly surmises that an individual calling to elicit help for another might not want to help. Not only does this appear overwhelmingly false, it is a negative approach, just when firm, in-charge, professional leadership-based action is most needed.

We can't physically make anybody do something over the phone they don't want to do. (The instruction for telephone-imposed "arm twisting" has yet to be developed.) American baseball legend Yogi Berra summed it up as only he can, "If people don't want to come out to the ballpark, how ya gonna stop 'em?" Then why suggest such inappropriate inaction to the caller as one of their choices?

There are three possible generic end actions to dispatch-instructed PAIs:

1. **The caller does as instructed.**

2. **The caller says they are doing as instructed but doesn't.**

3. **The caller refuses to help.**

They always have the third option and "How ya gonna stop them?"

It has been our experience that when unprimed callers refuse to help, they usually have a fairly good reason to decline (the patient is obviously "gone" or long dead or they fear infection or involvement in third party situations).

Paramedics and EMTs don't ask people in the street if they want help. If the patient doesn't want help, they will usually say so. If the patient's condition prevents them from answering, they have implied their consent to be treated.

Similarly, the EMD shouldn't ask someone, who has no right to express the unspoken will of the patient, if they "want to help." If they really don't, they will decline or just not perform. We consider the failure to provide pre-arrival instructions when appropriate and possible to do so as "dispatcher malpractice." Asking permission only encourages such negligence.

(continued on 11.23)

Please Don't Ask Permission

(continued from 11.22)

I have literally heard dispatchers misuse a "permission" discussion to talk callers out of helping when, by policy, they were supposed to provide dispatch life support. Trained EMDs using medically sound and time-proven protocols should feel confident that their decisions, advice, and instructions are not only needed but wanted.

We don't answer the phone in the communication center by saying, "9-1-1 do you want help?" Then why start the "help" portion of our later message in a similarly weak way?

It is the official position of the Academy that:

PAIs are stop-gap emergency provisions that do not require informed consent of the provider (caller) and that delaying or confusing telephone treatment by asking permission is considered contrary to the ethic of emergency medical dispatch and may result in determined negligence or liability for the dispatcher and center advocating uninformed inaction. ❦

Fig. 11-13. "Please, Don't Ask Permission," revision of an article by J. Clawson, originally published in the JNAEMD.[116]

Important roles of a quality assurance program are to identify deficiencies in training and to identify inappropriate freelancing. Consistent use of standard protocols is as important as having the standards in the first place. Inconsistent (often called arbitrary) action can be exposed in court, damaging the credibility of the defendant dispatch system. It is often used to paint a damaging picture of such systems, regardless of whether that image is deserved.

The greatest risk of exposure from inconsistency is when dispatchers use protocols on their own, without training, supervision or system-wide implementation. The obvious way to prevent this risk is to assure consistent use of the system through initial training, continuing education, supervision, and quality assurance.

Although it may be generally reasonable to fear the risk of liability, trying to provide a shield from it by making *no* selective decisions is shortsighted. The following quote refers to physician selectivity in ordering diagnostic tests. The principles of the statement obviously apply to EMD prioritization:

Liability Risk Examined: One area... examined was whether or not use of a screening protocol increases risk of liability. According to current legal standards, a physician is considered negligent when he fails to exercise reasonable care and skill in patient evaluation and treatment. A physician who fails to obtain an X-ray out of carelessness could be held negligent if harm resulted, but the omission of an X-ray based on selectivity in ordering diagnostic tests is not negligent, provided the physician's decision is consistent with the patient's clinical presentation.[115]

With priority dispatch, as with anything else, one is expected to prepare reasonably and in accordance to the national standards. According to a respected newsletter on EMS legal issues, the EMS dispatcher's conduct will be less vulnerable to charges of careless or reckless judgment where priority dispatch is in place. Similarly, EMS employers can point to such protocols as a system of risk management in an area where human error and its dire consequences are clearly foreseeable. When an EMD goes beyond protocol parameters (for any reason), medical control and quality assurance should detect this and respond immediately.

Requiring the caller's permission before giving Pre-Arrival or Post-Dispatch Instructions. Requiring the caller's permission before giving instructions is inappropriate in the medical dispatch environment. This all-too-common practice has probably evolved from the field practice of obtaining actual or **informed consent** (asking the patient's permission prior to exam or treatment). However, the dispatch environment is different. The caller has already asked for help by calling for help on an emergency line. The caller is in no position to make an *informed* decision regarding the care of the patient. In fact, asking the caller's permission places the right to deny emergency care with someone other than the patient. The EMD is trained, and obligated by duty, to offer help to those in crisis. If the caller cooperates, as they most often do, the patient may benefit. If the caller refuses to cooperate, (they generally have a good reason for doing so), the EMD has done his job as expected and is not liable for any untoward outcome. The medical dispatcher is responsible for offering help to those in need but should not attempt to force help on those not willing (see **Official Position of the Academy** at the end of figure 11-13).

The concept of **implied consent** is more applicable in the EMD environment. In medicine, implied consent is a legal term used to describe consent as related to the unconscious patient or the patient who is otherwise incapable (mentally or physically) of making rational decisions about her/his care. A sound process of determining a patient's level of competence is impractical and unnecessary in the pre-arrival phase. Consent is generally implied based on the call for help and certainly implied in the case of the unconscious or "not alert" patient and should be always assumed at dispatch for the patient exhibiting priority symptoms. The EMD provides instruction to the caller, who, in turn, must be the agent of change for the patient. In a practical sense, a patient refuses the caller (the agent) not the remote EMD (the advisor).

> **"If people don't want to come out to the ballpark, how ya gonna stop 'em?"**
> —Yogi Berra

Never ask callers, "Do you want to help?" This gives them a chance to decline just when their help could be crucial to patients. After all, didn't they just call and ask for help? When the EMD begins Pre-Arrival or Post-Dispatch Instructions, the caller has three possible actions:

1. Do as the EMD suggests.

2. Only pretend to do as instructed.

3. Openly refuse to help.

When callers refuse to help, they may have a good reason—just don't put such an idea in their heads by asking permission. Who knows how the previous scenario, from a Florida city, might have turned out (see figure 11-12). Obviously, there was no protocol in effect here at the time.

EMDs who are using medically sound protocols should feel confident that their decisions, advice and instructions are not only needed, but wanted. Be a leader.

Omission of Pre-Arrival or Post-Dispatch Instructions. The EMD should *always* give Pre-Arrival or Post-Dispatch Instructions, if possible and appropriate. Permission discussions that essentially talk the callers out of helping are unacceptable within the current medical dispatch standard of care and practice. Asking

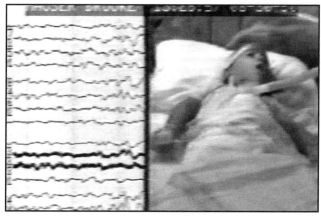

Fig. 11-14. Failure to provide pre-arrival instructions may have contributed to 14 month-old Brooke Hauser's brain damage and subsequent death.

permission is now considered dispatcher malpractice. In the dispatch realm, the Pre-Arrival Instructions in the MPDS for life-threatening situations are designed in user-friendly script form, graphically designed for optimal on-line application. Without these scripts, even experienced personnel might inadvertently omit a step or fail to follow the appropriate sequence of actions. It has happened. The results can be disastrous. Even the post-dispatch instructions, which are more generic than dispatch life support scripts, are carefully designed for the most accurate and appropriate use. Omission of pre-arrival instructions clearly belongs among the dispatch danger zones if, for no other reason, that providing them has become an international standard of care. The following transcript (fig. 11-16) demonstrates why. Brooke Hauser was eventually revived, and she lived in a vegetative state for 15 months before she died.

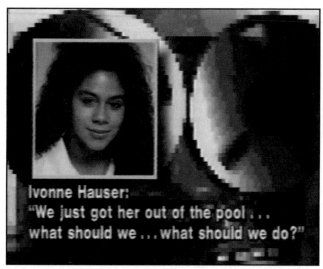

Ivonne Hauser:
"We just got her out of the pool . . . what should we . . . what should we do?"

Fig. 11-15. Ivonne Hauser, Brooke Hauser's 13 year-old sister, pleads with the calltaker for phone advice which never comes (see fig. 11-16).

Brooke Hauser Case (4:05 elapsed time)

Dispatcher: **911, is this an emergency?**
Caller: Yes, I…there's a baby drowned.

Dispatcher: **Pardon me?**
Caller: I think she's dead.

0:08
Dispatcher: **Ma'am, I can't hear you. Where are you at?**
Caller: 420…420 N.W. 70th Street.

0:12
Dispatcher: **What's the problem there?**
Caller: Um, she drowned in the pool.

0:18
Dispatcher: **Who did?**
Caller: My, my baby sister. She's…she's a twin and uh, she's…she's one years old.

Dispatcher: **Okay.**
Caller: Please hurry.

0:21
Dispatcher: **All right we're on the way. Stay on the line with me.**
Caller: Okay, please hurry she's dead. She's been in there for ten minutes I think. Oh my god.
Dispatcher: **Okay, stay on the line with me.**
Caller: (unintelligible screams)

Dispatcher: **Is there someone there to…Is there someone there?**
Caller: What?

0:35
Dispatcher: **Is there someone there to help her that knows CPR?**
Caller: My grandmother, but she doesn't know any…she doesn't know CPR.

0:39
Dispatcher: **Okay, how old is the child?**
Caller: She's, she's one year old and we don't hear her heart beat. She's turning blue. Oh my god, please. Please help.

0:46
Allocator: Engine 4, Rescue 44. Respond, respond to a baby drowning at 420 N.W. 70th Street.

Dispatcher: **We're on the way ma'am, we're on the way. Stay on the phone with me.**
Caller: Oh my god.

1:00
Dispatcher: **Stay on the phone with me. You say she's been in the pool? Do you know how long?**
Caller   I think for about like five or ten minutes. I'm not sure. (caller starts crying)

Allocator: (unintelligible) Fire, dispatch.

Dispatcher: **Stay on the line with me ma'am. Calm down. They're on the way.**
Dispatcher 2: **Are any parents there?**
Caller: No, my grandmother's here.

Dispatcher 2: **How old are you?**
Caller: I'm tw…um, 13.

1:23
Dispatcher: **This is your sister that's in the pool?**
Caller: Yes, we just got her out. I don't… what should, what should we do?

Dispatcher 2: **Okay. She's out of the pool?**
Caller: Yes.

Dispatcher 2: **Okay, hold on.**
Dispatcher: **Okay, stay on the line, ma'am. There's, there's… it… there's no one there that knows CPR. Is that correct?**
Caller: No.

1:32
Dispatcher: **Okay, then all you can do is wait for the rescue. They'll be there real shortly.**
Caller: I think she's dead.

Dispatcher: **Relax ma'am. The rescue will be there real shortly.**
Allocater: 503, standby for this one.

1:50
Dispatcher: **There's no movement at all, no breath?**
Caller: No, nothing. We found her floating in the pool.

Dispatcher: **Found her floating in the pool?**
Caller: Yes.

(continued on 11.26)

Brooke Hauser Case (4:05 elapsed time)

2:15

Dispatcher: **Okay, ma'am. The rescue's going to be on the way.**

Caller: Okay. Oh, my god. Her lips are turning...oh, she's got blood, she's got blood going out of her nose, and oh... her...her lips are turning purple.

Dispatcher: **Okay ma'am, their on the way.**

Allocator: Dispatch to Rescue 44.

Rescue 44: **44, go ahead.**

2:41

Allocator: Patient is a one-year-old child with under...at the bottom of the pool for approximately 5 minutes. She's not breathing at this time. Blood coming of out of the ear.

Caller: (crying) I don't know.

3:00

Dispatcher: **Stay on the line with me ma'am. The rescue should be there real shortly. Is there one... anyone out to see the rescue unit?**

Caller: My sister. Megan, go outside!

3:15

Dispatcher: **Make sure that she can flag them out. We're going to have a police and a fire unit.**

Caller: (crying) Oh no.

Dispatcher: **Take a deep breath now, relax. Does your sister see the rescue unit? They should be there real shortly.**

Caller: (crying) She's not breathing.

3:52

Rescue 44: **44's arrived. Rescue 44 will be (unintelligible) command.**

Dispatcher: **Okay, ma'am.**

Caller: Yes.

Dispatcher: **Okay, the rescue unit is out front there. You can hang up.**

Caller: Okay, thank you.

4:05

Dispatcher: **Uh huh, bye.**   🕇

Fig. 11-16. Brooke Hauser case.

Ellis Case (partial transcript)

Ellis: Okay listen, tell me, what are the compressions to breaths? Please, you...

Dispatcher: **You are asking me?**

Ellis: Yes.

Dispatcher: **I...I can't give you that information.**

Ellis: You don't know how many breaths you give, and then...

Dispatcher: **No ma'am.**

Ellis: ... the compressions? Isn't that what you're supposed to know? To tell us "okay give five breaths for every compression?"

Dispatcher: **Let me get the information for you.**

Ellis: Thank you. She doesn't know how many breaths...

Dispatcher: **How many is he giving? What is he doing?**

Ellis: Oh, the ambulance is pulling in right now.

Dispatcher: **Okay, I'm going let you off the line now, okay?**

Ellis: All right, bye.

Dispatcher: **Bye.**   🕇

Fig. 11-17. Tina Ellis, the mother of a one-year-old drowning victim, is unable to get any advice from a CPR-trained dispatcher instructed by her management not to provide telephone help. Sacramento area, California, 1991.

Boff Case—First Call (1:52 elapsed time)

Dispatcher: Fire Department.

Boff: Yes, I'd like to have an ambulance at (his address), please.

Dispatcher: What's the problem, sir?

Boff: I don't know and if I knew I wouldn't be calling you all.

Dispatcher: Are you the one that needs the ambulance?

Boff: No I am not, it's my mother.

Dispatcher: I want to let you speak to the nurse. *[Nurse Billie Myrick]*

Boff: Oh bullshit!

Myrick: And what is the problem there?

Boff: I don't know, if I knew I wouldn't be needing…

Myrick: Sir, I… would you answer my questions, please. What is the problem?

Boff: She is having difficulty in breathing. *[Constitutes clear identification of a priority symptom and possibly the chief complaint.]*

Myrick: How old is this person?

Boff: She is 60 years old.

Myrick: Where is she now?

Boff: She is in the bedroom right now.

Myrick: May I speak with her please?

Boff: No you can't. She can't… she seems like she is incoherent.

Myrick: Why is she incoherent?

Boff: How the hell do I know?

Myrick: Sir, don't curse me.

Boff: Well, I don't care, you… those stupid ass…. ass questions you're asking. (pause, confusion in background) Give me someone that knows what they're doing. Why don't you just send an ambulance out here?

Myrick: Sir, we only come out on life-threatening emergencies, okay?

Boff: Well, this is a life-threatening emergency.

Myrick: Hold on, sir, I'll let you speak with my officer.

Green: Hello.

Boff: Yes, what do I have to do to get an ambulance out to this house?

Green: You have to answer the nurse's questions.

Boff: All right, what are they before she dies? Would you please tell me what the hell you want?

Green: Well, I'll tell you what, if you cuss one more time, I am going to hang up the phone.

Boff: Well, I'll tell you what, what if it was your mother in there and can't breathe? What would you do?

Green: (yelling) You answer that nurse's questions and we'll get you some help.

Boff: Having difficulty in breathing. She cannot talk…

Green: (interrupting) All right, she's not going to… (audible phone click) she's back on there… and don't you cuss her again.

Myrick: Okay, sir, I need to talk to her still.

Boff: You can't, she is incoherent.

Myrick: Let me talk to her, sir.

Boff: (in the background, to Fleming) Will you please tell her that she is incoherent, that she cannot talk? (to nurse) She cannot talk at all.

Myrick: (yelling) Why!?

Boff: (now yelling back) Well, how am I supposed to know?

(continued on 11.28)

Boff Case—First Call (1:52 elapsed time)

(continued from 11.27)

Myrick: (yelling louder) Well then, give her the phone!

Boff: (in the background to Fleming) Give her the phone in there. Give her the phone in there for the chief. I know she can't talk, but they want to talk to her, but she can't talk. (again to the nurse) Forget it, I'll call an amb... a hospital around here, okay?

Myrick: (flippantly) Okay, bye. ⚜

Fig. 11-18a. Boff Case—the first of 2 calls received at 9-1-1.

Boff Case—Second Call (0:26 elapsed time)

Myrick: Are you same one now that I was talking to earlier?

Fleming: No, that was my roommate.

Myrick: A-ha. Why can't I talk to the lady?

Fleming: She cannot talk.

Myrick: Why?

Fleming: She is inco... I mean, she is just out of it. *[Breathing problems and altered level of consciousness mentioned as priority symptoms.]*

In fact, he is going in there now, he thinks she's dead.

Myrick: What do you mean by "out of it"?

Fleming: (in the background, Boff is saying she is dead) She is incoherent.

Boff: She is dead now. Thank you ma'am. Would you please send an ambulance? (pause) Would you please send an ambulance here! ⚜

Fig. 11-18.b Boff Case—the second of 2 calls received at 9-1-1.

This case speaks for itself. Ironically, this agency had been debating the pros and cons of an EMD system complete with pre-arrival instructions. Rather than following the negative example of agencies that deny any wrong-doing and fight losing battles against such apparently well-founded lawsuits, this city moved rapidly to implement a full priority dispatch program. It is reported that Ivette Hauser withdrew the lawsuit stating, "They can't bring Brooke back, but they've done everything they can." However, she didn't drop the issue behind the suit. Ms. Hauser founded Parents Against Negligent Dispatch Agencies (**PANDA**), an organization dedicated to changing the standards of many other communication centers who don't help in those critical first minutes by providing pre-arrival instructions.

Let me talk to the patient. In some of the most classic legal cases on record, the dispatchers have made the mistake of asking to speak with the patient. If a medical problem has been identified by the caller, nothing is gained by asking to speak with the patient. Review of these cases often reveals that the dispatcher did so in an attempt to *disprove* the caller's information. This is just another form of judging the integrity of the caller.

The most well-known case to arise in the history of medical dispatch occurred in January 1984, in Dallas, Texas.[16,117]

A 40 year-old man, Larry Boff, called for an ambulance for his stepmother, who was having difficulty breathing. When the calltaker could not get a clear chief complaint (or so he thought), he referred the call to the nurse, Billie Myrick, for screening. Following is a transcript of the infamous call that brought international attention (and spirited debate) to medical tried calling a nearby hospital, but it couldn't send an ambulance. Boff's friend, Dennis Fleming, then made a second call to the Fire Department.

Eight minutes later an ambulance was finally dispatched. It arrived to find Boff's stepmother already dead. The lawsuit that was subsequently filed for several hundred thousand dollars in damages, was eventually settled out of court for an undisclosed sum, reportedly for less than $50,000 based on causation and other undisclosed issues.

One fatal error in the Dallas incident was that the supervising Captain became more concerned about the caller's use of relatively mild profanity than the nature of the call itself. Another major error was that the nurse *screened out* the call entirely instead of sending someone to investigate. After all, the caller reported a woman exhibiting two priority symptoms. But obviously, *Myrick did not believe the caller and she did not follow her own protocols.* There may be times when it seems relevant to speak with certain patients, but the EMD must do it out of honest concern for the patient and not to *prove the caller wrong.*

This case also illustrates the point that an EMD must not make assumptions about whether the caller is telling the truth or being deceptive. The only exception to this principle is concerning rescuer safety. In very rare instances, an EMD may need to consider a scene unsafe until law enforcement or specialized HAZMAT personnel arrive and secure the scene, even if the caller says that scene is safe.

The EMD's First Law of Scene Safety

When in doubt, don't send them in (to an unsafe scene).

The EMD cannot wait for the lay public to learn the right medical words that signal a real problem. Nor can the EMD ever disregard a call for help because the interaction has been obnoxious or insulting when the message is clear that a problem exists. In the Lam case,

the report was of terrible pains in her back and stomach and later, problems in her chest. The latter is a priority symptom, as is incoherence (Boff case) and difficulty breathing (Archie case).

Attitude problems. The call-screening nurse in the Boff case displayed a disagreeable attitude. Just reading this transcript sheds some light on the contributing factor of attitude. But hearing the inflection and tone of her voice on audiotape leaves no doubt.

Job burnout in dispatch personnel can lead to profound managerial regret. Inappropriate attitudes cannot be tolerated in this profession. Dispatcher personalities must be appropriately matched with the demands of the dispatch office. In fact, the nurse in Dallas had already been reported twice by the supervising nurse screener for a questionable attitude, possibly based on built-up stress. As usual, there were several factors that contributed to the evolution of that unfortunate event.

Inappropriate behavior and errors must be avoided. But the reality is that dispatchers sometimes behave unprofessionally. Dispatching *is* highly stressful. But even from the isolated and stressful environment of dispatch, there are many interpersonal communication strategies that can be used to demonstrate the EMD's interest in the caller's concerns. For example, the old adage about nice physicians not getting sued is appropriate here. Someone perceived as nice is less likely to be sued than one who is rude. Medical control and the quality improvement system must bear some of the responsibility for ensuring that errors do not occur.

Hendon Case — (partial transcript excerpt)

Dispatcher: Hello?

Dispatcher: Hello? What's your address?

Dispatcher: Hello? What's your address?

4:03

Dispatcher: Do you need a police out? Cause if you're playing on the ph... if you're playing on the phone, officer's gonna come and take you to jail.

[Time passes as the dispatcher continues to ask caller for information.]

Dispatcher: Do you need an ambulance out?

Dispatcher: Hello?

Dispatcher: Hello? Do you need a...

Dispatcher: Hello?

Dispatcher: Do you need a police out?

4:39

Dispatcher: Hello? I'm gonna hang up if you don't tell me what's the problem.

[For more complete transcript see Hendon Case, Chapter 8: Time-Life Priority Situations.]

Fig. 11-19. The Hendon Case—partial transcript excerpt of 55 minute call.

Preconceived notions and imposed negative impressions. Attitudes, preconceived notions and prejudices regularly get dispatchers into trouble. Dispatchers sit in a non-visual world, where the only clues about a situation are via telephone. It is easy to develop inappropriate and negative impressions about a call by considering the part of town where it comes from, or by drawing conclusions about the caller's ability to provide information based on their accent, vocabulary, or vocal inflection. Boff's voice was argumentative and whining. In the Archie case, Hiles told the dispatcher on his second call about his, "little black girlfriend." (Although unrelated to this statement, this case was tried under civil-rights law based on the "special relationship" allegation.) The calltaker in the Lam case referred to David Lam, then a freshman at UCLA, as, "the young boy." EMDs must be exceedingly careful in their telephone demeanor not to base their responses on the behavior of others. Only rarely does anyone get a second chance to make a good impression.

> **Rarely does anyone get a second chance to make a good impression.**

The EMD's First Rule of Demeanor

"De-meanor" the dispatcher, "de-meanor" the caller.

Closely tied to attitude problems are preconceived notions which are equally deadly for a dispatcher. A case in Georgia involved one of the longest audiotapes in the library of EMD dispatch danger zone examples. For a full 55 minutes, the dispatch center listened to a caller do nothing but grunt repeatedly. Initially, the dispatcher asked what was wrong, but the caller still only grunted. At first, when the caller didn't seem to be cooperating, the dispatcher got frustrated and angry. She went to the point of threatening the caller, saying, "You could go to jail if you don't stop this."

To her credit, the dispatcher finally realized something was truly amiss, and summoned the supervisor. However, no efforts to trace the call or try to identify the caller's location were made for almost nine minutes. At no time was any effort made to see if the caller could answer questions through signalling yes or no (perhaps by tapping or grunting). Although the dispatcher, and then the supervisor, did not hang up (even though it was threatened several times), neither was very proactive. Finally, they traced the call, but when they got the address, they sent a police cruiser without a medical unit backup in violation of their own policy.

Then began an unfortunate series of miscommunications. As it happened, one of the police officers responding to the call was a long-term veteran with his own attitude problems. He recognized that he and his rookie partner had been sent to what he recalled was the residence of a "drunk." They found signs of life (such as lights on and car in the driveway), but no one answered their knocks. They looked through the windows but could see nothing. The rookie suggested they investigate more and perhaps break in, but first the sergeant asked dispatch, "Do you still have the reporting party on the phone?" The dispatcher said, "Yes, but he's refusing to come to the door." Perhaps they thought the dispatchers had achieved better communication, but this was not the case. The case was terminated because no one communicated well.

A day later, the caller's son found the caller on the floor, having suffered a severe stroke. When his condition finally improved, he could report that he had called, not one time, but also several hours previously. On the first call, the dispatchers had hung up. While it does not make a difference, the veteran police officer responding to this incident was incorrect, the caller was not habitually intoxicated, but a recovered alcoholic sober for years. Unfortunately for this large southern U.S. county, the caller was also a retired judge.

Another example of inappropriately judging the caller involves a call from a pay phone in a run-down section of a large California city, where the caller stated, "There's a guy laying here. He can't see or can't breathe or something!" The calltaker classified this as a 32-B-3 (unknown situation, third party.) The case was reviewed. When the calltaker was confronted with the possibility that the call should have been coded as a 6-C-1 (difficulty breathing, v10.0), he bridled at the suggestion, stating, "Listen to this guy, he's an idiot. He doesn't have a clue. Look where he's calling from."

In this situation, the calltaker ignored sufficient information to properly prioritize the call because this calltaker judged the information on extra non-sensical information provided by the caller and from where the call originated. The lesson is for the calltaker to listen carefully for any information that indicates the call may be a high priority, and not to judge the caller's ability to provide information based on communication skills, class, race, location, etc. Remember, even those who may be under the influence of alcohol or other drugs may still be able to recognize an emergency!

> ### The EMD's First Rule of Caller Judgment
>
> The EMD is never allowed to judge the integrity of the caller.

The preconceived notion that people with alcohol-related problems are somehow less deserving of help and quality care is rampant in emergency work. So are other prejudices. Personal prejudices or impressions cannot be allowed to influence the performance of the EMD's critical duties, and it does not matter whether these negative thoughts result from the stress of a situation, or from the EMD's personal system of beliefs.

> ### ! Authors' Note
>
> A colleague of ours has referred to this judgment as "the Sacrament of EMS"—implying a dispatcher-determined worthiness to receive help.

Never judge the caller. The accuracy of the caller's information can be best assessed by those on the scene, who can make any necessary changes to the response or resources using judgment gained from the responder's greater training and experience.

> ### The EMD's Second Rule of Caller Judgment
>
> Let's replay that tape for the ladies and gentlemen of the jury.

Misinterpretation of the caller's complaint. Correct classification of calls is not as easy or straightforward as it seems. However, it is an essential task so the EMD can send the appropriate assistance. The most consistent way to correctly interpret caller complaints is to follow the dispatch protocol.

We have seen those dispatch centers who have EMD-trained personnel and are using a protocol system incur much less attention from the legal community than those without.[111]

Problems at shift change. Coordinating part (or all) of an EMS system requires concentration. The system is vulnerable when one EMD is detaching from the task and another prepares to take charge. EMDs must use extra caution when shifting their dispatch positions so as not to forget important, undone tasks.

For example, in one U.S. west coast city, the dispatcher at the primary public safety answering point (not the ambulance service) received a call from a woman who had found her husband collapsed. During interrogation, the dispatcher asked her, "How long has he been down?" Her answer was, "I haven't seen him for a couple of hours."

The dispatcher notified the secondary public safety answering point at the ambulance service without transferring the caller. The EMD at the ambulance service tried to call the primary public safety answering point for some clarification, but the dispatcher who had taken the call had just gone off duty. The new dispatcher, just starting the shift, did not know the needed information. In the end, *no ambulance was sent.* Instead, the sheriff's coroner arrived about 90 minutes after the woman's initial call for help. She was rather distraught. The patient died. The case was settled out of court. The couple had been in separate parts of their home, and just hadn't interacted in a while. Later, it was determined that his collapse may have occurred around the time she called. But none of this was clarified during her call for help—and the original interrogator had long since gone home.

The dispatch danger zones described above have been identified during the evolution of priority dispatch in response to consistently observed errors and omissions. These unacceptable behaviors are often as detrimental to patients as they are to the systems. Now that the dispatch danger zones are known, communities and dispatchers can take steps to prevent these inappropriate activities from actually causing harm.

Insurance Aspects of EMD

The issue of whether the provision of pre-arrival and post-dispatch instructions have achieved the level of "standard of care" is finally made clear by the rejection of an insurance application for 9-1-1 liability coverage. The following statement is included in a 1995 letter from Ryan Insurance of Kingston, New York (see Appendix C for full copy of the letter):

Thank you for your assistance on the application for 9-1-1 liability coverage. I have heard back from the insurance company underwriter and am sorry to report that a coverage quotation will not be forthcoming at this time as your system does not currently give pre-arrival medical instruction to callers needing this service. The company has in the past been made aware of situations where the caller requested medical advice, and was told that was beyond the system capabilities. The resulting worsened condition quickly turned into a liability claim against the system operators. It seems the currently running television shows depicting 9-1-1 situations which include pre-arrival instruction have caused the general public to expect this service from all 9-1-1 operations.

As predicted 10 years ago, the insurance industry is now beginning to codify and thereby, require that standards be in place for medical dispatching before underwriting these activities.[118]

In their "Underwriting Guidelines for EMS Insurance Program,"[119] Medical Transportation Insurance Professionals of Scottsdale, Arizona, weights 5 to 10 percent of its approval process on whether:

Communication Center utilizes MEDICAL PRIORITY DISPATCH and dispatchers are certified by the National Academy of Emergency Medical Dispatch.

This is determined by the following section of their "Application for EMS Insurance Program":[120]

Indicate whether or not <u>all</u> communication center dispatch personnel are trained in:

a. Medical Priority Dispatching?   ❏ *No* ❏ *Yes*

b. System Status Management?   ❏ *No* ❏ *Yes*

c. Certified by the National Academy of Emergency Medical Dispatch?   ❏ *No* ❏ *Yes*

Risk managers and governmental attorneys pay close heed to these trends as external validation of the standards of care and practice within high-risk industries.

Emergency Medical Vehicle Collisions

Currently, most lawsuits in EMS stem not from patient care, but from emergency vehicle collisions. They come in the wake of emergency medical vehicle collisions and secondary collisions.[22, 121] Reducing the numbers of emergency vehicles on the road—especially those traveling in the

> **Though boys throw stones at frogs in sport, the frogs do not die in sport, but in earnest.**
> **—Greek proverb**

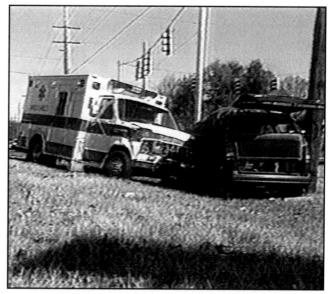

Fig. 11-20. Double fatal EMVC involving a daycare van full of children, Chesterfield, Virginia—responding HOT on an earache.

emergency mode—should be a critical priority to anyone concerned about liability.[24, 122, 123, 124] The destruction and carnage caused when an emergency vehicle crashes contradict such vehicles' purpose for being on the road. The best way to address the inevitable legal scrutiny that accompanies an emergency vehicle collision is to ensure that the emergency vehicle was traveling in an appropriate manner and speed, given the patient's situation and roadway circumstances, and that it was being operated with due regard for the safety of others.[24, 25, 125, 126, 127, 128, 129]

James O. Page framed the actual psychology of this issue when he stated:

What is the likelihood you'll get sued? Let's start by putting things in proper perspective. By far the greatest legal hazards facing EMTs arise from ambulance vehicle accidents. For some reason or other, we don't like to talk about ambulance vehicle accidents, even though most of them are preventable. Instead, we are fascinated—in a morbid kind of way—with the whole subject of "medical malpractice."[130]

If an EMD can determine that a call can safely be handled by sending less than a maximal response, preferably COLD, so much the better. Being able to send less than a maximal response, and having the ability to send that response without lights-and-siren (running COLD) is an excellent way to reduce the risk to the field providers, the patient, and most importantly, to the greater public.[37, 123, 131] Safe, decreased use of lights-and-siren certainly minimizes general legal liability. In fact, in Salt Lake City, Utah, fleet management data showed a 78 percent decrease in emergency medical vehicle collisions after the full implementation of the EMD program.[132]

Nesbit's Law of Mechanical Devices

And there's a dreadful law here… it was made by mistake, but there it is—that if anyone asks for machinery, they have to have it, and keep on using it.

An interesting side effect of HOT response is the wake-effect, which occurs when a vehicle collision appears to be caused by the passage of an emergency vehicle, but does not actually involve the emergency vehicle itself. A study published in the *Journal of Prehospital and Disaster Medicine* indicated that wake-effect collisions happen more frequently than emergency medical vehicle collisions, possibly by a factor of four or five, multiplying the negative effects of HOT responses gone wrong.[13] Perhaps lyricist Billy Joel, in his appropriately titled hit song, "Don't Ask Me Why," was calling to the EMS community about the wake-effect problem when he sang, "You are still a victim of the accidents you leave."

Does driving HOT (lights-and-siren) really make all that much difference anyway? Richard Hunt, et al.,[36] measured the time taken for each of 50 urban ambulance transports using lights-and-siren. They also timed a paramedic who drove an ambulance over identical routes but without lights-and-siren (each simulated transport was matched to the corresponding lights-and-siren transport with respect to the time of day and day of the week; the driver was instructed to obey the speed limit, traffic laws, and traffic signs). On average, lights-and-siren transports arrived 43.5 seconds earlier than the corresponding simulated transports. 22 percent of the lights-and-siren transports were up to 2 minutes and 49 seconds slower, 2 percent took the same amount of time, and 76 percent of the lights-and-siren runs were up to 2 minutes and 42 seconds faster than the corresponding simulated transports (there was one outlier that arrived 5 minutes earlier than the corresponding simulation).

Hunt, et al., concluded that "the 43.5 second mean time savings does not warrant the use of lights-and-siren during ambulance transport, except in rare situations or clinical circumstances." Douglas Kupas, et al.,[128] examined whether avoiding lights-and-siren had any deleterious effects on patient outcomes. 92 percent

! Authors' Note

We routinely receive correspondence like the following from EMD-Instructor David Lloyd of Bethlehem, Pennsylvania:

I attended the EMD-Q class with two of my staff. We all were impressed with the program and they have had their batteries recharged and they are working towards developing a viable quality management program for the City of Bethlehem.

I was surprised to learn from the attendees that so many of them are operating with EMD but are not utilizing non-lights-and-siren responses. It was great news to hear about the Salt Lake Center attaining it Accreditation as a Center of Excellence and that they will be responding without lights-and-siren to bravo calls. Bethlehem EMS has been running non-lights-and-siren on bravos for about one year now, with no negative patient outcomes or complaints, due to "slow" response. The public has been basically unaware of the change in policy. We are hoping to begin non-lights-and-siren responses for some charlie calls in the near future. I would like to take on this project with the local teaching hospital in the hope that they will support the concept and perhaps do a formal research paper on it. It is our goal to someday run lights-and-siren for probable delta calls only.

There is still a lot of work to be done in EMD. In my teaching this year, from polling my students I found out that students in four of my classes have been involved in recent emergency medical vehicle collisions and that two of the students had been involved in crashes with fatalities. The good news has been that I have been hearing from the students that as a result of the EMD classes, some of the fire departments are looking at non-lights-and-siren responses for some of their fire (non-EMS) calls!

I would like to thank you for the opportunity to teach EMD this past year. It is something I truly enjoy and it is something that I believe will make a difference to our patients.

December 13, 1997

First Law of Medical Dispatch   Protocol 32

First, do no harm.

(1,495 out of 1,625) of transports during their study were transported without lights-and-siren. While 47 percent of these non-lights-and-siren transports involved patients who required, and received, ALS interventions, only 13 patients (less than 1 percent) actually worsened during transport and none suffered any worsened outcome related to non-lights-and-siren transport.

> **Hunt, et al.,**[36] **concluded that the 43.5 second mean time savings does not warrant the use of lights-and-siren during ambulance transport, except in rare situations or clinical circumstances.**

> **Kupas, et al.,**[128] **found that less than 1 percent of patients actually worsened during transport and none suffered any worsened outcome related to non-lights-and-siren transport.**

In addition to decreasing collisions, prioritizing calls also reduces attrition of prehospital personnel through burnout. It is an emotional strain to respond HOT (lights-and-siren) unnecessarily to numerous calls that don't require it (see Chapter 1: The *First*, First Responder for more information). Sending the right responders, *in the right way*, will help ensure that dispatchers don't violate the first law of dispatch.

In 1997, the Salt Lake City Fire Department initiated an internal study to evaluate the post-arrival urgency of all BRAVO-level calls. Out of a total of 9,608 BRAVO runs only 72 (<1%) resulted in HOT transports to the hospital. Using the fire department Medical Director's EMS patient condition score (5 = alive/stable; 4 = alive and critical; 3 = died in ER; 2 = worked and pronounced on scene; 1 = dead on arrival), only 14 were scored as less than a 5 and only 14 received any ALS treatment subsequent to the initial BLS BRAVO response. Based on this data, as of January 1st, 1998, the fire department amazingly began responding to all BRAVO-level calls COLD (see Appendix A.13)! A year later they shared information comparing the all HOT BRAVO response year 1997 with the all COLD BRAVO response year 1998. The data in figure 11.21 shows total average response times and differences between the two years for all BLS engine company first responder units. They are now in the fourth year of BRAVO (in addition to ALPHA) COLD responses.

As a student of the MPDS would know, the largest group of BRAVO calls in any system are 29-Bs (Traffic/Transportation Accidents) with various injuries excluding MAJOR INCIDENT, HIGH MECHANISM, HAZMAT, pinned victims, and not alert patients. This program appears to be working safely and has reduced the numbers emergency vehicles running HOT by approximately 48% (based on 9,608 BRAVO out of 19,737 total EMS runs in the study year).

Development of State Regulations for EMDs

Adapting state regulations for EMS personnel or creating new statutes to add EMD training standards, certification, and protocol use was a predictable event in EMS evolution.[39] There appeared to be then (early 1980s) and stills appears to be now, no rationale for the EMD not being a regulated medical and EMS professional. The case, however, is certainly much stronger today. National standards documents abound. At the simplest level, as a colleague once stated, "An EMD can save you faster, or kill you deader, than a paramedic or EMT. Certify them."

Since that time, a patchwork quilt of varying rules and regulations and public safety/EMS statutes slowly

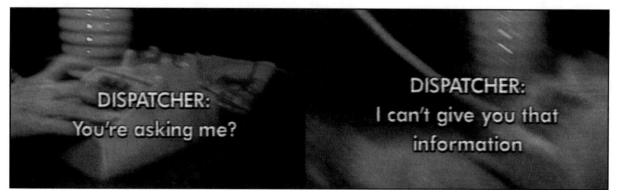

Fig. 11-21. Ellis Case—Uncertified dispatcher's response to the mother requesting CPR advice in a toddler drowning case as shown on television special "Lives on the Line" KTVX, 1992.

BLS Response Times: 1997 (HOT) vs. 1998 (COLD)								
	T-1	T-5	T-8	E-6	E-4	E-10	E-13	E-2
1997	5:04	5:04	5:17	5:18	5:14	5:43	5:39	5:04
1998	5:31	5:40	5:17	5:19	5:19	6:13	5:28	5:18
Diff.	+:27	+:36	:00	+:01	+:05	+:30	-:11	+:14

Fig. 11-22. Salt Lake City Fire Department BLS response time study on BRAVO-level calls.

emerged that have begun to address this important issue. Currently only 18 states have legislation regarding EMD regulation. However, a National Academy-sponsored state-by-state survey revealed that 59% of states are currently planning to regulate. Interestingly, 35% of the states indicated an interest in moving their dispatching systems toward accreditation. The consensus among the states is that the **NHTSA**'s core curriculum for EMD is cited as the minimum standard that any national standard-setting organization, such as NAEMD, must meet to have its curriculum, training, certification, recertification, and instructor training recognized.

ASTM's Standard Practice for EMD Management (F 1560-90) set the standard for states to establish EMD recognition links with credible national-standard-setting organizations:[44]

Reciprocal certification shall be established between certifying agencies and organizations having programs that meet the requirements contained in this practice and Practice F 1552.

One of the most difficult issues for state EMS regulators to understand is that the training an EMD initially receives must by based heavily on the specific protocol that the EMD's agency has approved and adopted. Generic training in the general issues of EMD—importance of PAIs, medical/legal, professionalism, etc.—while good, are not sufficient to train an EMD to an acceptable level of proficiency in the standard 3-day course. A good analogy is the aircraft pilot. While every pilot must obtain a basic understanding of the principles of flight (i.e., Aeronautics 101), without additional, specific and detailed "how to" training in the piloting of the specific aircraft they are to safely and efficiently fly (i.e., a 747, helicopter, or the Space Shuttle), they will likely fail. The protocol of each organization's choosing may be very

different than another's, requiring protocol-specific training, understanding, and scenario drilling for each to be used correctly. Again ASTM clarifies:[44]

The diversified EMDPRS protocols require specific training and knowledge in their proper use, therefore, the Emergency Medical Dispatcher wishing reciprocal certification must receive formal training on the specific EMDPRS that is used for the certification being sought and as used within the employing medical dispatch agency.

In this way, a "one-size-fits-all" state-level testing program cannot possibly incorporate, account for, and rapidly adapt to the varied specific protocols available today. The one-size-fits-all examination only works at the national standard-setting organization level for those organizations utilizing a unified protocol that is, therefore, not a moving target for standardized testing.

The States of Maryland and North Carolina have developed excellent regulatory models of how to move otherwise recalcitrant EMS and public safety providers forward toward a standardized implementation of EMD systems that recognize the Academy. New Hampshire, Delaware, the District of Columbia have done is in another way having formally adopted the full National Academy EMD program as did the Canadian provinces of Quebec and British Columbia.

In 1994, The National Association of State EMS Directors issued a position paper on the direction of state EMD standards:

WHEREAS, a key component of an EMS system is that of EMD; and

WHEREAS, other components of the EMS system have had standards enacted under legislative authority, including those for training and certification of prehospital basic, intermediate, and advance life-support personnel who function on EMS response units; and

WHEREAS, there have been significant developments in the field of EMD, including specialized training programs to train dispatchers to interrogate callers, prioritize calls, and provide pre-arrival initial treatment instructions to caller in emergency situations; and

WHEREAS, there is an expectation by the public that when they call for emergency medical help, a properly trained dispatcher will handle their call regardless of where they are located in the nation; and

WHEREAS, EMD programs meeting appropriate standards have been shown to result in more effective dispatch and the saving of lives; and

WHEREAS, organizations such as the National Association of Emergency Medical Services Physicians (NAEMSP), the National Heart, Lung, and Blood Institute (NHLBI), and the National Highway Traffic Safety Administration (NHTSA) have endorsed the development and adoption of standards for emergency medical dispatch; and

WHEREAS, national consensus standards (American Society of Testing Materials) have been developed for EMD; and

WHEREAS, most states do not yet have legislative authority to enact standards for EMD; and

WHEREAS, there is a need to take affirmative action in order to ensure that citizens throughout the nation have the benefit of EMD programs meeting accepted standards;

NOW, THEREFORE BE IT RESOLVED that the NASEMSD supports the enactment of legislation at the state level related to standards for EMD including the training and certification of EMD personnel, with appropriate medical oversight and in coordination with the EMS system.

In late 2000, the National Academy established a Special Task Group to undertake the development of Model State EMD legislation and regulations. Members of the Academy's Board of Certification together with six former and current State EMS Directors, as of this printing, are finalizing these documents to be distributed

> **! Authors' Note**
>
> **The Academy does not advocate immunity for organizations**, because, in its experience, immune organizations have a tendency not to achieve an acceptable level of care. The Academy feels that holding those who make mistakes responsible for their actions will better motivate individuals and organizations to achieve an acceptable level of care and conduct. The Academy advocates adopting a total quality management program, one that attempts to reduce risk through proactive measures. Being proactive and using a quality management program has clearly proven successful for EMDs and their respective systems and patients.

to interested agencies, public support organizations, and state and provincial EMS and health departments.

For example, as early as 1982, a movement began in Utah to create state rules and standards for EMDs which would result in a standardized priority dispatch system. However, imposing requirements for specific training and certification was nearly impossible because of political forces and complaints about costs.[39] Nonetheless, some early results were achieved:

> *Dispatchers serving as medical providers are not required to be certified as Emergency Medical Dispatchers, but are encouraged to voluntarily seek training and certification through a department-approved course.*[133]

The drive to achieve certification has been bolstered by the standard-setting document developed by ASTM, titled, "Standard Practice for Emergency Medical Dispatch" (designation F-1258-95). Clause 4.7, reads:

> *The EMD must be certified through either state government processes, or by professional medical dispatch standard-setting organizations.*[54]

Similarly, the NAEMSP position paper states, "Minimum training levels must be established, standardized, and all EMDs must be certified by governmental authority."[20] The Academy's training and certification is currently officially recognized by 34 U.S. states and Puerto Rico, as well as by several Canadian provinces and Australian states, and 27 U.K. ambulance service NHS trusts.

Two Simple Safeguards

Still, a few agencies persist in believing that it is still too risky not to send a maximal response. One could suggest that these concerned agencies could still comfortably adopt a protocol that does not always call for a maximal response, provided the system emphasizes to the caller to call back if the situation changes before help arrives (see Appendix C).

Secondly, with rare and approved exceptions, every call for help should be evaluated by an appropriately trained, out-of-hospital care provider or team.

Priority dispatching is not a process of screening out some callers so they get no help at all. Basic life support providers can handle many everyday emergencies. Interestingly, in Salt Lake City, Utah, once the system was in place, the fire department discovered that in 33.4 percent of the cases, emergency fire department responses were not necessary and were safely eliminated. Instead, the private ambulance company, with both basic life support EMTs and transport capability, could handle the majority of ALPHA calls safely, successfully, appropriately, and *alone.*[3]

It is the sincere hope of those who advocate priority dispatch concepts that others will realize the distinct advantages of adhering to the international standard that has evolved for EMD. With all the advice available for correctly implementing a comprehensive dispatch system, no one wants the consensus offered by an often unpredictable group—the jury.

Summary

The waning reluctance over implementing priority dispatch has emanated from people whose thought processes are based on red herrings—those "what if" situations that arise once in thousands (if not millions) of calls. In the end, when priority dispatch is clearly defined, explained, implemented, and carefully followed, its legal basis proves to be remarkably sound. Pre-Arrival Instructions are not only safe to give but are a moral necessity and, potentially, a legal necessity. Approved training with Academy certification of medical dispatch personnel provides a standard for professional conduct. In many cases, it may also provide governmental immunity to those who are certified and perform their functions wisely and in good faith. A unified system of proven priority dispatch protocols greatly reduces arbitrary decision-making and provides a standard that is legally but, more importantly, ethically defensible.

Perform your duties well while always caring about those whose terrified moments and painful days are entrusted to you and you will seldom go wrong.
—Anonymous physician

From Dumb to Dumber

Departments must intelligently dispatch 9-1-1 calls to avoid problems—even lawsuits

One of America's major fire departments has lost several multimillion dollar lawsuits over its dispatching on medical emergencies. The problem started years ago when the city actively encouraged citizens to dial 9-1-1 for police, fire, and medical emergencies, without conditions or exceptions. Nationwide, 9-1-1 has become the universal symbol for help.

The city in question bought one set of protocols (flip cards). It then modified the cards and attempted to train its dispatchers about how to use them for calls requesting medical assistance. If used properly, the protocols would guide the interrogation process so the dispatcher could send emergency resources based on medical condition and need. Also, the protocols could guide dispatcher in providing post-dispatch (prearrival) instructions to callers while emergency units responded.

The fire department in the opening example has provided emergency ambulance service for many years. For most of those years, the city's leaders treated that service as a stepchild, responding to its need for more resources only when a publicized crisis occurred. Thus, as the public caught on to 9-1-1, demand for ambulance service increased much faster than the number of ambulances. So, the dispatchers became the pressure point. They started deciding who would get an ambulance and who wouldn't. For those who didn't qualify, the dispatchers offered a phone number for private ambulances.

Denying emergency ambulance service is always risky, but the risk can be managed by using time-tested protocols, thoughtful dispatcher training,

(continued on 11.40)

EMD Risky Business

The Risks Associated With the Failure To Correctly Implement A Formal Emergency Medical Dispatch Program

This article started with a conversation I had with a colleague. We were commiserating with each other about our increasingly heavy workload as providers of expert witness testimony in 9-1-1 EMS dispatch lawsuits. The stories would just curl your hair ... failure to dispatch EMS resources to life-threatening emergencies, delays of as long as 40 minutes in dispatching EMS resources even after repeated calls for help ... dispatchers refusing the caller's pleas for CPR instructions ... the list just goes on and on. I see the lawyers, and those of us who assist them, as kind of like a clean-up squad. We didn't create the mess, but we help sort it out, bring some sense of closure to the survivors and try to do what we can to make sure that such a tragedy doesn't reoccur. These tragedies are inflicted on an unsuspecting public by the very agencies that are duty bound to help them.

My colleague and I ended our conversation by wishing that the entities responsible for providing 9-1-1 EMS dispatch services to the public would put us out of the expert witness business. Unfortunately we both know that in all too many cases, some 9-1-1 EMS dispatch agencies will do the right thing only when it becomes demonstrably cheaper than doing the wrong thing. I frequently listen to agency officials moan about how they were just unlucky, and that the horrible EMS dispatch incident could have happened anywhere, and that it really wasn't anybody's fault. I don't feel one bit sorry for them. I hope the taxpayers hold them accountable for wasting their money, and I go home and sleep the sleep of the just.

The courts are the ultimate venue for grieving families who want to find someone to blame for the needless loss of their loved one. They sue for negligence ... and municipalities and agencies responsible for dispatching EMS resources incur astronomical costs in both defending themselves and paying out huge sums in punitive damages. The most visible and recent example is the City of Chicago. Juries have found against the City in a number of relatively recent 9-1-1 dispatch-related lawsuits. In Gant vs. City of Chicago the family of a deceased asthmatic, 19 year old Douglas Gant, sued

for $10 million after having to call 9-1-1 three times for an ambulance and failing to receive pre-arrival instructions from a dispatcher on each occasion. The jury awarded the plaintiffs $50 million dollars! Although a judge recently set aside the jury award as excessive (a lesser amount will be determined), the jury's decision demonstrates how they felt about the story they heard at trial. In Cooper vs. City of Chicago the jury awarded $3.06 million to the family of a man who bled to death from a leg ulceration. Chicago Fire Department dispatchers had refused two requests for an ambulance response.

Chicago is certainly not alone. Los Angeles, Dallas, New York and a host of other cities, large and small, have had "high profile" EMS dispatch incidents that wound up in court. The costs of the bad publicity that arises from these tragedies are two-fold. We now know that such suits cause other suits ... people read the horrific newspaper article, recall their own similar experience and start looking around for an attorney. The cost of undermining the public's faith in 9-1-1 systems is incalculable but real. It is both ludicrous and tragic because the solution exists that can absolutely prevent these tragedies from occurring. And yet they go on and on.

Twenty years ago Emergency Medical Dispatch was just a good, albeit unproven, idea. Simply stated, formalized Emergency Medical Dispatch programs utilize trained EMDs (Emergency Medical Dispatchers) to ask the right questions of 9-1-1 callers for EMS assistance; to send the appropriate resources; and to tell the caller what to do prior to the arrival of EMS resources. Over the course of the last twenty years, however, something very important has happened. The theory and practice of Emergency Medical Dispatch have been validated in the peer reviewed medical literature. Studies have been published in such peer-reviewed journals as Prehospital Emergency Care and the Annals of Emergency Medicine that demonstrate the efficacy of formal emergency medical dispatch programs. Dispatchers who answer the public's calls to 9-1-1 for EMS assistance are performing a medical task. Nationally recognized EMS expert and attorney James O. Page has stated that there is an evolving legal duty to provide dispatchers with the tools they

(continued on 11.39)

EMD Risky Business

(continued from 11.38)

need to perform their medical tasks safely, competently and effectively. Although this article may be somewhat provocative, it is really intended as friendly advice to 9-1-1 EMS dispatch agencies.

There is no longer any valid excuse for failing to correctly implement a formal Emergency Medical Dispatch program. The textbooks have been written, the practice standards are published, and all of the relevant national organizations that have anything to do with EMS and public safety telecommunications have publicly expressed their support for the implementation of such programs. The American Society for Testing and Materials (ASTM), the National Association of EMS Physicians, and the National Institute of Health, to name but a few, have all published standards documents on Emergency Medical Dispatch. If a given 9-1-1 EMS dispatch agency has not implemented a formal Emergency Medical Dispatch program it is misallocating EMS resources, exceeding national res-ponse time performance standards, causing needless emergency vehicle crashes, and needlessly jeopardizing and losing lives. The agency is, literally, a tragedy waiting to happen.

When the tragedy inevitably occurs, all of the texts, published practice standards, medical res-earch, and national organization support documents will be presented as plaintiff's exhibits. Nationally recognized emergency medical dispatch experts will be interviewed by the local news media to explain how the tragedy could have been avoided. Agency representatives will be closely questioned about their knowledge of Emergency Medical Dispatch programs and will be required to explain why they haven't implemented one. The agency's existing emergency medical dispatch policies, procedures, and practices will be compared to the published texts and national standards documents.

About the only thing worse than not implementing a formal Emergency Medical Dispatch

program at all, is implementing one and then not adhering to it. It is not unknown for 9-1-1 EMS dispatch agencies to implement the program on paper only. In other instances agencies have not provided the ongoing management support to ensure that the Emergency Medical Dispatch program is conducted properly. 9-1-1 EMS dispatch agencies will spend money on emergency medical dispatch—one way or the other. The money can be spent defending the agency against negligence suits, or the money can be spent doing what the agency should have done in the first place. There is an old medical axiom that says, "Prevention is always the best and cheapest medicine."

There are a variety of options available for agencies that choose to implement formal Emergency Medical Dispatch programs. I encourage agency officials to closely examine those options. Agency decision-makers should review the texts, the practice standards and the published medical research. Keep in mind that, given the sheer volume of the public's demand for EMS service, bad choices will inevitably reveal themselves. Agencies and agency officials are ultimately responsible and accountable for the Emergency Medical Dispatch program choices that they make.

For those agency officials who choose to continue to visit unnecessary harm on both the EMS system and the public let me conclude by saying, on behalf of those of us on the clean-up squad, I look forward to meeting you. ⚜

In a twenty-five year career in EMS, Fred Hurtado served as an EMT, Paramedic, EMS administrator and manager, emergency medical dispatch consultant and state EMS official. In 1997 Mr. Hurtado left the public sector and started his own computing and Internet solutions company. He is frequently called upon to provide expert witness testimony in EMS and Emergency Medical Dispatch-related lawsuits.

Fig. 11-23. "EMD Risky Business?" by Fred Hurtado, reprinted with permission of *9-1-1 Magazine*, first published in October 2001.

From Dumb to Dumber

(continued from 11.37)

good supervision, ongoing training, and a quality management program. In the city we're talking about, the dispatchers received the flip cards but not much else. Before long. Some of the dis-patchers began freelancing, trying to apply the protocols from memory, if at all. If asked, most couldn't locate the training manual issued to them when hired.

Because the number of ambulances didn't keep up with population growth and demand, the dispatchers were instructed to ration them to only those cases that involved "life-or-death emer-gencies." Their unskilled managers and supervisors criticized and disciplined quickly but rarely dis-pensed any positive feedback for jobs well done. Meanwhile, a culture of discourtesy, disrespect, and impatience evolved in the dispatch center. It became an angry place and the unhappiness began to affect how employees treated callers.

The protocol (Flip) cards all bear the boldly printed words, "When in doubt—send." In several cases over a period of years, where the facts about the caller's information should have raised doubts, dispatchers deviated from the protocols and denied ambulance service to dying people. When that happened, the dead person's survivors usually got mad. The most effective tool they had was a law-suit. After a few of those lawsuits cost the city some really big bucks, the people in charge went from dumb to dumber. They looked to the city's lawyers for advice on how to dispatch.

Prompted by the lawyers, the fire department now sends too many resources on most calls. These days, it's not uncommon to have a street filled with fire apparatus, ambulances, and staff cars for a relatively minor medical emergency. The fire-fighters know this over-reaction make no sense to anybody but the city's lawyers.

The whole concept of prioritized emergency medical dispatching (EMD) was carefully designed to provide the appropriate response—without undue denials of service and without unnecessarily tying up too many resources. If prioritized EMD has a fault, it is the assumption that all public officials would be smart enough to implement and operate the system as it's supposed to operate.

In many places, the people in charge are smart enough to make prioritized EMD work and keep it working the way is should. Their success makes is easy to criticize those other places. Sadly, in too many of those other places, the dispatch center is controlled by people who seem to have been pro-moted or elected beyond their levels of com-petence. When incompetent leaders allow the system to go haywire, people get hurt and lawsuits occur.

When the lawsuits create a crisis, the leaders—oftentimes at the suggestion of their lawyers—overreact. Why must we make it so difficult? The public has been offered a service they can access by merely dialing three digits (9-1-1). They accept that offer more than anybody expected. So, there are two possible solutions: 1) revoke the offer, or 2) manage the demand for service intelligently. There's no politician foolhardy enough to revoke the offer, so that leaves only one option

The key word: intelligently. Dispatch centers cannot be a dumping ground for hand-me-down managers and supervisors. Dispatchers cannot be treated as disposable employees. The concept of prioritized EMD cannot be created as an optional procedure.

If dispatch errors cause big-buck lawsuits, employ a simple solution. Utilize a current, nation-ally standardized emergency medical dispatch program, learn how to do it right, treat dispatchers as professionals and train them accordingly, select and train good supervisors, and implement a con-tinuous quality management program.

If those simple tasks are more than your organ-ization can master, keep the checkbook handy. You'll need it. ❦

James O. Page is the publisher/editor-in-chief of JEMS (Journal of Emergency Medical Services) and Fire/Rescue Magazine. His career in the fire service spans more than 40 years and he has served as a chief officer in three California departments. An attorney, author of several books, and frequent lecturer on fire- and EMS-related topics, he was the first recipient of the IAFC's "James O. Page EMS Achievement Award" 1995.

Fig. 11-24. "From Dumb to Dumber" reprinted with permission of James Page, published in *Fire Rescue Magazine, August 2001.*

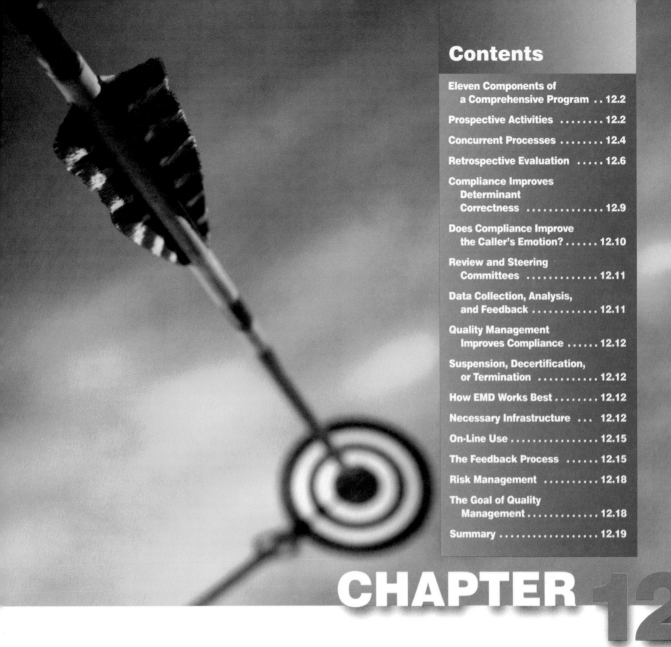

Contents

CHAPTER 12

Quality Management

Chapter Overview

This chapter reviews essential functions that constitute a comprehensive and effective quality management program. Unlike various other EMD programs that may include training and the discretional use of a set of interrogation guidelines, priority dispatch is a structured systems approach to emergency medical dispatching. Priority dispatch includes the most advanced quality management process in EMD as well as in EMS and public safety in general.

We must touch his weakness with a delicate hand. There are some faults so nearly allied to excellence that we can scarcely weed out the faults without eradicating the virtue.

—*Oliver Goldsmith*

No other prehospital medical activity is subjected to a similar level of performance evaluation or quantification of practitioner performance as emergency medical dispatch. The successful implementation of priority dispatch occurs with the establishment and ongoing operation of each activity within this comprehensive quality management process. This chapter explains why quality management activities are essential and how they should be structured for optimal effectiveness.

Quality management and medical control are essential for the safe and efficient use of any EMD program.[44, 134] As with other components of the EMS system, priority dispatch initially had little in the way of formalized quality management processes. However, over the years, much has been learned about the components, interactions, and functions of an effective EMD quality management process. The success of the quality management approach that follows has been and continues to be demonstrated in a rapidly increasing number of U.S. and international EMD communication centers.[44]

The cornerstone of an effective quality management program begins with one of the system's basic components—the recording of every activity of the EMD by the communication center's audio logging system. These records of case evaluation and patient care can be compared to a performance standard for evaluation and quantification. In no other part of prehospital care delivery is a practitioner's activity as precisely documented on each encounter. This unique feature of EMD activity provides an unequaled opportunity to implement a quality management process that takes full advantage of W. Edwards Deming's principles of quality management using statistical process control.[136, 137, 138]

Eleven Components of a Comprehensive Program

Eleven key components or activities must exist or occur within the quality management process for its successful operation.[134] These components are organized into three basic categories:

- **Prospective** quality management activities that occur before the activity begins

- **Concurrent** quality management activities that occur as the activity is taking place

- **Retrospective** quality management process that occurs after the activity is completed

The goal of quality management is to minimize variance or variation in expected outcomes (response determinant selection) and improve the quality of each activity as defined by the standard. Quality standards will vary by each identified activity. For example, minimum compliance to the protocol scores have been developed by the Academy for each component of priority dispatch as a standard measure of quality for communication centers that want to become accredited as Centers of Excellence (see Appendix A).[139] To become eligible for accreditation, the agency must present documentation that demonstrates the center's EMDs are complying with or following the protocol 90 to 95 percent of the time, depending on the activity being measured. The center's leadership must therefore establish the acceptable minimum percent compliance to the protocol score for EMD performance, and clearly communicate that standard to all EMDs.

To improve any process and its outcome, the process must be evaluated. Is the process working as it should? Think of priority dispatch as a map for finding the right EMS response. By following the map's directions, the EMD will end up in the right place. If the EMD fails to identify the caller's needs, s/he cannot hope to provide the right directions. Priority dispatch is a systems approach designed to minimize variation in EMD decision-making (clinical determinant coding), given a set of conditions identified through caller interrogation. In other words, with priority dispatch there is less chance of ending up in the wrong place. Each of the following activities is an essential component of a comprehensive quality management process. The careful implementation and maintenance of this process will minimize responder risk and provide sound medical direction in the form of resource response, Post-Dispatch or Pre-Arrival Instructions.

The following activities exist in almost all quality management programs and are organized into prospective, concurrent and retrospective processes. These functions are essential to the safe and medically prudent provision of EMD and constitute the foundation of priority dispatch. The success of the quality management program relies on the completeness and integration of each activity.

Prospective Activities

These activities occur before the center begins taking calls using priority dispatch, and establish the "baseline" from which quality assurance measurements are taken. They include:

- Selection and Implementation of the EMD Protocol

- EMD Candidate Selection and Evaluation

- EMD Candidate Orientation Programs

- Initial EMD Training

- EMD Certification

Selection and Implementation of the EMD Protocol. The Priority Dispatch protocol is the standard operating procedure that dictates the functions an EMD performs to manage a medical emergency remotely. Compliance to protocol and its ongoing evolution occur as a result of the quality management process. An effective program focuses on how well people are doing (and how the program can be improved), not just on the end results. The EMD protocol must not only conform to current medical practice standards, but its design, in wording and structure, must also facilitate compliance to the protocol. Graphic design

elements, layout, and physical accessibility are important factors in how efficiently the EMD uses the protocol tool. Priority dispatch is a "living" tool that is updated as the need is shown.

EMD Candidate Selection and Evaluation. A good chef always cooks with high-quality ingredients, and dedicated dispatchers are essential ingredients to correct priority dispatching. Effective employee selection depends on the ability of the organization to successfully identify necessary skills, personality traits and aptitudes and match those characteristics to job requirements.[140] Unfortunately, in many systems the communication center has become a "dumping" ground for those who could not or would not perform in other areas of the organization. However, today's mission-critical environment requires the hiring and

---

EMD Entry-Level Selection Criteria

6.1.0 **Each emergency medical dispatch agency shall adopt a formal written policy delineating the selection procedures for individuals to be employed as EMDs. It must address the ability to:**

1.1 Read and write at a high school graduate or GED level;

1.2 Perform those clerical skills as delineated by the employing agency;

1.3 Perform verbal skills in a clear and understandable manner, in the required language or languages established as necessary to that EMD agency;

1.4 Perform alphanumeric transcription skills necessary to correctly record addresses, locations and telephone numbers; and

1.5 Demonstrate competency in basic telecommunications skills as required by the employing or training agency.

6.2.0 **Selection criteria should also include the following:**

2.1 A clear attribute of helpfulness and compassion toward the sick or injured patient and the caller advocate;

2.2 The ability to clearly guide callers in crisis through application of necessary interrogation procedures and the provision of telephone pre-arrival instructions;

2.3 The ability to learn and master the skills, philosophy and knowledge required to successfully complete the training process;

2.4 The ability to efficiently and effectively organize multiple tasks and complicated situations and activities;

2.5 The ability to handle the levels of emotional stress present in caller/patient crisis intervention, death and dying situations, call prioritization and triage, and multiple tasking;

2.6 The ability to function within the team framework of public safety and EMS systems; and

2.7 The ability to elicit and assimilate caller information and then to prioritize and appropriately consolidate and summarize this information in a format used to inform and direct public safety responders.

Fig. 12-1. Excerpt from ASTM F 1560-94: Standard Practice for EMD Management.[44]

training of people who possess a variety of technological skills and multi-tasking aptitudes. It is vital to select people with the emotional and psychological ability to handle this unique environment effectively (see fig.12-1).

A careful job analysis and necessary skills list can be used to create a selection process that will ensure that the most qualified applicants are selected. Even the smallest EMS system should have a comprehensive hiring process that includes multiple interviews, assessment centers, background and reference checks, and other hiring procedures as allowable by law.

EMD Candidate Orientation Programs. A comprehensive orientation program is the first step in the training process.[140] It formally introduces the employee to the organization and its culture. The orientation should include a comprehensive overview of the entire public safety and EMS system in addition to the communication center's role. A structured and accountable probationary process will ensure the new employee receives the information needed to conform to agency policies, and create a record of the employee's initial performance.

The probationary process should include assigning a preceptor to answer questions and provide performance feedback. The probationary process should also include opportunities to expose probationary employees to the realities of the dispatch environment. New employees should visit with the prehospital and hospital personnel they will be working with. They should also ride along with EMS, fire, and law enforcement personnel to develop an understanding of the public-safety environment. Finally, this probationary process must include the capacity for remediation or termination if the candidate is unable to function effectively.

Initial EMD Training. In many centers, training typically consists only of having new employees sit with the most senior personnel, often learning to make the same mistakes as their predecessors. Proper training should provide a thorough introduction to emergency medical dispatching, the use of the priority dispatch protocol, and an opportunity to role-play using the protocol system. This training must be specific to the exact protocol selected for use. Generic-type training is unfortunately still too common in the industry and clearly lacks enough protocol-specific information to allow a new EMD to go on-line immediately and safely. The EMD's training for efficient and effective use of the MPDS has evolved from a disproportionate amount of "why" to a more effective and useful "how."

Initial training should include a demonstration of the behaviors and habits necessary to master medical dispatch, with regular practice and performance evaluation. Incorrect behaviors or techniques are difficult to correct once they become the norm rather than the exception. The EMD should have ample instruction and practice in the presence of a instructor or preceptor using all required protocol and equipment.

EMD Certification. Certification of personnel by a nationally recognized and respected certifying organization provides an external and unbiased evaluation of the practitioner's skills and knowledge necessary to competently function as an EMD.[44, 141] Although agency-based training may provide essentially the same course content, having it provided by an EMD instructor who is extensively trained, certified, and monitored by a national organization minimizes claims that the "fox is guarding the hen house." Academy certification demonstrates that the EMD has met or exceeded all established requirements and standards. Additionally, formally monitored certification ensures that the instructional format is presented in a consistent manner and provides for reliable assimilation of curriculum improvements by the certified membership.

Concurrent Processes

These activities start occurring once the center begins taking calls using priority dispatch. They include:

- Medical Director involvement

- Continuing dispatch education

- EMD recertification

Medical Control and Medical Director Involvement. Priority Dispatch was among the first EMS programs to formally incorporate a framework for both medical control and quality management. Medical control is an active, involved role that requires leadership and dedication by the physician medical director. This term is slowly being replaced with the term "medical oversight" as the concept of medical control and quality management merge. Within the context of EMS, the medical director is much more than an advocate for competent clinical care. S/he must become familiar with the processes that result in the provision of that care. The National Association of EMS Physicians' Position Paper on EMD defines medical control by asserting that:

EMS physician(s) are responsible for the provision of education, training, protocols, critiques, leadership, testing, certification, decertification, standards, advice, and quality control through an official authoritative position within the prehospital EMS system.[20]

The position paper further clarifies that:

The trained Emergency Medical Dispatcher (EMD) is an essential part of a prehospital EMS system. Medical direction and control for the EMD and the dispatch center also constitutes part of the prescribed responsibilities of the Medical Director of the EMS system. The functions of emergency medical dispatching must include the use of predetermined questions, pre-arrival telephone instructions, and pre-assigned response levels and modes.[20]

Thus, it is important that medical directors become thoroughly familiar with each component of the EMD system through early involvement in its implementation. To thoroughly familiarize the medical director as well as other system administrators with priority dispatch concepts and operation, the Academy maintains a National Leader's Seminar. Being "medical dispatch literate" is also a requirement in Academy Accreditation. Even if many of the described quality management functions of a medical director are delegated to others, to achieve optimal performance, the communication center must have an involved and a committed physician to provide effective medical oversight. Ultimately, a physician-patient relationship is created when the EMD attempts to determine the patient's chief compliant, thus responsibility for patients and their welfare rests with the medical director and EMD until the patient is under the care of on-scene providers.[142]

The medical director plays an essential role in the configuration of the EMS system's response to each of the 296 determinant codes. Resource deployment with respect to clinical capability and response code should be developed by the medical director and dictated by medical practice standards (not tradition and anecdotal beliefs). Because the medical priorities of dispatch are largely modeled after the emergency department physician experience, many emergency physicians readily accept the concepts of prioritization as medically appropriate and are strong supporters of this approach.

Physician direction for EMDs is strongly supported by the American Society for Testing and Materials (ASTM) in its F1560-94 document "Standard Practice for Emergency Medical Dispatch Management."[44] In the ASTM document describing and defining medical dispatch (F1258-95), there is an important reference to medical direction.[54] There, the physician must attend to:

The management and accountability for the medical care aspects of an emergency medical dispatch program including: the medical monitoring oversight of the training of the EMD personnel; approval and medical control of the operational emergency medical dispatch priority reference system; evaluation of the medical care and Pre-Arrival Instructions rendered by the EMD personnel; direct participation in the EMD system evaluation, quality assurance, and quality improvement process and mechanisms; and, responsibility for the medical decisions and care rendered by the EMD and emergency medical dispatch program.

ASTM further stipulates that:

Provision of EMS physician medical direction [should occur] regardless of whether the EMD function is carried on in a free-standing EMS communication center or a consolidated public-safety answering point or communication center.[54]

Thus, physician medical oversight is unquestionably a standard of care in non-EMS-based medical dispatch centers, such as law enforcement and the fire service.

Continuing Dispatch Education. Continuing dispatch education (CDE) is to recertification what initial training is to certification. This process should include a rotating curriculum that covers all of the EMD's continuing education needs, as well as topics that are identified through quality improvement unit processes as needing special attention.

> **Employees with good morale and current knowledge are less likely to handle a situation poorly.**

Through protocol compliance scoring, the system identifies and quantifies EMD activities that are not meeting the standard either collectively or at the individual EMD level. The objectives of a continuing education program include:[44]

First Law of Medical Control at Dispatch

A safe and sound protocol is the EMS physician's authorization for the EMD to practice dispatch life support-based medicine. Without it there would be no emergency medical dispatch as we currently know it.

- Developing a better understanding of telecommunications and the EMD's roles and responsibilities

- Enhancing on-line skills related to the provision of pre-arrival instructions and emergency telephone procedures within the scope of practice of EMD

- Improving skills in the proper application of all components of Priority Dispatch, including interrogation and prioritization

- Creating opportunities for discussion, skill practice, and critique of skill performance

- Maintaining an understanding of the evolving science of medical dispatching methods

An effective program addresses performance deficiencies identified through case review and enables EMDs to refresh and improve seldom-used skills. Other activities that should be considered include classroom lectures, EMS field experience, involvement in EMD-relevant research, and attendance at professional conferences.[44]

Self-enrichment bolsters confidence, and as an EMD learns from new information and reinforces existing knowledge, there is an increase in morale. Employees involved in effective continuing education programs will recognize management's interest in and commitment to the quality of their job performance. In addition, a comprehensive continuing dispatch education program will reduce risk to the agency. Employees with good morale and current knowledge are less likely to handle a situation poorly. As Mark Twain said more than a century ago, "Talent is useless without training, thank God."

EMD Recertification. Recertification ensures that EMDs, through on-line use and CDE requirements, maintain a minimum competency level by successfully completing the EMD recertification exam.[143] Initial Academy certification is for two years, as recommended by ASTM. However, individual states, regions, and provinces vary in terms of their recertification requirements.

To recertify with the Academy, the EMD must:

- Demonstrate continued knowledge of emergency medical dispatch by passing a 50 question (open book) correspondence exam with a score of 80 percent or higher.

- Maintain a current CPR certification (or dispatch life support equivalent).

- Verify completion of at least 24 hours of continuing dispatch education (in addition to CPR) during the two-year recertification period.

Continuing education should be spread among several areas to provide diversity in the educational experience. For this reason, the Academy allows a maximum number of hours in each of the following categories to be counted toward EMD recertification.

1. **National Journal of Emergency Dispatch,** CDE Article review and quiz are included in each issue. Max: 8 credit hours (4 per year).

2. **Workshops and Seminars related to EMS,** preferably to the required skills of an EMD; i.e., airway management, review of essential skills, scenarios, medical-legal issues, computer-aided dispatch, stress reduction, refresher courses, etc. Max: 16 credit hours (8 per year).

3. **Multimedia educational products** which illustrate and review proper emergency care and EMD procedures. Titles are restricted to those that are EMS, preferably EMD-related, and should be written on the application. Max: 16 credit hours (8 per year).

4. **Quality Assurance case review,** planning, and analysis of issues or findings identified by dispatch Q.A., theoretically or in practice. Max: 8 credit hours (4 per year).

5. **Local planning and management meetings,** including general organization for disaster, mass casualty, and HAZMAT. Max: 8 credit hours (4 per year).

6. **Teaching the general public** any topic within the scope of basic EMD/EMS relations. Synopsis of subjects taught should be included with application. Max: 4 credit hours (2 per year).

7. **Protocol Review of the MPDS,** especially College of Fellows updates or new versions. Max: 4 credit hours.

8. **Miscellaneous.** Max: 4 credit hours.

Retrospective Evaluation

These activities start occurring as soon as the center begins processing calls using priority dispatch. They include:

- Case Review and Performance Feedback
- Data Collection, Analysis, Feedback
- Suspension, Decertification, or Termination

Case Review and Performance Feedback. (Where the rubber meets the road). If there was ever a case of "getting what you pay for" it lies in the case review process.[144] Case review starts with an evaluation of individual cases, but should also include the implementation of three oversight committees responsible for ongoing review of system performance. These committees—the Quality Improvement Unit, the Medical Dispatch Review Committee (MDRC) and MPDS Steering Committee—also develop and implement changes to the policies and procedures that govern how the protocol will be used within the communication center in an ongoing effort to correct system deficiencies.

The process of reviewing cases should be conducted in the quality improvement unit by EMD case reviewers who are medically trained ALS-level providers, preferably with a communication background or orientation. These specially trained EMD quality improvement specialists (EMD-Qs) listen to audio tapes of selected calls and compare the EMD's actions to the protocol, keeping track of whether all the questions were asked, whether they were asked as written and whether the EMD deviated from the protocol. Quantification of the case review is accomplished through the completion of a Case Review Template, which permits an objective compliance scoring of the case. Each component of the protocol is assigned a weighted value based on the relative value of the activity as it relates to the entire EMD process. The scoring formula standard is maintained by the Academy's Board of Accreditation (see Case Review Template, Appendix A). EMD performance is tracked as a percent compliance to protocol score.

! Author's Note

The Academy approved this new standard in 1997 as it relates to large communication centers. This was a significant change from the previous fixed case review percentage of 7 percent[44] and was based on an Academy study project measuring the ability of three large centers to demonstrate the effectiveness of the 3 percent scale in reaching high compliance and accreditation. Metro Dade, Miami Fire Rescue and Integraph Public Safety/Melbourne have all achieved Center of Excellence accreditation.

In 1999, the Board of Accreditation clarified the case review standard for the low volume centers. The official standard is now 3% or 5 calls/EMD/month which ever is greater.

Measuring compliance to protocol. The ability to precisely quantify EMD activity is one of the most powerful features of priority dispatch. Combined with other operational data such as call processing times, shift lengths, and outcome studies, the protocol can be studied. However, to effectively use compliance to protocol data, a sufficient number of cases must be reviewed to make statistical inferences regarding the population. Based on the Board of Accreditation's updated standards for case review, the Academy recommends that each center review 25 cases per week or 3 percent of call volume, whichever is greater. The fixed 25 calls per week become an increasing 3 percent at an annual case load of approximately 43,000 calls.[145] Staffing levels of the quality improvement unit must, therefore, reflect anticipated workload.

> **The power of accurate observation is commonly called cynicism by those who have not got it.**
> **—George Bernard Shaw**

In the development of minimum case review parameters, two requirements of the sampled data must be met. First, the sample size must be sufficient to validate inferences regarding the population. Second, each EMD must receive a sufficient amount of feedback to legitimize the

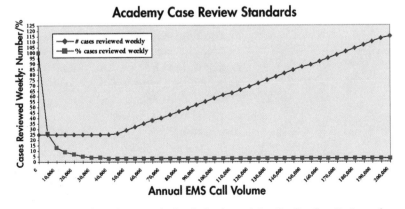

Academy Case Review Standards

- # cases reviewed weekly
- % cases reviewed weekly

Cases Reviewed Weekly: Number/%

Annual EMS Call Volume

Fig. 12-2. Revised Academy standard scale for determining Quality Case Review volumes.

process from the her/his point of view. In addition to an Academy Medical Dispatch Case Evaluation Form, an authorized software application called AQUA™ (Advanced Quality Assurance) utilizes the format and protocol compliance scoring formula maintained and evolved by the Board of Accreditation of the Academy.

The six protocol components evaluated and scored consist of:

1. **Primary Case Entry interrogation.** Questions designed to determine and verify incident location and callback phone number, type of presenting condition, and life-threatening conditions, e.g., respiratory or cardiac arrest identification; the EMD's evaluation component analogous to the field responder's primary survey.

2. **Chief Complaint selection.** Choosing one of the predefined Chief Complaint categories based on information gathered during initial interrogation, e.g., breathing problems or heart problems; the dispatcher's evaluative component, analogous to the field responder's preliminary working diagnosis.

3. **Secondary Key Question interrogation.** Closed-ended questions specific to each Chief Complaint category that establishes the appropriate clinical

---

A Real Tough Time Breathing (1:48 elapsed time)

Caller:	…eighty-nine years of age and she is having a real tough time breathing.
EMD:	**Okay, what address sir?**
Caller:	158 Herbert Avenue.

0:07
EMD:	**Okay, and the phone number there?**
Caller:	(caller repeats phone number)
EMD:	**And you are there with her?**
Caller:	I am here with her.

0:13
EMD:	**Is she conscious?**
Caller:	She is conscious.

0:15
EMD:	**Is she breathing?**
Caller:	Yes, but she's having a really tough time breathing.

0:19
EMD:	**And how old did you say she was?**

0:22
Caller:	She's eighty-nine years of age.
EMD:	**Is she able to talk to you at all?**
Caller:	Yes, she can talk to me but she has a tough time talking because it affects her breathing.
EMD:	**Okay, is she alert?**
Caller:	Yes, uh huh.
EMD:	**Is she sweaty or changing color?**
Caller:	She is not sweaty, no.
EMD:	**Okay.**

Caller:	But she can't stand either. She cannot get up.
EMD:	**Does she have any heart problems?**
Caller:	Yes, she does.

0:46
EMD:	**And does she have asthma?**
Caller:	No, I don't believe she has asthma.

0:53
EMD:	**Okay, and she is having a real hard time breathing?**

→   *[EMD initiates dispatch in CAD]*

Caller:	Yes, uh huh. She's a…there is a nurse that comes down to see her and I tried to get in touch with her but, a, she can't breathe right now. I mean really had tough time, so I thought I better call these people…

1:00
EMD:	**Oh, yeah… we'll get some help out to her. What I'd like you to do though, sir, is to allow her to assume the most comfortable position that she can. And then if her condition worsens in any way at all, can you call me back immediately for further instructions?**

1:20
Caller:	I sure will.

(continued on 12.9)

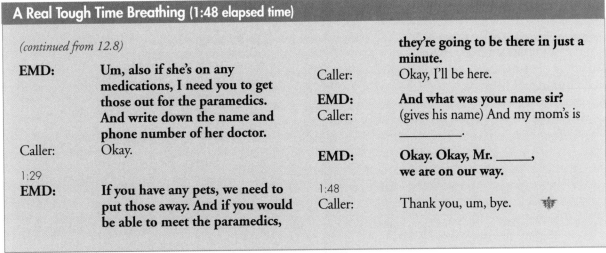

A Real Tough Time Breathing (1:48 elapsed time)

(continued from 12.8)

EMD:	Um, also if she's on any medications, I need you to get those out for the paramedics. And write down the name and phone number of her doctor.
Caller:	Okay.
1:29	
EMD:	If you have any pets, we need to put those away. And if you would be able to meet the paramedics,

	they're going to be there in just a minute.
Caller:	Okay, I'll be here.
EMD:	And what was your name sir?
Caller:	(gives his name) And my mom's is _____.
EMD:	Okay. Okay, Mr. _____, we are on our way.
1:48	
Caller:	Thank you, um, bye.

Fig. 12-3. "A Real Tough Time Breathing," Salt Lake Fire Department, 1997.

code and response mode of system resources; the EMD's evaluation component analogous to the field responder's secondary survey.

4. **Determinant Code selection.** Choosing the most appropriate determinant and assigning responding units using the relevant pre-assigned response code.

5. **Post-Dispatch Instructions provision.** Delivering generalized instructions related to the Chief Complaint containing basic first aid, cautionary statements, and verifications whenever possible and appropriate.

6. **Pre-Arrival Instructions provision.** Delivering scripted instructions regarding verification and management of cardiac arrest, choking, childbirth, and maintenance of ABCs.

Other elements of priority dispatch that can be included in the review process are:

- Call-processing times

- Whether information was relayed to field crews correctly

- How well the EMD interacts with other agencies

- EMD attitudes and customer service

- EMD communication skills and overall impression portrayed to the caller

The following case demonstrates excellent protocol compliance while the EMD maintains a caring profes-

sionalism. Even with a moderately, rambling caller, the EMD sends the case for dispatch at the 53 second mark following a full interrogation that included primary and secondary survey.

Compliance Improves Determinant Correctness

The ability to scientifically study the protocol is a function of comparing compliance to protocol scores with observed outcome. An example of this type of system investigation follows with a review and discussion of Los Angeles City Fire Department EMD data obtained shortly after the comprehensive implementation of priority dispatch in 1989.

In a review of 3,210 cases which had been scored using an earlier version of the case review scoring process just described, the LAFD data provided some very interesting results regarding the impact of non-compliance on the correct selection of a response determinant code. Each case was placed in one of four categories by reviewing two parameters. Those were:

1. Did the EMD ask all the primary interrogation (Case Entry) questions?

2. Did the EMD ask all the relevant secondary interrogation (Key) questions?

Each reviewed case was then placed in one of four categories consisting of various compliance to protocol combinations based on whether "all" (100%) or "less than all" (< 100%) of the questions were asked (see fig. 12-4).

Los Angeles City Fire Department Protocol Compliance Data

Entry Question/Key Question Compliance (%)	Question Totals	Compliance Level	Determinant-Level Correctly Chosen	
→ 100 / 100	1,943	Full	1,811	93.2 % ←
<100 / 100 *or* 100 / <100	1,023	Partial	722	75.5 %
<100 / <100	244	Low	89	36.5 %
	3,210		2,672	83.2 %

Fig. 12-4. Los Angeles City Fire Department quality assurance data demonstrating the relationship of protocol compliance to correct determinant-level selection, 1989-1990.

The results revealed that when compliance was less than 100 percent for both categories, the correct determinant had been chosen only 36.5 percent of the time. When compliance for primary interrogation was 100 percent, but was less than 100 percent for secondary interrogation, correct Determinants were chosen 74.5 percent of the time. When compliance was less than 100 percent for Case Entry, but 100 percent for Key Questions, the correct determinant was chosen 82.2 percent of the time. When compliance on both the Case Entry and Key Questions was *100 percent*, the correct determinant was selected *93.2 percent* of the time.

In the group 100 percent compliant on both initial and secondary interrogation, only 6.8 percent were found on review to have selected an "incorrect" response determinant. However, in nearly all of those cases (6.0 of the 6.8 percent), the dispatcher effectively overrode the recommended response to the next higher level, possibly in keeping with the Second Law of Dispatch: "When in doubt, send them out," or always err in the direction of patient safety. Only 0.8 percent of those cases were found to be significantly incorrect, either dispatching more than one level too high or sending too little.

Does Compliance Improve the Caller's Emotion?

The misconception that the caller is too upset may be related to a common belief expressed by some dispatchers, "The caller made me crazy." There is data that suggests that this relationship may actually be the other way around. The stratified compliance data from Los Angeles when compared with the ECCS of the caller provides a valuable explanation.

We have speculated that the caller may actually be "evaluating" the caller in some subconscious way. Their "scoring" system might pose the following questions:

1. Have I reached a **helper** or a **hinderer**?
2. Have I reached a **professional** or an **amateur**?
3. Have I reached a **leader** or someone who is **just as confused as I am**?

Los Angeles City Fire Department Protocol Compliance and PAI Provision Data

Entry Question/Key Question Compliance (%)	Compliance Level	Provision of PAIs when possible and appropriate	
→ 100 / 100	Full	89.7%	←
<100 / 100 *or* 100 / <100	Partial	64.0%	
<100 / <100	Low	52.5%	

Fig. 12-5. Los Angeles City Fire Department quality assurance data demonstrating the relationship of protocol compliance to provision of pre-arrival instructions, 1989-1990.

If the caller perceives that they have reached any of the latter, what would you suspect would happen to their emotional content. If you said it would become higher, you are probably right (see fig. 12-6).

The three compliance groups suggest an increase in emotional content (and a decrease in cooperation) associated with a decrease in compliance. Just who is making whom crazy?

Review and Steering Committees

The second quality management committee specific to actual case review is the Medical Dispatch Review Committee.[144] This group—a combination of personnel with a variety of operational and communication expertise and responsibility—establishes an appropriate review process for the system.[44] The committee reviews the detailed work conducted by the quality improvement unit, and their recommendations regarding corrective action. This committee serves at the "middle-management level." It is typically tasked with developing corrective responses when compliance to protocol percent scores fall below pre-established limits.

> ## ! Author's Note
>
> Any proposal for protocol changes must ultimately be approved by the submitting agency's MPDS Steering Committee and Medical Director before submission to the Academy's Council of Standards.

The third committee is the MPDS Steering Committee. This committee is responsible for approving policies and procedures developed by the Review Committee. It comprises upper-level management, such as chiefs, deputy chiefs, CEOs, owners, communication center directors, medical director, etc. It is also responsible for strategic planning and the development of broader policy and position statements. These oversight processes are essential for true excellence.

Data Collection, Analysis, and Feedback

Perhaps the most powerful and poorly understood feature of priority dispatch is the "unified" medical protocol that lies at the heart of the system. The term unified is used to describe the protocol since each of the more than 2,200 licensed users operate the exact same protocol without modifications or changes. The use of a unified protocol at thousands of locations creates an opportunity for multiple-site replication with respect to scientific investigation—an often unattainable goal in prehospital research. Only through predictable use (compliance to protocol) and multiple-site replication can cause-and-effect relationships be validated. The local customization of an EMD protocol eliminates the ability of any organization to externally validate the safety and effectiveness of the protocol. The value of multiple-site replication is best illustrated in the following calculation. There are more than 88 million permutations mathematically possible of the current priority dispatch question-and-answer combinations. Any potential errors that occurred as a result of an individual center's changes to the protocol could remain undetected until it caused an error in system response or patient evaluation or treatment.

It is estimated that the MPDS processes over 30 million calls annually. Because 2,400 locations use the same protocol, if a change does result in an error, it will be quickly identified by the users. Furthermore, the protocol is regularly reviewed and scrutinized by hundreds of medical directors each year and routinely compared to local, national, and international standards of care.

As each EMS system collects data from the case review process, the results should be entered in a database or spreadsheet for further analysis. Once a statistically valid sample of that system's population is gathered, a lower

Los Angeles City Fire Department Protocol Compliance and ECCS Data

Compliance (%)	Compliance Level	Emotional Content Cooperation Score
→ 100 / 100	Full	1.11 ←
<100 / 100 *or* 100 / <100	Partial	1.23
<100 / <100	Low	1.33

Fig. 12-6. Los Angeles City Fire Department Quality Assurance data demonstrates the relationship of protocol compliance to the caller's emotional content and cooperation level, 1989-1990.

"control limit" or minimum compliance score must be established and approved by the Steering Committee. This score is used to identify individual cases that require review. The data analysis process must be capable of creating an "exception" report that immediately notifies the communication center's administration of protocol compliance scores that fall below an established percentage (i.e., 75 percent average compliance). In addition, management needs reports on communication center activity and summaries of average compliance scores.[144] This data can be shared with each EMD as feedback to provide them with an objective assessment of their performance, in addition to providing them with specific information regarding their performance on each portion of the protocol. The success of this approach in modifying EMD behavior was revealed in a study, conducted by members of the Academy, of a U.S. communication center that comprehensively implemented priority dispatch in 1993.[26]

> **Things do not turn up in this world unless someone turns them up.**
> **—James A. Garfield**

Quality Management Improves Compliance

Prior to the introduction of a quality management process into the medical dispatch arena, pre-arrival instructions were given sporadically in most centers. The EMDs staffing these early centers were often unsure about the validity, safety, and probably, more realistically, their support from upper-level management of their provision of PAIs.

Without the collection and evaluation of this data, communication center managers would be unable to verify their personnel's compliance to protocol or the policies and procedures that govern the provision of EMD. While there is a place for real-time (concurrent) observation of EMD activity and real-time feedback in identifying the level of EMD performance subjectively, concurrent review cannot replace the careful and much more objective retrospective review process. Such a process must sample an adequate number of cases, be consistent, objective, and sufficiently randomized to be statistically significant (see fig. 12-7).[26]

Suspension, Decertification or Termination

In well-managed communication centers, managers can expect that only about one out of 20 EMDs will

ultimately be unresponsive to constructive feedback and retraining. Having exhausted proactive and improvement-based processes to prod refractive individuals, those not willing to comply with the protocol (and thus practice safe and efficient dispatch-life-support-based medicine), must face discipline and, ultimately, termination (see Appendix: Quality Improvement Case Review and Remediation Actions Policy example).

Used only as a last resort, the ability to decertify, suspend or terminate personnel must be available to systems managers. The doctrine of foreseeability places a burden on center managers to act when substandard performance has been identified. Whether substandard performance is unintentional is not relevant. If the agency does not act to correct the behavior it is negligent. In some cases, following multiple efforts to remediate, the manager may have only one choice remaining. The records identifying and reporting the actions of a substandard (and potentially harmful) EMD must be complete and in order. The medical director should be involved in all clinical aspects of required due process. An exceptional feature of the MPDS quality assurance process is its clear objectivity of use which removes the uncertainty from management's ultimate decision in disciplinary actions. Most protocol compliance issues boil down to this—you either did it, or you didn't.

How EMD Works Best

Quality management occurs with the skillful coordination and administration of each of the 11 components of quality management just described.[26, 134] The combined effect of these programs is intended to promote continual improvement of the service. Good quality management includes a lot of positive reinforcement, rather than focusing only on the delivery of punitive measures for substandard work. Quality management bridges the working life span of the EMD. It starts with hiring, and doesn't end until the retiring, firing, or expiring of the dispatcher. An effective quality management program inspires dispatch personnel to achieve high levels of performance. Without continual re-evaluation and renewal, any program, regardless of how comprehensive the initial training and education, maybe, will result in skill and outcome degradation.

Necessary Infrastructure

Priority dispatch starts with the selection, orientation, and training of the EMD candidate. The EMD training program teaches the prospective EMD both the medicine and use of the protocol. Certification

The Impact of a Comprehensive Quality Management Process on Compliance to Protocol

Study Hypothesis

Discussion regarding the Emergency Medical Dispatcher's (EMD's) ability to effectively use EMD medical triage systems has been increasing in the EMS and public safety literature. However, most (if not all) of the published literature on these systems lack adequate quantification of protocol or process compliance by EMDs.

This study retrospectively reviewed the results of quality management activities to measure the impact of these activities on compliance to protocol. The authors hypothesized that a properly designed and uniformly applied quality management process, which included quantification of protocol compliance and feedback to EMDs, would result in improved compliance to protocol.

Methods

A combined police-fire-EMS dispatch center in the Pacific Northwest internally evaluated its medical dispatch process. Quantification of compliance to the protocol, before and after provisions of performance feedback to the EMDs was studied by comparing the EMD's online performance to a grading standard following a review of audio-taped cases. The review process was validated through a randomized second review of selected cases by a "master" reviewer and the results were quantified using a scoring formula.

Results

Compliance data for each of six main components of the protocol, as well as a total compliance score, were analyzed for statistical significance using a two-tailed Z-test of sample means. Shown here are weighted mean compliance scores in the months preceding and following performance feedback.

In general, a P-value of 0.05 means results are "statistically significant" and indicates there is only one chance in twenty (5 percent) that the results were obtained purely by chance. Compliance to three protocol components (Key Questions, Response Level, and PDIs) as well as the total score, increased by more than ten percent (with a statistical probability that the observed improvements were wrong of less than 0.1 percent: $P<0.001$); compliance to the chief complaint component of the

protocol increased by 7.5 percent ($P=0.01$); and compliance to the case entry component of the protocol increased by almost 10 percent ($P=0.05$).

Protocol Component	Before Feedback	After Feedback	P Value
CE	92.3	98.6	p = .002
CC	89.9	91.6	p = .271
KQ	65.8	96.2	p < .0001
Level	79.6	93.3	p < .0001
PDIs	40.8	95.8	p < .0001
PAIs	92.9	100.0	p = .005

	Sept.	Oct.	Feedback begins	Nov.	Dec.
CE	92.3	87.4	|	97.2	98.6
CC	89.8	87.3	|	94.9	91.6
KQ	65.8	73.4	|	89.3	96.2
PDI	40.8	75.4	|	93.8	95.8
PAI	92.9	95.2	|	99.0	100.0
Level	79.6	81.8	|	99.0	93.3
Total	79.1	80.4	|	93.3	97.4

Blue indicates compliance at Accreditation standards.

The only area of protocol compliance that did not increase in a statistically significant fashion was provision of PAI's. The most likely reason for this is that there was little room for improvement in the compliance to the PAI component of the protocol because it was at over 95 percent even before performance feedback was provided to the EMDs.

(continued on 12.14)

Legend for Table (above)

CE	=	Case Entry (primary survey)
CC	=	Chief Complaint
KQ	=	Key Questions (secondary survey)
PDI	=	Post-Dispatch Instructions
PAI	=	Pre-Arrival Instructions
Level	=	Response Determinant Coding

The Impact of a Comprehensive Quality Management Process on Compliance to Protocol

(continued from 12.13)

Effect of Feedback on Determinant Drift:

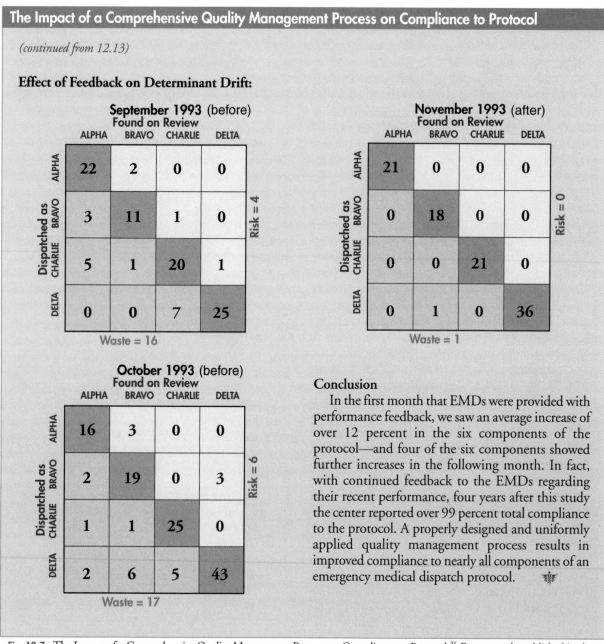

September 1993 (before)
Found on Review

Dispatched as	ALPHA	BRAVO	CHARLIE	DELTA	
ALPHA	22	2	0	0	
BRAVO	3	11	1	0	Risk = 4
CHARLIE	5	1	20	1	
DELTA	0	0	7	25	

Waste = 16

November 1993 (after)
Found on Review

Dispatched as	ALPHA	BRAVO	CHARLIE	DELTA	
ALPHA	21	0	0	0	
BRAVO	0	18	0	0	Risk = 0
CHARLIE	0	0	21	0	
DELTA	0	1	0	36	

Waste = 1

October 1993 (before)
Found on Review

Dispatched as	ALPHA	BRAVO	CHARLIE	DELTA	
ALPHA	16	3	0	0	
BRAVO	2	19	0	3	Risk = 6
CHARLIE	1	1	25	0	
DELTA	2	6	5	43	

Waste = 17

Conclusion

In the first month that EMDs were provided with performance feedback, we saw an average increase of over 12 percent in the six components of the protocol—and four of the six components showed further increases in the following month. In fact, with continued feedback to the EMDs regarding their recent performance, four years after this study the center reported over 99 percent total compliance to the protocol. A properly designed and uniformly applied quality management process results in improved compliance to nearly all components of an emergency medical dispatch protocol. ☙

Fig. 12-7. The Impact of a Comprehensive Quality Management Process on Compliance to Protocol.[26] From a study published in the *Annals of Emergency Medicine,* 1998.

ensures that the candidate is competent in the protocol's use (other training would also include basic telecommunications, CAD, radio and procedural training).

Concurrently, management selects, trains, and implements the QM oversight infrastructure. Personnel are appointed to oversight committees (quality improvement unit, Review and Steering Committees), which are multi-disciplinary action groups that can change and approve dispatch policies and procedures. These committees must also create and approve an implementation timeline, reaching consensus on the start-up

date for use of priority dispatch. As the date for start-up approaches, changes to policies and procedures must be developed, reviewed and approved by the Review and Steering Committees. Before implementation, the individual or group responsible for the development and provision of continuing education should begin orienting personnel to the policies and procedures essential to the correct use of priority dispatch. Other activities include medical director review and approval of priority dispatch and the assignment of an EMS resource response to each of the determinant codes.

On-Line Use

Following EMD training and medical direction approval of the protocols, agency management must decide when the EMD will begin using the protocol. Essentially there are two common approaches. The first is to allow the dispatchers as they become EMD certified to begin using the protocol individually. The second is to wait until all of the dispatchers are certified and schedule a date and specific time to begin using the protocol. In this case, protocols should be placed in the center for "review and familiarization" purposes but should be specially authorized for use by those already certified in cases in which PAIs are clearly needed.

> Computers are worthless. They can only give you answers.
> —Pablo Picasso

Each method or approach has unique advantages and disadvantages that should be considered in the context of the operating environment and patient care objectives. A written plan that outlines and justifies the specific method chosen will minimize any potential liability from inequality of care. Considerable attention must be given to such issues as unit response with respect to determinant codes, skill degradation, policies specific to protocol use, political issues and media notification.

The Feedback Process

Medical dispatch case review must begin at the same time the EMDs begin using priority dispatch. EMD performance feedback, as well as cases reviewed from the first day of protocol use, boosts protocol compliance. The presence of an EMD instructor or EMD-Q™ on the communication floor, in those centers that start using Priority Dispatch at a scheduled date and time, can increase EMD confidence as well as identify gross performance problems. Calls can be reviewed as soon as they are completed, providing immediate feedback to the EMD on the first day.

A properly implemented case review process can shift the quality management paradigm from a punitive process toward a more positive, productive one. The theme of quality management should include "Let's

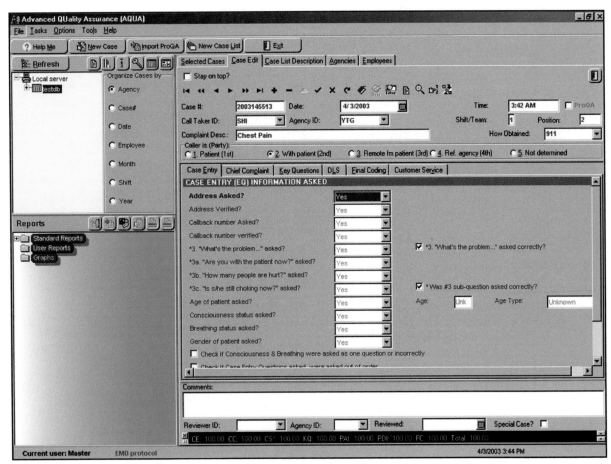

Fig. 12-8. Automated compliance reporting software data entry screen (AQUA™ v.4.0 ©1992-2001 MPC).

catch them doing it right!" As part of the case review process, the system should have a procedure for acknowledging exemplary EMD performance. Positive reinforcement in the initial implementation of priority dispatch can significantly increase the confidence of the EMD in following the protocol. Improving compliance to the protocol leads, ultimately, to improved patient care.

The end result of case review in systems with high compliance to protocol is the identification of what are called the "elements of success." These constitute identifiable features of performance and protocol that occur on cases with successful outcomes, control of difficult situations, and increased customer satisfaction. Superior compliance to the protocol is similar to playing a record at the right speed with a clean needle. The music that the recording musicians intended you to hear is clear and beautiful. It is the same with compliance to protocol, which, done right, results in outcomes that were intended by the protocol designers.

The data gleaned from the case review process is analyzed in the quality improvement unit, which results in the creation of several compliance reports. Each

component (i.e., Case Entry, Chief Complaint selection, Key Questions, Post-Dispatch Instructions, Pre-Arrival Instructions, and final coding) of the protocol f   o   r each Chief Complaint must be regularly analyzed to identify performance problems. In addition to the data gleaned from the EMDs' use of the protocol, other reporting components to the quality management process should include field feedback reports, incident reports, and procedures for requesting clarification regarding the protocol. Field feedback reports, from pre-hospital and hospital personnel, assist the medical director in the further refinement of the EMS resource response. The results of this analysis are reviewed as part of an ongoing quality improvement process which improves EMD performance through education and EMD process change.

The development of continuing education programs are in response to the educational needs identified through compliance to protocol data analysis and as a function of meeting routine educational needs. Automated reporting systems simplify compliance reporting. With the provision of continuing education and performance

---

Guidelines for Risk Management in an EMD Quality Assurance Program

A comprehensive program for managing the quality of care includes not only quality assessment, but quality-assurance risk management activities, designed to assist medical directors, dispatch supervisors, and EMDs in modifying practice behavior found to be deficient by quality assessment, to protect the public against incompetent practitioners, as well as to modify structural, resource, or protocol deficiencies that may exist in the medical dispatch system.

These 10 guidelines should be utilized in any medical dispatch system, whether private or governmentally operated, and whether conducted by medical directors, administrators, supervisors, peers, or government authorizing agencies:

1. **The general policies and processes to be utilized in any quality-assurance activity should be co-developed and concurred with by the professional EMDs, whose performance will be scrutinized and should be objectively and impartially administered.** Such initial involvement with and commitment to ongoing objectivity is critical to ensuring continued participation and cooperation with the program.

2. **Any remedial quality-assurance related to an individual EMD should be triggered by concern for that individual's overall practice, rather than by deviation from specified criteria in single cases.** Because of the inherent variability of patients and incidents, judgment as to the competence of specific dispatchers should be based on an assessment of their performance with a number of patients and not on the examination of single, isolated cases, except in extraordinary circumstances.

3. **The institution of any remedial activity should be preceded by discussion with the EMD involved.** There should be ample opportunity for the EMD to explain observed deviations from accepted practice patterns to supervisors, professional reviewers, and/or the medical director, before any remedial or corrective action is decided on.

(continued on 12.17)

Guidelines for Risk Management in an EMD Quality Assurance Program

(continued from 12.16)

4. **Emphasis should be placed on education and modification of unacceptable practice patterns, rather than on sanctions.** The initial thrust of any quality-assurance activity should be toward helping the EMD correct deficiencies in knowledge, skills, or technique, with practice restrictions or disciplinary action considered only for those not responsive to remedial activities.

5. **The quality-assurance system should make available the appropriate educational resources needed to effect desired practice modifications.** Consistent with the emphasis on assistance, rather than punitive activity, the medical-dispatch quality-assurance program should have the capability of offering or directing the EMD to the educational activities needed to correct deficiencies, whether they be peer consultation, continuing education, retraining or self-learning, and self-assessment programs.

6. **Feedback mechanisms should be established to monitor and document needed changes in practice patterns.** Whether conducted under the same auspices or separately, linkages between a quality-assurance system and a quality-assessment activity should allow for assessment of the effectiveness of any remedial activities instituted by or for an EMD.

7. **Restrictions or disciplinary actions should be imposed on those dispatchers not responsive to remedial activities, whenever the EMD's supervisor and/or appropriate medical control deem such action necessary to protect the public.** Depending on the severity of the deficiency such restrictions may include loss of certification.

8. **The imposition of restrictions or discipline should be timely and consistent with due process.** Before a restriction or disciplinary action is imposed, the EMD affected should have full understanding of the basis for the actions, ample opportunity to request recon-

sideration and to submit any documentation relevant to the request, and the right to meet with those considering its imposition. However, in cases where those considering the imposition of restrictions or discipline deem the dispatcher to pose an imminent hazard to the health of patients, personnel, or the public at large, such restrictions or disciplinary actions may be imposed immediately. In such instances, the due-process rights noted above should be provided and documented on an expedited basis.

9. **Quality-assurance systems for medical dispatch should be structured and operated so as to ensure immunity for those conducting or applying such systems who are acting in good faith.** To ensure the active, unfettered participation of all parties in the review process, all case reviews and the documents and opinions generated by them should be structured, if possible, for protection from subpoena and legal discovery. This incident-review protection is common in most hospitals and medical review environments. Reviewing state and federal legislation, as well as pertinent court decisions, as the basis for developing comprehensive guidelines on immunity in review activities is essential.

10. **To the fullest degree possible, quality assurance systems should be structured to recognize care of high quality, as well as correcting instances of deficient practice.** The vast majority of practicing, professionally trained EMDs provide care of high quality. Quality assurance systems should explore methods to identify and recognize those treatment methodologies, procedures, and protocols that consistently contribute to improved patient outcomes, system efficiency, and safety. Information on such results should be communicated to the medical-control community and dispatch-agency administrations. EMDs providing high- and consistent-quality care should be rewarded. Commendations, awards, advancements, and other forms of positive reinforcements are important facets of quality assurance.

Fig. 12-9. This dispatch-oriented philosophy of risk management within a quality-assurance program[134] is derived from the Guidelines for Quality Assurance from the Council on Medical Service of the American Medical Association.[148]

feedback to the EMDs, the quality management cycle is complete. The remaining activities that are related to making changes to the protocols occur in conjunction with the Academy.

One of the most powerful features of priority dispatch is its use of a "uniform protocol."[146, 147] The inability of users to "customize" the protocol does not mean that the protocol is stagnant in its evolution. Since its inception the protocol has had more than two thousand changes to its design, content, and syntax. Changes to the protocol result from the submission of "Proposal for Change" forms (see page A.5) that users send to the Academy mean compliance scores in the months preceding and following performance feedback (see Appendix C). The Council of Standards carefully reviews each request and evaluates supporting data. With literally thousands of priority dispatch users, the potential to identify and recommend changes that may significantly enhance the protocol occur on a continual basis. This far outweighs any benefit that might be achieved by permitting uncontrolled local modification of the protocol and, therefore, the loss of this unique, unified feature of priority dispatch. Version 11 is evidence of the success of this process.

Risk Management

Don Jones, a noted EMS expert and attorney, has said, "Risk is always there. We determine if we want more risk or less risk." The outcome of a comprehensive quality management program is the management of risk to the patient and the subsequent risk exposure or liability that results

> **Risk is always there. We determine if we want more risk or less risk.**
> **—Don Jones**

from a substandard system res-ponse to the delivery of patient care. The comprehensive orientation of quality management activities review not only the delivery of medicine, but the operational activities that are necessary to provide that care (see fig. 12.9).[148]

The Goal of Quality Management

The elemental or fundamental goals of a good quality improvement program for EMDs are four-fold and are essentially the same for any aspect of organizational endeavor:

1. **To ensure that all employees understand policy, practice, procedure, and protocol.** This requires

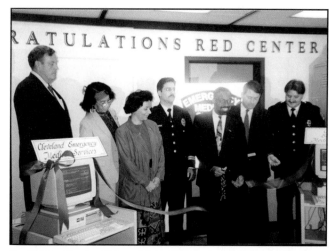

Fig. 12-10. Cleveland Mayor Michael White cuts the ribbon at the Center of Excellence Accreditation and new CAD system dedication ceremony, May 4, 1993, while EMS Commissioner Bruce Shade smiles.

system wide education including both training and orientation by appropriately trained and certified instructors. Educating recruits is easy if a comprehensive orientation program is in place. In addition, there must be an effective system of notifying current practitioners of new developments in protocol science, as well as new policies and procedures, and ample opportunity for them to receive answers to questions that might arise.

2. **To ensure that all employees comply with policy, practice, procedure, and protocol.** Assuring compliance is the most essential challenge in EMD management. No organization can afford to have a supervisor hover over line personnel 24 hours a day, nor is that a good work practice. Line personnel must be guided and motivated to want to do the job right. High-quality companies know that compliance with the policies, practices, and procedures of an organization relies on good leadership and guidance. Optimally, management has a vision that transcends "quality assurance accounting."

Quality assurance accounting—which involves data collection and number crunching—is essential, but is only a piece in the larger framework of a comprehensive quality management program. Successful programs also promote proper values among communication center personnel, instilling the desire to practice the craft of dispatching and

EMD's First Rule of Quality Management
Without quality assurance there is no quality improvement.

> ### Corollary to the EMD's First Rule of Quality Management
>
> Without quality management, how does an EMD know when they are doing a good job? No one says anything.

remote patient care appropriately on their own. Case tape studies, using the case review process, are great for this. Other audit-type programs can also help the quality improvement coordinator account for whether dispatch personnel are doing their jobs the way they should.

3. **To determine if policy, practice, procedure, and protocol themselves are safe, efficient, and effective.** What may seem like a good idea on paper or during planning may not translate to the working console. To be effective, written policies and protocols must work. Sometimes this is not evident until one uses the procedure in question at length. Subsequent fine-tuning increases the degree of quality, especially in an environment of continuous improvement. What is deemed correct at one point may change; the system merits frequent re-evaluation, especially if those using it raise concerns. Dispatch personnel often contribute valuable suggestions when they feel included in the evaluation process and sense that their views will be respected. On a larger scope, when there is a formal recommendation for protocol improvement made by seasoned, well trained EMDs, supported with proper data, a process of evaluation and approval is then conducted by the Council of Standards within the Academy's College of Fellows. This scientific, uniform process allows for continual refinement and improvement of the protocols.

These improvements are then implemented by all centers using the unified system. This maintains consistency while sharing valuable improvement among all "users."

4. **The final goal is to fix what is missing (understanding, compliance, safety, efficiency, or effectiveness).** If compliance is substandard or if the policies, practices, procedures, and protocols seem for some reason to be incorrect, changes are made through performance feedback, retraining, improvement of protocol, and discipline. One way organizations can avoid much of this is by developing a hiring process that draws in new line personnel with "the right stuff."

Summary

Dispatching is not a job for just anyone. EMDs must have the ability to handle complex situations at a rapid pace (multi-tasking) and have the ability to appropriately deal with human beings in great distress (empathize).

Guiding the implementation and application of priority dispatch demands flexibility and awareness by the quality improvement coordinator. That person's tasks must be integrated within the framework of the organization, and must be genuinely and whole-heartedly supported by top administration. Without this essential backing, even the finest quality improvement coordinator is unlikely to be able to function effectively.

> **If you don't have time to do it right, when will you have time to do it over?**

No, you don't have to do this. Survival is not compulsory.

—*W. Edward Deming*

Contents

CHAPTER 13

The Evolution *of* EMD

Chapter Overview

The genesis of EMD processes used by medical dispatchers to interrogate callers and determine the need for dispatch life support and system response was occurring in several locations simultaneously in the 1970s.[1] At that time, new pressures resulting from increased availability and use of 9-1-1 in the EMS and public safety environment served as the catalyst needed to change inefficient and unsafe dispatch practices. The growing demand for modern emergency medical services has continued to fuel this process.

This need to evolve has effectively called the question to choose between either a disarrayed, every-system-for-itself future versus a unified standard. Using a scientific method-based evaluation and change process, the National/International Academy of Emergency Medical Dispatch grew to manage a full range of medical dispatch standards as the preeminent professional organization for EMD worldwide.

> *The art of progress is to preserve order amid change and to preserve change amid order.*
>
> — *Alfred North Whitehead*

In the mid-1980s the city of Detroit began a well-funded citywide advertising campaign to jolt public awareness not to call 9-1-1 unless a true emergency existed. After billboard, radio, and television ads were run, the outcome was an unpleasant surprise to both the politicians and public safety officials. Calls to 9-1-1 rose more than five percent!

In the late 1970s, the Dallas Fire Department tried a different approach to managing the increasing 9-1-1 call volume. Assistant Chief Bill Roberts issued a white paper, "EMS Dispatch—Its Use and Misuse."[149, 150] This document identified that the dispatch center was central to the appropriate management of emergency calls and that if the determination of 9-1-1 problem severity could be safely accomplished, calls could be successfully "triaged" (see fig. 3-1).[149, 150]

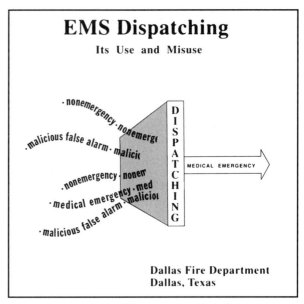

Fig. 13-1. Cover of early "white paper" on EMS dispatching by Bill Roberts et al., 1978.[149]

> **The knowing of this is a humble revelation, that even one's goals are a step on the road, and not their true destination.**
> **—A. Seaton**

The result was the implementation of a screening program begun in 1980 and staffed by nurses. It was based on Debra Cason's master's thesis work at Texas Women's University titled, "Telephone Triage of Emergency Patients by a Nurse." Although it was first used with apparent success, the program was eventually dropped after the Boff "no send" disaster embroiled that city in 1984 (see Boff case transcript in Chapter 11: Legal Aspects of EMD).

An early protocol-based solution called the Illinois Advisory Flip File was designed in the late 1970s by Karen Kabat, RN and Daniel VonBerg. It is no longer in widespread use. In addition, various locally devised protocols have been used in several places throughout the world.[151]

The concept of formal dispatch prioritization was created in 1976 and underwent major developmental and design work in 1977. The first working protocol prototype was introduced into the Alarm Office of the Salt Lake City Fire Department in 1978 for "use, comment, and review." The actual on-line implementation took place a few hours after the first EMD course ended there Sept. 14, 1979. Two other participants in the initial Utah training experience, Davis County Sheriff's Office and Gold Cross Ambulance, also initiated use of the system at that time.[2]

In 1980, a copy of the protocol found its way to Aurora, Colorado, seeding development of the first MPDS protocol variant. Other seeds ended up in Montana and the Stockton/Sacramento area of California by way of early EMD training courses. In 1981, the Journal of Emergency Medical Services published an article on "priority medical dispatch." As a result, hundreds of public safety agencies requested the third edition of MPDS along with various EMD training aids. By 1990, several thousand sites were using some form or edition of priority dispatch.[2] By 1982, the MPDS protocols were in use in one form or another in Baltimore County, Maryland; Grand Island, Nebraska; and Prescott and Mesa, Arizona. Each reported their successes in print.[4, 12, 152, 153]

While there are various versions of priority dispatch, essentially only two significantly divergent EMD philosophies have evolved. There are several variants of protocol-based systems available, but the introduction of a guidelines-based process in the 1990s raised significant quality management liability and patient care issues.

A comparison provides valuable insight into several very Darwinian-like principles of EMD evolution and adaptation represented by the very divergent processes of guidelines versus protocols.

Around 1990, a set of EMD guidelines was developed by Linda Culley and Suzie Funk. Dubbed "criteria-based dispatch" (CBD), these guidelines were not described or designed as protocols.[154] Cully and Funk argued that adherence to protocols was not necessary when trained dispatchers used this system. Rather, there was an emphasis on dispatching responses off of "key words"

How I "Discovered" Protocols

In 1975, I was an intern at Charity Hospital of Louisiana at New Orleans. After a few months, I found myself working in the large medical clinics at Charity. The "clinics" were much different than anything I had experienced in my limited medical practice to date, especially compared to my medical student experience back in the relatively sedate setting of the University of Utah Medical Center in Salt Lake City. Sick people came to Charity—lots of them. For the patients, clinic began as early as 6 a.m. Not that we saw the patients quite that early, but since clinic was "first come, first served," 100 to 150 patients had generally been waiting in the queue several hours each morning.

Upon entering any of the small evaluation rooms, each intern was confronted with stacks of patient charts leaning high upon the wall at the back of each work table—and I mean thick charts. Most adult patients at Charity, if not born there, had received all their medical care at CHNO. That often represented 50 to 70 years of medical documentation for each patient in Hypertension clinic. In addition to "High Blood Clinic" as it was called, other clinics included "Sugar Clinic" (diabetes) and "Pus Clinic" (surgical follow-up).

After a few weeks "working the clinics," I became increasingly frustrated. Each patient I evaluated and treated seemed to be a new experience. I knew as a physician, albeit a very new one, that I should be able to "figure out" what to do with each patient. After all, this is what I had trained for years to do. However, I often couldn't remember what I had done for a similar patient two hours, two days, or two weeks before.

I sensed I was moving too slowly and patients weren't getting their money's worth from me (even though Charity's medical care was basically "free" at the time).

At one point, my growing despair drove me to seriously consider quitting to return to Salt Lake and become a paramedic with several of my friends at Gold Cross Ambulance. Late one morning, as "High Blood Clinic" ended, I confronted the senior resident on the LSU service, Dr. J. V. Jones, an imposing, stocky fellow from Baylor.

"Look J.V." I said, "I think I'm killing people here. How do you keep it all straight, patient after patient, with all these complaints, symptoms, lab values, medications and everything?"

He slowly put his arm around me, laughed, and said, "Clawson, that's why I'm the resident and you're the intern." I was definitely caught off guard, but then I was given some needed advice. He opened his coat, revealing an inner pocket from which he pulled a set of worn, dog-eared 4 by 6 inch cards held together with a dirty rubber band, and said, "What you need, my man, is a protocol."

"Protocol?" I frowned, "You mean a cookbook?" They had warned me at Utah, that cookbooks were bad. "You're a doctor now. You should be able to figure it out yourself." Silently for a moment, he turned, pointing toward the now empty, but trashed, waiting room of a hundred folding chairs, and said, "Cook book, my ass! At the Big Free, Clawson, you can't live without 'em."

Needless to say, I was a bit shocked. For the next 10 minutes, he sat down and showed me through his "protocols" which he lent me overnight. I made a set and went to clinic the next day with a different feeling— a bit skeptical, but definitely curious. Soon I was having a very new and remarkable experience. Things went smoother and faster, and my time was better spent gleaning the necessary information from the patient rather than reinventing common medical care. In a short time, I found myself, leaning out of my little evaluation room, much happier, and much more often, calling spiritedly to the next of dozens of patients still waiting, "Mary Jones, come on down!"

Not everybody should have to learn the hard way that there are certain times and places for protocol use within the patient evaluation and care process regardless of where you practice your medicine. I guess, in a way, the first life I ever "saved" with a protocol was my own.   ❊

Fig. 13-2. "How I 'Discovered' Protocols" by J. Clawson.

based on certain symptoms. The following is a representation of discretionary "vital points" questions for abdominal pain listed in a set of CBD guidelines from the U.K.:

1. Is the patient short of breath?

2. Does it hurt to breathe?

3. Can the patient talk in full sentences?

4. Has the patient vomited?

5. What does the vomit look like?

6. Are the patient's bowel movements different?

7. How would you describe them?

8. Is the pain above or below the naval [sic]?

9. Is the patient wearing a medical alert tag?

10. Is the patient pregnant?

11. Has she felt weak and dizzy?

12. Has there been any vaginal bleeding?

13. Has her period been very heavy or too soon?

14. How does the patient feel when he/she sits up?

15. Does the patient have any medical/surgical history?

The proponents of these guidelines explained at a conference in 1992 that, "There is no requirement to ask these (vital points) questions if a dispatch criteria is volunteered by the caller." Suggested questioning was necessary only when a key word was not readily identified.

Several program assumptions for the guidelines were listed in explanatory material[155] and include:

1. *It is the criticalness of illness or injury that should be the determining factor for level of response, therefore we need to elicit those same critical criteria from the caller.*

2. *Dispatchers are professionals and therefore capable of using their intelligence, ability, and experience to elicit information from callers.*

3. *Emergency calls vary greatly and dispatchers should be allowed to use flexibility in how they obtain information from the caller.*

4. *Information comes to the dispatcher in many ways, upset and frantic callers do not easily adhere to a given set of questions.*

Several of the CBD developmental concepts were based on a survey of local area paramedics who reportedly urged, "Don't ask so many questions," and "Let the patient tell you what's wrong." In addition, the statement that seems to be at the core of this program is "Guidelines give dispatchers flexibility" with the most common example of this summarized by "Things never fit into pre-determined questions."

Initial emphasis on a non-proprietary approach by this group has subsequently changed as an increasing number of different versions of these guidelines have appeared in various centers. Its proponents state it is okay to modify these guidelines in any way for local use, suggesting (but not requiring) medical approval for such changes. While the basis of a protocol approach to EMD is usually accompanied by advice to strictly adhere to them, criteria-based guidelines are not.

The Critical Selection of an EMD Program

There is now widespread agreement in public safety circles that EMDs must be provided with specific tools and training to enhance their role in the patient care process. But what kind of tools and training should be employed to best understand and master the use of those tools? Should the medical dispatcher's "scope of practice" be tightly defined or loosely structured?

The ASTM "Standard Practice for EMD" states:

The protocols for inquiry, response, and resource coordination are essential and must not be modified based on an individual's possible experiences as a responder.[54]

The difference lies in whether medical dispatchers should use protocols or guidelines.[156] There are fundamental medical and functional differences between the structure and core philosophies of guidelines as compared to protocols. With this in mind, it is essential that EMD managers and physician medical directors exercise due regard and diligence in the evaluation and ultimate selection of a medical dispatch program.

Understanding how these programs differ will help all parties in the selection process appreciate how these intrinsic differences may affect patient evaluation and care.[157] To do so requires a careful, detailed comparison of various dispatching systems, including the methodology for delivering each through its associated training curricula and systematic quality management processes.

In 1989, the National Association of EMS Physicians published its position paper on emergency medical dispatching.[20] The following year the American Society for Testing and Materials set forth the "Standard Practice for Emergency Medical Dispatch" in the Annual Book of ASTM Standards.[158] These documents have contributed significantly to a developing "standard of care" and "standard of practice" for EMDs. EMS system managers who are considering the implementation of an EMD program should review them. Each document takes the position that medically appropriate protocols should be used by EMDs in the medical dispatch decision-making process.

> **There are fundamental medical and functional differences between the structure and core philosophies of guidelines as compared to protocols.**

NAEMSP defines its requirement for a medical dispatch system as a "medically approved system used by a medical dispatch center to dispatch appropriate aid to medical emergencies."[20] This includes:

1. Systematized caller interrogation questions;

2. Systematized pre-arrival instructions;

3. Protocols that match the dispatcher's evaluation of the illness or injury type and severity with vehicle response mode and configuration.[20]

ASTM standards state, "The emergency medical dispatch priority reference system directs the EMD to complete a full, programmed interrogation" and "the protocols for inquiry, response, and resource coordination are essential and must not be modified based on an individual's possible experiences as a responder."[54]

The implication in each of these documents is that the EMDs should follow a structured, predetermined interrogation process in order to activate predetermined response levels and modes and as the basis for providing medical instructions.

Just Listen or Actively Ask? Proponents of the guidelines approach to medical dispatching say that the dispatcher should listen rather than interrogate. The criteria-based dispatching model contains no structured questions that a medical dispatcher is required to ask.

The first listed fundamental of this guideline process is, "No required or mandatory questions; suggested questions are provided in training and appear on guideline cards."[155]

At the 1992 Emergency Cardiac Care Conference in Seattle, a physician advisor to the program developers of the initial guidelines-based system, explained that the "questions" or "vital points" portion of the guidelines can be completely eliminated at the discretion of each user, adding that, "Things never fit nicely into predetermined questions." This approach to evaluating medical calls for assistance has emphasized a high reliance on "the thinking, intelligent" attributes of the CBD dispatcher, which protocol systems somehow "fail to recognize."

> **A structured interrogation ensures that the dispatcher always accomplishes the four basic objectives of medical dispatch evaluation.**

Protocol proponents, however, point out that the caller's perception of the "needs" of the medical dispatcher is limited at best. In the vast majority of cases, the caller simply says something to the effect of "just send help!" A structured interrogation ensures that the dispatcher always accomplishes the four basic objectives of medical dispatch evaluation:

1. The identification of the proper **response configuration** (who goes) and mode (how they respond);

2. The identification of the **presence of conditions** that may require pre-arrival instructions;

3. The collection of information that will **assist responders** in preparing for and addressing the call;

4. The collection of information that will assist in **ensuring the safety** of patients, bystanders, responders, and the caller.

Advocates of the guidelines approach to dispatching claim that it treats the dispatcher as an "intelligent human being who is capable of exercising good medical judgment." However, the practice of prehospital medicine (indeed, the practice of any type of time-critical medicine) is not guideline- or judgment-driven—it is protocol-driven. For example, physicians follow the ACLS protocol for patients in cardiac arrest until there is time and room in the process to make more subjective decisions based on judgment and experience. Judgment by all prehospital care providers is a function of deciding which protocol applies and how to apply it in specific situations.

This initially entails recognizing (and at times interpreting) what the caller is saying in response to specific questions or during evaluations and treatments. EMDs shouldn't invent interrogation "on-the-fly." This doesn't mean EMDs are robots. The EMD's subjective intelligence becomes essential in *synthesizing* this information into action on the patient's behalf. The actions of emergency medical dispatchers need to be structured and prioritized just as the actions of paramedics and EMTs are structured and prioritized, based on defined, medically approved protocols.[29, 157]

> **History will remember the master of synthesis.**
> —Norm Dinerman, M.D.
> EMS philosopher

"You Shall" or "You May If You Want." With the refinement of modern EMS systems has come widespread appreciation of the need for medical quality improvement. As with hands-on caregivers, continuous review of the individual EMD's performance is essential.

The fundamental issue in the retrospective review of the performance of prehospital care personnel is compliance to established prehospital care protocols. Retrospective quality assurance of EMDs is impractical, if not objectively impossible, in a guidelines-oriented medical dispatch system. Simply stated, a protocol says, "You shall," while a guideline says, "You may if you want." Because protocols require compliance to a predefined set of behaviors, it is possible, after the fact, to determine precisely the extent of compliance.

A guideline, on the other hand, does not require compliance and allows for (or even sanctions) deviation at the discretion of the individual practitioner. Retrospective reviewers of dispatcher adherence to guidelines, therefore, must be prepared to examine and debate an infinite number of reasons or conflicting sets of reasons why the guideline might not have been followed. Every case review will thus involve the evaluation of significant subjective judgments, making quantification of performance difficult, comparisons of one EMD's performance to another's strained, creating mistrust of the quality management process by the EMDs and adding to frustration of managers attempting to quality assure these moving targets.

Unfortunately, experience has shown that, in far too many cases, individual discretion, when applied by EMDs, has been inappropriate and even medically unsound. At the very least in such systems, it remains inconsistent and, at times, dangerously arbitrary.

Years of quality assurance review of medical dispatch tapes reveal that unstructured interrogation—at the heart of the "guidelines" approach to dispatching—may lead to the dispatcher asking irrelevant and time-consuming questions that fail to identify the basic problem. Such call-taking anarchy has earned a not-so-flattering name: Dodge City dispatching. As in the lawless Dodge City of the American Wild West, "Do what you want to do, to whomever you want, whenever you want to do it." Indeed, although the written versions of the guidelines approach (CBD) have been around for several years, the open-ended concept upon which they are based may have been in existence much longer.

> **Such calltaking anarchy has earned a not-so-flattering name: Dodge City dispatching.**

Many years ago this similar process of unstructured interrogation was identified when dispatchers applied their own questioning randomly until a "positive" answer was obtained. After making a "hit" (as these "positive" answers were first called in the mid 80's) dispatchers, sensing they were "hot on the trail," asked a series of related questions. The following case transcript demonstrates this approach (see fig.13-3). The patient in this case died. Reportedly no lawsuit ensued.

This case represents a consistently observed, risky pattern in unstructured interrogation (the "guidelines" approach). One irrelevant question ("Has she been drinking?") leads to a process known, in medical dispatch terminology, as **side-cycling**, a lateral deviation from the usual vertically listed key question objectives, that is common among dispatchers who function without specific protocols. The dispatcher in this case got off the main track and allowed a bias—that the patient was merely drunk and passed out—to creep into the decision-making. Biases can, as this case shows, cause a dispatcher practicing without a set protocol structure, to "lead" a caller along inappropriate information-gathering pathways.

Observe how the dispatcher continued asking questions even after the caller reported a priority sign representing unconsciousness. The dispatcher kept asking irrel-

Unstructured Discretionary Interrogation Case

First Call

Caller 1: Um, hello. Can I have you come over to my house?

Dispatch: What's the address?
Caller 1: (given by caller)

Dispatch: (repeated to caller)
Caller 1: Yes.

Dispatch: What's the problem?
Caller 1: She started throwing up in the night and then everybody tried to wake her up and she wouldn't. She just kept snoring and just kept lying there and wouldn't wake up.

Dispatch: Okay, who is this? Is this your sister or something?
Caller 1: No, it's my mom.

Dispatch: It's your mom? How old is your mother?
Caller 1: Um, she's 48

Dispatch: And how old are you?
Caller 1: I'm 10.

Dispatch: Okay, is this a house or an apartment?
Caller 1: House.

Dispatch: Okay, do you know, she wasn't throwing up blood was she?
Caller 1: I don't know, let me see. Dad, was she throwing up blood?

Father: (unintelligible)

Caller1: No, just throw-up.

Dispatch: Okay, and you can't, you can't wake her up now, right?
Caller 1: Uh uh.

Dispatch: Has she been drinking tonight, do you know?
Caller 1: Yeah.

Dispatch: She has? [The "hit" moment] ←
Caller 1: Uh huh.

Dispatch: Does she get sick when she drinks very much?
Caller 1: Yeah.

Dispatch: Okay, what's your phone number?
Caller 1: (given by caller)

Dispatch: Okay, we'll have them right there, alright?
Caller 1: Okay.

The first call was terminated and no paramedics were sent. BLS ambulance responding.

Second Call

Caller 2: Did you send paramedics to (gives address)?

Dispatch: They are on the way. How is your mother doing? Or is it your mother?
Caller 2: Well, uh, it's my aunt and I don't know, I ain't there, but they said they haven't been there yet.

Dispatch: Ah, well um, apparently it sounds like she's been drinking a lot and she's passed out. Um, do you know any more information?
Caller 2: They said her lips are turning blue?

Dispatch: They are? Okay, we'll send them right, we'll send, send... Excuse me. We'll step them up. They'll be there in about one minute, Okay? Thank you. You're not there then?
Caller 2: I'm over... (unintelligible).

Dispatch: It's only been about three or four minutes. Thank you. Bye, bye.

Second call terminated. Dispatch initiated a call to the responding unit.

Dispatch: Ambulance, dispatch.
Ambulance: Go ahead.

Dispatch: Ambulance you are responding red-lights-and-siren.

Ambulance: 10-4.

Dispatch: ETA? Ambulance, dispatch. ETA? Ambulance, dispatch.
Ambulance: Our ETA is two minutes.

Dispatch: 0227.

(continued on 13.8)

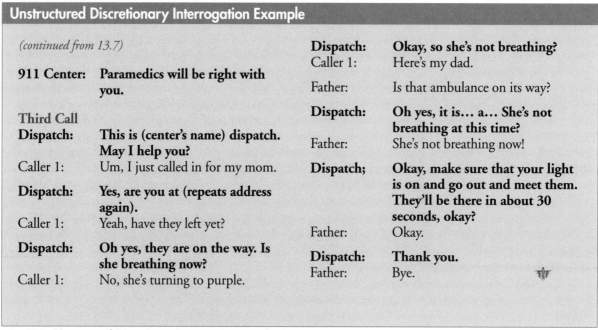

Fig. 13-3. Unstructured Discretionary Interrogation example, circa 1983.

evant and unimportant questions until an answer just happened to match what the dispatcher "expected" to hear. These *hits* are analogous to getting a bite when fishing. This type of "fishing" for irrelevant information is common for dispatchers not functioning under specific protocols. A dispatcher functioning under a specific protocol would only be concerned with the level of consciousness of the patient, and would have easily recognized the primary problem here—an unconscious woman.

> **Dispatchers should not be allowed to introduce significant personal bias by concocting questions "as-they-go."**

In a protocol EMD system, medical dispatchers are prompted, in a verifiable, repeatable manner, to ask for information that they *need to know*, not what would merely be interesting to know. Such a system protects the EMD from being swayed by personal bias, prejudice, and intolerance.

For the same reason lawyers are over-ruled when "leading" a witness, dispatchers should not be allowed to introduce significant personal bias by concocting questions "as-they-go" (i.e., there must be a dispatch-valid "reason" why the dispatcher asked them).

Does Field Work Equal Phone Work? Proponents of the guidelines approach advocate using field-experienced EMTs and paramedics to do emergency medical dispatching. The belief is that they can appropriately apply their field interrogation and basic life support treatment skills to the medical dispatch activity.

However, this fails to take into account the nonvisual nature of medical dispatching.[20] Most EMTs and paramedics can relate to the problem of having a physician suddenly appear at a prehospital scene. Often, the physician functions inadequately (despite a greater level of training and knowledge) because he or she is "out of context." This same problem exists comparing dispatch care with field care. The training of paramedics and EMTs is based on having patients in front of them, where they can "look, listen, and feel." Dispatch is different. EMDs cannot look or feel. The medical dispatcher not only can't see the patient, but is frequently talking to someone "representing" the patient (e.g., a bystander or a relative). Specifically designed protocols help the medical dispatcher overcome the limitations inherent in assessing and "treating" people over the telephone.[54]

A study done in 1996 by the Medical Care Research Unit of the University of Sheffield (U.K.) attempted to compare CBD guidelines to priority dispatch in two centers that first implemented these programs in the U.K.[159] The study reported that it was difficult to compare a discretionary process with a more formal protocolized one; however, it was possible to compare the mandatory and vital interrogation parts of CBD to their equivalents in priority dispatch.

The findings are revealing. The priority dispatch-based Derbyshire center was functioning at high compliance levels—collecting or verifying all the mandatory and vital information in over 95 percent of its cases (Academy accreditation level), while the CBD-based Essex center was only collecting or verifying mandatory and vital information in 40 percent of its cases.

To not verify the location 15 percent of the time nor breathing and consciousness in 50 percent of all calls handled by a control center using CBD is staggering, yet similar results occur reproducibly in centers utilizing this type of system. The data lead to a conclusion not ventured by the Sheffield researchers: it is evident that where discretion plays a major role in the performance of a dispatch "system," the operators (EMDs) do not, indeed cannot, move efficiently between discretionary and formal use in interrogation (or between discretionary and formal parts of the system). This is why, even though certain areas of CBD are "mandatory," dispatchers trained to use this system often fail to comply.

> **Protocol without compliance is a bowl of Jell-O™...**
> **...without the bowl.**
> **—Joseph Ryan, M.D.**

An ominous statement by the Sheffield researchers appears in a discussion of their data:

Plainly in the CBD system, earlier questions relating to the main complaint meant that these questions were often considered redundant, and it is difficult to make any judgement about whether their omission was a failure of the system or reflected the success of having a more flexible approach.[159]

Evolutionary Dead End—Protocols Without Process

In 1993, Sheila Q. Wheeler, the preeminent expert in nurse telephone triage, stated:

Telephone triage is both art and science, a synthesis of human intuition and artificial intelligence. Artificial intelligence parallels the thought processes, logical steps, rules and intuition used in problem-solving. The same process is used in "computer diagnostics" to help physicians think through diagnostic and treatment decisions. Like artificial intelligence systems, protocols help to analyze and classify symptoms.[160]

> **We are what we repeatedly do. Excellence, then, is not an act, but a habit.**
> **—Aristotle**

Protocols, Wheeler advises, have four functions:

1. **Problem-solving.** Protocols are expert systems on paper or computer that guide one through the processes of interview, assessment, and decision making, comparable to having an expert at one's side.

Frequency of questions asked, CBD versus MPDS: Sheffield Study				
Questions Vital/Mandatory	**Criteria-Based Dispatch (CBD)**		**Priority Dispatch (MPDS)**	
	n.	**%**	**n.**	**%**
Confirm Location	53	85.5	62	100.0
Age and Sex	50	80.6	60	96.8
Breathing and Consciousness	31	50.0	60	96.8
All vital questions	25	40.3	59	95.2

Fig. 13-4. Stratified random sample (124 calls) Essex (CBD) versus Derbyshire (MPDS), U.K., 1997[159]

2. **Structure.** Protocols organize vast amounts of information for consideration by the decision-maker. They determine what constitutes significant information.

3. **Risk Management Safeguard.** Protocols show the interrelationship of various data, forcing consideration of all possible decision choices and safeguarding against stereotyping.

4. **Reconstructive.** In some institutions, especially gatekeeper systems, nurses must defend their dispositions. Protocols can help reconstruct the decision-making process.

Wheeler wisely added, "Protocols must be well-designed, comprehensive, standardized, and actively used by staff."

The early visionary, Aristotle, made a statement over two thousand years ago that applies to this discussion: "We are what we repeatedly do. Excellence, then, is not an act, but a habit."

The selection and adoption of an EMD protocol is analogous to choosing whether or not your agency will follow the American Heart Association's Advanced Cardiac Life Support (ACLS) protocol or develop their own. An EMD protocol is the medicine that the dispatch center will practice. That medicine can be developed scientifically, though a controlled consensus process, or anecdotally from a single medical director's perspective. Therefore, when considering the selection of a potential protocol, there are several important elements to evaluate when conducting an EMD protocol-by-protocol medical evaluation:

> **Protocols must be well-designed, comprehensive, standardized, and actively used by staff.**

1. The use of questions listed in paraphrase or "two-word" form demonstrates lack of current knowledge of how "on-the-fly" construction of full questions (from incomplete paraphrases) can introduce interrogator bias and result in different answers from the same paraphrase. We have identified at least seven ways the paraphrase "Chest Pain?" has been converted into a complete question (e.g., "Does he have chest pain?" vs. "He doesn't have chest pain, does he?").

2. Inconsistencies in wording, style, formats, treatments, determinants, and coding between various cards or sections of the protocol are readily visible in protocols formulated by committees and reflect a lack of critical editing. More than an occasional typo, misspelling, or format error should be a signal regarding the care and attention used in initially creating or maintaining protocols.

Factors Resulting in EMD Evolutionary Dead Ends

There are several factors that cause guidelines or protocols to enter an evolutionary dead end:

1. Initial developmental enthusiasm is often like a "supernova" in consistency. That is, there is an initial flurry of activity with early interest and attention to detail. This is followed by a much longer, if not indefinite, epoch of contentment with the end product. The product eventually stagnates due to lack of interest.

2. Often a "project mentality" exists during implementation, and, after the initial rough road of start-up smoothes out, little attention is formally paid to the results. Quality improvement processes are seldom in place, thus giving a false impression of program success, especially in regard to dispatcher compliance to protocol. As it usually goes with projects, another quickly takes its place—such as auto-defibrillation, critical incident stress debriefing, or primary care—and the once front-burner "EMD project" languishes like yesterday's news.

3. The failure to formally network with other similar protocol users is practically a universal omission. While occasional "ideas" or opinions are bounced around via the mail or the Internet, there is no official process to review or approve such "ideas." Thus, there is no organized, consistent cross-pollination. This "all's well here" attitude fosters an ingrown complacency in systems that have no organized methodology to learn of the successes or failures of others. And it's merely chance that determines if the failures happen to them.

Factors Resulting in EMD Evolutionary Dead Ends

(continued from 13.10)

4. Many systems administrators think they have an "EMD program" while all they really have is the provision of PAIs alone. In one U.S. state, the term "EMDing a call" widely means giving pre-arrival instructions. Without the protocol-driven ability to routinely and accurately identify patients needing pre-arrival instructions, the dispatcher often enters the fray based on a "gut" feeling when a situation "seems" like a serious one. Many a baby with a febrile seizure has been "CPR saved" by a dispatcher using this sort of non-system. (Just watch early reruns of "Rescue 9-1-1.")

5. The inability to compare protocol codes or data with other systems because of dissimilar programs contains significant EMD system management drawbacks and limitations. Systems with different codes have little ability to compare results. Even if dispatch code descriptions are similar, the methodology used to determine them is quite likely different. In addition, unique codes can "lock" the data into individual systems. What evolves is, again, an ingrown system.

6. Lack of expert input from many experienced users into the development and on-going refinement of the protocols creates a home-grown atmosphere surrounding protocol evolution. Ownership often plays a big part in local dispatch protocol development. The involvement in a managed consensus process that can consistently improve the protocols over time is very difficult for many.

7. Development of dispatch protocols by people without significant dispatch-relevant emergency medical knowledge and experience can create inappropriate responses and treatments. EMT-level developed protocols commonly exhibit a distinct over-emphasis on treatment to the exclusion of the evaluation that justifies the recommended treatment.

8. Lack of a protocol validation or testing process before going on-line after local protocol modifications that are generally done sporadically along the way. This requires a quality assurance program in-and-of itself.

Fig. 13-5. Factors Resulting in EMD Evolutionary Dead Ends.

3. The statement that "these aren't protocols, they're guidelines" should be a red flag to a potential user. Careful, professional compliance to protocol has been shown, time and time again, to be necessary for safe, efficient, and effective use. Guidelines are clearly not equivalent to protocols in the on-line world of medical dispatching and routinely result in the illusion of their actual "use."

> "Flexibility" is an excuse for not doing it right.
> —Gwyn Pritchard

4. The claim that "you (not necessarily meaning informed medical control) can tailor these protocols to fit your center" is little more than pandering to those who poorly understand the value of carefully constructed and expertly maintained protocols.

5. Finding handwritten alterations on previously printed protocols is the EMD equivalent of finding duct tape on the space shuttle's O-rings. Protocols are never changed on-line but only by an organized process of careful review and expert consensus managed by nationally-based organizations. Such locally written changes reflect an "oops, better fix it" attitude whenever a "zebra" is spotted at dispatch.

6. Lack of internal quality assurance within the agency, group, or company producing or selling "protocols" significantly reduces their reliability. Inquire about specific mechanisms used to modify or routinely up-date their protocols. Require an explanation of their internal quality improvement mechanisms for protocols, translations, software, curricula, etc. Ask how often this is done and by whom.

Nursing quality assurance expert Carolyn Smith-Marker best summarized these issues when she stated in regards to the nature of patient care and practice:

Nurses can function according to defined purposeful expectations or by intuition. A nursing system can operate in a designated manner or haphazardly. Patient care can be delivered by design or by impulse and habit. Standards either exist or they do not. If they exist, they must be detailed, consistent and comprehensive or they will be shallow, irrelevant and worthless.[161]

> **The use of guidelines is a dispatch placebo.**
> **—A. J. Heightman**

The Evolution of Organized Standards for EMD

In the mid-1980s, there were several dozen variations and different types of EMD systems. Unfortunately, no central forum was available to share problems and successes. There was a dearth of published articles on protocol specifics in the medical literature and those few that were published lacked any comparative descriptions or compliance data. EMD in that era could be described basically as two events—EMD training and selecting a protocol. Virtually no MPDS or other protocol modification, improvement, and management processes existed. In essence, EMD as an evolving standard was in disarray.

In February 1987, about 40 people attended an initial meeting of a fledgling group called the North American EMD Network in Anaheim, California. The meeting concluded with a vague call for more sharing of information on EMD protocol and process, but no insight emerged on how to accomplish that on a formal or even regular basis. It was becoming clear, however, that some form of organization was needed. The early "failure" of the Network caused a more in-depth examination of the structural scope and organization necessary for such an association to be meaningful and successful.

> **Standards either exist or they do not. If they exist, they must be detailed, consistent and comprehensive.**
> **—Carolyn Smith-Marker**

Using the American Heart Association's Emergency Cardiac Care Committee and parts of several EMS associations as examples, a new organizational design emerged— an "academy." The idea of an academy embodies the membership and political aspects of an association but further encompasses an academic standards-setting framework. On December 1, 1988, the National Academy of Emergency Medical Dispatch was formally launched.[146]

> **On Dec. 1, 1988, the National Academy of Emergency Medical Dispatch was formally launched.**

The DNA of Dispatch—Origins of the College of Fellows

1953 was the year of a remarkable discovery—a red letter day in science—the discovery by Francis Crick and James Watson of the double helix structure of DNA within the human chromosome.[162] We finally learned how one spiral chemical chain creates or "replicates" itself and, thus, how life is perpetuated in a predetermined non-arbitrary way. Frogs give birth to frogs, snakes give birth to snakes. Unfortunately, if the order or "code" of these genetic chemical units is defective, mutations can appear—two-eyed frogs become three-eyed frogs or frogs that can't jump.

Through its simplicity and eons of proven effectiveness, nature can provide a model for a better understanding of the apparently unrelated process of medical dispatch evolution. For many years, 9-1-1 requests were processed by a dispatcher with no applicable training and no structured protocol—in essence, no plan. This absence of a formal plan means that no reliable reproduction of that "plan" can exist. Similar, if not exact, problems were handled differently by different dispatchers in the same center or differently by the same dispatcher from one call to the next.

> **It is the mark of an educated mind to be able to entertain a thought without accepting it.**
> **—Aristotle**

Compare this "Dodge City dispatching" chaos with the orderly, effortless, near-perfect replication of living cells that DNA provides in countless functioning plants and animals. There is little (or no) resemblance. In Dodge City they shot from the hip. In cells there is a plan.

Priority dispatch protocols were designed for a specific purpose: to ensure that the right thing is sent to the right place, in the right way, at the right time. This is the most important reason these protocols exist.

The prioritization of response and the orderliness of evaluation and treatment is the true value of such protocol "plans." Now, more than ever, patient care is being impacted by new methods of mobile medical resource management in the prehospital setting. Pre-planning of emergency responses is becoming an essential science in a health care environment that stresses the efficiency as well as the economy of care.

To keep with the analogy, just as DNA determines the successful replication of life, dispatch determinant codes, or dispatch "DRGs" (diagnosis-related groups), form the replicative basis of priority dispatch protocols. DRGs are a universal type of medical coding system used by hospitals and clinics to medically classify and, ultimately, bill patients. Obviously, how a dispatcher arrives at the decision to select a given "DRG" is just as important as the resultant code itself, since selection of the wrong code may result in sending either too many or too few resources. This can be more simply defined as *risk vs. waste*.

From a dispatch standpoint, a pre-designed interrogation plan ensures reliable analysis of each new situation by the EMD following the plan. By following the plan, and only by following the plan, can outcomes be linked to the evaluation process so it can be studied, compared among different centers, and, therefore, improved over time.

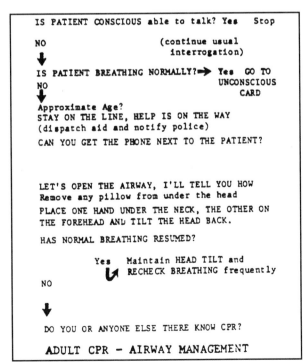

Fig. 13-6. Evolution of Pre-Arrival Instructions: Simple Linear type, circa 1982.

Like DNA replication, each plan must be followed to the letter or unforeseen consequences occur—such as the three-eyed frog. Imagine the genetic chaos that would be created if each cell had to "imagine," or guess what proteins to make, where they were to form, and in what order. We'd be lucky if any subsequent creatures based on these codes looked remotely the same as their parents, much less survived.

> A conclusion is the place where you get tired of thinking.
> —Arthur Block

In the same way, dispatch protocols must be followed in a given order; just using "chunks" of the plan doesn't work very well. Dispatch protocols are serial action plans, not arbitrary choices in a buffet line. Think of what would happen then if DNA was no more than this—in other words, only a "guideline."

Gene Sharing and Protocol Sharing— The Unified Protocol Model

According to the laws of genetic replication, each species can transfer minor genetic improvements to the next generation within that species. Orderly sharing of this genetic information causes improvement within the species in relatively short periods of time—stronger frogs and faster snakes. In the same way, by maintaining the same core plan (protocol structure and content), the actual experience of one communication center's use of the plan can be formally transferred to other centers that use the same plan.

> It was quite a mental shock to realize that such obsolescent protocols were still being used— proudly.

However, to continue the analogy, if the core plan of one dispatch center is, say, frog DNA and the core of another one close by is snake DNA, a new improved jumping adaptation in the frog protocol, won't, when mated with the snake, create a jumping snake. In fact, the frog and the snake can't mate at all.

One of the most important features of the MPDS as a *system* is the "unified protocol model." This means that all centers within each system use the same protocol and the same edition of that protocol. Years ago, this was seen as "restrictive" to the wide-open protocol-developing enthusiasm and freedom being experienced by new medical dispatch centers. And by the

> **The beauty of defined, quality-controlled, unified protocols is that every user leaps forward on the evolutionary chain at the same time sharing the success (and failures) of each collectively.**

mid-1980s, various versions of priority dispatch protocols were found in many places.

Unfortunately, no unified plan to assure orderly protocol improvement existed and many protocols were subsequently rewritten, modified, or just tweaked in some minor way. Yet as each center randomly "improved" their now unique protocol, what started out as the same protocol became increasingly different from center to center over time. Some groups eliminated questions based on the "too many questions" pressure found commonly in many centers. Some added expansive post-dispatch instructions. Some asked esoteric medical questions of the caller that on the surface might sound interesting to a medical novice but which, when examined in more depth, lacked clear dispatch-related objectives. In essence, without order, the protocols mutated.[147]

A personal experience by one of the authors (Clawson) in 1990 brought home the downside of such protocol "freedom." After giving the opening speech at the North Carolina State EMS Conference, a polite gentleman asked him to visit the local communication center. He pointed out his center was the first in the state to use the medical priority dispatch protocols.

Upon entering the dispatch room, the man pointed to the three stations and said, "See, Doc, there are your protocols—one, two, three." From a distance of about 20 feet away, however, something didn't look quite right. When asked how many cards were in each protocol set, a dispatcher on duty started counting them. The moment he stated, "29," it was clear what was wrong. This center had the 1981 version (3rd edition) of the protocols, the first version that was widely distributed. The version in use in 1990, however, was the 10th edition (32 cards).

The protocol they were using was now hopelessly out-of-date; it contained no treatment sequence cards (as the CPR, choking, and childbirth scripts were called back then) and was actually a potentially dangerous device.

What went wrong? This center had actually copied the protocol from a neighboring county that had originally obtained them, made some changes to the protocol initially, but then lost enthusiasm for any "updating." There were no attempts to secure updates. It was quite a mental shock to realize that such obsolescent protocols were still being used—proudly.

> **Sometimes you never know the sequence of events that must happen to bring you home.**
> **—James Lovell, Apollo 13**

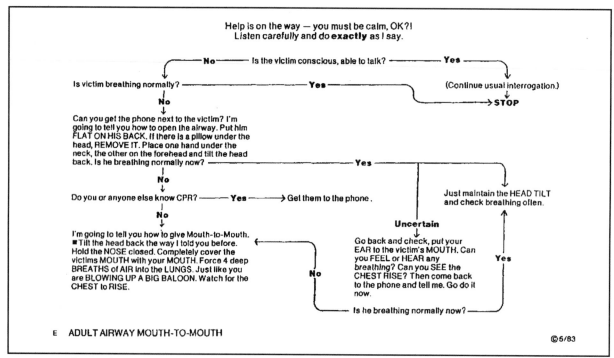

Fig. **13-7.** Evolution of Pre-Arrival Instructions: Complex Linear type, 1983. ©1978-2001 MPC.

After relating this strange but disturbing experience to the staff back home, colleagues in the logic division gave this disturbing lack of forward evolution a tongue-in-cheek nickname—the "Evolution of Fish." As in an evolutionary tree, if a certain edition of the protocol is introduced into a region without any process to maintain it, evolutionary stagnation sets in. That initial edition, the Research and Development staff irreverently called the "fish" version.

Each place originally using that same protocol makes their own modifications to their "fish." One center's fish quickly becomes a blue fish; another's, more slowly, a spotted fish; and yet another's a three-headed fish (after which they quit using their protocols stating that "they don't work very well"). But all in all, each version was still some form of a fish. None of the local efforts to modify ever went further than a year or so of "touching up" and never deeper than "scales" or "fins." And none of the "here-and-there" modifications to these protocols ever "genetically" crossed over to those used by other adjacent centers. Even sadder, none of these "fish" protocol varieties ever made any significant evolutionary "jumps" to become frogs, birds, horses or primate-class protocols. They just stayed fish (see fig. 13-7).

The beauty of defined, quality-controlled, unified protocols is that every user leaps forward on the evolutionary chain at the same time sharing the successes (and failures) of each collectively.

Some evolutionary advances are worth particular note. For priority dispatch one of the most significant advances was realized with the concept, creation and implementation of the scripted Pre-Arrival Instructions. For the first time, a truly "intelligent" system of providing instructions remotely with easy access to the necessary information, repeatable results, and controllable methods was available. Mike Smith recalls the circumstances behind this remarkable development in the following story (see fig. 13-8).

Imagine that a dispatch center in mythical East Eaglejaw, Manitoba, is using the same "protocol" as you. They experience a strange case that "tests" a rarely used logic path within the protocol containing a previously undetected weakness. The resulting problem causes a serious patient care failure. This center will likely attempt to fix that protocol—and quickly. But will they actually fix it? And will they fix it correctly? On a more global basis, will they get on the phone and call your center to warn you? Would they even know who you were? It would be even more unlikely that they would call the thousands of other dispatch centers in North America either, much less the myriad centers throughout the U.K., Germany, Italy, Finland, Spain, Austria, Switzerland, Australia, New Zealand, South America, Africa, and so on. Even if they did, would you believe them and make the change?

Without a systematic method of sharing information, each center has to wait until it encounters the same or similar problem and a tragedy occurs. This is the same reason that there are not 4,000, 14, or even four CPR, BLS, or ACLS protocols being used and locally modified at will. Before these core protocols were defined and accepted in the early 1970s, there were about a dozen different variations of CPR being used, and worse, the number of ACLS-like "protocols" in use then roughly equaled the number of hospital base-stations in North America—hardly scientific or even remotely controllable.

> **Without a systematic method of sharing information, each center has to wait until it encounters the same or similar problem and a tragedy occurs.**

But a unified system of a single core protocol, modified through a scientific method process, and routinely distributed to everyone, was functioning for these key protocolized areas of EMS. The same is done for medical dispatch protocols. For these reasons, the Academy initiated the College of Fellows.[146]

In the same way the heart associations and resuscitation councils maintain a core protocol for CPR, the College of Fellows of the Academy provides standardization, and, therefore, stability and reliability to EMD (see fig. 13-9). The College of Fellows is a unified, international scientific body of experts that maintains the integrity and credibility of the advanced MPDS protocols and related training and quality management processes. This is done through a pre-established process of reviewing and, where appropriate, approving proposed modifications and improvements to the protocols and standards.

From a mathematical standpoint, there are more than 88 million question and answer combinations in the computerized version of the Medical Priority Dispatch Protocol. This means that it would require 88 million *different* 9-1-1 calls to test every one of these potential decision pathways in the protocol—once. Obviously, some pathways get tested every day and some almost never in a given center.

Birth of the Pre-Arrival Instruction Grid

In Autumn 1989, I was approached by Dr. Clawson with a challenge. I had been working for the Academy for just a few months, and Dr. Clawson was president at the time. He asked if I could somehow rearrange, format, or improve on the pre-arrival instructions they had been using for almost 10 years.

Could it be improved? Perhaps, I thought. These pre-arrival instructions were a complex network of instructions and questions whose answers would lead to subsequent instructions and questions. They were arranged in a sprawling, branching fashion with lines wiggling all over indicating logical decision pathways. I understood why they were often called "Uncle Wiggley" charts. I took the project and went to my desk to work for awhile.

By the time the day was over, I had studied the logic, the presentations, and sensed that there might be a simpler way to present the them—one that was easier for the user to follow without compromising the medical logic. I asked Dr. Clawson, "Would you be upset if I came up with something that was totally different?" Perhaps a bit puzzled by my question, he responded, "No, I'll take as much improvement as you can offer."

Later that night, I continued at home working on the problem. There was inconsistency in positioning. It required the user to follow the little line marked "Yes" or "No" that winds to the next step with no anticipation of where it would end up. Each sequence of instructions had a completely different layout.

I had seen some software that Medical Priority had been developing for the Pre-Arrival Instructions. The computer screen had an instruction at the top with a question and a selection of answers at the bottom of the screen. The "Uncle Wiggley's" were logically the same, but the computer automatically *found* the next step for the user and presented it in a consistent format.

Finding the right instruction in an urgent moment is important, especially when a patient is relying on the next instruction for comfort, safety, or even life-saving advice. How should the instructions be organized? In a ring, in columns and rows, in clusters, or in no particular arrangement at all?

I decided that the layout of the instructions was best solved by a grid format. Some months earlier, I had read about how telephone keypads arranged

in a 3 x 4 grid allowed for rapid dialing and easier recall of phone numbers. It seemed natural to me that the human brain can easily perceive left and right, exterior and interior, and top and bottom, but it would be more difficult to discern multiple degrees of topness or leftness (see figures).

5 x 7 Grid

	Left		Middle		Right
Top	x	x	x	x	x
	x	x	x	x	x
Middle	x	x	x	x	x
	x	x	x	x	x
Bottom	x	x	x	x	x

3 x 3 Grid

	Left	Middle	Right
Top	x	x	x
Middle	x	x	x
Bottom	x	x	x

Once the format of a 3 x 3 grid was determined, I created a simple addressing system. There were 18 panels (two 3 x 3 grids), so I numbered them 1 through 18. The new design was simple, consistent, and more user-friendly. Instead of relying on the wiggly lines to guide the user through the logic pathways, all steps referenced a frame address. At any point in the sequence, the user could "jump" to another point and find it with ease.

Refining the product after that first draft was an extended process that was based on these two basic beliefs:

1. When there are many elements, mental-motor skills are more naturally suited for finding addresses in a predictable information "landscape" than following a network of winding lines.

2. The brain can perceive a combination of binary parameters (top/bottom, interior/exterior, left/right) more easily than it can perceive a value in a range.

Many subsequent decisions such as defining certain types of instructions with predictable placement, colorization, and answer determination were made in harmony with this new paradigm. ◈

Fig. 13-8. Birth of the Pre-Arrival Instruction Grid, Complex Non-Linear Type Panel Logic Script method by Michael Wayne Smith.

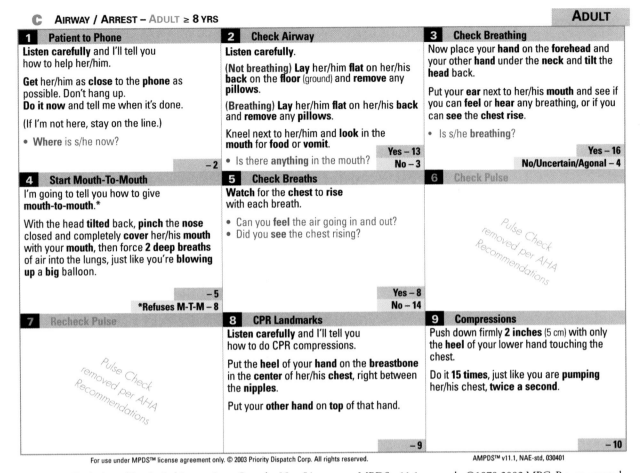

C   AIRWAY / ARREST – ADULT ≥ 8 YRS   **ADULT**

1 Patient to Phone

Listen carefully and I'll tell you how to help her/him.

Get her/him as **close** to the **phone** as possible. Don't hang up.
Do it now and tell me when it's done.

(If I'm not here, stay on the line.)

- **Where** is s/he now?

– 2

2 Check Airway

Listen carefully.

(Not breathing) **Lay** her/him **flat** on her/his **back** on the **floor** (ground) and **remove** any **pillows**.

(Breathing) **Lay** her/him **flat** on her/his **back** and **remove** any **pillows**.

Kneel next to her/him and **look** in the **mouth** for **food** or **vomit**.

- Is there **anything** in the mouth?   Yes – 13 / No – 3

3 Check Breathing

Now place your **hand** on the **forehead** and your other **hand** under the **neck** and **tilt** the **head** back.

Put your **ear** next to her/his **mouth** and see if you can **feel** or **hear** any breathing, or if you can **see** the **chest rise**.

- Is s/he **breathing**?   Yes – 16 / No/Uncertain/Agonal – 4

4 Start Mouth-To-Mouth

I'm going to tell you how to give **mouth-to-mouth.***

With the head **tilted** back, **pinch** the **nose** closed and completely **cover** her/his **mouth** with your **mouth**, then force **2 deep breaths** of air into the lungs, just like you're **blowing up** a **big** balloon.

– 5 / *Refuses M-T-M – 8

5 Check Breaths

Watch for the **chest** to **rise** with each breath.

- Can you **feel** the air going in and out?
- Did you **see** the chest rising?

Yes – 8 / No – 14

6 Check Pulse

Pulse Check removed per AHA Recommendations

7 Recheck Pulse

Pulse Check removed per AHA Recommendations

8 CPR Landmarks

Listen carefully and I'll tell you how to do CPR compressions.

Put the **heel** of your **hand** on the **breastbone** in the **center** of her/his **chest**, right between the **nipples**.

Put your **other hand** on **top** of that hand.

– 9

9 Compressions

Push down firmly **2 inches** (5 cm) with only the **heel** of your lower hand touching the chest.

Do it **15 times**, just like you are **pumping** her/his chest, **twice a second**.

– 10

For use under MPDS™ license agreement only. © 2003 Priority Dispatch Corp. All rights reserved.   AMPDS™ v11.1, NAE-std, 030401

Fig. 13-9. Evolution of Pre-Arrival Instructions: Complex Non-Linear type. MPDS, v11.1 protocols. ©1978-2002 MPC. Patents granted.

What does this all boil down to? Everyone involved with the MPDS—the designers who develop it, the public safety managers who select it, the medical directors who approve it, and the individual dispatchers who use it—makes a conscious and philosophical decision to trade personal or internal *control* of the dispatch protocol for an external, scientifically developed, method-based *process*. Frankly, most people do not have the time, or the expertise, to build a complex protocol in isolation.

> **The MPDS is the ACLS of dispatch.**
> —**Geoff Cady**

The MPDS is built on knowledge and experience that is wider in scope and deeper in content that could be generated by even the largest communication center. Nor do most people have the resources to maintain and update a protocol in response to changing medical practices and an evolving healthcare industry. This is the rationale for the mission and activities of the Council of Standards, a part of the Academy's College of Fellows.

The mission of the College of Fellows is: "To conduct an ongoing review of the current standards of care and practice in Emergency Medical Dispatch and evaluate the tools and mechanisms used to meet or exceed those standards."

If you obtained an MPDS protocol (version 10.0) in 1990, you received updates (at no charge) for nine years, all for the original cost outlay for the protocols. The process is continuous and designed to be perpetual.

As of this writing, the Academy now has approximately 32,000 currently certified members and 2,400 centers have obtained the current version of the MPDS. In addition, 71 centers have achieved Center of Excellence Accreditation. The potential of such a large "users' group" is being realized by a growing participation

> **My interest is in studying the deep essence of the protocol.**
> —**Marie Leroux**
> **Chairwoman**
> **Council of Standards**

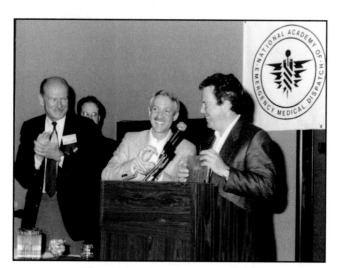

Fig. 13-10. William Shatner gets a standing ovation from Arnold Shapiro, producer of *Rescue 911* and James O. Page at the Academy's International Conference.

in the Council of Standards' controlled process for protocol evolution.

Like DNA, another nice thing about controlled, unified evolution in a medical priority dispatch protocol and system, is that the normal person out there, busily running his or her dispatch center or EMS agency, doesn't have to worry much about it. Because of the dedicated people participating in the Academy's diverse processes, it just happens. And the vast majority of the time, it happens remarkably well. Drs. Crick and Watson would be proud.

Summary

As a dedicated reader, you have carefully read hundreds of pages of information regarding EMD and priority dispatch. The science of medical dispatch has continued to evolve during the time we were writing (and you were reading) this textbook.

Since the first edition of the Principles of EMD in 1987, EMD has taken form as a comprehensive process. It will continue to evolve for decades to come as we begin a technology-rich 21st century. A thorough understanding and careful implementation of the concepts outlined in this text will provide a firm basis for using the inevitable future improvements brought by the forces of dispatch evolution we have tried to foster.[163]

> **Make no little plans. They have no magic to stir men's blood.**
> **—David Burham Hudson**

While the "things" of medical dispatch change and improve over time, the foundation for all of this is the personal dedication, drive, and ethic of the individual EMD. The EMD's professional and personal commitment to the public's safety, the correct care of patients, and empathetic service to every customer can never be replaced by technology or distilled to mere words on a page. EMD will continue to embody both the objective science as well as the subjective art of dispatch life support—the practice of remote medical care. Emergency Medical Dispatch is the earliest bridge between

---

! Authors' Note

Pluralizing the Academy: Formation of the expanded "Academies of Emergency Dispatch"

On the final morning of Navigator 2000, Dr. Jeff Clawson, founder of the National Academy of EMD and the MPDS, used the forum of the conference general session to announce a major expansion of the Academy's mission. With the introduction of the fire protocol, and with law enforcement protocols emerging, the Academy's mission was modified "To conduct an on-going review of the current standards of care and practice in EMD, Fire, Police, and other areas of public safety telecommunications and to evaluate the tools and mechanisms used to meet or exceed those standards."

With that in mind, the National Academy of EMD was pluralized to form the expanded National/International Academies of Emergency Dispatch. The NAED is comprised of three allied Academies with related programs and standards for Medical, Fire, and Police dispatching. Each Academy is formed from distinct boards and councils and staffed with experts from their respective fields, which allows them to embrace all elements of public safety, while continuing to provide outstanding, personalized service to each group.

To reflect and compliment the change in the Academy, Medical Priority Consultants, Inc. also evolved early in 2002 to allow for the addition of the fire and law enforcement protocols. Now known as Priority Dispatch Corporation, it oversees the graphic and computerized application of these new protocol logic programs as well as managing training and instruction development for each discipline.

the brink of despair and the hope of recovery. There is much more to EMD than saving lives. Every call is a plea for help, and the dedicated EMD can truly help people when they need it most. Be proud of your part in creating such meaningful change.

New and stirring things are belittled because if they are not belittled, the embarrassing question arises, why, then are you not taking part in them?

— *H. G. Wells*

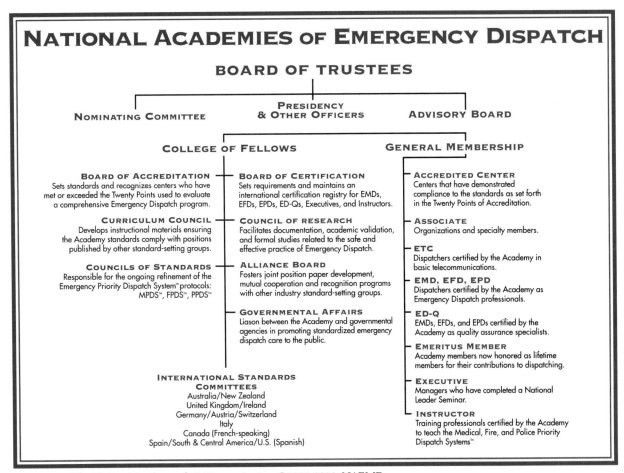

Fig. 13-11. The National Academy of EMD organization. ©1988-2003 NAEMD.

Contents

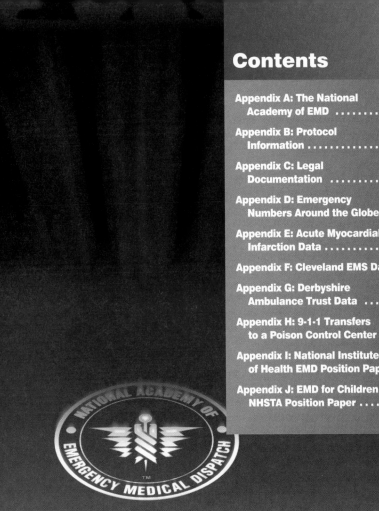

APPENDIX

National Academy Mission and Goals

Our mission is: "To advance and support the Emergency Medical Dispatch professional, and to ensure citizens in need of emergency, health, and social services are matched safely, quickly, and effectively with the most appropriate resource."

Our goals are: "To use and promote the fundamental principles of a scientific method in the pursuit of the mission."

"To advocate a single, scientifically defensible protocol which becomes the unifying standard under which all professional emergency medical dispatchers practice."

"To advance professionalism within the dispatch community by establishing and promoting an ethics policy as well as minimum standards for curriculum, instruction, certification, recertification, and accreditation of centers."

"To provide opportunities for members to improve themselves and their organizations through facilitation of communication, providing comprehensive information resources, and creating high-quality training and continuing dispatch education through seminars, publications, and other media designed to meet our members needs."

"To establish and promote a collegial, research-based culture that welcomes the expertise of many disciplines through the creation of standing committees, task forces, and subgroups which reach out to other organizations and advise the Academy."

"To be recognized as the authoritive, independent voice which represents the EMD and enhances the profession."

The National Academy of EMD Ethics Policy

The Academy is dedicated to promoting excellence in EMD by setting professional industry standards and recognizing the agencies and individuals who meet those standards. This recognition includes both the public and the EMS community and is communicated through public relations efforts, elegant Diplomas and Certificates, newspaper articles, and other professional publications and advertising.

The Academy encourages, advocates, and supports the proposition that "The community relies on the sound application of Priority Dispatch and imposes on the certified EMD an obligation to maintain professional standards of technical competence, morality and integrity." To accomplish this, the Academy's College of Fellows has unanimously adopted the following:

The Code of Ethics

1. Academy-certified EMDs should endeavor to put the needs of the public above their own.

2. Academy-certified EMDs should continually seek to maintain and improve their professional knowledge, skills and competence and should seek continuing education whenever available.

3. Academy-certified EMDs should obey all laws and regulations and should avoid any conduct or activity which would cause unjust harm to the citizens they serve.

4. Academy-certified EMDs should be diligent in the performance of their occupational duties.

5. Academy-certified EMDs should establish and maintain honorable relationships with their EMS peers and with all those who rely on their professional skill and judgment.

6. Academy-certified EMDs should assist in improving the public understanding of Emergency Medical Dispatch.

7. Academy-certified EMDs should assist in the operation of and enhance the performance of their dispatch systems.

8. Academy-certified EMDs should seek to maintain the highest standard of personal practice and also maintain the integrity of the National Academy of EMD by exemplifying this professional Code of Ethics.

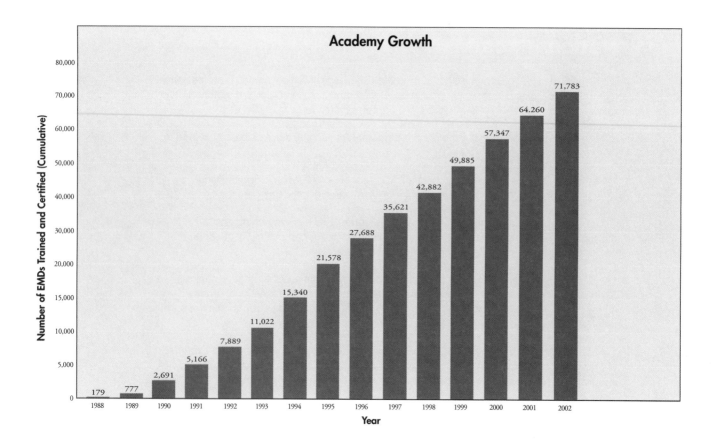

Academy Growth

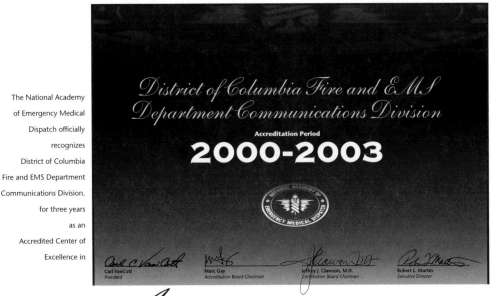

The National Academy of Emergency Medical Dispatch officially recognizes District of Columbia Fire and EMS Department Communications Division. for three years as an Accredited Center of Excellence in

District of Columbia Fire and EMS Department Communications Division

Accreditation Period

2000-2003

Emergency Medical Dispatch on this 27th day of January, 2000 for demonstrating compliance to the highest level of standards as set forth in the Academy's Twenty Points of Accreditation.

Carl VanCott
President

Marc Gay
Accreditation Board Chairman

Jeffrey J. Clawson, M.D.
Certification Board Chairman

Robert L. Martin
Executive Director

35TH CENTER OF EXCELLENCE

Accredited

THE TWENTY POINTS

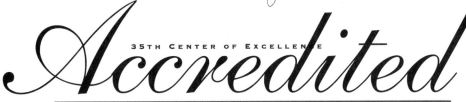

1 All medical dispatch call-taking and dispatching work stations.

2 Current Advanced MPDS licensing of each EMD position.

3 Current Academy certification of all EMD personnel.

4 How Academy certification will continue to be maintained.

5 Minutes from MDRC* and Steering Committee meetings (*Medical Dispatch Review Committee).

6 EMD quality assurance and improvement methodology.

7 EMD quality assurance and improvement database.

8 Numbers and percentages of randomly reviewed cases (per a sliding scale based on annual call volume).

9 Consistent, cumulative, MPDS case review at or above the following percentages:
• 95% — Case Entry protocol compliance,
• 95% — Chief Complaint selection accuracy,
• 90% — Key Question protocol compliance,
• 90% — Post-Dispatch Instruction protocol compliance,
• 95% — Pre-Arrival Instruction protocol compliance,
• 90% — Subdeterminant code selection accuracy,
• 90% — Cumulative overall score.

10 Correct quality assurance and improvement scoring and practices through independent Academy review of randomly assigned cases.

11 How EMS field personnel were oriented to the proper use of the MPDS

12 Use of field responder Medical Dispatch Feedback Reports.

13 Current Continuing Dispatcher Education (CDE) program functions.

14 How police and law enforcement received S.E.N.D. (Medical Miranda) pocket protocols and related inservice or video orientation.

15 Correct local configuration of all MPDS response assignments.

16 Field implementation of all MPDS response assignments.

17 How MPDS response assignments will be monitored and maintained.

18 Specific medical director oversight and controls.

19 Sharing of non-confidential data with the Academy for review.

20 Support of the Academy's Code of Ethics and practice standards.

Academy Accredited Centers of Excellence to Date:

1. Albuquerque Fire Department
2. Cleveland EMS
3. Calgary EMS
4. Clark County Regional Communications Agency
5. Derbyshire Ambulance NHS Trust
6. Urgences Sante
7. Shelby County/Memphis Fire Department
8. San Ramon Valley Fire Protection District
9. St. Louis EMS
10. Miami-Dade Fire-Rescue
11. Lancashire Ambulance NHS Trust
12. Staffordshire Ambulance NHS Trust
13. American Medical Response of Colorado
14. City of Miami Fire-Rescue
15. Salt Lake City Fire Department
16. Kent Ambulance NHS Trust
17. Fountain Police Communications
18. Colorado Springs Police Department
19. Intergraph Public Safety (Melbourne, Australia)
20. Rochester-Monroe County Office of Emergency Communications
21. Cumberland County Emergency Communications
22. South and East Wales Ambulance NHS Trust
23. AMR of Connecticut
24. Gaston County Telecommunications Center
25. American Medical Response of Evansville
26. Layton City Dispatch Center
27. San Diego Fire Life Safety Medical Services Enterprise
28. Fulton County Emergency Communications
29. El Paso County Sheriff's Office
30. New Hampshire Bureau of Emergency Comm.
31. Munroe Regional Medical Cntr. Ambulance Service
32. Mersey Regional Ambulance NHS Trust
33. AMR Pathways National Call Center
34. Sunstar Communications Center (Florida)
35. District of Columbia Fire & EMS Department Communications Division
36. Dauphin County Emergency Management Agency
37. Emergency Medical Services Authority— Eastern Division (Oklahoma City)
38. Emergency Medical Services Authority— Western Division (Tulsa, OK)
39. City of Austin EMS Communications
40. Welsh Ambulance Services NHS Trust, Church Village Control
41. Muskogee County EMS
42. South Yorkshire Ambulance NHS Trust
43. Nashville Fire Department Communications.
44. Centrale de Coordinations Sante de la Region de Quebec (03) Inc.
45. Minnehaha Metro Communications Sioux Falls
46. The Welsh Ambulance Service NHS Trust— Rhyl Control Room
47. The Welsh Ambulance Service NHS Trust— Caernarfon Control Room
48. M.D. Communications, Saskatoon (Saskatchewan)
49. Kent County Department of Public Safety
50. Welsh Ambulance Service NHS Trust Central and West Region
51. Dekalb County Public Safety Communications
52. Collier County Sheriff's Office
53. Citrus County Sherriff's Office
54. Regional Emergency Medical Services Authority
55. East Anglian Ambulance NHS Trust
56. Avon Ambulance NHS Trust
57. Groupe Alerte Sante Inc.
58. Richmond Police Department
59. Medstar Ambulance Inc.
60. Greater Manchester Ambulance
61. San Jose Fire Department Communications Center
62. American Medical Response
63. Pennington County 911
64. Two Shires Ambulance NHS Trust
65. Sussex County EOC Fire & Ambulance Call Board
66. American Medical Response
67. Bedfordshire & Hertfordshire Ambulance & Paramedic Service NHS Trust
68. Santa Clara County Communications
69. Centrale d'appels d'urgence Chaudiere-Appalaches (CAUCA)
70. Bernalillo County Communications Center
71. American Medical Response-Miami
72. AMR Los Angeles Metro Communications
73. Emergency Medical Care Inc.
74. New Castle Coundy Emergency Comm. Center.
75. Rural/Metro Ambulance (MedStar)
76. The London Ambulance Service NHS Trust
77. Kern County/Bakersfield City Emergency Communications Center
78. Centre d'Appel d'Urgence des Regions de l'Est du Quebec
79. Rehoboth Beach Police Department

Salt Lake City Fire Department Quality Improvement Case Review and Remediation Actions Policy

The Salt Lake City Fire Department is one of only a handful of public safety agencies who have acquired Center of Excellence certification from the National Academy of Emergency Medical Dispatch. To maintain accreditation, compliance to protocol must remain consistent with Academy requirements. Compliance is measured in six areas, and are as follows:

Case Entry	95%
Chief Complaint	95%
Key Questions	90%
Pre-Arrival Instructions	95%
Post-Dispatch Instructions	90%
Final Coding	90%

All EMDs who work for the Salt Lake City Fire Department must meet these job performance expectations. This document is meant to describe the action plan which will be followed whenever accreditation compliance (>90% overall) to the MPDS protocols is not maintained by a Fire Department Dispatcher.

Step 1: Coaching Stage

Taken the first month when an employees score drops below the required minimum performance level for a Center of Excellence EMD. Feedback from Quality Improvement Unit to employee's Supervisor documenting unacceptable compliance score performance. Supervisor meets with employee to discuss performance issues. Any number of possibilities are now at the supervisors disposal to assist employee in meeting expected performance (QIU involvement will be available, but not mandatory). This is designed to assist the employee in improving compliance score performance, and is not meant to be disciplinary. The employee has a month to improve protocol performance. If performance minimums are reached, no other action is needed or taken. If performance has not reached acceptable levels, a management performance review is scheduled, as provided below.

Step 2: Management Performance Review

After two months, if an employee does not meet expected performance minimums with regards to protocol performance, a management performance review

is initiated. At this point, remediation is required to change performance behavior. Included in this meeting will be: Employee, Employee's Supervisor, Communications Director, and Communications Battalion Chief.

Systematic Process or Overview:

- What is the problem?

- Why is it a problem?

- What are the Department's expectations?

- What can Management do to help employee reach those expectations?

- What are the consequences if these expectations are not met?

Due to the critical value the EMD plays in the delivery model of our EMS system, a shortened time frame of 6 consecutive shifts will be given to achieve expected compliance performance. If performance levels have reached appropriate compliance minimums, no other action is warranted and the process is reset to step 1 if necessary. If performance has not improved to accreditation standards, a pre-termination hearing is scheduled with Human Resources.

Step 3: Pre-determination Hearing

A pre-determination hearing will be held if performance is not yet corrected. Resource Development personnel, in addition to the employee's supervisor, the Communications Director, and the Division Battalion Chief will be present. The employee has the right to representation at this stage as well. Documentation of performance deficits will be provided by the QIU in addition to action plans that have been implemented to change employee performance. This hearing involves fact-finding processes that, when completed, will be turned over the Operations Deputy Chief for final action, which can include any measure of discipline up to, and including termination.

—Revised July 1, 1998

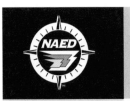

PROPOSAL FOR CHANGE – PROTOCOL

LOG NUMBER:

☐ **MPDS**   ☐ **FPDS**   ☐ **PPDS**   ☐ Other: _____   **DATE REC'D:**

Protocol Number(s) & Section(s) affected:_____

Protocol Version #:_____ **Language(s):**_____**Type(s):** _____

DESCRIPTION OF PROPOSED CHANGE

To the Academy: Please accept for your review the attached Proposal for Change to the protocol section and version noted above. SUMMARIZED as follows:

_____

_____

_____

_____

_____

_____

_____

I have included the following supportive material:

☐ Graphic or written description of proposed change

☐ Explanation of problem with current version

☐ Explanation of desired effect of proposed change

☐ References or copies of cited studies, articles, case transcripts, tapes, etc. (if applicable)

The number of attached pages is:_____ (indicate date and instructor/organization/agency on all papers)

I rate the necessity (URGENCY) for this change at: _____ (rate **1-10**, 1 = minimal, 10 = urgent)

RECOMMENDING CONTACT PERSON

Signature   Date Submitted

Full Name (please print)   Primary Phone Number

Title(s) or Academic Credentials   FAX and/or Alternate Phone Number

Organization/Agency Representing

Address for Correspondence

City   State/Prov./Shire   Zip/Postal Code   Country

OVERSIGHT APPROVAL

The Academy takes all proposals for change very seriously and enters them into a formally defined process for review. To expedite official approval, please recommend potential *solutions* whenever possible and attach approval signatures from your local Dispatch Review or Steering Committee(s) as appropriate.

Dispatch Review Committee Signature   Steering Committee Signature

Full Name (please print)   Full Name (please print)

©2002 NAED 9 DEC 2002

SETTING THE COURSE FOR EMERGENCY DISPATCH WORLDWIDE

Protocol Information

Determinants per Protocol

Protocol	Number of Determinants
1	6
2	11
3	12
4	10
5	4
6	6
7	12
8	9
9	9
10	8
11	4
12	9
13	5
14	8
15	9
16	5
17	10
18	8
19	12
20	5
21	9
22	4
23	13
24	11
25	6
26	31
27	10
28	8
29	11
30	7
31	10
32	4
33	10
Total	**296**

Key Questions per Protocol

Protocol	Required KQ (Optional)		Safety KQ (Optional)	
1	2	(2)		
2	4	(4)		(1)
3	7	(1)	2	
4	7		2	
5	4	(2)		
6	6	(1)		
7	4	(4)	1	(4)
8	6	(1)	4	(1)
9	1	(3)	1	(1)
10	6			
11	2	(1)		
12	5	(3)		
13	3			
14	3		1	
15	6	(2)	4	(2)
16	2	(1)		
17	6	(1)		
18	6			
19	7	(1)		
20	4	(1)		
21	5	(1)		
22	3		1	
23	4	(2)		(2)
24	3	(5)		
25	4	(1)	2	
26	4	(1)		
27	6		1	
28	5	(1)		
29	4	(3)		(2)
30	5	(1)		
31	2	(4)		
32	4	(1)		
33	7	(8)		
Total	**147**	**(56)**	**19**	**(13)**
Average KQ per protocol	**4.45**	**(1.7)**	**.6**	**(.4)**

Legal Documentation
Letter from James O. Page to Aurora Colorado Fire Department, Sept. 28, 1981

Dear Ms. Blackwood,

This is response to your letter of September 22nd. To the extent that my response deals with legal issues, I will respond in general terms, based on my understanding of the national experience (or lack thereof) with these similar issues. I presume that ultimately you will be guided by the advice of you local municipal legal counsel.

Specifically, your questions are as follows:

(1) What are the legal implications for dispatchers who have had only a twenty-one hour course in the use of this card system (your newly-instituted Medical Self-Help Dispatch Program), eleven hours of which included basic CPR and CPR Instructor's training, when they begin giving CPR instruction over the telephone, and the victim dies?

(2) If a dispatcher successfully gives CPR instruction, or any other aid, over the telephone to one individual, but is unable to give the same to another person who calls in because of a rash of alarms at the time of the call or other circumstances beyond his/her control, can the dispatcher be held liable?

(3) What is your professional opinion of the necessity and/or importance of such a program as this one?

On the subject of civil liablilty, as it relates to cardiopulmonary resuscitation (CPR), we have been quite vocal. For example, in September, 1977, in our EMS Action publication, we published an article entitled "CPR and Red Herring." Coincidentally, in the same issue, we published a story about the innovative dispatching system in Phoenix. Our article (about CPR) produced a heavy demand for reprints. Thus, we created a pamphlet entitled "CPR and the Law."

We feel that the legal issues (or non-issues) are very clear. A person who needs CPR is pulseless and non-breathing. That is the state of the victim at the time the call is received by the dispatcher. The dispatcher did not cause the victim to be a pulseless, non-breathing state. There is no way the victim can be made worse. If the effort to direct CPR by phone fails, the victim is no worse off then s/he was when the dispatcher received the call and offered assistance via CPR instruction. If the victim services (even for a brief period, or even in a vegetative state), s/he is better off than when s/he was

clinically dead. There can be no liability for a good faith effort that fails, of for leaving a person better off.

The length of the course undertaken by your dispatchers (in terms of hours) is relatively insignificant. In the unlikely event of a lawsuit, their performance in the particular care would be at issue, not the length of their training program. Millions of lay persons have learned to perform CPR competently in courses as short as three hours. Whether they took a three-hour course or a twelve-hour course is not significant from either legal or medical points of view. The issue is how well does the individual perform when called upon to respond in an actual emergency?

If a CPR-trained dispatcher permits his/her knowledge and skills to deteriorate (does not engage in periodic refresher training), and if that dispatcher issues inappropriate instructions to a caller, there could be cause for concern (more medical and ethical than legal, in my opinion). For example, if the dispatcher fails to follow the protocol for airway, breathing, and circulation, and thereafter instructs the caller to perform CPR. If the victim simply has fainted, there could be legal difficulty.

The New Jersey case of In re Roy (362 A2d589 (1976)) may be illustrative... In that case, untrained police officers and volunteer ambulance personnel performed a technique on Mrs. Roy that was described as "vigorous pounding on the chest." As the medical examiner reported, Mrs. Roy had merely fainted and had not suffered a heart attack. The autopsy revealed that her death was caused by the thoroughly unskilled rescue effort. Had the police officers and ambulance personnel been properly trained, they would have known enough to conduct the essential airway, breathing, and circulation checks before initiating their resuscitative effort, and they would have known how to support the victim's vital functions without causing fatal injuries.

It should be noted that the Roy case is not a CPR case. The defendants were not trained in CPR and they did not perform CPR as it was taught them (in 1974) or now. Certainly, your dispatching personnel, despite their present concerns, would find the Roy case shocking. And certainly, with their recent training and the excellent protocols they have to work from, they shouldn't be worried about themselves directing a caller to commit such a disastrous act.

As I mentioned in our phone conversation, I personally feel that the highly successful "medical self-help" program introduced by the Phoenix Fire Department may have started a process which will redefine a municipality's duty to its citizens. Similarly, the "Emergency Medical Dispatch Priority Card System" created by Dr. Jeff Clawson in association with the Salt Lake City Fire Department, may have further advanced the municipality's duty. In other words, I can foresee a day when a citizen might allege that the municipality (which maintains a full-time public safety dispatching service) was negligent for failing to implement and operate such a service.

Professors Prosser and Keeton, in their book on "The Law of Torts," stated in regards to the issue of duty that "Changing social conditions lead constantly to the recognition of new duties. No better general statement can be made, than that the courts will find a duty where, in general, reasonable men should recognize it and agree that it exists" (p. 359). Since the Dispatch Priority Card System first gained national visibility (JEMS, vol. 6, No. 2, February, 1981), numerous municipalities have inquired about the article and the Salt Lake City system it describes. It is apparent that this additional measure of life-saving service will become more prevalent ("changing social conditions"), thus leading to the recognition of a new duty upon municipalities to implement the service where feasible. Though there may have been no initial duty for a municipality to provide rescue and emergency medical services to its residents, it assumes certain duties when it offers those services to the public. To the extent that adjunctive advisory and/or life-saving services become widespread or prevalent among American municipalities, such services may constitute a new standard to which all similar municipalities (those with full-time public safety dispatching services) will be held.

The point is, while your dispatching personnel express anxiety over the posiblilty of liability for providing such a service, we may well see the day when a municipality faces allegations of negligence for not providing such a service. In view of the fact that implementation of this new level of service does not constitute a major expenditure to the municipality—and thus is basically an organizational/management/training issue, rather than a funding/taxation issue—I feel the case for a legal obligation (duty) to provide it becomes stronger.

With regard to your second question, I feel we need only to refer to one of the standard definitions of negligence. That is, failure in a particular situation to perform as a "reasonable man" would under the same or similar circumstances. What would a "reasonable man" do under the circumstances described in your question? Obviously, the dispatcher would continue to instruct or aid the first caller to a reasonable conclusion. The

alternative would be to "abandon" a patient who is known to be in life-threatening circumstance (discussed later).

The natural sequel to this question is whether the municipality would be negligent for failing to provide sufficient numbers of trained dispatchers to successfully deal with the ultimate contingency (numerous simultaneous alarms). Though it has been some time since I have researched this question, I have found that the courts traditionally have applied the standard of "reasonableness." That is, a public safety agency cannot be expected to incur the cost of always meeting the demands of extraordinary emergency situations (such as an unusual situation where numerous simultaneous alarms or requests for service are received).

For nearly a century, courts in this country have applied an "emergency rule" which Prosser discusses as follows: "the courts have been compelled to recognize that (a person) who is confronted with an emergency is not to be held to the same standard of conduct normally applied to one who is in no such situation" (p. 196). Having worked as a dispatcher in a busy urban fire department, I know there are occasional situations where this "emergency rule" would apply.

As we discussed in our phone conversation, "abandonment" has been legally defined as the unilateral termination of a physician-patient relationship by the physician, without the patient's consent and without giving the patient sufficient opportunity to secure the services of another competent physician. As to whether this responsibility (and potential liability) could attach to agents or surrogates of the physician—such as paramedics, or dispatchers operating under a physician's protocols—there is no case law (simply because there have been no cases).

In my opinion, wrestling with this question of possible "abandonment" and whether it applies to non-physicians is a waste of time. The denial of service, refusal to accept calls, failure to provide advice, etc. always would be judged as to the "reasonableness" of the action under the circumstances prevailing at the time of the incident in question. Unless you can anticipate that one or more of your employees will act unreasonably, thus subjecting the municipality to liability, I wouldn't be concerned. If you can anticipate that one or more of your employees will act unreasonably, you have a legal obligation to protect the public from the actions of that employee (through training, discipline, discharge, etc.).

Although you did not pose a question concerning imputed negligence (response superior), it seems an appropriate topic for consideration. That is, if an employee (such as a dispatcher) was negligent in the conduct of her/his duties under you Medical Self-Help Dispatch Program, would the municipality ultimately be responsible for the injured person, and likewise obligated to indemnify the employee for his/her losses (legal expenses, judgement, settlement, etc.)? This question would be answered by Colorado statutes with which I am not familiar.

Finally, my professional opinion. After years of arriving "too late" at the scenes of hundreds of life-threatening emergencies, it is difficult for me to offer a detached and unemotional opinion. Throughout the U.S., we have spent billions of dollars constructing systems to respond to medical emergencies and we have done little to cure the deadly four minute gap at the front of the system. While we race through city traffic to get to the scene, a brain dies for lack of CPR (oxygen). Frankly, I don't understand how any public safety or health care worker can accept these recurring tragedies without actively seeking a solution to the "response time" problem which proves fatal in so many cases.

More than 20 million Americans have been trained to perform CPR, and it has been estimated that another 80 million are interested in learning the technique. These millions of trained lay rescuers are performing the techniques hundreds (if not thousands) of times throughout the country each day. Yet, in the eight years since the American Heart Association and the American Red Cross endorsed the concept of training the public we haven't heard of a single lawsuit (successful or unsuccessful) against a trained CPR rescuer who performed the technique on a person who needed it.

The statistical proof as to the effectiveness of bystander-initiated CPR is beyond question. As greater numbers of fire and police departments initiate "first responder" programs—to get professional rescuers to the scene as quickly as possible—we can expect the survival statistics to climb. And, finally, communities such as Aurora are beginning to fill the deadly four-minute gap by providing invaluable medical self-help instruction via telephone.

I have personally witnessed the innovative Phoenix "Lifeline"system—and it is saving lives! I have investigated the Salt Lake City program and I feel it is a natural evolution of the Phoenix concept. In my opinion, your City is to be commended for your quick but thorough adaptation of this important service.

In summary, I suppose the concerns which have been expressed over supposed legal hazards are little more than a "red herring" issue. Of greater concern to me is the collective attitude which places such unwarranted fears on a higher plane than the compulsion for human service——especially saving lives.

In 1975, I wrote a book entitled, Emergency Medical Services for Fire Departments (National Fire Protection Assn.). In it, largely based on my own experience as a dispatcher and supervisor of dispatchers, I included the following:

One effective method of obtaining understanding and cooperation from dispatching personnel is to allow them to spend a tour of duty as an observer on an EMS unit. Long periods of time confined to a switchboard tend to deprive the dispatcher—communicator of perspective of field problems. Nothing can cure this common problem faster than a period of first-hand observation of the real world at its worst.

I suspect your problem may be one of narrow perspective, rather than legal hazards.

I apologize for the length of this response. I feel that your undertaking is very important and must not be sidetracked by unrealistic anxiety. As you know, our organization is funded by several leading pharmaceutical companies, and we are pleased to be able to assist you as part of your program of public service. If additional questions occur, I hope you will feel free to call on us again.

Sincerely,

James O. Page, J.D.
Executive Director
The ACT Foundation

Letter used with the permission of James O. Page, J.D.

California Liability Limitation Statues, Chapter 9, Effective Jan. 1, 1997

1799.100. In order to encourage local agencies and other organizations to train people in emergency medical services, no local agency, entity of state or local government, or other public or private organization which sponsors, authorizes, supports, finances, or supervises the training of people, or certifies those people, excluding physicians and surgeons, registered nurses, and licensed vocational nurses, as defined, in EMS, shall be liable for any individual damages alleged to result from those training programs.

1799.102. No person who in good faith, and not for compensation, renders emergency care at the scene of an emergency shall be liable for any civil damages resulting from any act or omission. The scene of an emergency shall not include emergency departments and other places where medical care is usually offered.

1799.104 (a) No physician or nurse, who in good faith gives emergency instructions to an EMT-II or mobile intensive care paramedic at the scene of an emergency, shall be liable for any civil damages as a result of issuing the instructions.

(b) No EMT-II or mobile intensive care paramedic rendering care within the scope of his duties, who in good faith and in a non-negligent manner, follows the instructions of a physician or nurse shall be liable for any civil damages as a result of following such instructions.

1799.105 (a) A poison control center which (1) meets the minimum standard for designation and operation established by the authority pursuant to Section 1798.180, (2) has been designated a regional poison control center by the authority, and (3) provides information and advice for no charge on the management of exposures to poisonous or toxic substances, shall be immune from liability in civil damages with respect to the emergency provision of that information or advice, for acts or omissions by its medical director, poison information specialist, or poison information provider as provided in subdivisions (b) and (c).

(b) Any poisonous information specialist or poison information provider who provides emergency information and advice on the management of exposures to poisonous or toxic substances, through, and in accordance with, protocols approved by the medical director of a poison control center specified in subdivision (a), shall only be liable in civil damages, with respect to the emergency provision of that information or advice, for acts or omissions performed in a grossly negligent manner or acts of omissions not performed in good faith. This subdivision shall not be construed to immunize the negligent adoption of a protocol.

(c) The medical director of a poison control center specified in subdivision (a) who provides information and advice on the management of exposures to poisonous or toxic substances, where the exposure is not covered by an approved protocol, shall be liable only in civil damages, with respect to the emergency provision of that information or advice, for the acts of omission performed in a grossly manner or acts of omission not performed in good faith.

This subdivision shall neither be construed to immunize the negligent failure to adopt adequate approved protocols nor to confer liability upon the medical director for failing to develop or approve a protocol when the development of a protocol for a specific situation is not practical or the situation could not have been reasonably foreseen.

1799.106. In addition to the provisions of Section 1799.104 of this code and of Section 1714.2 of the Civil Code and in order to encourage the provision of emergency medical services by firefighters, police officers or other law enforcement officers, EMT-I, EMT-II, or EMT-P, a firefighter, police officers or other law enforcement officers, EMT-I, EMT-II, or EMT-P who renders emergency medical services at the scene of an emergency shall only be liable in civil damages for acts or omissions performed in a grossly negligent manner or acts or omissions not performed in good faith. A public agency employing such a firefighter, police officers or other law enforcement officer, EMT-I, EMT-II, or EMT-P is not liable.

Salt Lake City EMS Abuse Ordinance
Sec. 14-2-8. Purpose. Whereas the City has experienced repeated calls from citizens for emergency medical services when there exists no real emergency. Further, responding to such non-emergency calls requires the use of men and equipment so that they are not readily available in the event of a real emergency. Therefore, the purpose of this ordinance is to reduce such abuse and the use of emergency medical services provided by Salt Lake City Corp.; thus keeping men and equipment available for use in real emergency situations, conserving energy and reducing costs.

Sec. 14-2-8.1. Unlawful request of service.

(a) Any person who shall request the Salt Lake City Fire Department emergency medical system to respond unnecessarily, falsely, capriciously or for non-emergency situations shall be guilty of a misdemeanor and may be punished by a fine of up to $299 or six months in jail or both such fine and imprisonment.

(b) For the purpose of this section non-emergency situations shall be the following: Alcohol intoxication, minor lacerations, minor contusions and sprains, minor illnesses, insect and animal bites not deemed emergencies, rashes, skin disorders, hives without dyspnea (difficulty of breathing), home delivery to avoid doctor and hospital services, venereal disease, patients seeking non-emergency transportation, forehead and scalp lacerations only, cold syndrome, sore throat, earache,

hiccough, nervousness, anxiety, toothache, minor bruises, non-life threatening overdoses, non-life threatening
self-inflicted injuries.

State of Utah EMS Act (Abuse Section)

Sec. 26-8-15. Violation of chapter a misdemeanor.
Calling ambulance when not needed a misdemeanor.

(1) Any person who violates this chapter is guilty of
a class B misdemeanor.

(2) Any person who willfully summons an
ambulance or emergency response vehicle or
reports that one is needed when such person
knows that the ambulance or emergency
response vehicle is not needed is guilty of a
class B misdemeanor.

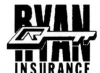

Robert J. Ryan, Inc.
95 Schwenk Drive
P.O. Box 3995
Kingston, New York 12
914/338-6000
FAX 914/331-0006

Robert J. Ryan, Jr., CIC
President

January 13, 1995

[Names removed]

RE: 911 Professional Liability Coverage

Dear

Thank you for your assistance on the application for 911 liability
coverage. I have heard back from the insurance company
underwriter and am sorry to report that a coverage quotation will
not be forthcoming at this time as your system does not currently
give pre-arrival medical instruction to callers needing this
service. The company has in the past been made aware of
situations where the caller requested medical advice, and was told
that was beyond the system capabilities. The resulting worsened
condition quickly turned into a liability claim against the system
operators. It seems the currently running television shows
depicting 911 situations which include pre-arrival instruction
have caused the general public to expect this service from all 911
operations.

I understand that the plans are for this to be implemented soon.
I strongly encourage that action and will be more than happy to
resubmit your system for quotation consideration upon the
implementation of this service.

Thank you for your continued assistance and please let me know of
your time frame when decided.

Sincerely,

Kevin M. Roach
Account Executive

KMR/19472

THOMAS J. TALLON
CHIEF OF FIRE DEPARTMENT

SALT LAKE CITY CORPORATION
FIRE DEPARTMENT

DEEDEE CORRADIN
MAYOR

To: All Fire Department Personnel
From: Tom Tallon, Fire Chief
Subject: Fire Department Response On Bravo Calls
Date: 23 December, 1997

For over a year now, the Salt Lake City Fire Department has been evaluating our response and subsequent treatment of Bravo level EMS calls within Salt Lake City. Our research has shown that the time savings we realize for these calls does not outweigh the danger of responding in a lights-and-siren mode. The fact that 52.3% of lawsuits against EMS agencies are produced by Emergency Medical Vehicular accidents certainly points out the inherent dangers surrounding 10:39 responses. Now that our dispatch center is one of only 15 Accredited Centers of Excellence worldwide has bolstered our confidence that we can change our responses to previously identified EMS situations.

Given this information, on Thursday, January 01, 1998, our Department will respond to all Bravo calls in a non-lights and siren (10:40) mode. In this matter, we hope to increase safety for our firefighters and citizens alike. The Officer in charge of the apparatus may, at their discretion, respond 10:39 if they feel patient care and/or safety dictates a Hot response. Some of the situations which may warrant a lights-and-siren response would include; environmental conditions, dispatch updates which indicate condition changes, exaggerated out of district responses, or extreme border responses within given district. We ask for your continued support in evaluating this new era of EMS response in our community. We are the first department in the country to implement a measure as bold as this. If you begin to see problems, please contact your Battalion Chief with a feedback report.

Respectfully,

Tom Tallon, Chief
Salt Lake City Fire Department

Emergency Numbers from around the Globe	
Argentina	101
Australia	000
Austria	144
Belgium	900, 100, 101, 112
Brazil	190
Canada	911
Columbia	12, 123
Costa Rica	911
Croatia	112, 92, 93, 94
Cypress	112, 199
Czech Republic	155, 150, 154, 158, 112
Denmark	000, 112
Egypt	912644
Estonia	001, 01, 112
European Alliance	112
Finland	112
France	17, 112, 15, 17, 18
Germany	112, 110
Greece	100, 166, 199, 112
Hong Kong	999
Hungary	04, 104, 105, 107, 112
Iceland	0112
India	102
Ireland	999, 112
Isle of Man	999
Israel	100
Italy	118, 112, 113, 115
Jamaica	119
Japan	119, 110
Latvia	01, 02, 03, 04, 112
Malta	196, 199, 112
Mexico	080
Moldovia	901, 902, 903
Moscow	051
Netherlands	008, 0611, 112
New Zealand	111
Nigeria	112
Norway	113, 110, 112, 113
Panama	911
Philippines	599011
Poland	999, 997, 998, 112
Portugal	112, 115
Romania	961
Slovak Republic	150, 155, 158, 112
Slovenia	112, 985
South Africa	112
Singapore	999
Spain	112, 061, 080, 532
Sweden	112
Switzerland	117, 119, 144, 112, 143
Thailand	2815051, 191
Turkey	112, 110, 155, 156
United States	911
United Kingdom	999, 112
Venezuela	169

Many countries have moved to triple digit emergency numbers such as 9-9-9 or 0-0-0 in an attempt to simplify access to emergency resources.

Additionally, the European community is working towards establishing a uniform emergency number. The number currently under discussion is 1-1-2.

If you have any information regarding the addition of new emergency numbers, or changes to the emergency numbers listed above, please contact the Academy.

Acute Myocardial Infarction Data

The Centers for Disease Control (CDC) in Atlanta, Georgia, maintains a number of health and mortality databases in its "CDC-Wonder" system. One of these, compressed mortality, tracks counts and rates of death by age (seventeen categories), race (white/black/other), gender, year, state and county of residence, and underlying cause. Causes of death are stored as ICD (international classification of disease) codes.

ICD code 410 covers acute MI. The fourth digit identifies the location of the infarction. For example, 410.0 is an infarction of the anterolateral wall, 410.2 an infarction of the inferolateral wall, and 410.3 an infarction of the inferoposterior wall. ICD code 410.8 covers a variety of less common infarction sites, and 410.9 is a "catch-all" for any unspecified sites of acute MI. Codes 410.0 to 410.9 cover just acute MI, so other heart-related diseases, such as hypertensive disease (401-405) or other forms of chronic ischemic heart disease such as coronary atherosclerosis (414) would be excluded from a search for 410.0 to 410.9.

We searched the CDC-Wonder database for all reports of ICD code 410.0 to 410.9 inclusive. These records were reported by age, gender, and year for the sixteen-year period from 1979 to 1994. Data were imported into Microsoft Excel and reformatted as shown in panel A (male) and B (female).

Male and Female MI Deaths

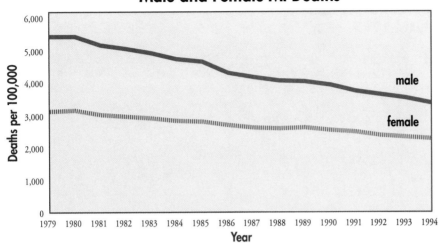

Figure 1

Deaths < 35 Years Old

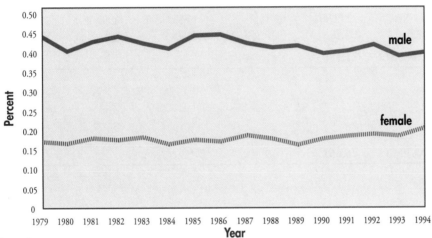

Figure 2

Deaths < 45 Years Old

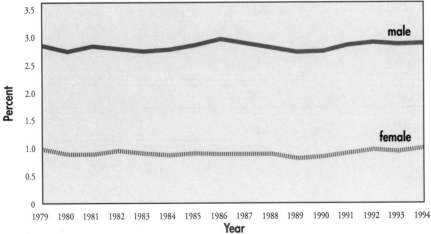

Figure 3

	Total	87,203	100.0%

Cleveland Emergency Medical Services
Master Dispatch Analysis, 1995

Determinant Level	Incidents Level	Calls Level
DELTA	32,534	37.3%
CHARLIE	16,136	18.5%
BRAVO	24,814	28.5%
ALPHA	13,719	15.7%

1 ABDOMINAL PAIN/PROBLEMS   2, 847 incidents   3% of all complaints

DETERMINANT LEVEL	INCIDENTS/ LEVEL	PERCENT/ CHIEF COMPLAINT	DETERMINANT CODES	INCIDENTS/ CODE	PERCENT/ CODE
CHARLIE	**1,186**	**41.7%**			
			1-C-0	9	0.32%
			1-C-1	563	19.78%
			1-C-2	483	16.97%
			1-C-3	60	2.11%
			1-C-4	71	2.49%
ALPHA	**1,661**	**58.3%**			
			1-A-1	1,661	58.34%

2 ALLERGIES/HIVES/MED REACTIONS/STINGS   672 incidents   1% of all complaints

DETERMINANT LEVEL	INCIDENTS/ LEVEL	PERCENT/ CHIEF COMPLAINT	DETERMINANT CODES	INCIDENTS/ CODE	PERCENT/ CODE
DELTA	**62**	**9.2%**			
			2-D-1	25	3.72%
			2-D-2	34	5.06%
			2-D-3	3	0.45%
CHARLIE	**254**	**37.8%**			
			2-C-1	254	37.80%
BRAVO	**267**	**39.7%**			
			2-B-1	267	39.73%
ALPHA	**89**	**13.2%**			
			2-A-1	89	13.24%

3   ANIMAL BITES/ATTACKS   230 incidents   < 1% of all complaints

DETERMINANT LEVEL	INCIDENTS/ LEVEL	PERCENT/ CHIEF COMPLAINT	DETERMINANT CODES	INCIDENTS/ CODE	PERCENT/ CODE
DELTA	43	18.7%			
			3-D-1	34	14.78%
			3-D-4	2	0.87%
			3-D-5	2	0.87%
			3-D-6	5	2.17%
BRAVO	93	40.4%			
			3-B-0	2	0.87%
			3-B-1	82	35.65%
			3-B-2	9	3.91%
ALPHA	94	40.9%			
			3-A-1	80	34.78%
			3-A-2	14	6.09%

4   ASSAULT/RAPE   7,228 incidents   8% of all complaints

DETERMINANT LEVEL	INCIDENTS/ LEVEL	PERCENT/ CHIEF COMPLAINT	DETERMINANT CODES	INCIDENTS/ CODE	PERCENT/ CODE
DELTA	1,232	17.0%			
			4-D-1	196	2.71%
			4-D-2	218	3.02%
			4-D-3	350	4.84%
			4-D-4	468	6.47%
BRAVO	5,559	76.9%			
			4-B-1	3,207	44.37%
			4-B-2	167	2.31%
			4-B-3	2,185	30.23%
ALPHA	437	6.0%			
			4-A-1	316	4.37%
			4-A-2	121	1.67%

5   BACK PAIN (NON-TRAUMATIC)   671 incidents   1% of all complaints

DETERMINANT LEVEL	INCIDENTS/ LEVEL	PERCENT/ CHIEF COMPLAINT	DETERMINANT CODES	INCIDENTS/ CODE	PERCENT/ CODE
DELTA	9	1.3%			
			5-D-1	9	1.34%
CHARLIE	35	5.2%			
			5-C-0	8	1.19%
			5-C-1	27	4.02%
ALPHA	627	93.4%			
			5-A-1	572	85.25%
			5-A-2	55	8.20%

6   BREATHING PROBLEMS   12,116 incidents   14% of all complaints

DETERMINANT LEVEL	INCIDENTS/ LEVEL	PERCENT/ CHIEF COMPLAINT	DETERMINANT CODES	INCIDENTS/ CODE	PERCENT/ CODE
DELTA	8,032	66.3%			
			6-D-0	9	0.07%
			6-D-1	2,894	23.89%
			6-D-2	996	8.22%
			6-D-3	4,133	34.11%
CHARLIE	4,084	33.7%			
			6-C-1	2,576	21.26%
			6-C-2	1,275	10.52%
			6-C-3	233	1.92%

7   BURNS/EXPLOSIONS   376 incidents   < 1% of all complaints

DETERMINANT LEVEL	INCIDENTS/ LEVEL	PERCENT/ CHIEF COMPLAINT	DETERMINANT CODES	INCIDENTS/ CODE	PERCENT/ CODE
DELTA	45	12.0%			
			7-D-0	1	0.27%
			7-D-1	12	3.19%
			7-D-3	3	0.80%
			7-D-4	29	7.71%
CHARLIE	129	34.3%			
			7-C-0	1	0.27%
			7-C-1	16	4.26%
			7-C-2	112	29.79%
BRAVO	40	10.6%			
			7-B-0	1	0.27%
			7-B-1	39	10.37%
ALPHA	162	43.1%			
			7-A-1	154	40.96%
			7-A-2	8	2.13%

8   CARBON MONOXIDE/INHALATION/HAZMAT   107 incidents   < 1% of all complaints

DETERMINANT LEVEL	INCIDENTS/ LEVEL	PERCENT/ CHIEF COMPLAINT	DETERMINANT CODES	INCIDENTS/ CODE	PERCENT/ CODE
DELTA	40	37.4%			
			8-D-1	20	18.69%
			8-D-2	8	7.48%
			8-D-3	10	9.35%
			8-D-4	2	1.87%
CHARLIE	32	29.9%			
			8-C-1	32	29.91%
BRAVO	35	32.7%			
			8-B-1	35	32.71%

9   CARDIAC/RESPIRATORY ARREST   2,054 incidents   2% of all complaints

DETERMINANT LEVEL	INCIDENTS/ LEVEL	PERCENT/ CHIEF COMPLAINT	DETERMINANT CODES	INCIDENTS/ CODE	PERCENT/ CODE
DELTA	1,717	83.6%			
			9-D-1	1,704	82.96%
			9-D-2	13	0.63%
BRAVO	337	16.4%			
			9-B-1	337	16.41%

10   CHEST PAIN   7,480 incidents   9% of all complaints

DETERMINANT LEVEL	INCIDENTS/ LEVEL	PERCENT/ CHIEF COMPLAINT	DETERMINANT CODES	INCIDENTS/ CODE	PERCENT/ CODE
DELTA	4,531	60.6%			
			10-D-0	1	0.01%
			10-D-1	140	1.87%
			10-D-2	297	3.97%
			10-D-3	4,093	54.72%
CHARLIE	2,447	32.7%			
			10-C-1	1,064	14.22%
			10-C-2	1,110	14.84%
			10-C-3	16	0.21%
			10-C-4	257	3.44%
ALPHA	502	6.7%			
			10-A-1	502	6.71%

11   CHOKING   555 incidents   1% of all complaints

DETERMINANT LEVEL	INCIDENTS/ LEVEL	PERCENT/ CHIEF COMPLAINT	DETERMINANT CODES	INCIDENTS/ CODE	PERCENT/ CODE
DELTA	418	75.3%			
			11-D-1	196	35.32%
			11-D-2	208	37.48%
			11-D-3	14	2.52%
ALPHA	137	24.7%			
			11-A-1	137	24.68%

12 CONVULSION/SEIZURES   3,967 incidents   5% of all complaints

DETERMINANT LEVEL	INCIDENTS/ LEVEL	PERCENT/ CHIEF COMPLAINT	DETERMINANT CODES	INCIDENTS/ CODE	PERCENT/ CODE
DELTA	2,305	58.1%			
			12-D-1	1,964	49.51%
			12-D-2	329	8.29%
			12-D-3	12	0.30%
CHARLIE	365	9.2%			
			12-C-0	20	0.50%
			12-C-1	46	1.16%
			12-C-2	105	2.65%
			12-C-3	83	2.09%
			12-C-4	111	2.80%
BRAVO	201	5.1%			
			12-B-0	12	0.30%
			12-B-1	189	4.76%
ALPHA	1,096	27.6%			
			12-A-1	1,096	27.63%

13 DIABETIC PROBLEMS   1,402 incidents   2% of all complaints

DETERMINANT LEVEL	INCIDENTS/ LEVEL	PERCENT/ CHIEF COMPLAINT	DETERMINANT CODES	INCIDENTS/ CODE	PERCENT/ CODE
DELTA	323	23.0%			
			13-D-0	3	0.21%
			13-D-1	320	22.82%
CHARLIE	764	54.5%			
			13-C-1	585	41.73%
			13-C-2	179	12.77%
ALPHA	315	22.5%			
			13-A-1	315	22.47%

14 DROWNING (NEAR)/DIVING ACCIDENT   37 incidents   < 1% of all complaints

DETERMINANT LEVEL	INCIDENTS/ LEVEL	PERCENT/ CHIEF COMPLAINT	DETERMINANT CODES	INCIDENTS/ CODE	PERCENT/ CODE
DELTA	30	81.1%			
			14-D-1	20	54.05%
			14-D-2	2	5.41%
			14-D-3	3	8.11%
			14-D-4	4	10.81%
			14-D-5	1	2.70%
BRAVO	6	16.2%			
			14-B-1	6	16.22%
ALPHA	1	2.7%			
			14-A-1	1	2.70%

15	ELECTROCUTION		51 incidents		< 1% of all complaints

DETERMINANT LEVEL	INCIDENTS/ LEVEL	PERCENT/ CHIEF COMPLAINT	DETERMINANT CODES	INCIDENTS/ CODE	PERCENT/ CODE
DELTA	26	51.0%			
			15-D-1	5	9.80%
			15-D-2	7	13.73%
			15-D-3	4	7.84%
			15-D-4	2	3.92%
			15-D-5	5	9.80%
			15-D-6	1	1.96%
			15-D-7	2	3.92%
CHARLIE	25	49.0%			
			15-C-1	25	49.02%

16	EYE PROBLEMS/INJURIES		283 incidents		< 1% of all complaints

DETERMINANT LEVEL	INCIDENTS/ LEVEL	PERCENT/ CHIEF COMPLAINT	DETERMINANT CODES	INCIDENTS/ CODE	PERCENT/ CODE
DELTA	6	2.1%			
			16-D-1	6	2.12%
BRAVO	91	32.2%			
			16-B-0	1	0.35%
			16-B-1	90	31.80%
ALPHA	186	65.7%			
			16-A-1	90	31.80%
			16-A-2	96	33.92%

17	FALLS/BACK INJURIES (TRAUMATIC)		4,384 incidents		5% of all complaints

DETERMINANT LEVEL	INCIDENTS/ LEVEL	PERCENT/ CHIEF COMPLAINT	DETERMINANT CODES	INCIDENTS/ CODE	PERCENT/ CODE
DELTA	1,423	32.5%			
			17-D-0	2	0.05%
			17-D-1	175	3.99%
			17-D-2	639	14.58%
			17-D-3	326	7.44%
			17-D-4	281	6.41%
BRAVO	1,517	34.6%			
			17-B-0	11	0.25%
			17-B-1	117	2.67%
			17-B-2	114	2.60%
			17-B-3	1,275	29.08%
ALPHA	1,444	32.9%			
			17-A-1	1,096	25.00%
			17-A-2	348	7.94%

18   HEADACHE   729 incidents   1% of all complaints

DETERMINANT LEVEL	INCIDENTS/ LEVEL	PERCENT/ CHIEF COMPLAINT	DETERMINANT CODES	INCIDENTS/ CODE	PERCENT/ CODE
CHARLIE	519	71.2%			
			18-C-0	1	0.14%
			18-C-1	42	5.76%
			18-C-2	92	12.62%
			18-C-3	199	27.30%
			18-C-4	179	24.55%
			18-C-5	6	0.82%
ALPHA	210	28.8%			
			18-A-1	210	28.81%

19   HEARTH PROBLEMS   177 incidents   < 1% of all complaints

DETERMINANT LEVEL	INCIDENTS/ LEVEL	PERCENT/ CHIEF COMPLAINT	DETERMINANT CODES	INCIDENTS/ CODE	PERCENT/ CODE
CHARLIE	117	66.1%			
			19-C-0	1	0.56%
			19-C-1	17	9.60%
			19-C-2	91	51.41%
			19-C-3	8	4.52%
BRAVO	14	7.9%			
			19-B-1	14	7.91%
ALPHA	46	26.0%			
			19-A-1	46	25.99%

20   HEAT/COLD EXPOSURE   119 incidents   < 1% of all complaints

DETERMINANT LEVEL	INCIDENTS/ LEVEL	PERCENT/ CHIEF COMPLAINT	DETERMINANT CODES	INCIDENTS/ CODE	PERCENT/ CODE
DELTA	32	26.9%			
			20-D-1	32	26.89%
CHARLIE	6	5.0%			
			20-C-1	6	5.04%
BRAVO	64	53.8%			
			20-B-1	31	26.05%
			20-B-2	33	27.73%
ALPHA	17	14.3%			
			20-A-1	17	14.29%

21	HEMORRHAGE/LACERATIONS		3,421 incidents		4% of all complaints

DETERMINANT LEVEL	INCIDENTS/ LEVEL	PERCENT/ CHIEF COMPLAINT	DETERMINANT CODES	INCIDENTS/ CODE	PERCENT/ CODE
DELTA	**1,109**	**32.4%**			
			21-D-0	1	0.03%
			21-D-1	1,051	30.72%
			21-D-2	55	1.61%
			21-D-3	2	0.06%
BRAVO	**1,813**	**53.0%**			
			21-B-0	1	0.03%
			21-B-1	1,812	52.97%
ALPHA	**499**	**14.6%**			
			21-A-1	499	14.59%

22	INDUSTRIAL/MACHINERY ACCIDENTS		43 incidents		< 1% of all complaints

DETERMINANT LEVEL	INCIDENTS/ LEVEL	PERCENT/ CHIEF COMPLAINT	DETERMINANT CODES	INCIDENTS/ CODE	PERCENT/ CODE
DELTA	**18**	**41.9%**			
			22-D-0	1	2.33%
			22-D-1	6	13.95%
			22-D-2	11	25.58%
BRAVO	**25**	**58.1%**			
			22-B-1	25	58.14%

23	OVERDOSE/INGESTION/POISONING		2,220 incidents		3% of all complaints

DETERMINANT LEVEL	INCIDENTS/ LEVEL	PERCENT/ CHIEF COMPLAINT	DETERMINANT CODES	INCIDENTS/ CODE	PERCENT/ CODE
DELTA	**256**	**11.5%**			
			23-D-0	1	0.05%
			23-D-1	242	10.90%
			23-D-2	13	0.59%
CHARLIE	**777**	**35.0%**			
			23-C-0	1	0.05%
			23-C-1	360	16.22%
			23-C-2	189	8.51%
			23-C-3	69	3.11%
			23-C-4	79	3.56%
			23-C-5	15	0.68%
			23-C-6	64	2.88%
BRAVO	**1,187**	**53.5%**			
			23-B-0	14	0.63%
			23-B-1	1,173	52.84%

24 PREGNANCY/CHILDBIRTH/MISCARRIAGE   3,189 incidents   4% of all complaints

DETERMINANT LEVEL	INCIDENTS/ LEVEL	PERCENT/ CHIEF COMPLAINT	DETERMINANT CODES	INCIDENTS/ CODE	PERCENT/ CODE
DELTA	1,142	35.8%			
			24-D-0	3	0.09%
			24-D-1	72	2.26%
			24-D-2	38	1.19%
			24-D-3	713	22.36%
			24-D-4	310	9.72%
			24-D-5	6	0.19%
CHARLIE	1,395	43.7%			
			24-C-0	12	0.38%
			24-C-1	1,383	43.37%
BRAVO	234	7.3%			
			24-B-0	1	0.03%
			24-B-1	225	7.06%
			24-B-2	8	0.25%
ALPHA	418	13.1%			
			24-A-1	171	5.36%
			24-A-2	247	7.75%

25 PSYCHIATRIC/SUICIDE ATTEMPT   1,346 incidents   2% of all complaints

DETERMINANT LEVEL	INCIDENTS/ LEVEL	PERCENT/ CHIEF COMPLAINT	DETERMINANT CODES	INCIDENTS/ CODE	PERCENT/ CODE
DELTA	39	2.9%			
			25-D-0	2	0.15%
			25-D-1	37	2.75%
CHARLIE	871	64.7%			
			25-C-1	54	4.01%
			25-C-2	676	50.22%
			25-C-3	141	10.48%
BRAVO	133	9.9%			
			25-B-0	1	0.07%
			25-B-1	132	9.81%
ALPHA	303	22.5%			
			25-A-1	303	22.51%

26 SICK PERSON (SPECIFIC DIAGNOSIS)   6,146 incidents   7% of all complaints

DETERMINANT LEVEL	INCIDENTS/ LEVEL	PERCENT/ CHIEF COMPLAINT	DETERMINANT CODES	INCIDENTS/ CODE	PERCENT/ CODE
CHARLIE	1,556	25.3%			
			26-C-0	19	0.31%
			26-C-1	721	11.73%
			26-C-2	816	13.28%
BRAVO	705	11.5%			
			26-B-0	7	0.11%
			26-B-1	698	11.36%
ALPHA	3,885	63.2%			
			26-A-1	3,083	50.16%
			26-A-2	802	13.05%

27 STAB/GUNSHOT WOUND   1,901 incidents   2% of all complaints

DETERMINANT LEVEL	INCIDENTS/ LEVEL	PERCENT/ CHIEF COMPLAINT	DETERMINANT CODES	INCIDENTS/ CODE	PERCENT/ CODE
DELTA	1,635	86.0%			
			27-D-0	1	0.05%
			27-D-1	1,486	78.17%
			27-D-2	43	2.26%
			27-D-3	61	3.21%
			27-D-4	44	2.31%
BRAVO	263	13.8%			
			27-B-1	188	9.89%
			27-B-2	1	0.05%
			27-B-3	74	3.89%
ALPHA	3	0.2%			
			27-A-1	3	0.16%

28 STROKE (CVA)   1,077 incidents   1% of all complaints

DETERMINANT LEVEL	INCIDENTS/ LEVEL	PERCENT/ CHIEF COMPLAINT	DETERMINANT CODES	INCIDENTS/ CODE	PERCENT/ CODE
CHARLIE	672	62.4%			
			28-C-0	7	0.65%
			28-C-1	523	48.56%
			28-C-2	142	13.18%
BRAVO	180	16.7%			
			28-B-0	5	0.46%
			28-B-1	175	16.25%
ALPHA	225	20.9%			
			28-A-1	225	20.89%

29 TRAFFIC ACCIDENTS		10,054 incidents	12% of all complaints		
DETERMINANT LEVEL	INCIDENTS/ LEVEL	PERCENT/ CHIEF COMPLAINT	DETERMINANT CODES	INCIDENTS/ CODE	PERCENT/ CODE
DELTA	**4,331**	**43.1%**			
			29-D-0	6	0.06%
			29-D-1	1,682	16.73%
			29-D-2	1,468	14.60%
			29-D-3	258	2.57%
			29-D-4	466	4.64%
			29-D-5	246	2.45%
			29-D-6	195	1.94%
			29-D-7	10	0.10%
BRAVO	**5,707**	**56.8%**			
			29-B-1	3,579	35.60%
			29-B-2	2,128	21.17%
ALPHA	**15**	**0.1%**			
			29-A-1	15	0.15%

30 TRAUMATIC INJURIES, SPEFICI		2,737 incidents	3% of all complaints		
DETERMINANT LEVEL	INCIDENTS/ LEVEL	PERCENT/ CHIEF COMPLAINT	DETERMINANT CODES	INCIDENTS/ CODE	PERCENT/ CODE
DELTA	**273**	**10.0%**			
			30-D-0	3	0.11%
			30-D-1	185	6.76%
			30-D-2	7	0.26%
			30-D-3	78	2.85%
BRAVO	**1,322**	**48.3%**			
			30-B-0	8	0.29%
			30-B-1	1,152	42.09%
			30-B-2	162	5.92%
ALPHA	**1,142**	**41.7%**			
			30-A-1	856	31.28%
			30-A-2	286	10.45%

| 31 | UNCONSCIOUS/FAINTING (NON-TRAUMATIC) | | 4,200 incidents | | 5% of all complaints |

DETERMINANT LEVEL	INCIDENTS/ LEVEL	PERCENT/ CHIEF COMPLAINT	DETERMINANT CODES	INCIDENTS/ CODE	PERCENT/ CODE
DELTA	**3,093**	**73.6%**			
			31-D-0	1	0.02%
			31-D-1	2,412	57.43%
			31-D-2	99	2.36%
			31-D-3	581	13.83%
CHARLIE	**902**	**21.5%**			
			31-C-0	5	0.12%
			31-C-1	485	11.55%
			31-C-2	149	3.55%
			31-C-3	35	0.83%
			31-C-4	205	4.88%
			31-C-5	23	0.55%
ALPHA	**205**	**4.9%**			
			31-A-1	205	4.88%

| 32 | UNKNOWN PROBLEM (MAN DOWN) | | 5,385 incidents | | 6% of all complaints |

DETERMINANT LEVEL	INCIDENTS/ LEVEL	PERCENT/ CHIEF COMPLAINT	DETERMINANT CODES	INCIDENTS/ CODE	PERCENT/ CODE
DELTA	**364**	**6.8%**			
			32-D-0	12	0.22%
			32-D-1	352	6.54%
BRAVO	**5,021**	**93.2%**			
			32-B-1	2,383	44.25%
			32-B-2	562	10.44%
			32-B-3	2,076	38.55%

**Derbyshire Ambulance Services
Master Dispatch Analysis, 1995**

Determinant Level	Incidents Level	Calls Level
DELTA	11,705	33.4%
CHARLIE	6,086	17.3%
BRAVO	12,027	34.3%
ALPHA	5,256	15.0%
OMEGA	23	0.1%
TOTAL	**35,090**	**100%**

| **1** | **ABDOMINAL PAIN/PROBLEMS** | | **892 incidents** | | **3% of all complaints** |

DETERMINANT LEVEL	INCIDENTS/ LEVEL	PERCENT/ CHIEF COMPLAINT	DETERMINANT CODES	INCIDENTS/ CODE	PERCENT/ CODE
CHARLIE	**455**	**51.0%**			
			1-C-1	245	27.47%
			1-C-2	132	14.80%
			1-C-3	27	3.03%
			1-C-4	51	5.72%
ALPHA	**437**	**49.0%**			
			1-A-1	437	48.99%

| **2** | **ALLERGIES/HIVES/MED REACTIONS/STINGS** | | **97 incidents** | | **< 1% of all complaints** |

DETERMINANT LEVEL	INCIDENTS/ LEVEL	PERCENT/ CHIEF COMPLAINT	DETERMINANT CODES	INCIDENTS/ CODE	PERCENT/ CODE
DELTA	**13**	**13.4%**			
			2-D-0	1	1.03%
			2-D-1	4	4.12%
			2-D-2	8	8.25%
CHARLIE	**25**	**25.8%**			
			2-C-1	25	25.77%
BRAVO	**18**	**18.6%**			
			2-B-1	18	18.56%
ALPHA	**41**	**42.3%**			
			2-A-1	41	42.27%

3   ANIMAL BITES/ATTACKS   62 incidents   < 1% of all complaints

DETERMINANT LEVEL	INCIDENTS/ LEVEL	PERCENT/ CHIEF COMPLAINT	DETERMINANT CODES	INCIDENTS/ CODE	PERCENT/ CODE
DELTA	16	25.8%			
			3-D-1	7	11.29%
			3-D-3	1	1.61%
			3-D-6	8	12.90%
BRAVO	32	51.6%			
			3-B-1	12	19.35%
			3-B-2	20	32.26%
ALPHA	14	22.6%			
			3-A-1	8	12.90%
			3-A-2	6	9.68%

4   ASSAULT/RAPE   806 incidents   2% of all complaints

DETERMINANT LEVEL	INCIDENTS/ LEVEL	PERCENT/ CHIEF COMPLAINT	DETERMINANT CODES	INCIDENTS/ CODE	PERCENT/ CODE
DELTA	208	25.8%			
			4-D-1	57	7.07%
			4-D-2	44	5.46%
			4-D-3	82	10.17%
			4-D-4	25	3.10%
BRAVO	550	68.2%			
			4-B-1	213	26.43%
			4-B-2	30	3.72%
			4-B-3	307	38.09%
ALPHA	48	6.0%			
			4-A-1	42	5.21%
			4-A-2	6	0.74%

5   BACK PAIN (NON-TRAUMATIC)   180 incidents   1% of all complaints

DETERMINANT LEVEL	INCIDENTS/ LEVEL	PERCENT/ CHIEF COMPLAINT	DETERMINANT CODES	INCIDENTS/ CODE	PERCENT/ CODE
DELTA	8	1.7%			
			5-D-1	1	0.56%
CHARLIE	7	3.9%			
			5-C-1	7	3.89%
ALPHA	172	95.6%			
			5-A-1	158	87.78%
			5-A-2	14	7.78%

6   BREATHING PROBLEMS   2,982 incidents   8% of all complaints

DETERMINANT LEVEL	INCIDENTS/ LEVEL	PERCENT/ CHIEF COMPLAINT	DETERMINANT CODES	INCIDENTS/ CODE	PERCENT/ CODE
DELTA	1,705	57.2%			
			6-D-1	224	7.51%
			6-D-2	324	10.87%
			6-D-3	1,157	38.80%
CHARLIE	1,277	42.8%			
			6-C-1	717	24.04%
			6-C-2	370	12.41%
			6-C-3	190	6.37%

7   BURNS/EXPLOSIONS   344 incidents   1% of all complaints

DETERMINANT LEVEL	INCIDENTS/ LEVEL	PERCENT/ CHIEF COMPLAINT	DETERMINANT CODES	INCIDENTS/ CODE	PERCENT/ CODE
DELTA	142	41.3%			
			7-D-0	2	0.58%
			7-D-1	129	37.50%
			7-D-2	2	0.58%
			7-D-3	3	0.87%
			7-D-4	6	1.74%
CHARLIE	27	7.8%			
			7-C-0	1	0.29%
			7-C-1	6	1.74%
			7-C-2	20	5.81%
BRAVO	130	37.8%			
			7-B-1	130	37.79%
ALPHA	45	13.1%			
			7-A-1	25	7.27%
			7-A-2	20	5.81%

8   CARBON MONOXIDE/INHALATION/HAZMAT   38 incidents   < 1% of all complaints

DETERMINANT LEVEL	INCIDENTS/ LEVEL	PERCENT/ CHIEF COMPLAINT	DETERMINANT CODES	INCIDENTS/ CODE	PERCENT/ CODE
DELTA	29	76.3%			
			8-D-1	2	5.26%
			8-D-2	3	7.89%
			8-D-3	17	44.74%
			8-D-4	7	18.42%
CHARLIE	2	5.3%			
			8-C-1	2	5.26%
BRAVO	7	18.4%			
			8-B-1	7	18.42%

9 CARDIAC/RESPIRATORY ARREST — 662 incidents — 2% of all complaints

DETERMINANT LEVEL	INCIDENTS/ LEVEL	PERCENT/ CHIEF COMPLAINT	DETERMINANT CODES	INCIDENTS/ CODE	PERCENT/ CODE
DELTA	**660**	**99.7%**			
			9-D-0	1	0.15%
			9-D-1	649	98.04%
			9-D-2	10	1.51%
BRAVO	**2**	**0.3%**			
			9-B-1	2	0.30%

10 CHEST PAIN — 4,355 incidents — 12% of all complaints

DETERMINANT LEVEL	INCIDENTS/ LEVEL	PERCENT/ CHIEF COMPLAINT	DETERMINANT CODES	INCIDENTS/ CODE	PERCENT/ CODE
DELTA	**2,244**	**51.5%**			
			10-D-0	3	0.07%
			10-D-1	62	1.42%
			10-D-2	157	3.61%
			10-D-3	2,022	46.43%
CHARLIE	**2,082**	**47.8%**			
			10-C-1	1,084	24.89%
			10-C-2	180	4.13%
			10-C-4	818	18.78%
ALPHA	**29**	**0.7%**			
			10-A-1	29	0.67%

11 CHOKING — 166 incidents — < 1% of all complaints

DETERMINANT LEVEL	INCIDENTS/ LEVEL	PERCENT/ CHIEF COMPLAINT	DETERMINANT CODES	INCIDENTS/ CODE	PERCENT/ CODE
DELTA	**140**	**84.3%**			
			11-D-1	49	29.52%
			11-D-2	78	46.99%
			11-D-3	13	7.83%
ALPHA	**26**	**15.7%**			
			11-A-1	26	15.66%

12 CONVULSION/SEIZURES — 1,297 incidents — 4% of all complaints

DETERMINANT LEVEL	INCIDENTS/ LEVEL	PERCENT/ CHIEF COMPLAINT	DETERMINANT CODES	INCIDENTS/ CODE	PERCENT/ CODE
DELTA	663	51.1%			
			12-D-1	529	40.79%
			12-D-2	133	10.25%
			12-D-3	1	0.08%
CHARLIE	96	7.4%			
			12-C-1	5	0.39%
			12-C-2	46	3.55%
			12-C-3	19	1.46%
			12-C-4	26	2.00%
BRAVO	104	8.0%			
			12-B-1	104	8.02%
ALPHA	434	33.5%			
			12-A-1	434	33.46%

13 DIABETIC PROBLEMS — 569 incidents — 2% of all complaints

DETERMINANT LEVEL	INCIDENTS/ LEVEL	PERCENT/ CHIEF COMPLAINT	DETERMINANT CODES	INCIDENTS/ CODE	PERCENT/ CODE
DELTA	288	50.6%			
			13-D-1	288	50.62%
CHARLIE	210	36.9%			
			13-C-1	179	31.46%
			13-C-2	31	5.45%
ALPHA	71	12.5%			
			13-A-1	71	12.48%

14 DROWNING (NEAR)/DIVING ACCIDENT — 16 incidents — < 1% of all complaints

DETERMINANT LEVEL	INCIDENTS/ LEVEL	PERCENT/ CHIEF COMPLAINT	DETERMINANT CODES	INCIDENTS/ CODE	PERCENT/ CODE
DELTA	5	31.3%			
			14-D-1	3	18.75%
			14-D-3	1	6.25%
			14-D-4	1	6.25%
CHARLIE	1	6.3%			
			14-C-1	1	6.25%
BRAVO	8	50.0%			
			14-B-2	8	50.00%
ALPHA	2	12.5%			
			14-A-1	2	12.50%

15 ELECTROCUTION   **19 incidents**   **< 1% of all complaints**

DETERMINANT LEVEL	INCIDENTS/ LEVEL	PERCENT/ CHIEF COMPLAINT	DETERMINANT CODES	INCIDENTS/ CODE	PERCENT/ CODE
DELTA	14	73.7%			
			15-D-1	3	15.79%
			15-D-2	5	26.32%
			15-D-3	2	10.53%
			15-D-4	1	5.26%
			15-D-5	1	5.26%
			15-D-7	2	10.53%
CHARLIE	5	26.3%			
			15-C-1	5	26.32%

16 EYE PROBLEMS/INJURIES   **81 incidents**   **< 1% of all complaints**

DETERMINANT LEVEL	INCIDENTS/ LEVEL	PERCENT/ CHIEF COMPLAINT	DETERMINANT CODES	INCIDENTS/ CODE	PERCENT/ CODE
DELTA	16	19.8%			
			16-D-1	16	19.75%
BRAVO	33	40.7%			
			16-B-1	33	40.74%
ALPHA	32	39.5%			
			16-A-1	26	32.10%
			16-A-2	6	7.41%

17 FALLS/BACK INJURIES (TRAUMATIC)   **5,042 incidents**   **14% of all complaints**

DETERMINANT LEVEL	INCIDENTS/ LEVEL	PERCENT/ CHIEF COMPLAINT	DETERMINANT CODES	INCIDENTS/ CODE	PERCENT/ CODE
DELTA	898	17.8%			
			17-D-0	1	0.02%
			17-D-1	101	2.00%
			17-D-2	371	7.36%
			17-D-3	275	5.45%
			17-D-4	150	2.98%
BRAVO	2,870	56.9%			
			17-B-1	1,350	26.78%
			17-B-2	114	2.26%
			17-B-3	1,406	27.89%
ALPHA	1,274	25.3%			
			17-A-1	1,136	22.53%
			17-A-2	138	2.74%

18   HEADACHE   165 incidents   < 1% of all complaints

DETERMINANT LEVEL	INCIDENTS/ LEVEL	PERCENT/ CHIEF COMPLAINT	DETERMINANT CODESCODE	INCIDENTS/ CODE	PERCENT/
CHARLIE	93	56.4%			
			18-C-0	1	0.61%
			18-C-1	9	5.45%
			18-C-2	11	6.67%
			18-C-3	38	23.03%
			18-C-4	32	19.39%
			18-C-5	2	1.21%
ALPHA	72	43.6%			
			18-A-1	72	43.64%

19   HEARTH PROBLEMS   452 incidents   1% of all complaints

DETERMINANT LEVEL	INCIDENTS/ LEVEL	PERCENT/ CHIEF COMPLAINT	DETERMINANT CODES	INCIDENTS/ CODE	PERCENT/ CODE
DELTA	3	0.7%			
			19-D-1	3	0.66%
CHARLIE	160	35.4%			
			19-C-1	23	5.09%
			19-C-2	135	29.87%
			19-C-4	2	0.44%
BRAVO	236	52.2%			
			19-B-1	236	52.21%
ALPHA	53	11.7%			
			19-A-0	1	0.22%
			19-A-1	52	11.50%

20   HEAT/COLD EXPOSURE   8 incidents   < 1% of all complaints

DETERMINANT LEVEL	INCIDENTS/ LEVEL	PERCENT/ CHIEF COMPLAINT	DETERMINANT CODES	INCIDENTS/ CODE	PERCENT/ CODE
DELTA	2	25.0%			
			20-D-1	2	25.00%
BRAVO	6	75.0%			
			20-B-1	3	37.50%
			20-B-2	3	37.50%

| 21 | HEMORRHAGE/LACERATIONS | | 1,480 incidents | | 4% of all complaints |

DETERMINANT LEVEL	INCIDENTS/ LEVEL	PERCENT/ CHIEF COMPLAINT	DETERMINANT CODES	INCIDENTS/ CODE	PERCENT/ CODE
DELTA	315	21.3%			
			21-D-0	1	0.07%
			21-D-1	273	18.45%
			21-D-2	32	2.16%
			21-D-3	9	0.61%
BRAVO	878	59.3%			
			21-B-1	878	59.32%
ALPHA	287	19.4%			
			21-A-1	287	19.39%

| 22 | INDUSTRIAL/MACHINERY ACCIDENTS | | 43 incidents | | < 1% of all complaints |

DETERMINANT LEVEL	INCIDENTS/ LEVEL	PERCENT/ CHIEF COMPLAINT	DETERMINANT CODES	INCIDENTS/ CODE	PERCENT/ CODE
DELTA	11	25.6%			
			22-D-1	2	4.65%
			22-D-2	9	20.93%
BRAVO	32	74.4%			
			22-B-1	32	74.42%

| 23 | OVERDOSE/INGESTION/POISONING | | 1,502 incidents | | 4% of all complaints |

DETERMINANT LEVEL	INCIDENTS/ LEVEL	PERCENT/ CHIEF COMPLAINT	DETERMINANT CODES	INCIDENTS/ CODE	PERCENT/ CODE
DELTA	140	9.3%			
			23-D-1	125	8.32%
			23-D-2	15	1.00%
CHARLIE	630	41.9%			
			23-C-1	298	19.84%
			23-C-2	62	4.13%
			23-C-3	82	5.46%
			23-C-4	8	0.53%
			23-C-5	5	0.33%
			23-C-6	175	11.65%
BRAVO	709	47.2%			
			23-B-1	709	47.20%
OMEGA	23	1.5%			
			23-Ω-1	23	1.53%

24 PREGNANCY/CHILDBIRTH/MISCARRIAGE   1,150 incidents   3% of all complaints

DETERMINANT LEVEL	INCIDENTS/ LEVEL	PERCENT/ CHIEF COMPLAINT	DETERMINANT CODES	INCIDENTS/ CODE	PERCENT/ CODE
DELTA	298	25.9%			
			24-D-0	1	0.09%
			24-D-1	23	2.00%
			24-D-2	3	0.26%
			24-D-3	128	11.13%
			24-D-4	140	12.17%
			24-D-5	3	0.26%
CHARLIE	55	4.8%			
			24-C-1	55	4.78%
BRAVO	624	54.3%			
			24-B-1	620	53.91%
			24-B-2	4	0.35%
ALPHA	173	15.0%			
			24-A-1	73	6.35%
			24-A-2	100	8.70%

25 PSYCHIATRIC/SUICIDE ATTEMPT   355 incidents   1% of all complaints

DETERMINANT LEVEL	INCIDENTS/ LEVEL	PERCENT/ CHIEF COMPLAINT	DETERMINANT CODES	INCIDENTS/ CODE	PERCENT/ CODE
DELTA	19	5.4%			
			25-D-1	19	5.35%
CHARLIE	172	48.5%			
			25-C-1	9	2.54%
			25-C-2	131	36.90%
			25-C-3	32	9.01%
BRAVO	101	28.5%			
			25-B-1	101	28.45%
ALPHA	63	17.7%			
			25-A-1	63	17.75%

26 SICK PERSON (SPECIFIC DIAGNOSIS)   1,608 incidents   5% of all complaints

DETERMINANT LEVEL	INCIDENTS/ LEVEL	PERCENT/ CHIEF COMPLAINT	DETERMINANT CODES	INCIDENTS/ CODE	PERCENT/ CODE
CHARLIE	314	19.5%			
			26-C-1	189	11.75%
			26-C-2	125	7.77%
BRAVO	625	38.9%			
			26-B-1	625	38.87%
ALPHA	669	41.6%			
			26-A-1	486	30.22%
			26-A-2	183	11.38%

27 STAB/GUNSHOT WOUND — 70 incidents — < 1% of all complaints

DETERMINANT LEVEL	INCIDENTS/ LEVEL	PERCENT/ CHIEF COMPLAINT	DETERMINANT CODES	INCIDENTS/ CODE	PERCENT/ CODE
DELTA	39	55.7%			
			27-D-1	27	38.57%
			27-D-3	2	2.86%
			27-D-4	10	14.29%
BRAVO	31	44.3%			
			27-B-1	10	14.29%
			27-B-3	21	30.00%

28 STROKE (CVA) — 509 incidents — 1% of all complaints

DETERMINANT LEVEL	INCIDENTS/ LEVEL	PERCENT/ CHIEF COMPLAINT	DETERMINANT CODES	INCIDENTS/ CODE	PERCENT/ CODE
CHARLIE	192	37.7%			
			28-C-1	140	27.50%
			28-C-2	52	10.22%
BRAVO	134	26.3%			
			28-B-1	134	26.33%
ALPHA	183	36.0%			
			28-A-1	183	35.95%

29 TRAFFIC ACCIDENTS — 2,713 incidents — 8% of all complaints

DETERMINANT LEVEL	INCIDENTS/ LEVEL	PERCENT/ CHIEF COMPLAINT	DETERMINANT CODES	INCIDENTS/ CODE	PERCENT/ CODE
DELTA	1,921	70.8%			
			29-D-1	1,027	37.85%
			29-D-2	699	25.76%
			29-D-3	5	0.18%
			29-D-4	77	2.84%
			29-D-5	56	2.06%
			29-D-6	53	1.95%
			29-D-7	4	0.15%
BRAVO	787	29.0%			
			29-B-1	787	29.01%
ALPHA	5	0.2%			
			29-A-1	5	0.18%

30   TRAUMATIC INJURIES, SPEFICIC   2,351 incidents   7% of all complaints

DETERMINANT LEVEL	INCIDENTS/ LEVEL	PERCENT/ CHIEF COMPLAINT	DETERMINANT CODES	INCIDENTS/ CODE	PERCENT/ CODE
DELTA	196	8.3%			
			30-D-1	104	4.42%
			30-D-2	4	0.17%
			30-D-3	88	3.74%
BRAVO	1,204	51.2%			
			30-B-1	1,058	45.00%
			30-B-2	146	6.21%
ALPHA	951	40.5%			
			30-A-1	854	36.32%
			30-A-2	97	4.13%

31   UNCONSCIOUS/FAINTING (NON-TRAUMATIC)   2,035 incidents   6% of all complaints

DETERMINANT LEVEL	INCIDENTS/ LEVEL	PERCENT/ CHIEF COMPLAINT	DETERMINANT CODES	INCIDENTS/ CODE	PERCENT/ CODE
DELTA	1,577	77.5%			
			31-D-1	1,206	59.26%
			31-D-2	123	6.04%
			31-D-3	248	12.19%
CHARLIE	283	13.9%			
			31-C-1	108	5.31%
			31-C-2	57	2.80%
			31-C-3	10	0.49%
			31-C-4	41	2.01%
			31-C-5	67	3.29%
ALPHA	175	8.6%			
			31-A-1	175	8.60%

32   UNKNOWN PROBLEM (MAN DOWN)   3,041 incidents   9% of all complaints

DETERMINANT LEVEL	INCIDENTS/ LEVEL	PERCENT/ CHIEF COMPLAINT	DETERMINANT CODES	INCIDENTS/ CODE	PERCENT/ CODE
DELTA	135	4.4%			
			32-D-0	3	0.10%
			32-D-1	132	4.34%
BRAVO	2,906	95.6%			
			32-B-1	1,416	46.56%
			32-B-2	209	6.87%
			32-B-3	1,281	42.12%

9-1-1 Transfers to the
Utah Poison Control Center, 1994

For non-intentional poisonings in children 1 through 11 years of age, the MPDS protocols allow for referral of the telephone call to a poison control center. In 1994, the Utah Poison Control Center (UPCC) evaluated those calls that were referred by Emergency Medical Dispatchers in Utah to the Utah Poison Control Center. The following is a report on those poisoning calls diverted to the UPCC from emergency medical dispatchers.

The UPCC recorded 408 calls transferred from 9-1-1 operators in 1994. Of these, 405 were regarding actual poisoning exposures. The remaining three were information requests only. Of the 405 poisoning exposures, 4 were classified as chronic exposures. The majority of poisonings transferred to the UPCC were managed at home with telephone follow-up.

The following is a summary of the poisoning exposures transferred to the UPCC from emergency medical dispatchers.

Month of Call	Number	Percent
January	32	7.8
February	31	7.6
March	30	7.4
April	26	6.4
May	30	7.4
June	40	9.8
July	37	9.1
August	54	13.2
September	31	7.6
October	33	8.1
November	23	5.6
December	41	10.0
Total	**408**	**100.0**

The distribution of calls transferred from EMDs by month is more variable than all calls to the UPCC in 1994.

County	Number	Percent
Box Elder	2	0.5
Cache	17	4.2
Carbon	1	0.2
Davis	17	4.2
Duchesne	3	0.7
Grand	1	0.2
Iron	3	0.7
Morgan	1	0.2
Piute	1	0.2
Rich	1	0.2
Salt Lake	263	64.5
Summit	3	0.7
Tooele	3	0.7
Uintah	1	0.2
Utah	32	7.8
Wasatch	1	0.2
Washington	18	4.4
Weber	34	8.3
Unknown county	6	1.5
Total	**408**	**100.0**

Compared to all calls to the UPCC in 1994, calls transferred from EMDs were more likely to originate from Salt Lake and Weber Counties.

Caller Location	Number	Percent
Own residence	346	85.4
Other residence	25	6.2
Workplace	12	3.0
Health care facility	1	0.2
School	4	1.0
Public area	3	0.7
Other	13	3.2
Unknown	1	0.2
Total	**405**	**100.0**

Compared to all poisoning exposures reported to the UPCC in 1994, referrals from EMDs were more likely to originate from other residence or other locations.

Reason for Poisoning Exposure

Reason	Number	Percent
Unintentional		
General	274	67.7
Environmental	7	1.7
Occupational	5	1.2
Therapeutic Error	13	3.2
Misuse	14	3.5
Bite/sting	11	2.7
Food poisoning	6	1.5
Subtotal	**330**	**81.5%**
Intentional		
Suicide	48	11.9
Misuse	6	1.5
Abuse	7	1.7
Unknown	2	0.5
Subtotal	**63**	**15.5%**
Other		
Tampering	2	0.5
Malicious	2	0.5
Subtotal	**4**	**1.0%**
Adverse Reaction		
Drug reaction	7	1.7
Food reaction	1	0.2
Subtotal	**8**	**1.9%**
TOTAL	**405**	**100.0**

Compared to all poisoning exposures reported to the UPCC in 1994, calls transferred from emergency medical dispatchers were more likely to be regarding individuals who were attempting suicide.

Age Category by Management Site

Age Category	Managed On-Site #	Managed On-Site %	Referred to HCF #	Referred to HCF %	Total #	Total %
0–11 months	19	76.0	6	24.0	25	6.2
12–23 months	60	75.0	16	20.0	80	19.8
24–35 months	68	74.7	21	23.1	91	22.5
3–5 years	47	87.0	4	7.4	54	13.3
6–12 years	17	89.5	2	10.5	19	4.7
13–19 years	7	25.9	17	63.0	27	6.7
20–59 years	39	41.1	50	52.6	95	23.5
60+ years	5	83.3	1	16.7	6	1.5
Unknown adult	4	50.0	4	50.0	8	2.0
Total	**266**	**65.7**	**121**	**29.9**	**405**	**100.0**

Compared to all poisoning exposures reported to the UPCC in 1994, calls transferred from EMDs were more likely to need medical intervention in a health care facility (HCF). In addition to those referred to a HCF by the UPCC, an additional 13 patients went to a HCF on their own. Of those that were referred by the UPCC to a HCF, 20 refused to go. The disposition of patients managed in a HCF refers to those patients that actually arrived in a HCF and includes those who went in on their own.

Disposition of Patients Managed in a HCF

Disposition	Number	Percent
Treated and released	90	78.9
Admitted to critical care	5	4.4
Admitted to non-critical care	5	4.4
Admitted to a psychiatry unit	8	7.0
Lost to follow-up	6	5.3
Total	**114**	**100.0**

Compared to all poisoning exposures reported to the UPCC in 1994, calls transferred from emergency medical dispatchers were more likely to be treated and released from the emergency department.

Medical Outcome

Outcome	Number	Percent
No effect	167	41.2
Minor effect	158	39.0
Moderate effect	21	5.1
Major effect	1	0.2
Not followed, non-toxic exposure	24	5.9
Not followed minor toxicity expected	5	1.2
Not followed, potentially toxic	16	4.0
Unrelated effect	11	2.7
Confirmed non-exposure	2	0.5
Total	**405**	**100.0**

Compared to all poisoning exposures reported to the UPCC in 1994, calls transferred from emergency medical dispatchers were more likely to minor or moderate effect from the poisoning exposure.

Top Five Substance Categories Involved

Category	Number	Percent
Household Cleaning Substances	63	15.6
Analgesics	51	12.6
Personnel Care Products	36	8.9
Hydrocarbons	24	5.9
Antidepressants	17	4.2
Total	**191**	**47.2**

Summary

Compared to all poisoning exposures reported to the UPCC in 1994, there was a higher rate of exposures to cleaning substances, analgesics, hydrocarbons and antidepressants involved in calls transferred from emergency medical dispatchers.

The Medical Priority Dispatch System's direct transfer process only applies to children 1 to 11 years. There were 242 (59.7%) poisoning exposures in this age group, 93% of whom were between the ages of 1 and 5 years. The most common substances involved in poisonings in this age group included cleaning substances, household (19.0%), cosmetics and personnel care products (12.4%), analgesics (8.3%), hydrocarbons (7.0%) and foreign bodies, toys (3.7%). The majority of poisoning exposures (78.5%) were managed at home with telephone follow-up. All but one exposure was unintentional. The majority of children had no affect (49%) or a minor effect (36%). Four children had a moderate

outcome, in four the outcome was unrelated to the poisoning exposure and in two children it was later discovered that a poisoning had not occurred.

Children less than one-year are excluded from direct referral by the MPDS to a poison control center. In 1994, 25 calls regarding children less than one year old were transferred to the UPCC. Of these, 64% were between the ages of 9-11 months. The most common substance categories involved in exposures included plants (20%), cleaning substances (12.0%), rodenticides (8%) and cosmetics and personal care items (8%). The majority of children were managed at home (76%) with telephone follow-up. No effect was documented in 56%, minor effect in 32%. One child experienced a moderate effect of drowsiness and a positive chest x-ray following the ingestion of a furniture polish. Two children who ingested non-toxic substances and were asymptomatic were not followed.

Individuals 12 years and older accounted for 130 (32.1%) of calls diverted from 911 operators in 1994. The majority of these were female (65%). The reason for poisoning exposure in this age group was unintentional (45.4%), intentional (46.2%), other (2.3%) and adverse effect (6.2%). The majority of this age group was referred to a health care facility for treatment (52.3%). An additional 7 (5.4%) were not referred to a health care facility, but went to one on their own. The most common substance categories involved in poisonings in this age group were analgesics (21.5%), cleaning substances (10.0%), antidepressants (8.5%), alcohols (7.7%), and bites and envenomations (6.2%). The majority of patients in this age group developed a minor effect (45.4%) from the poisoning exposure. In addition, 26.2% developed no effect, 12.3% a moderate effect and one individual developed a major (life-threatening) effect from the exposure. The UPCC was unable to follow-up 7.7% of poisonings which were potentially toxic and 4.6% of outcomes were unrelated to the exposure.

It would be expected that calls to emergency medical dispatchers would be of a more serious nature and may be more likely to need referral to a health care facility. However, a significant portion of those individuals that were diverted to UPCC were managed at home with telephone follow-up. This translates to a significant savings in health care dollars. In addition, emergency medical vehicles can be used for the transport of other seriously ill patients.

Reprinted with permission of the Utah Poison Control Center.

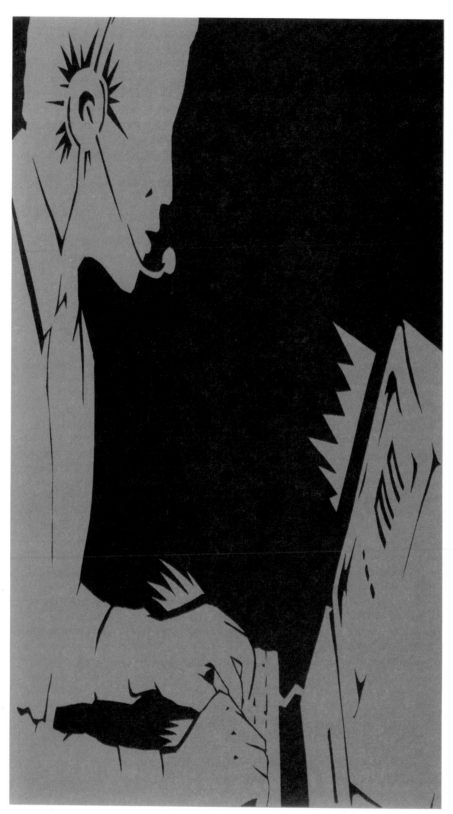

Emergency
Medical
Dispatching:

Rapid
Identification
and Treatment
of Acute
Myocardial
Infarction

U.S. DEPARTMENT OF
HEALTH AND HUMAN
SERVICES

Public Health Service
National Institutes of Health
National Heart, Lung and
Blood Institute

NIH Publication No. 94-3287
July 1994

NATIONAL INSTITUTES OF HEALTH
National Heart, Lung, and Blood Institute

TABLE OF CONTENTS

Coronary heart disease (CHD) continues to be the leading cause of death in the United States despite a remarkable decline in CHD mortality over the last 30 years. The National Heart, Lung, and Blood Institute estimates that as many as 1.25 million people will experience an acute myocardial infarction (AMI) in 1993, and nearly 500,000 will die.

The importance of early treatment has been underscored in the last decade with the results from clinical trials of thrombolytic therapy demonstrating mortality reductions with earlier treatment. Out-of-hospital sudden cardiac death is an ever-present threat, further highlighting the importance of early recognition and treatment.

However, a fundamental barrier to timely treatment is delay—at the level of the patient, the emergency medical services (EMS) system, and the emergency department. In June 1991, the National Heart, Lung, and Blood Institute launched the National Heart Attack Alert Program (NHAAP) with the goal of reducing AMI morbidity and mortality, including sudden cardiac death. The NHAAP Coordinating Committee was formed to help develop, implement, and evaluate the program. This committee is composed of representatives of 39 national scientific, professional, governmental, and voluntary organizations interested in lowering AMI morbidity and mortality through professional, patient, and public education.

The importance of the EMS system for cardiac care has been highlighted in the American Heart Association's recent guidelines for cardiopulmonary resuscitation and emergency cardiac care where early access to EMS is identified as the first link in the chain of survival for cardiac arrest. The chain of survival concept has been expanded to include patients with symptoms and signs of AMI.

Emergency medical dispatching has been recognized as a vital part of the early access link in the chain of survival for cardiac arrest. The potential important role for emergency medical dispatchers (EMD's) in the prehospital care of patients with symptoms and signs of an AMI, as well as patients with cardiac arrest, is the underlying assumption of this paper.

Thus, while emergency medical dispatching is a broader topic than AMI and cardiac arrest, this paper represents a consensus of its potential contribution to the seamless prehospital identification and treatment of patients with AMI, including cardiac arrest, as well as a consensus of the critical issues and recommendations for medical dispatch protocols, processes, training and certification, and quality control and improvement.

Nevertheless, it should be noted that there is a paucity of research related to outcomes associated with emergency medical dispatching. Only through evaluation research can the optimal EMD processes and protocols, associated with specified outcomes, be elucidated.

Claude Lenfant, M.D.
Director
National Heart, Lung, and
Blood Institute

**INTRODUCTION
TO EMERGENCY
MEDICAL
DISPATCHING**

The American Heart Association (AHA) has proposed the concept of a "chain of survival" for victims of cardiac arrest.[1] The chain of survival includes four links, each of which must be robust to ensure maximal survival rates.[2] The components of the chain are:

1. Early access to the emergency medical services (EMS) system

2. Early cardiopulmonary resuscitation (CPR), either by bystanders or first-responder rescuers

3. Early defibrillation by first responders, emergency medical technicians, or paramedics

4. Early advanced life support.

Although the chain of survival was initially conceptualized for cardiac arrest victims, patients with an acute myocardial infarction (AMI) also benefit from the chain-of-survival approach to emergency cardiac care in the community.[3]

The first link of the chain of survival (early access) encompasses several major actions that must occur rapidly. Among these are recognition of the symptoms and signs of the AMI by the patient and bystanders, notification of the EMS system (often by use of the 9-1-1 emergency telephone number), recognition of a cardiac emergency by the medical dispatcher, and activation of available EMS responders. Each action is a part of the early access link.[2]

During the past 15 years, the public has been educated to use the 9-1-1 emergency telephone number to summon help for a range of emergencies, from minor problems to life-threatening conditions.[3,4] The value of the 9-1-1 system is probably increased if there is a qualified professional—the emergency medical dispatcher (EMD)—to process emergency medical calls.[2,5]

An EMD is a trained public safety telecommunicator with the additional training and specific emergency medical knowledge essential for the efficient management of processing 9-1-1* calls and other emergency medical communications.[6] EMD's can perform some important functions that may enhance the efficiency and effectiveness of prehospital care for AMI patients. They can elicit symptoms from callers to determine if a heart attack is possibly occurring[7,8] and activate appropriate EMS responders to deal with the AMI patient.[9] Dispatchers can also provide 9-1-1 callers with instructions for how to care for the possible AMI patient until help arrives—including CPR, if necessary.[7,10-16] Effective emergency medical dispatching has the goal of sending the right EMS resources to the right person, at the right time, in the right way, and providing the right instructions for the care of the patient until help arrives.

This goal can be ideally accomplished through the trained EMD's careful use of a protocol that contains the following elements:[6,17,18]

1. Systematized caller-interrogation questions that are chief-complaint specific

2. Systematized prearrival instructions

---

* or a 7-digit emergency access telephone number in those areas without 9-1-1 service.

3. Protocols that determine vehicle response mode and configuration based on the EMD's evaluation of injury or illness severity

4. Referenced information for dispatcher use.

The impact of well-trained, medically managed EMD's on the early care of potential heart attack victims is believed to be potentially beneficial. Five elements seem to be key to an effective emergency medical dispatch program:

- Use of medical dispatch protocols

- Provision of dispatch life support (see definition below)

- EMD training

- EMD certification

- Emergency medical dispatch quality control and improvement processes.

This paper discusses each of these elements and makes some recommendations for improving emergency medical dispatching in the United States. Local, county, and State governments have a responsibility to ensure that 9-1-1 and emergency medical dispatch centers are staffed by qualified EMD's. This involves including emergency medical dispatching as part of a community's assessment of its EMS needs, and designating resources that are indicated, to serve the welfare of its citizens.

Two documents on emergency medical dispatching that have been developed by nationally authoritative agencies are:

ISSUES AND RECOMMENDATIONS FOR EMERGENCY MEDICAL DISPATCHING

- The ASTM's "Standard Practice for Emergency Medical Dispatch"[6]
- The National Association of EMS Physicians' (NAEMSP) position paper, "Emergency Medical Dispatching."[17]

The recommendations set forth in these documents are believed to be appropriate, and all EMS systems are encouraged to implement them as much as possible. Rather than repeating or superceding the points made in those documents, this paper addresses emergency medical dispatching issues with an emphasis on care of the AMI patient and reiterates the recommendations that are relevant for an emergency medical dispatching system to effectively handle the AMI patient.

The ASTM is also currently developing two additional documents on emergency medical dispatching. It is anticipated that these standards will parallel many of the recommendations contained in this paper. These documents are:

- The ASTM F-1552 "Standard Practice for Training, Instructor Qualification and Certification Eligibility of Emergency Medical Dispatchers"[19]
- The ASTM F-1560 "Standard Practice for Emergency Medical Dispatch Management."[20]

It should be noted that few well-constructed, objective, published studies exist that address the components or the effectiveness of components of emergency medical dispatching. This is in large part due to the difficulty in defining, as well as determining, those patient outcomes or improvements in patient conditions that are a result of emergency medical dispatching. The patient's condition can deteriorate during the time it takes a prehospital provider to arrive at the scene. Outcome parameters based on the EMS personnel's initial patient findings are not well defined for most prehospital problems other than cardiac arrest and critical trauma. To guarantee that outcomes actually result from the use of a given protocol, a study must demonstrate high compliance to that protocol by the dispatchers. Studies must clearly identify the exact protocol or specific part of the protocol that is undergoing evaluation. The need for further studies regarding the training and retraining, quality control and improvement of EMD's, and the benefit and optimum configuration of prehospital EMD protocols is a general recommendation of this paper.

Medical Dispatch Protocols

Effective EMD practice is based on the consistent use of medically approved dispatch protocols. These protocols are a written system of procedures for the evaluation of, response to, and provision of care to emergency patients.[13] A written dispatch protocol system directs the EMD to complete a chief-complaint-specific, preplanned interrogation of the 9-1-1 caller to accurately assess and act on the medical emergency.[6] A dispatch protocol requires the EMD to interrogate the caller to identify the demographics, characteristics, and general medical problem of the patient and to determine the status of consciousness and breathing. This is followed, when appropriate, by a more specific systematized interrogation related to the reported general medical problem, selected by the EMD from among protocol choices that cover all possible presenting medical emergencies. Systematized interrogation is an essential component of a comprehensive medical dispatch protocol, even for those systems not prioritizing between advanced life support (ALS) and basic life support (BLS) calls.[5]

The dispatcher interrogation process has four important purposes:

1. Provide the EMD with the information needed to make a correct decision regarding initial unit response, including type of EMS personnel required and use of lights and siren

2. Enable the EMD to determine the presence of conditions or situations requiring prearrival instructions

3. Enable the EMD to provide responders with prearrival information for planning of, and preparation for, on-scene patient care activities

4. Assist in ensuring the safety of the patient, the responders, the caller, and other bystanders.

Use of a medical dispatch protocol helps the EMD to avoid making a faulty "diagnosis" of the medical emergency and incorrect dispatching decisions. When EMD's fail to use medical dispatch protocols, they may be prone to make an assessment of the situation based on inadequate information. The EMD may fail to identify the patient's chief complaint and, therefore, may provide inadequate response or advice. EMS literature provides many examples of the adverse outcomes and legal problems arising from such faulty dispatch practices.[21,22]

The issue of patient and bystander denial of or inability to recognize heart attack symptoms is commonly encountered at dispatch.[13]

Medical dispatch protocols should include standardized response classifications based on the EMD's structured assessment of the medical urgency of the incident and indicate the level of EMS response needed. These response classifications should be based on recognized medical symptoms and the type of incident.[9,23-25] In systems that vary levels of response, dispatch protocols should specify which situations require an ALS versus a BLS response. This is important in those EMS systems that are "tiered" and allow rapid response by a level of EMS personnel appropriate for the seriousness of the emergency as determined by the EMD (e.g., ALS personnel are dispatched for life-threatening emergencies). Medical dispatch protocols may also specify which situations require a lights-and-siren response to the scene and which do not. With EMS vehicle-related accidents in the United States reported to have been 2,400 for ambulances in 1990,[26] it is medically unsound and managerially unsafe to require lights-and-siren response on all incidents.[27-29]

Response classifications will vary from one EMS system to another based on the type of system resources, response limitations, traffic patterns, and geography of their service areas. Response configurations often become more complex for larger or more sophisticated systems.[23-25] It must be stressed that decisions regarding response assignments are a responsibility of medical management and should be subject to the approval of the medical director of an EMS system.[6,11,12]

Ideally, standardized response classifications should be based on a uniform coding system. This would assist in consistency of use, statistical comparison, and scientific research across EMS systems that use the same medical dispatch protocols.[9]

The non-English-speaking caller poses an ever-increasing challenge for many dispatch centers, especially those in large urban centers. This issue has three basic solutions: 1) sufficient staffing of EMD's with multilingual capability where a center's constituency has demonstrated frequent use of a particular language or languages other than English; 2) secure access to a language-interpreting service such as that provided by one of the major long distance carriers; and 3) provision of medical dispatch protocols in commonly encountered languages. At the time of publication of this paper, alternate language versions of protocols used in the United States are available in Spanish, French, and German.

It is recommended that emergency medical dispatch protocols:

- Be medically approved

- Be uniform throughout each EMS jurisdiction

- Use standard response classification codes to facilitate scientific comparison and study among systems using the same protocols

- Be followed consistently and nonarbitrarily by all EMD's, except when additional clarification is needed

- Delineate the types of cases requiring an ALS versus a BLS response (especially in tiered systems) and the types of cases requiring use of lights and siren from those that do not.

Dispatch Life Support

Dispatch life support encompasses the knowledge, procedures, and skills used by trained EMD's to provide care through prearrival instructions to callers. It consists of those BLS and ALS principles that are appropriate for application by EMD's. Dispatch life support forms the basis for establishing the content and application methodology for prearrival instructions used by medical dispatchers.[30] The NAEMSP[17] has also defined dispatch life support (see the definitions that follow).

Prearrival instructions differ from the less well-specified telephone aid, and the differences between them form the basis of recommendations for standardization of EMD training and practice (including dispatch life support):

Prearrival Instructions. Prearrival instructions are medically approved, written instructions given by trained EMD's to callers that help provide necessary assistance to the victim and control of the situation prior to the arrival of EMS personnel. Prearrival instructions are read word for word by the EMD to the fullest extent possible.

The necessity to routinely provide prearrival instructions has been addressed by the NAEMSP: "Pre-arrival instructions are a mandatory function of each EMD in a medical dispatch center. . . .Standard medically approved telephone instructions by trained EMD's are safe to give and in many instances are a moral necessity."[17] The failure to provide prearrival instructions, when possible and appropriate, is currently being litigated in the Nation's courts as a form of dispatcher negligence. It is interesting to note that one of the most significant obstacles to the establishment of prearrival instructions, and medical dispatch protocol systems in general, has been the notion that agencies can be successfully sued for engaging in such activities. It appears that there has never been a dispatcher negligence lawsuit filed for the provision of medically sound prearrival instructions. There are a significant number of lawsuits recently completed or in progress for which the omission of prearrival instructions (or "dispatcher abandonment," as the legal terminology describes it) has been alleged.

The nature of prearrival instructions is such that they must be provided in a timely manner, over the telephone, and without the benefit of practice or visual verifications. Thus, it is important that EMD's carefully adhere to protocols for the provision of telephone-instructed treatment in a standard, nonarbitrary, and reproducible way.

Box 1. Application of Emergency Medical Dispatching Principles to the Patient With Suspected AMI and Cardiac Arrest

Emergency medical dispatching principles, as operationalized in medical dispatch protocols and prearrival instructions, can be readily applied to the potential AMI and cardiac arrest patient. For all patients, key questions are asked as to whether the patient is reported to be unconscious and not breathing to ascertain if a cardiac arrest has occurred. For example, the answer "I'm not sure" regarding breathing status given by a second-party caller (someone who can see or easily access the patient) is assumed to mean "no"; therefore, a maximal response, preferably ALS/paramedics, would be sent immediately. The key questions, then, also determine the most appropriate level of response. If a cardiac arrest has been verified, first responders can be given the chief complaint, approximate age, the status of consciousness and breathing, and the dispatch response code, facilitating preparation for possible use of an automated external defibrillator. Prearrival instructions in the case of a cardiac arrest would entail dispatcher-assisted CPR.

For a patient with chest pain, additional dispatcher interactions with the caller are recommended to overcome caller or patient denial or to validate that the caller's descriptions of symptoms and signs may represent the presentation of a heart attack. Specifically, the dispatcher may ask the caller if the patient has severe indigestion; tightness; heavy pressure; constricting band and crushing discomfort in the chest with the spread of these feelings to the arms, jaw, neck, or back; as well as the presence of nausea or sweating. Verification of these symptoms directs the dispatcher to advise the responders so that their functions at the scene can be expedited. Prearrival instructions in these cases would include correct positioning of the patient, instructions for vomiting, and instructions to monitor very closely and to call back if the patient's condition worsens.

Telephone Aid.

Telephone aid, as defined herein, consists of "ad libbed" instructions provided by either trained or untrained EMD's. Telephone aid differs from dispatch life support in that the instructions provided to the caller are based on the dispatcher's previous training in a procedure or treatment but are provided without following a scripted prearrival instruction protocol. This method exists because either no protocols are used in the medical dispatch center or protocol adherence is not required by policy and procedure (e.g., the dispatcher is "trained" in CPR and thus describes to the caller, to the best of his or her verbal ability, how to do CPR).

As noted in the section (above) on prearrival instructions, dispatchers must carefully adhere to written protocols.

Unfortunately, coupled with a growing interest and effort within public safety agencies to provide some type of telephone instructions to callers, many agencies are "allowing" dispatchers to ad lib instructions. There appears to be a significant difference between dispatch life support-based prearrival instructions and telephone aid. Telephone aid, as defined, may only ensure that the dispatcher has attempted to provide some sort of care to the patient through the caller but does not ensure that such care is correct, standard, and medically effective or even necessary in the first place.

Telephone aid often causes the following predictable errors:

1. Failure to correctly identify conditions requiring telephone intervention and therefore prearrival instructions in the first place (e.g., "saving" an infant having a febrile seizure who was incorrectly identified as needing CPR due to failure to follow protocols that are medically designed to verify need—verify breathing, pulse, etc., before potentially dangerous dispatcher-invasive treatments such as compressions are initiated).

2. Failure to accurately identify the presence of interim symptoms and signs (or the lack of them) during the in-progress provision of telephone intervention (e.g., dispatchers who ad lib CPR sequences often miss important patient verifiers that cannot be seen by the dispatcher, such as watching for the chest to rise).

3. Failure to perform (describe or teach) multistep procedures, such as CPR care, in a consistent and reproducible fashion regardless of which dispatcher in a center provides such help (e.g., quality assurance review of these types of cases often reveals that dispatchers in the same center [or even the same dispatcher] perform care differently each time if they are not following scripted prearrival instruction protocols closely).

Telephone aid, as defined, often provides only the illusion of correct help via telephone without predictably ensuring consistent and accurate instructions to all callers. Telephone aid, therefore, is usually considered an inappropriate and unreliable form of dispatcher-provided medical care.

Medical dispatch practice must be safe, competent, and effective. The systematic use of medically preapproved protocols will help to ensure that the dispatcher performance is structured and reproducible and can be objectively measured.

In light of the important differences between prearrival instructions and telephone aid, and to improve standardization of EMD training and practice, it is recommended that:

- Dispatch life support be adopted nationwide as an essential concept of emergency medical dispatch

- Dispatch life support be standardized

- Prearrival instructions be provided from written protocol scripts for all medical emergencies.

Medical Dispatcher Training

Formal EMD training contributes to the safe and effective performance of the medical dispatcher's role in EMS.[11]

Guidelines for the core content of EMD courses are currently being standardized by the ASTM.[19] These guidelines will provide direction for the training (and certification) of EMD's regarding appropriate decisions about EMS responses in a safe, consistent, and nonarbitrary manner. Within the context of this broad goal, current EMD training is generally at least 24 hours in length (e.g., three 8-hour days). A typical course consists of an overview of dispatching objectives and basic dispatch techniques, concentrating on known problem areas.

The role of the EMD is defined, and the concepts of medical dispatching are discussed in detail. The medical dispatch protocol in use by the sponsoring EMS agency is learned, with emphasis on interrogation skills, protocol compliance, and the provision of prearrival instructions. Common medical problems are reviewed, with an emphasis on interrogation specifics for each type of problem, and the relevance and relationship of listed prearrival instructions. Throughout the training, the importance of identifying the presence or absence of symptoms (such as "chest pain") during interrogation is emphasized, rather than making a judgmental diagnosis of "heart attack." The medical significance of the various levels of urgency for each chief complaint and its resultant response is clarified to give the student the ability to prioritize quickly the various types of incidents confronting EMD's daily. Often, courses use mock case drills to give the dispatcher a hands-on feel of protocol performance.

A formal examination to test student understanding and assimilation of the curriculum should be administered at the completion of an EMD course. This enables formal certification in jurisdictions requiring or allowing it.[6,17,31]

It is recommended that EMD training:

- Be required of all medical dispatchers

- Be consistent in core curriculum content nationally

- Be based on the medical dispatch protocol selected and approved by the sponsoring agency's physician medical director, allowing for practice use of the protocol by the EMD trainee.

Medical Dispatcher Certification

Given the very important role of the dispatcher in the chain of survival, certification should become governmentally mandated throughout the United States.[6,17,31]

Certification should include requirements for continuing education and recertification. Continuing education programs should incorporate formal written and practical tests. Continuing education and recertification allow EMS agencies to formally promote and ensure the ongoing quality of EMD performance. Certification also establishes processes for decertifying individuals who cannot meet minimum standards. There have been no studies to determine the optimal frequency or process of recertification; therefore, expert panels have recommended that EMD's should be recertified every 2 to 4 years.[6] At least 12 hours per year of continuing education should be required for EMD recertification.[20,31]

It is recommended that EMD certification:

- Be required of all EMD's through either State government processes or professional medical dispatch standard-setting organizations

- Require continuing education and recertification as components of a continuing certification process.

Medical Dispatch Quality Control and Improvement

Each EMS system should have in place a comprehensive quality improvement program. Four goals in the quality control and improvement of medical dispatch activities are that:

1. Dispatchers understand medical dispatch policy, protocol, and practice

2. Dispatchers comply with medical dispatch policy, protocol, and practice

3. Deficiencies in understanding and compliance with medical dispatch policy, protocol, and practice among dispatchers be corrected

4. Medical dispatch policy, protocols, and practice be updated on a continuous basis to ensure that they are appropriate and effective.

A comprehensive quality control and improvement system for emergency medical dispatching has several components. Among these are selection of personnel; orientation; initial training; certification and recertification; continuing dispatch education; physician medical direction; data generation; case review and performance evaluation; correction of performance problems (risk management); and decertification, suspension, or termination.[32] These components of medical dispatcher quality improvement are essential for maintaining the type of employment environment necessary to ensure safe and effective patient evaluation and care.

One of the most important areas of quality control/improvement is that of case review and performance evaluation.[32] Between 7 and 10 percent of each EMD's cases should be randomly reviewed.[20] The review of random cases ensures that each dispatcher's current practice (especially compliance with protocol) is determined.[33] In addition, the review of out-of-the-ordinary cases (both excellent and problematic) is important. These cases are often identified by sources external to the dispatch center. The involvement of EMS field personnel in reporting incidents that appear to represent dispatch-related problems can be very helpful in strengthening the performance and policy evaluation process.

These case reviews should serve as the basis for periodic dispatcher performance evaluation. The cumulative level of compliance to protocol of each medical dispatcher should be evaluated and compared with preset levels of acceptable practice. This provides an objective method of establishing thresholds of performance for these essential members of the EMS team. Corrective steps may include continuing education or disciplinary action.

In the absence of adequate case review and performance evaluation, it has been shown that dispatcher compliance to protocol deteriorates and is generally under 50 percent.[34]

Medical direction is an essential element in the overall assurance of quality performance of EMD's. Just as medical direction is uniformly recommended for emergency medical technicians and paramedics, the EMD requires careful attention and guidance. According to the NAEMSP, "The medical aspects of emergency medical dispatching and communications are an integral part of the responsibilities of the Medical Director of an EMS system. . . .Quality Improvement, Risk Management, and Medical Control and Direction are essential elements to the management of medical dispatch operations within the EMS system."[17]

It is recommended that ongoing medical dispatch quality control and improvement processes:

- Be in place for all medical dispatch centers
- Allow for random review of cases
- Require high-level compliance to protocol as a major factor in dispatcher performance evaluation
- Be the basis of dispatcher reeducation, feedback, discipline, and medical management
- Be carried out under the medical direction of a qualified physician.

SUMMARY

The EMD is a key member of the EMS team. EMD's may have a profound effect on the early care of potential heart attack victims. To ensure optimal emergency medical dispatching, this paper has made a number of recommendations, which are highlighted below:

- Each EMS system should utilize a set of written, medically approved dispatching protocols for the evaluation of, response to, and provision of care to the AMI patient. These protocols should be followed consistently and nonarbitrarily by all EMD's.

- Dispatch life support should be provided by each EMS system. EMD's should be required to use medically approved, written prearrival instructions to help callers provide aid to the AMI patient and control the situation prior to the arrival of EMS personnel.

- Every EMD should be formally trained, based on a nationally consistent core curriculum, with an emphasis on mastery of the dispatching protocol used by the sponsoring EMS agency.

- Certification should be required of all EMD's, either through State governments or professional medical dispatch standard-setting organizations. This process should also mandate continuing education and recertification.

- Every EMS system should have in place a system of continuous quality improvement for medical dispatching. This should include a random review of each EMD's cases. Periodic performance evaluations should be conducted with each EMD, with emphasis on the EMD's adherence to dispatching protocol.

- All aspects of emergency medical dispatching should be the ultimate responsibility of the EMS physician who provides medical direction for a given EMS system. That is, an EMS physician should be in an authoritative position to manage the medical care components of an EMD program, including overseeing training, selecting and approving dispatch protocols and prearrival instructions, and evaluating the EMD system.

These recommendations, if implemented, may result in improvement of emergency medical dispatching in general—and potentially better identification and treatment of patients with symptoms and signs of AMI, in particular.

1. Cummins RO, Ornato JP, Thies WH, Pepe PE. Improving survival from sudden cardiac arrest: the "chain of survival" concept. A statement for health professionals from the Advanced Cardiac Life Support Subcommittee and the Emergency Cardiac Care Committee, American Heart Association. Circulation 1991;83(5):1832-47.

2. American Heart Association, Emergency Cardiac Care Committee and Subcommittees. Guidelines for cardiopulmonary resuscitation and emergency cardiac care, II: adult basic life support. JAMA 1992;268(16):2184-98.

3. Becker LB, Pepe PE. Ensuring the effectiveness of community-wide emergency cardiac care. Ann Emerg Med 1993;22(2):354-64.

4. Roberts BG. EMS dispatching: its use and misuse. Dallas Fire Department internal report, 1978.

5. Cocks RA, Glucksman E. What does London need from its ambulance service? Br Med J 1993;306:1428-9.

6. American Society for Testing and Materials (ASTM). F 1258-90, Standard practice for emergency medical dispatch. In: Annual book of ASTM standards. Vol. 13.01, Medical Devices. Philadelphia: ASTM; 1991.

7. Clawson JJ. The hysteria threshold: gaining control of the emergency caller. J Emerg Med Serv 1986;11(8):40.

8. Eisenberg MS, Carter W, Hallstrom A, Cummins R, Litwin P, Hearne T. Identification of cardiac arrest by emergency dispatchers. Am J Emerg Med 1986;4(4):299-301.

9. Clawson JJ. Medical priority dispatch—it works. J Emerg Med Serv 1983;8(2):29-33.

10. Carter WB, Eisenberg MS, Hallstrom AP, Schaeffer S. Development and implementation of emergency CPR instruction via telephone. Ann Emerg Med 1984;13(Pt 1):695-700.

11. Clawson JJ. Dispatch priority training: strengthening the weak link. J Emerg Med Serv 1981;6(2):32-6.

12. Clawson JJ. Telephone treatment protocols: reach out and help someone. J Emerg Med Serv 1986;11(6):43-6.

13. Clawson JJ, Dernocoeur KB. Principles of emergency medical dispatch. Englewood Cliffs (NJ): Brady/Prentice Hall; 1988. 352 p.

14. Culley LL, Clark JJ, Eisenberg MS, Larsen MP. Dispatcher-assisted telephone CPR: common delays and time standards for delivery. Ann Emerg Med 1991;20(4):362-6.

15. Valenzuela T, Spaite D, Clark D, Meislin H, Sayre R. Estimated cost-effectiveness of dispatcher CPR instruction via telephone to bystanders during out-of-hospital ventricular fibrillation. Prehospital Disaster Med 1992;7(3):229-34.

16. Kellermann AL, Hackman BB, Somer G. Dispatcher-assisted cardiopulmonary resuscitation. Validation of efficacy. Circulation 1989;80:1231-9.

REFERENCES

17. National Association of Emergency Medical Services Physicians. Emergency medical dispatching [position paper]. Prehospital Disaster Med 1989;4(2):163-6.

18. Clawson JJ. Emergency medical dispatching. In: Roush WR, editor. Principles of EMS systems: a comprehensive text for physicians. Dallas: American College of Emergency Physicians; 1989;119-33.

19. American Society for Testing and Materials (ASTM). F-1552, Standard practice for training, instructor qualification and certification eligibility of emergency medical dispatchers. September 1994.

20. American Society for Testing and Materials (ASTM). F-1560, Standard practice for emergency medical dispatch management. September 1994.

21. Adams R. Lessons learned from Dallas. Firehouse 1984; May:12-4.

22. Clawson JJ. Priority dispatching after Dallas: another viewpoint. J Emerg Med Serv 1984;9(5):36-7.

23. Curka PA, Pepe PE, Ginger VF, Sherrard RC. Computer-aided EMS priority dispatch: ability of a computerized triage system to safely spare paramedics from responses not requiring advanced life support [abstract]. Ann Emerg Med 1991;20(4):446.

24. Kallsen G, Nabors MD. The use of priority medical dispatch to distinguish between high- and low-risk patients [abstract]. Ann Emerg Med 1990;19(4):458-9.

25. Stratton SJ. Triage by emergency medical dispatchers. Prehospital Disaster Med 1992;7(3):263-9.

26. National Safety Council. Accident facts. 1992 edition. p. 78,79.

27. Auerbach PS, Morris JA Jr, Phillips JB Jr, Redlinger SR, Vaughn WK. An analysis of ambulance accidents in Tennessee. JAMA 1987;258:1487-90.

28. Clawson JJ. The red-light-and-siren response. J Emerg Med Serv 1981;6(2):34-5.

29. Kupas DF, Jula DJ, Pino BJ. Patient outcome using medical protocol to limit "red lights and siren" transport [abstract]. J Emerg Med Serv/ Prehospital Care Forum 1993;18(3 Suppl):S-9.

30. Clawson JJ, Hauert SA. Dispatch life support: establishing standards that work. J Emerg Med Serv 1990;15(7):82-8.

31. Clawson JJ. Regulations and standards for emergency medical dispatchers: a model for state or region. Emerg Med Serv 1984;13(4):25-9.

32. Clawson JJ. Quality assurance: a priority for medical dispatch. Emerg Med Serv 1989;18(7):53-62.

33. Clawson JJ. Medical dispatch review: "run" review for the EMD. J Emerg Med Serv 1986;11(10):40-2.

34. Clawson JJ. Six month status report with evaluations and recommendations for the comprehensive medical priority dispatch system of the Los Angeles City Fire Department. Salt Lake City: Medical Priority Consultants, Inc; December 27, 1990. 21 p.

EMERGENCY MEDICAL DISPATCH FOR CHILDREN

WHERE ARE WE AND WHERE DO WE GO?

On June 16-17, 1998 a distinguished panel of Emergency Medical Dispatch (EMD) experts met in Washington, D.C. to discuss emergency medical dispatch for children. The meeting was jointly sponsored by the Emergency Medical Services for Children Program of the Health Resources and Services Administration (HRSA), the National Highway Traffic Safety Administration (NHTSA), and the Georgia Department of Human Resources, Office of Emergency Medical Services. The purpose of the gathering was to solicit expert opinion on the current status of EMD for children and directions for further development.

Objectives

The objective of this meeting was to consolidate the experiences of a number of nationally recognized EMD experts, together with data from a recent survey conducted by the Georgia Office of EMS, to address a number of questions about the ability of the nation's EMD system to respond to the needs of children. Specifically, the questions posed to the group included:

- Is our current EMD system capable of responding appropriately to 9-1-1 calls made by children and 9-1-1 calls about a sick or injured child?

- Is there a need for a specific pediatric dispatch card set?

- What are the greatest needs for further improvement of the nation's EMD system?

- What are the barriers to further development of the EMD system?

The Experts

The panel of EMD experts included pediatric emergency physicians, EMD educators, producers of EMD programs and card sets, representatives of the American Society for Testing and Materials, members of the National Academy of Emergency Medical Dispatch, and Federal and state program representatives.

Background and Significance

Organized emergency medical dispatch is a recent phenomenon in the United States. Twenty years ago less than 20 percent of the nation's population was covered by the emergency access system that we take for granted today—the 9-1-1 system. Today, nearly 90 percent of the nation is covered by this life-saving link to emergency care. And over these 20 years, our emergency access and dispatch system has grown as much in sophistication as it has in coverage. HRSA and NHTSA recognize that access and dispatch are the first links in the chain of emergency response and that the strength of our EMS system is dependent on rapid access to a skilled emergency medical dispatcher. This is especially true in responding to emergencies involving children, where special accommodations and skills may be needed to prevent or reduce a tragedy.

One of the first steps toward national recognition of the criticality of EMD was the development of a dispatcher training program for emergency medical technicians in 1976 by NHTSA. This was revised in 1983 and published as the *Emergency Medical Dispatch: National Standard Curriculum.*[1] During this same period, cities such as Phoenix, Arizona and Salt Lake City, Utah, began to develop structured protocol systems for providing pre-arrival information to callers requesting emergency medical assistance. The field grew rapidly in the early 1980s and in many locales, emergency medical services, and specifically emergency medical dispatch, joined fire and police services in the 9-1-1 public safety program.

The national consistency provided by the NHTSA *Emergency Medical Dispatch: National Standard Curriculum* was augmented in 1994 by the introduction of the American Society for Testing and Materials (ASTM) national standard for EMD programs. These standards were the product of the ASTM Committee on Emergency Medical Services (ASTM Committee F-30).[2]

Medical protocols were introduced to the EMD system early in its development. These commonly took the form of a structured set of reference cards for the dispatcher. Several proprietary card sets have been developed, addressing the 32 commonly occurring complaints

[1]*Emergency Medical Dispatch: National Standard Curriculum: Government Printing Office*
[2]*Annual Book of ASTM Standards, Vol 13.01*

EMERGENCY MEDICAL DISPATCH FOR CHILDREN

identified in the *Emergency Medical Dispatch: National Standard Curriculum*. In addition, local systems have developed and employed additional protocols to meet local needs.

Survey on Pediatric Emergency Medical Dispatch

With support from the HRSA Emergency Medical Services for Children (EMSC) program, the Georgia Office of EMS conducted a national survey of public service emergency communications directors to learn more about the current status of pediatric EMD.

This survey was conducted in 1997 to provide basic information about the perceptions of local system administrators concerning their capability to respond to pediatric emergencies. The surveys were sent to the Emergency Medical Services Director in each state and achieved a 50 percent response rate, with 25 of the 50 states completing the survey instrument. The survey contained four statements about the comfort level of communications officers in responding to calls from or concerning children:

■ Agencies in 17 of 25 states (68%) "Strongly Agreed" or "Agreed" that their communications officers were comfortable dealing with adults calling for medical help concerning adult patients.

■ Agencies in 17 of 25 states (68%) also "Strongly Agreed" or "Agreed" that their communications officers were comfortable dealing with adults calling for medical help concerning child patients.

■ Four agencies "Strongly Agreed" and 10 "Agreed" (56%) that their communications officers were comfortable dealing with children calling for medical help concerning adult patients.

■ Agencies in 10 states "Strongly Agreed"

or "Agreed" (40%) that their communications officers would feel comfortable dealing with children calling for medical help concerning child patients.

A majority of respondents also agreed with the following statements:

"A pediatric dispatch system designed to assist communications officers with injured or ill children in need of medical assistance would be of value to (their) system."

"A pediatric dispatch system designed to assist communications officers with child callers needing help for themselves or others would be of value to (their) system."

These findings suggest that while administrators feel that their communications officers are comfortable dealing with adult callers, they feel that their officers are much less comfortable when dealing with child callers. The cause of this concern appears to be centered not on the age of the emergent victim, but on the age of the caller. Not surprisingly, respondents also felt that technical assistance would be useful both for improving skills in handling cases involving pediatric victims, and for developing greater competence in handling child callers.

Expert Considerations and Recommendations

? *Is our current EMD system capable of responding appropriately to 9-1-1 calls made by children and 9-1-1 calls about a sick or injured child?*

Expert Opinion:

Consistent with the findings of the pediatric dispatch survey, the expert panel generally felt that the current system is adequately addressing the special dispatch needs related to children. The group emphatically recognized the criticality of accommodating the needs of children, citing a recent unpublished study by New York University Medical Center which focuses on the role of EMD on the out-

comes of pediatric patients and includes information on the influence of EMD on system resource utilization.

Specific comments from the group included:

"No one has been able to identify a pediatric problem to fix; EMD is working for children."

"I am not aware of a problem with the card sets, a pediatric-related inadequacy with them, or changes that would better facilitate pediatric care."

"We have heard nothing so far to suggest that there is a problem with the way EMD functions for children, no data, no stories, not even innuendo."

While expressing some confidence that the current system appears to adequately address the needs of children, the expert panel also stressed that continuous improvement in this area is critical. The panel also recommended that research be conducted to further assess the efficacy of pediatric EMD and offered a commitment to examine any evidence of problems that might arise.

? *Is there a need for a specific pediatric dispatch card set?*

Expert Opinion:

The question of the need for a specific pediatric dispatch card set elicited a strong response from the expert panel. The experts generally believed that the currently available card sets covering 32 common medical complaints are adequately meeting pediatric needs.

The panel felt that ongoing refinement of the protocol is necessary, and one expert pointed out that there have been 12 revisions to the National Academy of Emergency Medical Dispatch (NAEMD) protocols over the past 19 years to keep them current with state-of-the-art practice.[3] However, the group felt that developing an additional set of cards without specific

---

[3]*Medical Priority Dispatch System, 10.3, Salt Lake City, Utah*

EMERGENCY MEDICAL DISPATCH FOR CHILDREN

evidence of need, might unnecessarily complicate the protocols and result in a net negative effect on system performance. The panel also expressed a willingness to consider change or the addition of specific pediatric cards if any problems with EMD for children are identified.

? *What are the greatest needs for further improvement of the Nation's EMD system?*

Expert Opinion:

The expert panel identified two priority needs for further improvement of the EMD system. These relate to the consistency of local adherence to established protocols and the utilization of a continuous quality improvement program. The group pointed out that national standards have been developed to identify the essential elements of an effective EMD system. The ASTM Standard for EMD Management is explicit in calling for:

"...a comprehensive plan for managing the quality of care in the emergency medical dispatch system (that) must include careful planning, EMD program selection, proper system implementation, employee selection, training, certification, QA/QI, performance evaluation, continuing dispatch education, re-certification, and risk management activities..."[4]

The experts stressed that the overall quality of the national EMD system is dependent on the manner and degree to which these voluntary standards are implemented across the nation. Panelists felt that current implementation is highly variable. It was the observation of one participant that as few as 10 percent of EMD systems are fully and rigorously adhering to all EMD policies, practices, procedures, and protocols, and have a continuous quality improvement system in place that actively monitors and assesses a statistically significant percentage of EMD calls.

? *What are the barriers to further development of the EMD system?*

Expert Opinion:

The expert panel felt that one of the most serious barriers to further progress in EMD is a widespread assumption that strict adherence to standards is unnecessary. That is, system administrators and the communities they serve may believe that because they have adopted some of the elements of the EMD standard, they have adequately addressed this part of their system. Panelists felt that this false confidence may be preventing many system administrators from allocating sufficient attention and resources to EMD. The experts stressed that system administrators and the public need to be reminded of the importance of a comprehensive EMD system that adheres to the consensus-developed protocols and includes an effective continuous quality improvement program.

Another area for improvement identified by the expert panel is EMD training. The panel felt that while the *Emergency Medical Dispatch: National Standard Curriculum* has been widely accepted as the basic EMD training standard, its local application is variable. The experts felt that, in general, more attention needs to be directed at EMD training nationwide, and further, that the most appropriate way to identify specific local training needs is through an effective continuous quality improvement program.

Specific comments from the group included:

"Training and the purchase of cards are little more than events in the life of communications and dispatch."

"If you do not have a QI program in place assessing 3-5 percent of calls, you are not adhering to protocol. Not only must you create the protocol, you must see that it is followed."

Summary

The expert panel gathered to provide insights on the current status of EMD for children and directions for further development of EMD. The panel offered the following observations and recommendations:

- The expert panel believes that in general, the EMD system now in place across the country is meeting the needs of children.

- The panel recommends that maintaining adequate coverage for children and the community at-large will require an ongoing commitment to continuous quality improvement, research, and training.

- Based on available evidence, the panel does not believe that a specific pediatric dispatch card set is needed or appropriate.

- The panel believes that further research and continuous quality improvement is needed to determine if any problems with EMD for children might exist. The panel recommends that any evidence of problems be thoroughly addressed.

- The expert panel believes that the effectiveness of EMD across the nation is currently limited by variation in local implementation. The panel recommends that system administrators and the public be reminded of the criticality of a comprehensive EMD system, that conforms to national consensus standards.

- The panel recommends that local systems implement effective continuous quality improvement programs to identify performance problems, training needs, and areas for system refinement.

- The panel recommends that EMD training be more consistently implemented across the country.

[4]*Annual Book of ASTM Standards, Vol 13.01, F1560-94*

EMERGENCY MEDICAL DISPATCH FOR CHILDREN

Consensus Statement

A consensus position statement was prepared by the expert panel. The statement sets the stage for important and continued work that the panel believes needs to be pursued to maintain and improve the quality of the national EMD system.

We believe that appropriate emergency care for the Nation's children should be among the highest priority of those issues currently affecting our public safety medical dispatch systems. A major threat to children (and indeed to all 9-1-1 emergency callers) is the failure of public safety communications centers to implement and utilize medically approved, standardized protocols that clearly delineate the evaluation, dispatch services, information, and pre-arrival instructions provided to callers. This means that compliance to these protocols should be enforced. Only with continuous evaluative case review of EMD performance in dealing with children both as callers and patients will the definitive issues regarding children's special health needs and treatment issues be better understood and dealt with by medical dispatch protocol and training standards organizations.

The content of the protocols can only be assessed when correctly used and when cases are carefully monitored and evaluated by qualified medical personnel. This information is vital to determine whether the current content of these protocols meets the needs of the Nation's children. The content of these protocols must be reviewed by expertly staffed standards groups that contain public safety experts and physicians with medical dispatch expertise, including pediatricians. Local and untested modification of protocols should be discouraged, as the complexity of the protocols is often significantly underestimated. Medical dispatch organizations should be encouraged to place children's needs and priorities high on the list of ongoing concerns within their standards groups.

Public safety communications has long been understood to be a special hybrid between the medical community and the public safety establishment. The control of these dispatch pre-arrival systems is predominantly within the public safety arena. The medical control responsibility within EMD systems has been clearly identified as residing within the medical physician's realm. This dichotomy creates many of the traditional road blocks to assuring that individual EMD programs are functioning in a safe, efficient, and effective manner. Public safety management in concert with medical oversight physicians groups must embrace total quality management practices with adequate numbers of quality assurance case reviews as the core of this performance evaluation system.

Research support should be provided by appropriate governmental divisions, managed care organizations, or other funding sources to facilitate careful examination of issues facing children as prehospital patients.

Emergency medical dispatch is a critical element of the emergency medical services system. Health and safety professionals, together with community members and children's advocates, must continue to work to ensure that our emergency medical dispatch system is providing the best possible care for our children.

Participants

Jean Athey, Ph.D.
Director
Emergency Medical Services for Children

Charles D. Carter
Executive Director
National Communications Institute (NCI)

Jennifer Clarke
Communications Specialist
Georgia EMS for Children
Office of EMS and Injury Prevention

Jeff Clawson, MD
National Academy of Emergency Medical Dispatch

Captain Garry Criddle, R.N.
EMS Specialist
National Highway Traffic Safety Administration

Ej Dailey
Project Coordinator
Georgia EMS for Children
Office of EMS and Injury Prevention

Captain Brian Dale
Salt Lake City Fire Department &
National Academy of Emergency Medical Dispatch

David H. Fagin, MD
Director, Emergency Medicine
Emergency Department
Scottish Rite Children's Medical Center

Chuck Glass
EMD Consultant
American Society for Testing and Materials

Leigh Haislip
EMD Consultant

Patrick Lanzetta, MD
Medical Director
PowerPhone, Inc.

Patty Maher
EMD Program Manager
APCO

Paul Rasch
Manager
Training and Development
PowerPhone, Inc.

Paul Roman
EMD Consultant
American Society for Testing and Materials

Michael G. Tunik, MD
Assistant Professor of Clinical Pediatrics
Bellevue Hospital Center

Carl VanCott
Office of EMS
North Carolina Department of
Health and Human Services

Unnecessary Lights-and-Siren Use:
A Public Health Hazard

Jeff Clawson

Recent events trumpeted in the national news media have cast a recurring spotlight on the safety, effectiveness, and ethical use of lights and sirens in both emergency response and transport. While emergency-vehicle tragedies have punctuated the entire history of public safety's use of a HOT (lights-and-siren) response mode, the problem and its unfortunate extent have never before captured the attention of the general public as they have now.

Members of the vocal minority in the public safety community offer, in defense against these mounting questions and inquiries, a few familiar rationalizations:

- The motoring public's supposed indifference to their urgent responses (always claimed to be increasing).
- The argument that the public expects them to hurry to get there fast.
- The contention that there is a lawsuit waiting in the wings if they don't use a lights-and-siren mode during a response.
- The evolving technology of the automobile, with improved interior soundproofing, airtightness, stereo systems, and so forth.

Reprint from Public Management published by the International City/County Management Association (ICMA)

Rarely do we ever admit that we, the public safety community, might have a problem, and a major one at that. In a front-page article in the March 21, 2002, edition of *USA Today* the new head of the National Highway Traffic Safety Administration within the U.S. Department of Transportation, Dr. Jeffrey Runge, stated: "There are not a lot of data out there. It tells me there is not a huge safety problem."

Many experts seriously disagree. Every year, thousands are injured and hundreds killed, mostly needlessly, in an otherwise civilized society.

The incidence of emergency-vehicle collisions (EVCs) is not just a "problem" or even a "dilemma." It is a public health epidemic. If 70 deaths from anthrax or rabies were reported, the CDC would arrive in space suits and spend perhaps millions to mitigate the epidemic, if not actually to quell it. But the CDC is not the government agency responsible for this particular type of epidemic. Apparently, nobody is. Clearly, it doesn't take a scientist at the CDC to see that the 15,000 to 25,000 ambulance and rescue-vehicle accidents in the United States alone each year constitute a true public-safety disease of epidemic proportions.

Suggest that the problem may lie within the public safety community, and "patient care" and "we save lives" rationalizations spew forth like spurts of ink from a frightened octopus. The concept of reducing lights-and-siren use is just slightly more popular in our nation's fire and ambulance services than gun control is with the National Rifle Association. But unlike guns, the use of lights-and-siren is not protected by the second Amendment of the Constitution.

EMS expert, *JEMS* (*Journal of Emergency Medical Services*) publisher, and attorney Jim Page has stated in his *EMS Legal Primer*, "For some reason, most of us don't like to talk about ambulance accidents—even though most of them are

> # The incidence of emergency-vehicle collisions is not just a "problem" or even a "dilemma." It is a public health epidemic.

preventable. Clearly, the greatest legal hazards facing prehospital personnel arise from ambulance vehicle accidents." In addition, the financial payout by local governments for these recurrent tragedies is immense, often costing millions per incident.

This expenditure often eclipses, by several magnitudes, the medical and public-safety "malpractice" negligence awards in dollars lost. Government officials often are unaware of this impending risk because of persistent and blatantly false information routinely offered up by public safety leaders and personnel.

An examination of a long-existing and wide variety of misconceptions regarding lights-and-siren use within the public safety community reveals these mistaken beliefs:

1. Motorists can hear us.
2. Motorists can see us.
3. Motorists don't care about emergency vehicles and ignore them.
4. We can educate the motoring public to "get out of the way."
5. Fast can be safe.
6. Everyone's dying; we've got to hurry (response phase).
7. We really don't know how sick or hurt the patient is (transport phase).
8. We are more qualified than the professional dispatcher to decide when to use lights-and-siren to the scene.

9. We are more qualified than the emergency room staff to decide when to use lights-and-siren in transport.
10. Lights and/or sirens work effectively as warning devices.
11. Running with lights-and-siren saves lots of time.
12. I've never been in an accident before; therefore, they don't happen often, and one won't happen to me.

These are not only misconceptions, but myths—beliefs not supported by history or science—that are currently plaguing public safety personnel and their managers. Times are not just changing . . . they have changed. Here's what we now know:

1. The use of lights-and-siren does not routinely save significant time. In fact, several published studies show time saved to be less than a minute.
2. Time does not matter *much* in most incidents, and *not at all* in many. The vast majority of 911 calls are not time-sensitive emergencies, and most are not even emergencies at all.
3. Running HOT is a lot riskier than traveling routinely.
4. By correctly using sound emergency medical-dispatch protocols, we can identify the small population of time-critical patients at the time of their 911 calls. We can then appropriately extend the lights-and-siren safety net around *only* this small population of patients.
5. By correctly using sensible protocols (emergency-room or field-based), we can identify at the scene those patients actually needing HOT transport to the receiving hospital or trauma center.
6. For years, progressive agencies have safely responded COLD to a significant portion of their "emergency" calls.

7. Lawsuits for not responding lights-and-siren do not exist. In fact, there has never been a lawsuit in the history of the United States or Canada for not responding HOT.
8. The public does *not* always expect it. What citizens want is rationality in using these devices when this extreme practice can actually make a difference. In fact, it is not uncommon for a caller to ask for a COLD response in many situations.
9. Lots of mayhem occurs as a result of HOT response, and much of it, by anyone's definition of an emergency, is simply unnecessary. Historically, an amazing number of EMVCs (emergency medical-vehicle collisions) occur while running HOT to trivial or non-escalating "emergencies."
10. There is a significantly higher awareness of the correct use of lights-and-siren within the legal community. Dispatch tapes and records (and the clinical and operational decisions they portray) are routinely subpoenaed and commented on by an increasingly knowledgeable field of experts.
11. Widespread use of emergency medical-dispatch protocols to organize responses has created a *standard of practice* clearly separating the reasonable use of lights-and-siren mode, an often-dangerous special privilege, from its indiscriminate and potentially tragic misapplication. It is more than evident that "one size does *not* fit all" calls.
12. Special training of emergency-vehicle drivers (in EVOC and low-force driving) reduces collisions by educating the operators to a plethora of risks, predictable motorist behaviors, and the absolute necessity of exercising "due regard" during urgent response and transport.
13. Use of in-vehicle monitoring devices

("black boxes")—which record and sometimes warn errant drivers of excessive speed, unsafe movements and turns, heavy braking, and other non-optimal behaviors on the roadway—has been proven effective in the private ambulance-service community.

The Salt Lake City Fire Department has been responding COLD to all "Bravo" response codes. The biggest category within this group is the "traffic accident with injury" call (excluding defined "major traffic" incidents, high mechanisms of injury, hazmat incidents, extrications, and traffic accidents in which patients are reported "not alert"). This has been the department's response method for more than four years now, with nary a problem or complaint.

When the Salt Lake City Fire Department first fully implemented this dispatch-based response program in 1983—with 50 percent fewer units sent at all and even fewer HOT responses—its EMVC rate dropped an astounding 78 percent.

In 1994, the National Association of EMS Physicians, with the National Association of State EMS Directors, published the landmark position paper "Use of Warning Lights and Siren in Emergency Vehicle Response and Patient Transport." The author is not sure whether most EMS or public safety leaders and managers are even aware of this paper's standards and official, practice-setting recommendations, which are the following:

1. EMS medical directors should participate directly in the development of policies governing emergency medical-vehicle response, patient transport, and the use of warning lights-and-siren (L&S) mode.
2. The use of L&S during an emergency response to the scene and during patient transport should be based on standardized protocols that take into account situational and patient-

problem assessments.
3. EMS dispatch agencies should use an emergency medical-dispatch priority reference system that has been developed in conjunction with and approved by the EMS medical director to determine which requests for prehospital medical care require the use of warning lights-and-siren mode.
4. Except for suspected life-threatening, time-critical cases or cases involving multiple patients, L&S response by more than one EMV usually is unnecessary.
5. The use of emergency-warning L&S should be limited to emergency responses and emergency-transport situations only.
6. All agencies that operate EMVs or are responsible for emergency medical responders should institute and maintain educational programs in emergency-vehicle operation for EMV operators.
7. Emergency medical vehicle–related collisions occurring during an emergency response or transport should be evaluated by EMS system managers and medical directors.
8. A national reporting system for EMV collisions should be established.
9. cientific studies evaluating the effectiveness of warning L&S under specific situations should be conducted and validated.
10. Laws and statutes should take into account prudent safety practices both by EMS providers and by the monitoring public.
11. National standards for safe EMV operation should be developed.

The time has come to state, unequivocally and for the record, that we can no longer disregard the thousands of injuries and deaths caused by the indiscriminate use of lights-and-siren response. We must reexamine the when, where, how, and why of lights-and-siren use. Individual EMS field responders and emergency medical dispatchers (EMDs) must begin actively to question their managers about the irrational practice of responding HOT on all calls. In particular, EMDs should not be placed in the ethically ambiguous position of carrying out these clearly unsound response schemes.

So warned, elected officials, city and county administrators, and progressive public safety managers must act now, collectively, to prevent the recurring tragedies that are the antitheses of our mission: to help those in need when they need it most, by at least doing "no harm." The indiscriminate use of lights-and-siren mode is an outdated practice not supported by science, the medical community, or even the public we serve. To continue this unsafe and outdated practice is to violate Hippocrates' first law of medicine: "First, do no harm." **PM**

*Jeff J. Clawson, M.D., is a member of the Council of Standards, College of Fellows of the National Academy of Emergency Dis - patch, in Salt Lake City, Utah. He can be contacted at **800-960-6236** or **801-359-6916** or at **info@emergencydispatch.org**.*

Related articles on Lights and Siren Issues and Emergency Vehicle Accidents are available at www.emergencydispatch.org
(http://www.emergencydispatch.org/research.shtml)

- Is Ambulance Transport Time With Lights and Siren Faster Than That Without?
- Above All—Do No Harm
- The Wake Effect—Emergency Vehicle-Related Collisions
- The Maximal Response Disease—"Red Lights and Siren" Syndrome in Priority Dispatching
- Lights, Sirens and Liability
- Lights and Siren: A Review of Emergency Vehicle Warning Systems
- Dispelling Myths on Ambulance Accidents
- Patient Outcome Using Medical Protocol to Limit "Lights and Siren" Transport
- Running "HOT" and the case of Sharron Rose
- Use of Warning Lights and Siren in Emergency Medical Vehicle Response and Patient Transport (NAEMSP Position Paper)
- What a Waste When the System Fails

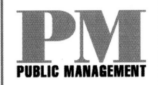

Web site: icma.org

Public Management
ICMA
(International City/County Management Association)
777 North Capitol Street
N.E., Suite 500
Washington, D.C. 20002-4201
(202) 962-3675

This reprint courtesy of *Public Management*

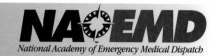

The National Academy of Emergency Medical Dispatch

Model EMD Legislation

Model Statute for the Regulation of Emergency Medical Dispatch Agencies and Emergency Medical Dispatchers

Over the last 25 years it has become widely recognized that the person who takes a telephone request for emergency medical assistance must be able to do more than take the address of the incident and then call the ambulance personnel on the radio and tell them where to go.

The modern Emergency Medical Dispatcher (EMD) must be able to quickly identify the seriousness of the problem, dispatch the appropriate response (from a single ambulance with no lights-and-siren to the "cavalry": police, fire truck, paramedics, and ambulance with sirens blaring), and provide life-sustaining medical instructions to the caller when necessary.

The EMD has become a medical professional that makes medical decisions about what care the patient needs, e.g., what medical resources to send to the patient, and a teacher of medical care over the telephone, what to do or not to do.

All other medical professionals are regulated by States for the purpose of assuring the public that those that provide the service are properly trained and supervised. This document provides a model that a State or Province can use to provide that same level of assurance for Emergency Medical Dispatchers and the agency that provides Emergency Medical Dispatch Services to the public.

This document was prepared for the National Academy of EMD by the Model EMD Legislation Task Force:

Tom Scott, Chair of the Task Force and President, Scott Consulting, Inc., and former State of Alaska EMS Director

Dia Gainor, State of Idaho EMS Director, and Chair of the National Association of State EMS Directors

Dan Manz, State of Vermont EMS Director, and past-Chair of the National Association of State EMS Directors

Joe Phillips, State of Tennessee EMS Director

Matt Anderson, State of Alaska EMS Director

Carol Biancalana, State of California Communications Dispatch Coordinator

Steve L'Heureux, Chair, Alliance Board, NAEMD, and EMD QA Director, State of New Hampshire Communication Center

Carl VanCott, President, NAED, and Director of Telecommunications, State of North Carolina

Carlynn Garcia, Associate Director, NAEMD and NAED, and Secretary of NENA, State of Utah Chapter

Jeff J. Clawson, M.D., Chair, Board of Certification, member College of Fellows and the Board of Trustees, NAEMD

The Model EMD Legislation document was approved by the Task Force on May 4th, 2001, and by the NAEMD Board of Trustees on June 1st, 2001. This Model EMD Legislation document does not necessarily reflect the views of all participants or any participant's State agency.

Justification

Each of the following national standards-setting organizations have identified that emergency medical dispatch is a critical component of an emergency medical services system:

- **American College of Emergency Physicians**[1]

- **American Heart Association**[2]

- **EMS for Children Program, Department of Health and Human Services**[3]

- **National Academy of Emergency Medical Dispatch**[4]

- **National Association of EMS Physicians**[5]

- **National Association of State EMS Directors**[6]

- **National Emergency Number Association**[7]

- **National Highway Traffic Safety Administration**[8]

- **National Institutes of Health**[9]

Furthermore, the ASTM F-30 Committee on Emergency Medical Services has published voluntary standards for emergency medical dispatch:

- **Standard Practice for Emergency Medical Dispatch** (F 1258)

- **Standard Practice for Training Instructor Qualification and Certification Eligibility of Emergency Medical Dispatchers** (F 1552)

- **Standard Practice for Emergency Medical Dispatch Management** (F 1560)

In spite of this national consensus, only 18 of the 50 states have legislation regulating Emergency Medical Dispatch. This document is designed to provide a framework for legislation and rules that will implement these national recommendations and standards. This document includes key components of legislation and rules with annotations regarding the need for specific language. The Academy is willing to assist with any additional information, including copies of the referenced documents. We hope you will find it useful.

Model EMD Legislation

Essential Areas and Elements for Safe, Efficient, and Effective Government Control

The Model Legislation Package approved by the National Academy of EMD contains the provisions for each State to regulate the individuals and agencies providing Emergency Medical Dispatch services to its citizens. The diversified Emergency Medical Dispatch Priority Reference System (EMDPRS) protocols used by EMDs today require specific training and knowledge in their proper use, therefore, the emergency medical dispatcher wishing certification must receive formal training in the specific EMDPRS that is used for the certification being sought and as used within the employing emergency medical dispatch agency. This document contains the following areas and elements, all of which are deemed essential to ensuring a complete process that ultimately results in the correct performance of EMDs and program management by EMD-provider agencies. A complete process as defined therein, must meet all applicable national standards for safe, efficient, and effective dispatch patient evaluation, patient care, and response decision-making as well as the equally safe, efficient, and effective deployment of EMS and public safety trained personnel and vehicles. The basic enabling legislation areas are:

- **Purpose**
- **Authority and Responsibility**
- **Recognition**
- **Definitions**

Within the area of **authority** and **responsibility** lie the 13 essential elements requiring regulation by the States. These are:

1. **Certification of EMDs and EMD agencies**
2. **Recertification of EMDs and EMD agencies**
3. **Training and EMD curriculum standards**
4. **Instructor standards**
5. **Continuing Dispatch Education standards**
6. **Approval of the EMDPRS selected by the EMD agency**
7. **Required use of an approved EMDPRS**
8. **Compliance standards for EMDPRS use**
9. **Quality Assurance (including random case review and performance reporting)**
10. **EMD program governing Policies and Procedures standards**
11. **Medical Direction and Oversight**
12. **Prevention of misrepresentation**
13. **Revocation and suspension of certification**

Within the area of **recognition** lie 5 essential elements to be addressed by the States in dealing with national standard-setting organizations. These are:

1. **Certification programs**
2. **Recertification programs**
3. **Continuing Dispatch Education programs**
4. **Instructor programs**
5. **Accreditation programs**

Within the area of **definitions**, the following should be addressed either within the legislation itself or within administrative rules. They may be present in other associated legislation such as EMS, EMT, and Paramedic, but must be consistent with the required meanings for EMD. If not, the suggested wording below should be used. These are:

"Advanced Life Support Provider"
"Continuing Dispatcher Education"
"Compliance to Protocol"
"Department"
"Dispatch Life Support (DLS)"
"Emergency Medical Dispatcher (EMD)"
"Emergency Medical Dispatching"
"Emergency Medical Dispatch Agency (EMD Agency)"
"Emergency Medical Dispatch Priority Reference System (EMDPRS)"
"EMD Medical Direction"
"EMD Medical Director"
"Pre-arrival Instructions"
"Post-dispatch Instructions"
"Quality Assurance and Improvement Program"
"Vehicle Response Mode"
"Vehicle Response Configuration"

Model State Emergency Medical Dispatch Act
enabling legislation for EMD regulation

Sec. 1. Short title.
This Act shall be known and may be cited as the "Emergency Medical Dispatch Act."

Sec. 2. Definitions.
"Advanced Life Support Provider" means a person that has been licensed or certified as an EMT-Intermediate, an EMT-Paramedic, a Registered Nurse, or a licensed physician in any State *[Territory, Province].* [this definition may not be necessary if identified elsewhere in the applicable EMS statute or rules]

"Call Routing" shall mean the reception of emergency calls where the purpose is to only determine the course of direction of routing (police, fire, medical) resulting in rapid transfer of medical callers to the EMD agency or EMD calltaker for emergency medical dispatching services.

"Compliance to Protocol" shall mean the adherence to the written text or scripts and other processes within the approved EMDPRS except that, deviation from the text or script may only occur for the express purpose of clarifying the meaning or intent of a question or facilitating the clear understanding of a required action, instruction, or response from the caller. EMD performance is determined by the evaluation of this compliance.

"Continuing Dispatcher Education" shall mean medical dispatch relevant educational experiences in accordance with standards set forth in national standards established for the practice for emergency medical dispatching (i.e., ASTM F 1560 Standard practice for Emergency Medical Dispatch, Section 13).

"Department" shall mean the Department of *[Health or agency with responsibility for certifying emergency medical personnel].*

"Dispatch Life Support (DLS)" shall mean the knowledge, procedures, and skills used by trained EMDs in providing care and advice through pre-arrival instructions and post-dispatch instructions to callers requesting emergency medical assistance.

"EMD Medical Direction" shall mean the management and accountability for the medical care aspects of an emergency medical dispatch agency including: responsibility for the medical decision and care advice rendered by the emergency medical dispatcher and emergency medical dispatch agency; approval and medical control of the operational emergency medical dispatch priority reference system (EMDPRS); evaluation of the medical care and pre-arrival instructions rendered by the EMD personnel; direct participation in the EMD system evaluation and continuous quality improvement process; and, the medical oversight of the training of the EMD personnel.

"EMD Medical Director" shall mean a licensed physician approved by the Department who provides EMD medical direction to the emergency medical dispatch agency and works with the local EMS medical director if not the same person.

Model EMD Legislation

"Emergency Medical Dispatcher (EMD)" shall mean a person trained to provide emergency medical dispatch services and is *[certified, licensed]* in accordance with this Act.

"Emergency Medical Dispatching" shall mean the reception, evaluation, processing, provision of dispatch life support, management of requests for emergency medical assistance, and participation in ongoing evaluation and improvement of the emergency medical dispatch process. This process includes identifying the nature of the request, prioritizing the severity of the request, dispatching the necessary resources, providing medical aid and safety instructions to the callers and coordinating the responding resources as needed but does not include call routing per se.

"Emergency Medical Dispatch Agency (EMD Agency)" shall mean any company, organization, or government agency that provides emergency medical dispatch services for emergency medical assistance, and is *[certified, licensed]* in accordance with this Act.

"Emergency Medical Dispatch Priority Reference System (EMDPRS)" shall mean a Department approved and EMD Medical Director approved system that includes: the protocol used by an emergency medical dispatcher in an emergency medical dispatch agency to dispatch aid to medical emergencies that includes: systematized caller interrogation questions; systematized dispatch life support instructions; and, systematized coding protocols that match the dispatcher's evaluation of the injury or illness severity with the vehicle response mode and vehicle response configuration; continuous quality improvement program that measures compliance to protocol through ongoing random case review for each EMD; and a training curriculum and testing process consistent with the specific EMDPRS protocol used by the emergency medical dispatch agency.

"National EMD Standard-Setting & Certification Organization (NESSCO)" An organization that provides and maintains a comprehensive EMD protocol and training system development process including a scientific methods-based standards improvement methodology. Such organizations must maintain current and up-to-date EMDPRS, curriculum, training, testing, certification, recertification, instructor, quality improvement, and accreditation programs and standards.

"Pre-arrival Instructions" shall mean the current, scripted medical instructions given in life threatening situations whenever possible

and appropriate, where correct evaluation, verification, and advice given by Emergency Medical Dispatchers is essential to provide necessary assistance and control of the situation prior to arrival of emergency medical services personnel. These protocols are part of an EMDPRS and are used as close to word-for-word as possible.

"Post-dispatch Instructions" shall mean case-specific advice, warnings, and treatments given by trained EMDs whenever possible and appropriate after dispatching field responders. These protocols are part of an EMDPRS.

"Quality Assurance and Improvement Program" shall mean a program approved by the medical director and administered by the EMD agency for the purpose of insuring safe, efficient, and effective performance of EMDs in regard to their use of the EMDPRS and patient care advice provided. This program shall include at a minimum, the random case review evaluating EMD performance, feedback of EMDPRS compliance levels to EMDs, related CDE retraining and remediation, and submission of compliance data to medical director and the Department.

"Vehicle Response Mode" shall mean the use of emergency driving techniques, such as warning lights-and-siren or routine driving response as assigned by the EMS agency and approved by the EMS Medical Director.

"Vehicle Response Configuration" shall mean the specific vehicle(s) of varied types, capabilities, and numbers responding to render assistance as assigned by the EMS agency and approved by the EMS Medical Director.

Sec. 3. Certificate Required.
(a) No person may represent herself/himself as an emergency medical dispatcher unless *[certified, licensed, accredited]* by the Department as an emergency medical dispatcher.
(b) No business, organization, or government agency may represent itself as an emergency medical dispatch agency unless the business, organization, or government agency is *[certified, licensed, accredited]* by the Department as an emergency medical dispatch agency.

Sec. 4. National Standards Required.
The Department shall use applicable national standards when developing the rules and requirements for emergency medical dispatchers and emergency medical dispatch agencies.

Sec. 5. Authority and Responsibilities.
The Department shall have the authority and responsibility to establish rules and requirements for the following pursuant to this Act:
(a) Require certification and recertification of a

person who meets the training and other requirements as an emergency medical dispatcher.
(b) Require certification and recertification of a business, organization, or government agency that operates an emergency medical dispatch agency that meets the minimum standards prescribed by the Department for an emergency medical dispatch agency.
(c) Establish a biannual recertification requirement that requires at least 12 hours of medical dispatch specific continuing education each year.
(d) Require minimum education and continuing education for the Emergency Medical Dispatcher which meet national standards.
(e) Require the EMD to follow the questions and decision-making processes within their EMDPRS in compliance to the written policies and procedures of their EMD agency as approved by the Department.
(f) Require the EMD to provide dispatch life support (including pre-arrival instructions) in compliance to the written text or scripts and other processes within the approved EMDPRS.
(g) Require the EMD agency to have in place Department-approved polices and procedures for the safe and effective use of the EMDPRS.
(h) Require the EMD to keep the Department currently informed as to the entity or agency that employs or supervises his/her activities as an Emergency Medical Dispatcher.
(i) Approve all EMDPRS protocols used by emergency medical dispatch agencies to assure compliance with national standards.
(j) Require that Department-approved emergency medical dispatch certification training programs shall be conducted in accordance with national standards and shall include a written examination approved by the Department that tests for competency in the specific EMDPRS taught in the approved certification training program.
(k) Require that Department-approved emergency medical dispatcher certification training programs shall be conducted by instructors that meet Department-approved qualifications.
(l) Require that the emergency medical dispatch agency be operated in a safe, efficient, and effective manner in accordance with national approved standards including but not limited to:

1) All personnel providing emergency medical dispatch services must be certified by the Department prior to functioning alone in an on-line capacity.

2) The use on every request for medical

Model EMD Legislation

assistance of a Department-approved emergency medical dispatch priority reference system (EMDPRS).

3) The EMD interrogating the caller and coding the incident must be the same EMD that gives the DLS instructions. The EMD dispatching the response may be another person.

4) Under the approval and supervision of the medical director, the establishment of a continuous quality assurance, improvement and management program that measures various areas of compliance to the EMDPRS through ongoing random case review for each EMD and provides feed back to the individuals and management of the EMS agency regarding the level of compliance and performance.

5) A case review process evaluating the EMD's compliance to various Department defined areas within the EMDPRS.

6) Reporting of EMDPRS performance and compliance data at Department approved intervals.

7) The appointment of a dispatch medical director to review and approve the EMDPRS, the EMD training program, quality assurance/improvement program, medical dispatch oversight committee(s), continuing dispatch education program, and the medical aspects of the operation of the emergency medical dispatch agency.

8) The agency shall have and use the most current version of the Department approved EMDPRS selected for use by the agency as defined by the Department.

9) The EMDPRS selected for use by the agency and approved by the Department,

including its questions, instructions, and protocols, shall be used as a whole and not piecemeal.

(m) Require that a person, organization, or government agency may not offer or conduct a training course that is represented as a course for emergency medical dispatcher certification unless the person, organization, or agency is approved by the Department to offer or conduct that course.

(n) Establish recognition and reciprocity between the Department and national standard-setting organizations having programs that meet the requirements contained in this Act and the rules established for it by the Department.

(o) Require each EMD, EMD agency, or recognized national standard-setting organization to report to the Department whenever an action has taken place that may require the revocation or suspension of a certificate issued by the Department.

Sec 6. Effective Dates.

The provisions of this chapter shall become effective on [within 2 years].

Sec 7. Penalties.

(a) Any person guilty of willfully violating or failing to comply with any provision of this Act or regulations set forth by the Department under Section 5 of this Act shall be fined not more than two hundred fifty dollars, or imprisoned not more than three months, or be both fined and imprisoned.

(b) Any agency or organization guilty of willfully violating or failing to comply with any provision of this Act or regulations set forth by the Department under Section 5 of this Act shall be fined not more than one thousand

dollars, or imprisoned not more than six months, or be both fined and imprisoned.

Sec 8. Grants (optional)

(a) The Department shall establish a grant in aid program to provide funds to government and non-profit agencies that provide emergency medical dispatch services for the purpose of initially implementing the provisions of this Act.

(b) The Department shall develop a statewide implementation plan and budget for submission to the legislature during the next regular session of the legislature.

WORKS CITED

1. American College of Emergency Physicians. *Physician Medical Direction of Emergency Medical Services Dispatch Programs*. Policy number 400201, October, 1998

2. American Heart Association, Emergency Cardiac Care Committee and Subcommittees. *Guidelines for cardiopulmonary resuscitation and emergency cardiac care*, October 2000.

3. EMS for Children Program, HRSA, USDHHS. *Emergency Medical Dispatch for Children*. June 1998.

4. National Academy of Emergency Medical Dispatch. Center of Excellence: The Twenty Points of Accreditation. 1993-2000.

5. National Association of EMS Physicians. "Position Paper: Emergency Medical Dispatching." *Prehospital and Disaster Medicine*. Vol. 4. No. 2. October-December 1989.

6. National Association of State EMS Directors, "Resolutions of the National Association of State EMS Directors: 1994." *Prehospital and Disaster Medicine*. 1995 Vol. 10:2, 124-125.

7. National Emergency Number Association. "Statement on EMD". *NENA News*. 2000.

8. National Highway Traffic Safety Administration. *EMS Agenda for the Future*. August 1996.

9. National Institutes of Health. *Emergency Medical Dispatching: Rapid Identification and Treatment of Acute Myocardial Infarction*. NIH Publications. 1994; No 94-3287.

Endorsed And Supported By :

(9-1-1
POLICE ★ MEDICAL ★ FIRE
EMERGENCY
NENA

NAEMT

N·A EMD

For More Information Please Contact:

National Academy of EMD

139 E. South Temple, Suite 530
Salt Lake City, Utah 84111 USA
USA/Canada: (800) 960-6236
International: (801) 359-6916
Fax: (801) 359-0996
Email: standards@naemd.org
Web: www.naemd.org

©2001 NAEMD

The National Academy of Emergency Medical Dispatch

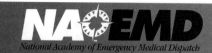

Model EMD Rules & Regulations
of the NAEMD Model EMD Legislation Program

Model Statute for the Regulation of Emergency Medical Dispatch Agencies and Emergency Medical Dispatchers

Over the last 25 years it has become widely recognized that the person who takes a telephone request for emergency medical assistance must be able to do more than take the address of the incident and then call the ambulance personnel on the radio and tell them where to go.

The modern Emergency Medical Dispatcher (EMD) must be able to quickly identify the seriousness of the problem, dispatch the appropriate response (from a single ambulance with no lights-and-siren to the "cavalry": police, fire truck, paramedics, and ambulance with sirens blaring), and provide life-sustaining medical instructions to the caller when necessary.

The EMD has become a medical professional that makes medical decisions about what care the patient needs, e.g., what medical resources to send to the patient, and a teacher of medical care over the telephone, what to do or not to do.

All other medical professionals are regulated by States for the purpose of assuring the public that those that provide the service are properly trained and supervised. This document provides a model that a State or Province can use to provide that same level of assurance for Emergency Medical Dispatchers and the agency that provides Emergency Medical Dispatch Services to the public.

This document was prepared for the National Academy of EMD by the Model EMD Rules and Regulations task force:

Leslee Stein-Spencer, Director State of Illinois EMS

Jim Lanier, Assistant Manager, Sunstar Communications Center, Pinellas County, Florida

Tom Scott, President, Scott Consulting, Inc., and former State of Alaska EMS Director

Greg Scott, EMD Quality Assurance Specialist, NAEMD

Steve L'Heureux, Chair, Alliance Board, NAEMD, and EMD QA Director, State of New Hampshire Communication Center

Jeff J. Clawson, M.D., Chair, Board of Certification, member College of Fellows and the Board of Trustees, NAEMD

Carlynn C. Garcia, Associate Director, NAEMD and NAED, and Secretary of NENA, State of Utah Chapter

©2001 NAEMD. All National and International copyrights reserved.

The Model EMD Rules and Regulations document was approved by the task force on October 4th, 2001, and by the NAEMD Board of Trustees on October 8th, 2001. This Model EMD Rules and Regulations document does not necessarily reflect the views of all participants or any participant's State agency.

National Academy of EMD
139 E. South Temple, Suite 530
Salt Lake City, Utah 84111 USA
(800) 960-6236 USA, (801) 359-6916 Int'l
standards@naemd.org, www.naemd.org

Justification

Each of the following national standards-setting organizations have identified that emergency medical dispatch is a critical component of an emergency medical services system:

- **American College of Emergency Physicians**[1]
- **American Heart Association**[2]
- **EMS for Children Program, Department of Health and Human Services**[3]
- **National Academy of Emergency Medical Dispatch**[4]
- **National Association of EMS Physicians**[5]
- **National Association of State EMS Directors**[6]
- **National Emergency Number Association**[7]
- **National Highway Traffic Safety Administration**[8]
- **National Institutes of Health**[9]

Furthermore, the ASTM F-30 Committee on Emergency Medical Services has published voluntary standards for emergency medical dispatch:

- **Standard Practice for Emergency Medical Dispatch (F 1258)**
- **Standard Practice for Training Instructor Qualification and Certification Eligibility of Emergency Medical Dispatchers (F 1552)**
- **Standard Practice for Emergency Medical Dispatch Management (F 1560)**

In spite of this national consensus, only 18 of the 50 states have legislation regulating Emergency Medical Dispatch. This document is designed to provide a framework for legislation and rules that will implement these national recommendations and standards. This document includes key components of legislation and rules with annotations regarding the need for specific language. The Academy is willing to assist with any additional information, including copies of the referenced documents. We hope you will find it useful.

Model EMD Rules & Regulations

MODEL EMD RULES & REGULATIONS
of the NAEMD Model EMD Legislation Program

I. Authority, Purpose, and Responsibilities

A. The authority to establish these Rules is provided to the Department by the State [*Territory, Province*] of _____ who shall issue and enforce such Rules once adopted.

B. The purposes of these Rules are:
1. To provide for the establishment of minimum standards to be met by those providing Medical Dispatch services in the State [*Territory, Province*] of _____ so as to protect and promote the health and safety of the people.

2. To establish standards for the training, continuing education, certification, recertification, protocol use and compliance, medical direction and oversight, and quality assurance, improvement, and management of dispatchers certifying as Emergency Medical Dispatchers within the State [*Territory, Province*] of _____.

C. The responsibilities included within these Rules shall be encompassed by the following specific areas:

1. Certification of EMDs and EMD agencies
2. Recertification of EMDs and EMD agencies
3. Training and EMD curriculum standards
4. Instructor standards
5. Continuing Dispatch Education standards
6. Approval of the EMDPRS selected by the EMD agency
7. Use of an approved EMDPRS
8. Compliance standards for EMDPRS use
9. Quality Assurance, Improvement, and Management (including random case review, scoring, and performance reporting)
10. EMD program governing Policies and Procedures standards
11. Medical Direction and Oversight
12. Prevention of misrepresentation
13. Revocation and suspension of certification

II. Definitions (as used in these Rules):

"Advanced Life Support Provider" means a person that has been licensed or certified as an EMT-Intermediate, an EMT-Paramedic, a Registered Nurse, or a licensed physician in any State [*Territory, Province*]. [*this definition may not be necessary if identified elsewhere in the applicable EMS statute or rules*]

"Call Routing" shall mean the reception of emergency calls where the purpose is to only determine the course of direction of routing (police, fire, medical) resulting in rapid transfer of medical callers to the EMD agency or EMD calltaker for emergency medical dispatching services.

"Compliance to Protocol" shall mean the adherence to the written text or scripts and other processes within the approved EMD-PRS except that, deviation from the text or script may only occur for the express purpose of clarifying the meaning or intent of a question or facilitating the clear understanding of a required action, instruction, or response from the caller. EMD performance is determined by the evaluation of this compliance.

"Continuing Dispatcher Education" shall mean medical dispatch relevant educational experiences in accordance with standards set forth in national standards established for the practice for emergency medical dispatching (i.e., ASTM F 1560 Standard practice for Emergency Medical Dispatch, Section 13).

"Department" shall mean the Department of [*Health or agency with responsibility for certifying emergency medical personnel*].

"Dispatch Life Support (DLS)" shall mean the knowledge, procedures, and skills used by trained EMDs in providing care and advice through pre-arrival instructions and post-dispatch instructions to callers requesting emergency medical assistance.

"EMD Medical Direction" shall mean the management and accountability for the medical care aspects of an emergency medical dispatch agency including: responsibility for the medical decision and care advice rendered by the emergency medical dispatcher and emergency medical dispatch agency; approval and medical control of the operational emergency medical dispatch priority reference system (EMD-PRS); evaluation of the medical care and pre-arrival instructions rendered by the EMD personnel; direct participation in the EMD system evaluation and continuous quality improvement process; and, the medical oversight of the training of the EMD personnel.

"EMD Medical Director" shall mean a licensed physician approved by the Department who provides EMD medical direction to the emergency medical dispatch agency and works with the local EMS medical director if not the same person.

"Emergency Medical Dispatcher (EMD)" shall mean a person trained to provide emergency medical dispatch services and is [*certified, licensed*] in accordance with this Act.

"Emergency Medical Dispatching" shall mean the reception, evaluation, processing, provision of dispatch life support, management of requests for emergency medical assistance, and participation in ongoing evaluation and improvement of the emergency medical dispatch process. This process includes identifying the nature of the request, prioritizing the severity of the request, dispatching the necessary resources, providing medical aid and safety instructions to the callers and coordinating the responding resources as needed but does not include call routing per se.

"Emergency Medical Dispatch Agency (EMD Agency)" shall mean any company, organization, or government agency that provides emergency medical dispatch services for emergency medical assistance, and is [*certified, licensed*] in accordance with this Act.

Model EMD Rules & Regulations

"Emergency Medical Dispatch Priority Reference System (EMDPRS)" shall mean a Department approved and EMD Medical Director approved system that includes:
the protocol used by an emergency medical dispatcher in an emergency medical dispatch agency to dispatch aid to medical emergencies that includes: systematized caller interrogation questions; systematized dispatch life support instructions; and, systematized coding protocols that match the dispatcher's evaluation of the injury or illness severity with the vehicle response mode and vehicle response configuration; continuous quality improvement program that measures compliance to protocol through ongoing random case review for each EMD; and a training curriculum and testing process consistent with the specific EMDPRS protocol used by the emergency medical dispatch agency.

"National EMD Standard-Setting & Certification Organization (NESSCO)"
An organization that provides and maintains a comprehensive EMD protocol and training system development process including a scientific methods-based standards improvement methodology. Such organizations must maintain current and up-to-date EMDPRS, curriculum, training, testing, certification, recertification, instructor, quality improvement, and accreditation programs and standards.

"Pre-arrival Instructions" shall mean the current, scripted medical instructions given in life threatening situations whenever possible and appropriate, where correct evaluation, verification, and advice given by Emergency Medical Dispatchers is essential to provide necessary assistance and control of the situation prior to arrival of emergency medical services personnel. These protocols are part of an EMDPRS and are used as close to word-for-word as possible.

"Post-dispatch Instructions" shall mean case-specific advice, warnings, and treatments given by trained EMDs whenever possible and appropriate after dispatching field responders. These protocols are part of an EMDPRS.

"Quality Assurance and Improvement Program" shall mean a program approved by the medical director and administered by the EMD agency for the purpose of insuring safe, efficient, and effective performance of EMDs in regard to their use of the EMDPRS and patient care advice provided. This program shall include at a minimum, the random case review evaluating EMD performance, feedback of EMDPRS compliance levels to EMDs, related CDE retraining and remediation, and submission of compliance data to the medical director and the Department.

"Vehicle Response Mode" shall mean the use of emergency driving techniques, such as warning lights-and-siren or routine driving response as assigned by the EMD agency and approved by the EMD Medical Director.

"Vehicle Response Configuration" shall mean the specific vehicle(s) of varied types, capabilities, and numbers responding to render assistance as assigned by the EMD agency and approved by the EMD Medical Director.

III. Authority and Responsibilities
The Department shall:

A. **Certify** and **recertify** any **person** who meets the responsibilities and requirements as an emergency medical dispatcher outlined in **VI/VII.**

B. Set **minimum training** requirements that meet national standards for Emergency Medical Dispatcher **certification.**

C. **Evaluate and approve** EMD training programs based on national standards.

D. Set **minimum recertification** requirements including continuing dispatch education requirements that meet national standards for Emergency Medical Dispatcher **certification.**

E. **Certify and recertify** any **agency** that meets the responsibilities and requirements as an EMD agency according to national standards.

F. **Approve National EMD Standard-Setting & Certification Organizations** for recognition by the Department, one or more of the following: EMD training, testing, certification, recertification, curriculum, instructor, and accreditation processes.

IV. Requirements for providing Emergency Medical Dispatch Services

A. Require **all agencies** who accept calls for EMS assistance from the public and/or dispatch emergency medical personnel **shall be certified** and **have an Emergency Medical Dispatch Priority Reference System (EMDPRS)** used by certified Emergency Medical Dispatchers as follows:

1. All EMDPRS protocols used by emergency medical dispatch agencies must be approved by the Department to assure compliance with national standards. Any EMDPRS approved by the Department, including its questions, instructions, codes, and protocols, shall be used as a whole rather than piecemeal.

2. Use of a Department-approved EMDPRS on every request for medical assistance.

3. Each EMD shall follow the questions and decision-making processes within their EMDPRS in compliance to the written policies and procedures of their EMD agency as approved by the Department.

4. Each EMD shall provide dispatch life support (including pre-arrival instructions) in compliance to the written text or scripts and other processes within the approved EMDPRS.

5. Each EMD agency shall have in place Department-approved polices and procedures for the safe and effective use of their approved EMDPRS.

Model EMD Rules & Regulations

6. The Department shall identify pre-approved, standardized EMDPRS's for selection and use by local EMD agencies.

B. **Certify and recertify** any **person** who meets the responsibilities and requirements as an emergency medical dispatcher outlined in **VI/VII**.

C. Set **minimum training** requirements that meet national standards for Emergency Medical Dispatcher **certification**.

D. **Evaluate and approve** EMD training programs based on national standards.

E. Set **minimum recertification** requirements including continuing dispatch education requirements that meet national standards for Emergency Medical Dispatcher **certification**.

F. **Certify and recertify** any **agency** that meets the responsibilities and requirements as an EMD agency according to national standards.

G. **Approve** any **National EMD Standard-Setting & Certification Organization** for recognition by the Department of one or more of the following: EMD training, testing, certification, recertification, curriculum, instructor, and accreditation processes.

V. EMD Student Eligibility

To be eligible to enter an EMD training program an individual shall meet the following requirements:

A. 18 years of age or older.

B. A high school diploma or general education equivalent.

VI. EMD Certification

The EMD shall be recommended to the Department for certification based on the successful completion and demonstration of the following:

A. 18 years of age or older.

B. A high school diploma or general education equivalent.

C. A current basic cardiac life support card issued by (or DLS equivalent to the standards of) the American Heart Association or American Red Cross for adult and pediatric cardiopulmonary resuscitation.

D. Successful completion of a Department-approved EMD training course.

E. Upon receipt of a completed certification application, the Department shall issue a certificate to applicants who successfully complete certification requirements. The certificate shall contain the following:

1. The name of the individual certified.

2. The certificate number.

3. The effective date of certification.

4. The date of expiration.

5. A statement that the individual named on the card has fulfilled the requirements for certification and is EMD certified statewide to use the specific EMDPRS for which the EMD was trained.

6. The effective date of the initial certification shall be the day the license is issued.

7. The certification shall be valid for two (2) years from the last day of the month in which it was issued.

F. One may not represent oneself, nor may an agency or business represent an agent or employee of that agency or business, as an emergency medical dispatcher unless certified by the Department as an emergency medical dispatcher.

VII. EMD Recertification

A. An EMD that meets the following qualifications prior to certification expiration shall be eligible for recertification by the Department:

1. Complete and submit an EMD recertification application.

2. Is currently certified by the Department as an EMD.

3. Completes twelve (12) hours per year of approved EMD Continuing Dispatch Education (CDE) for each year of the current certification.

4. Pay the fee established by the Dept.

OR

1. Submits proof of having successfully recertified as an EMD through an approved National EMD Standards-Setting & Certification Organization.

B. The Department shall issue a certificate to applicants who successfully complete recertification requirements. The certificate shall contain the following:

1. The name of the individual certified.

2. The certificate number.

3. The effective date of certification.

4. The date of expiration.

5. A statement that the individual named on the card has fulfilled the requirements for certification and is certified to use the EMDPRS listed on the certificate.

C. The effective date of the recertification shall be the day the license is issued. The recertification shall be valid for two (2) years from the last day of the month in which it was issued.

VIII. Continuing Dispatch Education

Minimum continuing education meeting national standards is required for the Emergency Medical Dispatcher.

A. Twelve (12) hours of approved medical dispatch-specific continuing education each year.

B. EMD Continuing Dispatch Education activities or courses shall meet the following objectives:

1. Clear relevance to the practice of emergency medical dispatch and related to the knowledge base or technical skills required for the practice of emergency medical dispatch care.

Model EMD Rules & Regulations

2. Development of a better understanding of telecommunications and the EMD's role and responsibilities.

3. Enhancement of on-line skills in pre-arrival instructions and in all emergency telephone procedures within the practice of EMD.

4. Improvement of skills in the use and application of all component parts of the EMDPRS including interrogation and prioritization.

5. Practice and critique skill performance.

C. Documentation of successful completion of the course or training shall contain the following information:

1. Name of participant.

2. EMD certification number.

3. Course title.

4. Provider name and address.

5. Date(s) of course.

6. Signatures of instructor(s) and/or course director.

7. Number of Continuing Dispatch Education hours.

D. Each agency shall maintain CDE records for the current recertification period for each EMD in their employment. EMDs not currently employed by an EMD agency must maintain their own records.

E. The Department may monitor local EMD agency CDE provider compliance with these standards.

IX. Recognition of other States, Territories, Provinces and National EMD Standard-Setting & Certification Organizations

A. The Department will issue a certificate to a person who has a valid certification as an EMD from another state, territory, or province or has a valid certification from an approved National EMD Standard-Setting & Certification

Organization (NESSCO) if the person provides the Department with the following:

1. Copy of the valid state, territory, province, or NESSCO certification for the specific EMDPRS (name, version number, and date of last revision).

2. Letter of good standing from their previous dispatch employer as applicable.

3. Pay the fee established by the Department.

B. A person who is certified or licensed in another state, territory, or province as an EMD, whose training is not equivalent to the requirements of these Rules, must complete the requirements for initial certification.

C. A person who is certified or licensed in another state, territory, province as an EMD, but who has not been trained to use the EMDPRS of the employing EMD Agency, must meet the qualifications for initial certification.

D. The Department shall issue a certificate to those individuals trained prior to adoption of these Rules upon submission to the Department of the following:

1. EMD training completion certificate obtained within the last two (2) years.

2. Verification that the training course meets recognized national standards.

X. Approval of National EMD Standard-Setting & Certification Organizations

A. National EMD Standard-Setting & Certification Organizations (NESSCOs) may submit a request for approval of program recognition.

B. Request must include documentation of EMDPRS used (name, version number, and date of last revision), curriculum used (name, version number, and date of last revision), training methodology for instructor certification, and submit the certification examination for review.

C. Agree in writing to keep current all materials initially submitted for approval.

D. Any curriculum submitted for approval must meet current national standards.

E. Upon approval, the Department shall issue a certification of recognition within _____ days of receipt of all requested program material.

F. Non-compliance with any requirements of program approval, use of any unqualified teaching personnel, or non-compliance with any other applicable provision of these Rules may result in suspension or revocation of program recognition by the Department. A recognized NESSCO so notified of any noncompliance shall have sixty (60) days from the date of such written notice to comply with these Rules.

XI. EMD Training Program Approval

A. EMD training programs must be based on a Department-approved EMDPRS and Department-approved curriculum that shall be submitted to the Department for approval prior to training.

B. The Department shall receive and review the following prior to approving an EMD training program:

1. A statement identifying the specific EMDPRS (name, version number, and date of last revision) to be taught by the training program.

2. A course outline.

3. Maintain a final written examination specific to the EMDPRS taught by the program to be made available to the Department on request.

4. Name and qualifications of the EMD instructor.

5. Name of the director or responsible person(s).

6. The address and phone number of training program headquarters.

Model EMD Rules & Regulations

C. A person, organization, or government agency may not offer or conduct a training course that is represented as a course for emergency medical dispatcher certification unless the person, organization, or agency is approved by the Department to offer or conduct that course.

XII. Approved EMD Training Program Requirements

A. Department-approved EMD certification training programs shall be conducted in accordance with national standards and shall include a written examination approved by the Department that tests for competency in the specific EMDPRS taught in the approved certification training program.

B. Department-approved EMD certification training courses shall be taught by Department-approved instructors.

C. Department-approved EMD certification training courses shall be a minimum of 24 hours in length.

D. EMD certification training courses shall provide returnable copies of the EMDPRS for students to utilize during the course.

E. Noncompliance with any requirement for program approval, use of any unqualified teaching personnel, or noncompliance with any other applicable provision of these Rules may result in suspension or revocation of program approval by the Department.

F. An approved EMD training program shall have sixty (60) days from date of such written notice to comply with these Rules.

XIII. EMD Training Program Approval Notification

A. The Department shall notify the training program submitting its request for training program provider approval within _____ days of receiving the request that:

1. The request has been received.

2. The request contains or does not contain the information requested in these Rules.

3. What information, if any, is missing from the request.

B. Program approval or disapproval shall be made in writing by the Department to the requesting training program provider after receipt of all required documentation.

C. If using a National EMD Standard-Setting & Certification Organization program which has had prior approval of the Department, the provider shall notify the Department of the dates that the program is to be taught.

D. If using a non-standard program, the provider shall submit a request for approval to the Department _____ days prior to the course start date.

E. Department-approved emergency medical dispatcher certification training programs shall be conducted by instructors that meet Department-approved qualifications.

XIV. EMD Agency Performance and Certification

The Department shall [*certify, license*] all EMD agencies who document compliance with the following minimum standards:

A. Each emergency medical dispatch agency shall be operated in a safe, efficient, and effective manner in accordance with national standards including but not limited to:

1. All personnel providing emergency medical dispatch services must be certified by the Department prior to functioning alone in an on-line capacity.

2. The Department-approved EMD-PRS shall be used on every request for medical assistance.

3. The EMD interrogating the caller and coding the incident must be the same EMD that gives the DLS instructions. The EMD dispatching the response may be another person.

4. Under the written approval and supervision of the medical director, each agency shall establish a continuous quality assurance, improvement, and management program that measures various areas of compliance to the EMD-PRS as defined in Section XVI.

5. An EMD medical director shall be appointed to review, approve, and oversee the following:

   a. EMDPRS
   b. EMD training program
   c. quality assurance/improvement program
   d. medical dispatch oversight committee(s)
   e. continuing dispatch education program

6. The agency shall have and use the most current version of the Department-approved EMDPRS selected for use by the EMD agency, approved in writing by the EMD medical director, as defined by the Department.

7. The EMDPRS selected for use by the agency and approved by the Department, including its questions, instructions, and protocols, shall be used as a whole and not piecemeal.

B. A business, organization, or government agency may not represent itself as an emergency medical dispatch agency unless the business, organization, or government agency is certified by the Department as an emergency medical dispatch agency.

OR

1. Is currently accredited by National EMD Standard-Setting & certification Organization with standards that equal or exceed those listed in Section X of these Rules.

C. The Department shall certify the EMD Agency that:

1. Completes an application form as prescribed by the Department.

Model EMD Rules & Regulations

2. Submit the documentation of compliance with the requirements of Section (A) above.

3. Pay the fee established by the Department.

D. Upon receipt of a completed certification application, the Department shall issue a certificate to applicants who successfully complete certification requirements. The certificate shall contain the following:

1. The name of the agency certified.

2. The certificate number.

3. The effective date of certification.

4. The date of expiration.

5. A statement that the agency named on the card has fulfilled the requirements for certification for using the EMDPRS listed in the application.

E. The effective date of the initial certification shall be the day the license is issued. The certification shall be valid for two (2) years from the last day of the month in which it was issued.

F. The Department may deny, suspend, or revoke the approval of an EMD agency for failure to comply these Rules.

XV. EMD Agency Recertification

A. The Department will issue a recertification to the EMD Agency that meets the following qualifications:

1. Currently certified as an EMD Agency by the Department.

2. Provides documentation that the Agency is using the most current version of the EMDPRS (name, version number, and date of last revision) used by the Agency.

3. Provides documentation of maintained compliance with the initial certification requirements.

4. Pay the fee established by the Department.

B. Upon receipt of a completed recertification application, the Department shall issue a certificate to applicants who successfully complete recertification requirements. The certificate shall contain the following:

1. The name of the agency recertified.

2. The certificate number.

3. The effective date of recertification.

4. The date of expiration.

5. A statement that the agency named on the card has fulfilled the requirements for certification using the EMDPRS listed in the application.

C. The effective date of the recertification shall be the day the [recertification or license] is issued. The recertification shall be valid for two (2) years from the last day of the month in which it was issued.

XVI. Quality Assurance, Improvement, and Management Program Requirements

Each EMD agency shall establish a continuous quality assurance, improvement, and management program that is approved by the EMD medical director and, at a minimum, shall include the following:

A. Documentation of the quality assurance case review process utilized by the EMD agency to identify EMD compliance to the EMDPRS.

B. Written approval of the EMD medical director.

C. Random case review at a minimum of 25 cases per week or 3% of the total EMS call volume, whichever is greater.

D. Regular feedback of performance results to all EMDs on at least a monthly interval.

E. Establishment of EMD performance scoring standards defined within the following areas contained in the EMDPRS:

1. Address, phone number, consciousness, breathing verification

2. Chief complaint/incident type selection

3. Systematized interrogation questions

4. Post-dispatch instructions

5. Pre-arrival instructions

6. Dispatch code selection

7. Overall or aggregate performance score

F. Establishment of minimum performance levels for each EMD performance scoring standard defined in Section (E) above.

G. Establishment of a record-keeping system, including report forms or a computer-based data management system, to permit storage and subsequent evaluation of case records to ensure EMD compliance with the EMDPRS, evaluation of protocol effectiveness, and timeliness of interrogation questions and dispatch functions. The database or record-keeping system must, at a minimum, be capable of storing compliance scores for each EMD performance area defined in Section (E).

H. Scores shall be kept and submitted to the Department for individual EMDs and the EMD agency cumulatively.

1. Reporting Quality Assurance/ Improvement EMD performance scores to the Department on a quarterly basis.

2. Includes interval scores for the reporting period and cumulative score for the latest one year period.

I. Establishment of medical dispatch oversight committee(s) that meet quarterly at minimum and submit agendas and minutes of meetings to the Department on request.

J. The findings of this QI program, when approved by the EMD medical director, functionally fall under the EMS and/or hospital "Medical Procedures and Studies Act" [equivalent] and is therefore not discoverable information or documentation.

Model EMD Rules & Regulations

XVII. Lapsed Certification

To be eligible for recertification when an EMD's certification has lapsed, the following requirements shall apply:

A. For a lapse of up to six (6) months, the individual shall meet all recertification requirements and pay any additional reinstatement fees established by the Department.

   1. The recertification period for lapsed certification reinstatements will be two (2) years from the original expiration date.

B. For a lapse of more than (6) months, the individual must attend and pass the entire twenty-four hour EMD certification course.

C. Hardship cases will be evaluated on an individual basis at the discretion of the Department.

XVIII. Instructor Requirements

A. Those who teach Emergency Medical Dispatchers shall meet training and certification requirements established by the Department to include:

   1. Minimally trained and certified to an ALS-provider level.

   2. Minimum of 3 years of prehospital field or hospital experience

   3. Written approval of the local medical director

B. The Department shall recognize EMD Instructors who are currently certified by an approved National EMD Standards-Setting & Certification organization.

C. A person may not teach an EMD certification course unless that person is certified or approved as an instructor by the Department to offer or conduct that course.

XIX. Discipline

A. Each EMD, EMD agency, or recognized National Standard-Setting & Certification Organization is required to report to the Department whenever an action has taken place that may require the revocation or suspension of a certificate issued by the Department.

B. Upon receipt of a complaint, the Department shall investigate any possible violations of this Act or related Rules and Regulations.

   1. The department shall evaluate all information submitted, and based on these findings, appropriate disciplinary action shall be taken.

   2. Any proceedings by the Department to deny, suspend, or revoke certification as an EMD or EMD Agency, or place any EMD or EMD Agency certificate holder on probation shall be conducted in accordance with this article and pursuant to the provisions of the [*Administrative Procedures Act or equivalent*].

   3. Based on the gravity of the findings, or upon a recommendation for suspension or revocation from a medical director of a local EMS or EMD agency, the Department may immediately suspend certification when there is evidence of a threat to the public health and safety.

XX. Refusal, Suspension, or Revocation of Certification

The Department may refuse to issue a certification or recertification, or suspend or revoke a certification for any of the following causes:

A. Conviction of any offense relating to the use, sale, possession, transportation of narcotics or dangerous drugs.

B. Being under the influence of alcohol or illegal use of drugs while on call or on duty as an Emergency Medical Dispatcher or while driving any emergency vehicle.

C. Fraud or deceit in applying for or obtaining a certification or recertification as an Emergency Medical Dispatcher.

D. Dishonorable, unethical, or immoral conduct including incompetence, patient abuse, theft, or dishonesty in the performance of duties and practice as an Emergency Medical Dispatcher.

E. Instructing procedures or skills beyond the level of certification.

F. Violation of any rules or laws pertaining to medical practice and medication administration.

G. Conviction of a felony.

H. Mental incompetence as determined by due process.

I. Continued lack of compliance to protocol after remediation as demonstrated through the EMD agency's quality assurance and improvement process.

J. Failure to comply with these Rules.

XXI. Refusal, Suspension, or Revocation of Agency Certification

A. The Department may refuse to issue an agency certification or recertification, or suspend or revoke a certification for failure to comply with these Rules.

WORKS CITED

1. American College of Emergency Physicians. *Physician Medical Direction of Emergency Medical Services Dispatch Programs.* Policy number 400201, October, 1998

2. American Heart Association, Emergency Cardiac Care Committee and Subcommittees. *Guidelines for Cardiopulmonary Resuscitation and Emergency Cardiac Care,* October 2000.

3. EMS for Children Program, HRSA, USDHHS. *Emergency Medical Dispatch for Children.* June 1998.

4. National Academy of Emergency Medical Dispatch. Center of Excellence: The Twenty Points of Accreditation. 1993-2000.

5. National Association of EMS Physicians. "Position Paper: Emergency Medical Dispatching." *Prehospital and Disaster Medicine.* Vol. 4. No. 2. October-December 1989.

6. National Association of State EMS Directors, "Resolutions of the National Association of State EMS Directors: 1994." *Prehospital and Disaster Medicine.* 1995 Vol. 10:2, 124-125.

7. National Emergency Number Association. "Statement on EMD". *NENA News.* 2000.

8. National Highway Traffic Safety Administration. *EMS Agenda for the Future.* August 1996.

9. National Institutes of Health. *Emergency Medical Dispatching: Rapid Identification and Treatment of Acute Myocardial Infarction.* NIH Publications. 1994; No 94-3287.

References of Works Cited

1. Zachariah BS, Pepe PE. The Development of Emergency Medical Dispatch in the USA: A Historical Perspective. *European Journal of Emergency Medicine.* 1995; 2:109-112.

2. Clawson J. Dispatch Priority Training—Strengthening the Weak Link. *Journal of Emergency Medical Services.* 1981; 6:32-36.

3. Clawson J. Medical Priority Dispatch—It Works! *Journal of Emergency Medical Services.* 1983; 8:29-33.

4. St. John DR, Shephard RD, Jr. Emergency Medical Services-Dispatch and Response. *Fire Chief,* August. 1983; 27:142-144.

5. Campbell JP, Gratton MC, Salomone JA, Watson WA. Ambulance Arrival to Patient Contact: The Hidden Component of Prehospital Response Time Intervals. *Annals of Emergency Medicine.* 1993; 22:1254-7.

6. Campbell JP, Gratton MC, Girkin JP, Watson WA. Vehicle-at-Scene-to-Patient-Access Interval Measured With Computer-aided Dispatch. *Annals of Emergency Medicine.* 1995; 25:182-6.

7. Keene K. Promises, Promises: Does EMD Really Work? *Journal of Emergency Medical Services.* 1990; 19:25-7.

8. Hoge P. 911 Offers Guiding Hand in an Emergency. *The Sacramento Bee.* 1990; July 16.

9. Keller R. 1989 EMS Salary Survey. *Journal of Emergency Medical Services.* 1989; 18:54-64.

10. Edwards H. Seven Injured as Ambulance, Truck Collide. *Salt Lake Tribune.* 1987.

11. Clawson J. Running 'Hot' and the Case of Sharron Rose. *Journal of Emergency Medical Services.* 1991; 16:11-13.

12. Willis D. Dispatch Program. *Journal of Emergency Medical Services.* 1988; 13:15-16.

13. Clawson J., Martin RL, Cady GA, Maio RF. The Wake Effect—Emergency Vehicle-Related Collisions. *Prehospital and Disaster Medicine.* 1997; 12:274-77.

14. Board of Curriculum NAEMD. *Emergency Medical Dispatch Course Manual* (19th Ed.). Medical Priority Consultants; Salt Lake City, UT. 1996.

15. Morris G. Medical Self-help. *Paramedics International.* 1977; 2:22-4.

16. Clawson J. Priority Dispatching After Dallas: Another Viewpoint. *Journal of Emergency Medical Services.* 1984; 9:36-37.

17. Eisenberg MS, Carter W, Hallstrom A, Cummins R, Litwin P, Hearne T. Identification of Cardiac Arrest by Emergency Dispatchers. *American Journal of Emergency Medicine* 1986; 4:299-301

18. George JE. EMS Triage. EMT *Legal Bulletin.* 1981; 5:2-4.

19. Clawson J. Isn't the AMPDS an Unnecessary Burden? *Journal of National Academy of EMD.* 1992;3.

20. National Association of Emergency Medical Services Physicians. Position Paper: Emergency Medical Dispatching. *Prehospital and Disaster Medicine.* 1989; 4:163-6.

21. National Academy of Emergency Medical Dispatch. Unpublished Study, Salt Lake City, UT. 1990.

22. DeLorenzo RA, Eilers MA. Lights and Siren: A Review of Emergency Vehicle Warning Systems. *Annals of Emergency Medicine.* 1991; 20:1331-34.

23. Clawson J. The Maximal Response Disease—Red Lights and Siren Syndrome in Priority Dispatching. *Journal of Emergency Medical Services.* 1987; 12:28-30.

24. Clawson J. The Red-Light-and-Siren Response. *Journal of Emergency Medical Services.* 1981; 6(2) 34-35.

25. National Association of Emergency Medical Services Physicians (NAEMSP) and the National Association of State EMS Directors (NASEMSD). Use of Warning Lights and Siren in Emergency Medical Vehicle Response and Patient Transport. *Prehospital and Disaster Medicine.* 1994; 9:133-36.

26. Clawson J, Cady G, Martin R, Sinclair R. The Impact of a Comprehensive Quality Management Process on Compliance to Protocol in an Emergency Medical Dispatch Center. *Annals of Emergency Medicine.* 1998; 32:578-584.

27. Kuehl A. Prehospital Systems and Medical Oversight, (2nd Edition). Mosby Lifeline; St. Louis, MS. 1994.

28. Roush WE. Principles of EMS Systems, (2nd Edition). American College of Emergency Physicians; Dallas, TX. 1994.

29. Clawson J, Martin RL, Lloyd B, Smith M, Cady G. The EMD as a Medical Professional. *Journal of Emergency Medical Services.* 1996; 21:69-72.

30. Griffiths K. A New Approach to System Abuse. *Paramedics International.* 1979; 4:23-27.

31. Clawson J. Emergency Medical Dispatch. In: Roush W, Ed. *Principles of EMS Systems.* (2nd Edition). American College of Emergency Physicians; Dallas, TX. 1994: 269-275.

32. Clawson J. Medical Miranda. *Journal of Emergency Medical Services.* 1985; 10:54-5.

33. Supreme Court of the United States. Miranda vs. Arizona. *384 U.S. 436 No.* 759. 1966.

34. Stratton S. Triage by Emergency Medical Dispatchers. *Prehospital and Disaster Medicine.* 1992; 7:263-9.

35. Clawson J. Avoiding Response Code Confusion. *Journal of the National Academy of EMD.* 1997; 8.

36. Hunt RC, Brown LH, Cabinum ES, Whitley TW, Prasad NH, Owens CF, Mayo CE. Is Ambulance Transport Time With Lights and Siren Faster Than That Without? *Annals of Emergency Medicine.* 1995; 25:507-11.

37. Page JO. For Whom the Siren Oinks. *Journal of Emergency Medical Services.* 1990; 15:6.

38. Leonard WH. What a Waste When the System Fails. *Ambulance Industry Journal.* 1991; 22:6-7.

39. Clawson J. Regulations and Standards for Emergency Medical Dispatchers: A Model for State or Region. *Emergency Medical Services.* 1984; 13:25-29.

40. Stout JL. System Status Management: The Strategy of Ambulance Placement. *Journal of Emergency Medical Services.* 1983; 8:22-32.

41. Clawson J. Telephone Treatment Protocols: Reach Out and Help Someone. *Journal of Emergency Medical Services.* 1986; 11 (6): 43-44.

42. National Institutes of Health. Emergency Medical Dispatching: Rapid Identification and Treatment of Acute Myocardial Infarction. **NIH Publications.** 1994; No. 94.

43. American Heart Association Emergency Cardiac Committee and Subcommittees. Guidelines for Cardiopulmonary Rescuscitation and Emergency Cardiac Care, II: Adult Basic Life Support. *Journal of the American Medical Association.* 1992; 268: 2184-98.

44. ASTM. American Society for Testing and Materials: Standard Practice for Emergency Medical Dispatch Management F1560 - 94. *Annual Book of ASTM Standards.* 1994.

45. Clawson JJ, Hauert SA. Dispatch Life Support: Establishing Standards that Work. *Journal of Emergency Medical Services.* 1990; 15:82-86.

46. Pritchard G. Airway Management in Difficult Situations. *Journal of the National Academy of EMD.* 1997; 8.

47. Koop CE. Surgeon General's Declaration. *Public Health Reports.* 1985; 100:557.

48. Newman M. Heimlich Maneuver Rescuscitated in Utah: Will Others Follow Suit? (CPR Citizen Section). *Journal Emergency Medical Association.* 1983; 8:46-7.

49. Campbell J. Layton Mom Says Thanks to Dispatcher. *Deseret News.* 1988; September 3.

50. Lyons P. Before You Call 911. *Ladies Home Journal.* 1995; May:60-63.

51. Caughron C, Folks M. Lives on the Line. *Sun Sentinel.* 1991; September 1.

52. Adams B. Baby, Dispatcher Beat Grim Odds. *Deseret News.* 1989; May 30.

53. Sneed D. 9-1-1 Dispatcher Calm in a Crisis, Saves Life Over Phone. *The Union.* 1990; February 23.

54. ASTM. American Society for Testing and Materials: Standard Practice for Emergency Medical Dispatch F1258 - 95. *Annual Book of ASTM Standards.* 1995.

55. National Association of State Emergency Medical Services Directors. Resolutions of the National Association of State Emergency Medical Services Directors: 1994. *Prehospital and Disaster Medicine.* 1994; 10:75-6.

56. American College of Emergency Physicians. Guidelines for Emergency Medical Services Systems. *Annals of Emergency Medicine.* 1988; 17:742-5.

57. Clawson J. Can't You Tell Me What To Do?! *Journal of the National Academy of EMD.* 1991; 2.

58. Clawson J. The Hysteria Threshold: Gaining Control of the Emergency Caller. *Journal of Emergency Medical Services.* 1986; 11:40.

59. Clawson J. The Psychological Components of Pre-Arrival Instructing. *Emergency Medical Dispatch Training Program.* Medical Priority Consultants, Salt Lake City, UT. 1986.

60. Estavanell J. The Use of Repetitive Persistence. *Journal of National Academy of EMD* 1998; 9.

61. Kannel WB, Abbott RD. Incidence and Prognosis of Unrecognised Myocardial Infarction: An Update on the Framingham Study. *New England Journal of Medicine.* 1984; 311:1144-1147.

62. National Center for Vital Statistics. Death Rates for 72 Selected Causes by Age, United States 1992. *Monthly Vital Statistics Report.* 1995; 43:37-9.

63. Criss E. Women and Heart Disease. *Journal of Emergency Medical Services.* 1997; 26:59-60.

64. Bates CK. Medical Risks of Cocaine Use. *Western Journal of Medicine.* 1988; 148:440-4.

65. Tokarski GF, Paganussi P, Urbanski R, Carden D, Foreback C, Tomlanovich M. An Evaluation of Cocaine-Induced Chest Pain. *Annals of Emergency Medicine.* 1990; 19:1088-91.

66. Flomenbaum NE, Silverman RE. A Case Of Ruptured Abdominal Aortic Aneurysm. *Case Studies in Cardiac Emergencies.* 1983; 4.

67. Apter AJ, LaVallee HA. How Is Anaphylaxis Recognized? *Archives of Family Medicine.* 1994; 3: 717-722.

68. Litovitz TL, Felberg L, White S, Klein-Schwartz W. 1995 Annual Report of the Americal Association of Poison Control Centers Toxic Exposure Surveillance System. *American Journal of Emergency Medicine.* 1996; 14:487-537.

69. Greenfield DP. Prescription Drug Abuse and Dependence: How Prescription Drug Abuse Contributes to the Drug Abuse Epidemic. Charles C. Thomas; Springfield, IL. 1995.

70. Dernocoeur K. Poison Control Centers: They Can Ease Your Load. *Journal of Emergency Medical Services.* 1986; 11(1) 65-70.

71. Chaffee-Bahamon C. and Lovejoy FH. Effectiveness of a Regional Poison Center in Reducing Excess Emergency Room Visits. *Pediatrics.* 1983; 72(2): 164-169.

72. Clawson J. Poison Control and the EMD. *Journal of National Academy of EMD.* 1990; 1.

73. Malcher F. A Call To Remember. *Santa Fe Bulletin (Monthly Bulletin of American Medical Services, Fresno, CA).* 1991; Autumn.

74. Dernocoeur K. Understanding Seizures. *Journal of Emergency Medical Services.* 1982; 7:28-35.

75. Wright S. The Child With Febrile Seizures. *American Family Practice.* 1987; 36:163-7.

76. Clawson J. Pediatric Seizures. *Journal of National Academy of EMD.* 1994; 5.

77. National Institute of Neurological Disorders and Stroke rt-PA Stroke Study Group. Tissue Plasminogen Activator for Acute Ischemic Stroke. *New England Journal of Medicine.* 1995; 333: 1581-87.

78. Fagan SC, Morgenstern LB, Petitta A, Ward RE, Tilley BD, Marler JR, Levine SR, Broderick JP, Kwiatowski TG, Frankel M, Walker MD. Cost-Effectiveness of Tissue Plasminogen Activator for Acute Ischemic Stroke. NINDS rt-PA Stroke Study Group. *Neurology.* 1998; 50:883.

79. Sternberg S. Overhaul Urged for Handling of Strokes. *USA Today.* 1997; November 24.

80. Pepe P, Zachariah B, Sayre M, Floccare D. Ensuring the Chain of Recovery for Stroke in Your Community. *Prehospital Emergency Care.* 1998; 2: 89-95.

81. National Institute of Neurological Disorders and Stroke. Proceedings of a National Symposium on Rapid Identification and Treatment of Acute Stroke. Marler J, Winters-Jones P, Emr M, Eds; Bethesda, MD. 1997.

82. Kothari R, Barsan W, Brott T, Broderick J, Ashbrock S. Frequency and Accuracy of Prehospital Diagnosis of Stroke. *Stroke.* 1995; 26:937-941.

83. Sinclair R, Marler J. Using EMD For Acute Stroke Identification. *Journal of National Academy of EMD.* 1998; 9.

84. National Academy Press. Injury in America: A Continuing Public Health Problem. Washington, DC. 1985.

85. Cassel CK, Nelson EA, Smith TW, Schwab CW, Barlow B, Gary NE. Internists' and Surgeons' Attitudes Toward Guns and Firearm Injury Prevention. *Annals of Internal Medicine.* 1998; 128:224-30.

86. Dernocoeur J. The Ten-Minute Goal. *Journal of Emergency Medical Services.* 1982; 7:51-52.

87. Beckerman B. Mammalian Animal Bites. *Emergency Medical Services.* 1997; 26:50-4.

88. Centers for Disease Control and Prevention. Dog-bite-related Fatalities-United States, 1995-1996. *Journal of the American Medical Association.* 1997; 278:278-9.

89. Seipp C. Laws With Teeth. *American Way.* 1989; September 15:102-7.

90. Hammond JS, Ward CG. Transfers from Emergency Room to Burn Center: Errors in Burn Size Estimation. *Journal of Trauma.* 1987; 27:1161-64.

91. Short By A Measure. *Journal of the Emergency Medical Services.* 1988; 13:25.

92. Centers for Disease Control and Prevention. Fatal Occupational Injuries-United States, 1980-1994. *Morbidity and Mortality Weekly Report.* 1998; 47: 297-302.

93. National Highway Traffic Safety Administration. Traffic Safety Facts 1995. National Center for Statistics and Analysis; Washington, DC. 1996.

94. Clark JJ, Larsen MP, Culley LL, Graves JR, Eisenburg MS. Incidence of Agonal Respirations in Sudden Cardiac Arrest. *Annals of Emergency Medicine.* 1992; 21:1464-7.

95. Information Sidebar. *USA Today.* 1998; February 26.

96. Kellerman AL, Hackman BB, Somes G. Dispatch-Assisted Cardiopulmonary Resuscitation-Validation and Efficacy. *Circulation.* 1989; 80:1231-9.

97. Borak J, Callan M, Abbott W. Hazardous Materials Exposure, Emergency Response and Patient Care. Prentice Hall; Paramus, NJ. 1990.

98. CHEMTREC. The Chemical Transportation Emergency Center can provide immediate, 24-hour information to public safety personnel involved in a hazardous materials situation. Call 800-424-9300 (202-483-7611 if in the District of Columbia or outside the continental United States, Puerto Rico, or the Virgin Islands).

99. United States Fire Administration. Stress Management: Model Program for Maintaining Firefighter Well-Being. *Fire Administrator.* 1991; 100:15-16.

100. Mitchell J. Critical Incident Stress, Videotape. *University of Maryland.* 1985.

101. Dernocoeur K. The "We Save Lives" Myth. *Journal of the Emergency Medical Services.* 1986; 11:6-8.

102. Dernocoeur K. Streetsense: Communication, Safety, and Control. Brady; Bowie, MD. 1985.

103. International Association of Fire Fighters. Guide To Developing Fire Service/Labor Assistance Programs. Washington, DC. 1992:3.

104. Benson H. The Relaxation Response. Random House; NY: 1992.

105. Girdano D, Everly G. Controlling Stress and Tension. Allyn and Bacon; Needham Heights. 1997.

106. Mitchell J, Resnik HLP. Emergency Response to Crisis. Robert J. Brady: Bowie, MD. 1981.

107. Dispatch Disasters. *EMS Magazine.* 1995:33-44.

108. Page-Keeton WE. Prosser and Keeton on the Law of Torts, (5th Edition). West Publishing Co; St Paul, MN. 1984.

109. Page JO. Personal correspondence with Wanda L. Blackwood. Aurora Fire Dept; Aurora, CO. 1981.

110. Eisenberg MS, Hallstrom AP, Carter WB, Cummins RO, Bergner L, Pierce J. Emergency CPR Instruction via Telephone. *American Journal of Public Health.* 1985; 75:47-50.

111. Hauert S. The MPDS and Medical-Legal Danger Zones. *Journal of the National Academy of EMD.* 1990; 1.

112. Lazar R. Dispatch and the Law: How to Avoid the 9-1-1 Litigation Blues. *Journal of Emergency Medical Services.* 1989; 14:35-40.

113. George JE. Failure to Dispatch: A Civil Rights Violation? *EMT Legal Bulletin.* 1988; 12:2-6.

114. Clawson J. Follow the Protocol and Avoid Liability. *Journal of the National Academy of EMD.* 1996; 7.

115. Tennant H. Screening at Yale-New Haven Hospital ED finds 14% of Post-traumatic X-rays Unneeded. *Emergency Department News.* 1985; January:10.

116. Clawson J. Please–Don't Ask Permission! *Journal of the National Academy of EMD.* 1991; 2.

117. Adams R. Lessons Learned from Dallas. *Firehouse May.* 1984.

118. Clawson J. Ambulance Accidents. *Journal of Emergency Medical Services.* 1988; 13:23.

119. Underwriting Guidelines for Emergency Medical Services Insurance Program. Medical Transport Insurance Professionals; Scottsdale, AZ.

120. Application for Emergency Medical Services Insurance Program. Medical Transport Insurance Professionals; Scottsdale, AZ.

121. Auerbach PS, Morris JA, Phillips JB, Jr., et al. An Analysis of Ambulance Accidents in Tennessee. *Journal of the American Medical Association.* 1987; 258:1487-90.

122. Why Fire Apparatus Gets Wrecked. *Volunteer Firemen, March.* 1935.

123. Clawson J. Limiting Lights and Siren Provides Safer Transport. *EMS Update.* 1996:6-7.

124. Wolfberg D. Lights, Sirens and Liability. *Journal of Emergency Medical Service.* 1996; 21:38-40.

125. Childs BJ, Ptacnik DJ. Emergency Ambulance Driving. Prentice Hall; Engelwood Cliffs, NJ. 1986.

126. Elling R. Dispelling Myths on Ambulance Accidents. *Journal of Emergency Medical Services.* 1989; 11:60-4.

127. Elling R, Guerin R. Ambulance Accident Prevention. Seminar Student Workbook. *NYS EMS Program Publication.* 1988; December.

128. Kupas D, Jula D, Pino B. Patient Outcome Using Medical Protocol to Limit "Lights and Siren" Transport. *Prehospital and Disaster Medicine.* 1994; 9:226-9.

129. Solomon SS. Ambulance Accident Avoidance. *Emergency.* 1985; 17:34-35, 44.

130. Page JO. EMS Legal Primer. JEMS Publishing. 1985.

131. George JE, Quattrone MS. Above All—Do No Harm. *EMT Legal Bulletin.* 1991; 15:2-6.

132. Utah Department of Fleet Management. Annual Report—Salt Lake City, UT. 1982.

133. State of Utah, Department of Health, Emergency Medical Dispatcher Regulations and Standards of the Utah Emergency Medical Services System Act. Title 26, Chapter 8, Utah Code Annotated 1953, as amended, effective July 1, 1983. Section 2.5.

134. Clawson J. Quality Assurance: A Priority for Medical Dispatch. *Emergency Medical Services.* 1989; 18:53-58.

135. Woollard M. Medical Priority Dispatch: The Benefits for the UK Ambulance Service. *Journal of the British Association of Immediate Care.* 1993; 16:29-31.

136. Deming WE. Out Of The Crisis. MIT Center for Engineering Study; Cambridge, MA. 1986.

137. Walton M. The Deming Management Method. Berkeley Publishing Group; NY. 1988.

138. George S, Weimerskirch A. Total Quality Management: Strategies and Techniques. Wiley; NY. 1994.

139. National Academy of Emergency Medical Dispatch. The 20 Points of Accreditation. 2000.

140. Zalar CM. Re-examining Quality Assurance. *Management Focus.* 1988; 3.

141. ASTM. American Society for Testing and Materials: Standard Practice for Training Instructor Qualification and Certification Eligibility of Emergency Medical Dispatchers F1552 - 94. *Annual Book of ASTM Standards.* 1994.

142. Polsky SS, Johnson JC. Continuous Quality Improvement in EMS. Roush W, Ed. *Principles of EMS Systems,* (2nd Edition). American College of Emergency Physicians; Dallas, TX. 1994.

143. Garcia D. EMD Recertification. *Journal of the National Academy of EMD.* 1994; 5.

144. Clawson J. Medical Dispatch Review: 'Run' Review for the EMD. *Journal of Emergency Medical Services.* 1986; 11.

145. Saalsaa R. Quality Assurance Case Review, Communication to Robert Martin, Board of Accreditation, NAEMD. 1996.

146. Clawson J. What is the NAEMD? *Journal of the National Academy of EMD.* 1993; 3.

147. Clawson J. The DNA of Dispatch. *Journal of Emergency Medical Services.* 1997; 23:55-57.

148. Council on Medical Service—American Medical Association. Guidelines for Quality Assurance. *Journal of the American Medical Association.* 1988; 259.

149. Roberts B. EMS Dispatching—Its Use and Misuse. Dallas Fire Department; Dallas, TX. 1978.

150. Paramedics International Interview. Dallas Paramedic System. *Paramedics International.* 1977; 2:10-39.

151. Slovis CM, Carruth TB, Seitz WJ, Thomas CM, Elsea WR. A Priority Dispatch System for Emergency Medical Services. *Annals of Emergency Medicine.* 1985; 14:1055-1060.

152. Nelson L. EMD "Coaching" Saves Lives. *Fire Service Today.* 1983; December: 32-33.

153. Murphy RB. Priority Dispatch System Effectiveness Proven. *APCO Bulletin.* 1983; 59.

154. Culley L, Eisenberg M, Horton C, et al. Criteria Based Dispatch Sends the Appropriate Providers to the Scene. *Emergency.* 1993; 23:29-32.

155. Criteria Based Emergency Medical Dispatch Training and Certification Course Manual. APCO Institute; South Daytona, FL. 1990.

156. Clawson J, Martin RL, et al. Protocols vs. Guidelines: Choosing a Medical Dispatch Program. *Emergency Medical Services.* 1994; 23:52-56.

157. Cocks RA, Glucksman E. What Does London Need From its Ambulance Service? *British Medical Journal.* 1993; 306:1428-9.

158. ASTM. American Society for Testing and Materials: Standard Practice for Emergency Medical Dispatch F1258 - 90. *Annual Book of ASTM Standards.* 1990.

159. Nicholl J, Gilhooley K, Parry G, Turner J, Dixon S. The Safety and Reliability of Priority Dispatch Systems. Medical Care Research Unit; Sheffield, UK. 1996.

160. Wheeler S. Telephone Triage: Theory, Practice & Protocol Development. Delmar; Albany, NY. 1993.

161. Smith-Marker C. Setting Standards for Professional Nursing. Mosby; Baltimore, MD. 1988.

162. Watson JD, Crick FHC. Molecular Structure of Nucleic Acids: A Structure for Deoxyribose Nucleic Acid. *Nature.* 1953; 171:737-8.

163. Larson RD. Emergency Medical Dispatch: Looking Back, Looking Ahead. *9-1-1 Magazine.* 1998; March-April:28-71.

164. Clawson J, Sinclair R. "Medical Miranda"— Improved Emergency Medical Dispatch Information from Police Officers, *Prehospital Disaster Medicine.* 1999; 4.3.

165. Clawson J, Sinclair R. The Emotional Content and Cooperation Score in Emergency Medical Dispatching, *Prehospital Emergency Care.* 2000; 5:1.

166. Bailey E, et al. The Use of Emergency Medical Dispatch Protocols to Reduce the Number of Inappropriate Scene Responses Made by Advanced Life Support Personnel, *Prehospital Emergency Care.* 2000; 4:2.

167. American National Bank & Trust Co., Special Adm'r for the Estate of Renee Kazmierowski, Deceased Appellant, v. City of Chicago, et al., Appellee; Illinois Supreme Court Decision docket no. 86215. November 1999.

168. Giffis S. Dictionary of Legal Terms: A Simplified Guide to the Language of Law. Barron's Educational Series, Inc., Woodbury, NJ. 1983.

169. National Academies of Emergency Dispatch. Emergency Telecommunicator Course Manual, Jones & Bartlett Publishing Co., Sudbury, MA, 2001.

170. Billettier A, et al. The Lay Public's Expectations of Pre-Arrival Instructions When Dialing 9-1-1, *Prehospital Emergency Care.* 2000; 4:3.

Glossary

Abandonment Unilateral termination of a patient-caretaker relationship by the caretaker where an adequate replacement for that caretaker has not been provided when this action results in some preventable harm.

ABCs See Airway, Breathing, and Circulation.

Abrasion Scraping or rubbing away of a surface. It is usually the result of traumatic injury.

Accredited Center of Excellence Centers that have achieved compliance to the highest level of standards as set forth in the Academy's Twenty Points of Accreditation.

ACE See Accredited Center of Excellence.

ACEP American College of Emergency Physicians.

ACLS See Advanced Cardiac Life Support.

Acuity Levels Defined non-critical situations that require a preassigned clinical transport capability as approved.

Acute Sharp, severe, or having rapid onset and short course; not chronic.

Acute Pulmonary Edema Excessive fluid within the lungs or respiratory system which causes serious difficulty breathing. May be fatal if untreated.

Additional Information Reference information in the Medical Priority Dispatch System™ containing classifications, categories, definitions, rules, axioms, and laws.

Advanced Cardiac Life Support (ACLS) Unified standard for care of cardiac emergencies including drugs, intubation, and other invasive procedures.

Advanced Life Support (ALS) Intervention that utilizes cardiac monitoring, advanced airways, and pharmacology for the treatment of life-threatening emergencies. This term refers to care given prehospital or in-hospital.

AI See Additional Information.

Automated Implanted (Internal) Cardiac Defubrillator (AICD) A small surgically-implanted battery-operated defibrillator for automatically correcting life-threatening heart rhythms in patient's with pre-existing heart disease.

Airway, Breathing, and Circulation Basic elements of the primary survey of patient evaluation; often referred to as the ABCs.

Allergens Substances and proteins that cause allergic reactions in animals, usually foreign to that organism.

Allergy Body's over-reaction to generally harmless substances. Allergies are classified according to how the body's cells react to the allergen. Allergies are also divided into acute and chronic.

ALPHA Response A response level outlined in the protocol as sending the closest basic life support unit COLD.

ALS See Advanced Life Support.

AMA American Medical Association.

Ambulance Officer See Emergency Medical Technician.

AMPDS Advanced Medical Priority Dispatch System.™ See Medical Priority Dispatch System.™

Amputation Traumatic or surgical removal of a part of the body, often a leg, arm, finger, or toe.

Anaphylactic Shock (Anaphylaxis) Decreased tissue perfusion occur-ring when the body is exposed to a substance (antigen) that causes a severe allergic reaction (antibody response). Symptoms include hives, pale and clammy skin, with a corresponding decrease in blood pressure. Can be rapidly fatal if untreated.

Angina Spasmodic choking or suffocative pain. Almost exclusively used to denote angina pectoris which refers to a heart-related chest pain.

Aorta The largest artery in the body, arising from the left ventricle of the heart,

Appendicitis Inflammation and infection of the appendix resulting in abdominal pain, nausea, and fever. Treated surgically. Not a prehospital emergency.

AQUA™ Advanced Quality Assurance Software Computer software based on the MPDS protocols utilizing expert system logic and quality assurance data analysis; an acronym for advanced quality assurance.

Aqueous Humor Clear fluid that moves with the eyeball.

Asthma Disease Characterized by a spasm of the bronchial tubes causing shortness of breath and wheezing.

ASTM Formerly the American Society for Testing and Materials. An international consensus-based standards setting organization for a wide variety of products and industries.

Average Response Time Pre-set period of time (set at a local, state, national, or international level) allowed for an appropriately qualified responder to reach the scene after initial receipt of the emergency call. Different times are set for different categories of requests for assistance (immediately life threatening, non-life threatening, etc.).

Axiom Important features that are actually the basis of many of the decision-making processes in priority dispatch. They are self-evident truths that need proof. They differ from rules in that they tell us *why*, rather than how we do things.

Basic Life Support (BLS) EMS procedures (airway positioning, external cardiac compression, and ventilation) to sustain viability of brain and heart in the abscence of pulse or breathing. The splinting, dressing, and other initial care covered in basic first-aid training; traditionally has not required medical oversight.

Benign Not harmful; describing a condition or disorder that is not a threat to health.

Bipolar Disease (manic/depression) A mental disorder characterized by dramatically alternating manic (high) and depressive (low) periods; has been linked to creative genius in some individuals; sometimes called manic-depression.

Biomedical Telemetry Electronic transmission of a patient's electrocardiogram and vital signs, coupled with two-way voice transmission, to a receiving emergency department's medical control nurse and/or physician facilitating concurrent patient care decision-making with the field crew.

BLS See Basic Life Support.

BRAVO Response A response level outlined in the protocol as sending the closest basic life support unit HOT or COLD, depending on the situation.

Breech During childbirth, the presentation of the umbilical cord, hands, feet, or buttocks first from the birth canal.

Breach of Duty Breaking a legal or moral obligation.

BRIDGE Protocol connection in the Medical Priority Dispatch System between the dispatch protocol and the pre-arrival instructions which provides verification of the correct chief complaint and dispatch life support necessity.

Burn Out Psychological condition caused by various factors with multiple symptomatic manifestations that results in personnel being unhappy and dissatisfied with their work. A state of fatigue or frustration brought about by devotion to a cause, way of life, or relationship. Also called cumulative stress reaction.

CAD Computer-aided dispatch. Public safety computer systems often linked to universal emergency service number systems that manage various functions of call-reception, unit status and resource deployment. Also referred to as command and control device.

Call Screening Process whereby trained dispatchers take requests for emergency services and prioritize the response of EMS resources to the most critical need. Always includes the option of "no response" or "no sending."

Cardiac Arrest Sudden cessation of heart functions or blood pumping ability universally resulting in death unless reversed by resuscitation.

Cardiopulmonary Resuscitation (CPR) Maintenance of cerebral perfusion during cardiac arrest, by the performance of closed-chest cardiac massage in conjuction with mouth-to-mouth (or similar variation) ventilation. This procedure can be performed with one or two persons.

CDE See Continuing Dispatch Education.

CEI See Critical EMD Information.

Central Dispatch Coalescence of dispatch services for multiple public-safety services into a single dispatch entity. Often includes police, fire, EMS, and at times, aero-medical functions.

Cerebrovascular Accident See Stroke.

CHARLIE Response A response level outlined in the protocol as sending the closest advanced life support unit COLD (or HOT), and basic life support transport COLD.

Chief Complaint Reason the patient is seeking medical care (in some cases only the mechanism or injury). It must contain sufficient information to allow categorization in one of the 33 defined chief complaints.

Chronic Disease or disorder that persists for long periods of time.

Chronic Bronchitis Excess release of mucus in the bronchi accompanied by a productive cough lasting for at least 3 months. Causative factors include cigarette smoking, air pollution, and chronic infections.

Chronic Obstructive Pulmonary Disease Disease process that decreases the pulmonary system's ability to perform ventilation. Chronic diseases responsible for this condition include asthma, bronchitis, and emphysema. Symptoms include persistent dyspnea on exertion (with or without chronic cough). Increased chest diameter and pursed-lip breathing are often seen in patients with more advanced forms of this condition. Also known as chronic obstructive lung disease, COAD, or COPD.

Clonic Phase (seizure) The second and longest physical phase of a grand mal seizure in which the major muscles of the body contract then relax in a rhythmic jerking cycle; preceded by a shorter tonic phase characterized by a sustained extension of the limbs.

COF See College of Fellows.

COLD Routine EMS unit driving response mode not using lights-and-siren.

College of Fellows Academy's formal standard-setting body, consisting of internationally recognized experts in EMS, EMD, and public safety telecommunications. The College of Fellows maintains the standards and integrity of the MPDS, the Academy's EMD certification curriculum, individual and agency recognition programs, Accreditation standards, and all aspects of dispatch life support. Contains seven expert boards and councils.

Coma State of unconsciousness from which the patient cannot be aroused.

Confidentiality The need to be kept secret or private; in EMD implies the necessity to not release or broadcast certain information about a patient's conditions, name, or illnesses unless approved by supervisors or by policy.

Consent Agreement, acquiescence, compliance.

Consolidated Dispatch See Central Dispatch.

Continuing Dispatch Education Continuing education program designed specifically for EMDs to develop a better understanding of telecommunications and of the EMD's roles and responsibilities; to enhance on-line skills in dispatch life support and in all emergency telephone procedures within the practice of EMD; to improve skills in the use and application of all component parts of the MPDS, including interrogation and prioritization; and to seek opportunities for discussion, skill practice, and critique of EMD skill performance.

Contusion Tissue injury with diffuse bleeding into subcutaneous tissue, causing discoloration under unbroken skin. Also known as a bruise.

Conventions Stylistic cues used in the Medical Priority Dispatch System to help the user find and identify needed information. Includes modifications of color, font, parentheses, symbols, and other visual differentiations.

Convulsions See Epileptic Seizures.

CPR See Cardiopulmonary Resuscitation.

Cranial Pertaining to the skull.

Critical EMD Information Vital reminders to the EMD regarding hazard warnings, non-scripted advice for callers, special notifications, and directions for when to stay on the line with callers.

Critical Incident Stress Stress reaction often experienced after a stressful emergency call or response.

Critical Incident Stress Debriefing Formal decompression, counseling, and discussion following an emotional EMS event.

Croup Viral infection of the respiratory tract that occurs primarily in infants and young children. Symptoms include hoarseness, fever, a distinct "barking" cough, and breathing distress from upper airway edema. The acute stage starts rapidly, most often occurs at night after bedtime.

Crowning In childbirth, the stage in which the baby's head can be seen.

CVA Cerebrovascular Accident. See Stroke.

Cyanosis Bluish or purplish discoloration of the skin as a result of poor oxygenation of the blood. May be due to poor oxygen transport capability, as in anemia, or acute blood loss, or to respiratory insufficiency that prevents oxygen from reaching the blood.

Decompression Sickness Syndrome occurring in the human body when nitrogen bubbles are formed in the bloodstream after rapid ascent from a depth. Prolonged diving time at depths below 30 feet causes saturation of the blood with nitrogen. If appropriate periods of time are not spent at different levels of ascent, this nitrogen comes out of solution in the blood forming bubbles, which cause blockage of various blood vessels. Symptoms include mild to severe joint pain (limb-bends), skin mottling and itching (cutaneous decompression sickness, or skin-bends), cyanosis, dyspnea, and substernal chest pain (pulmonary decompression sickness, or chokes). Also known as bends, caisson disease, compressed air illness, DCS, diver's paralysis.

Defendant Person, company, etc., against whom a claim or charge is brought in a court (opposed to plaintiff).

Defibrillation Sudden electrical or pharmacological depolarization of fibrillating cardiac cells in cases of ventricular tachycardia without pulses or ventricular fibrillation. This uniform repolarization briefly stops all cardiac activity allowing reset of the cardiac electrical system, so that viable cardiac electrical activity, if able, is allowed to resume. Also known as defib.

Dehydration Loss of water from the body.

DELTA Response A maximum response level outlined in the protocol as sending both basic and advances life support providers to the scene as fast as possible. Indicative of a critical trauma.

Diabetes A person with diagnosed diabetes of several different types that has problems with the cellular assimilation and combustion of sugar-like carbohydrates.

Diabetic Ketoacidosis Altered level of consciousness due to an inability of the body to use glucose for metabolism, as a result of absent or decreased insulin production. Late stages characterized by coma with dry, flushed skin and acetone breath odor; generally requires 12 to 36 hours of decreased insulin levels before becoming obvious.

Diaphragm Dome-shaped muscle that separates the chest cavity from the abdominal cavity. The diaphragm aids breathing by moving up and down. When breathing in, it moves down and increases the space in the chest. When breathing out, it moves up, decreasing the volume.

Direct Pressure Generally used to describe the application of pressure by hand against a bleeding artery or vein, in order to control bleeding. It is the most reliable method of hemorrhage control associated with the least amount of damage to tissues.

Dislocation Displacement of any part of the body from its normal position. This applies most often to a bone moved from its normal position with a joint.

Dispatch Means by which emergency resources can be directed to the scene of the illness or injury. Also a dispatch or communication center.

Dispatch Danger Zones Fifteen identified behaviors or situations that predictably result in medico-legal problems, negligent situations, and lawsuits within the dispatch center or its management organization.

Dispatch Life Support Knowledge, procedures, and skills used by trained EMDs in providing care through pre-arrival instructions to callers. It consists of those basic and advanced life support principles that are appropriate to application by medical dispatchers.

Dissecting Thoracic Aortic Aneurysm Progressive dilatation of a portion of the aorta at a weak point between the middle (tunica media) and outer (tunica adventitia) layers of the vessel wall.

Diuretic Medicine used for decreasing fluid in the circulatory system; often used in congestive heart failure treatment.

DLS See Dispatch Life Support.

Duty Legal relationship, between one or more individual and an individual or private or public organization, that requires that the person or organization with the duty to act, possess, and bring to bear that degree of care, knowledge, and skill that is usually exercised by reasonable and prudent practitioners under similar circumstances, given prevailing knowledge and available resources.

ECCS See Emotional Content and Cooperation Score.

ECHO Response A maximum response level outlined in the protocol as sending the closest apparatus/personnel of any kind HOT. Indicative of imminent death situations.

Eclampsia Seizures due to toxemia of pregnancy, which may occur up to two weeks after delivery.

Ectopic Pregnancy Pregnancy occurring in a woman's body other than in the cavity of her uterus (i.e., tubal).

Electrolytes Element or compound that, when melted or dissolved in water or other solvent, dissociates into ions (atoms able to carry an electric charge). Electrolyte amounts vary in blood plasma, in tissues, and in cell fluid. The body must maintain electrolyte balance to use energy. Potassium (K+) is needed to contract muscles and propagate nerve impulses. Sodium (Na++) is needed to maintain fluid balance. Some diseases, defects, and drugs may lead to a lack of one or more electrolytes.

Emboli Foreign objects such as bubbles of air or gas, bits of tissue, or blood clots that travel through the bloodstream until becoming lodged in a vessel.

EMD See Emergency Medical Dispatcher or Emergency Medical Dispatch.

EMDPRS Emergency Medical Dispatch Priority Reference System. The generic term for a medical priority dispatch protocol coined by the U.S. government.

Emergency Medical Dispatch Reception and management of requests for emergency medical assistance in an EMS system.

Emergency Medical Dispatcher (EMD) EMS personnel specifically trained and certified in interrogation techniques, pre-arrival instructions and call prioritization with a minimum of 24-hours training including techniques of airway and hemorrhage control, CPR, Heimlich manuever, and childbirth.

Emergency Medical Services (EMS) Collective term describing the many agencies, personnel, and institutions involved in planning for, providing, and monitoring emergency care. Frequently refers only to prehospital care.

Emergency Medical Technician (EMT) Medical provider who generally performs prehospital basic life support medical care. Roughly equivalent to Ambulance Officer (U.K.) and Qualified Ambulance Officer (Australia).

Emergency Medical Vehicle Collision (EMVC) Collisions involving emergency medical vehicles during lights-and-siren (HOT) responses and transports.

Emergency Rule From a medical-legal perspective, when one is faced with an extraordinary emergency situation, they are not held to the same standard of conduct as when not faced with such a situation.

Emotional Content and Cooperation Score Used to quantify the level of emotion and cooperation of the caller at the beginning of a call. Can also be used during case review to evaluate the success of caller management techniques.

Emphysema Pulmonary over-inflation and alveolar destruction, which causes loss of lung elasticity and poor exchange of gases. This condition is one of several chronic obstructive lung diseases such as asthma, asbestosis, black lung, bronchitis, chronic obstructive lung disease.

EMS See Emergency Medical Services.

EMT See Emergency Medical Technician.

EMT-A Emergency Medical Technician-Advanced.

EMT-P Emergency Medical Technician-Paramedic.

EMVC See Emergency Medical Vehicle Collision.

Envenomation The injection of a caustic or poisonous substance by one organism into another, often accomplished by fangs, spines, or stingers.

Epiglotitis Leaf-shaped structure located posterior to the base of the tongue. It covers the tracheal entrance as swallowing occurs but generally remains open to allow free passage of air into the lung.

Epilepsy Condition where seizures (generally of unknown cause) recur spontaneously for one year.

Epileptic Seizures Abnormal firing of brain cells creating a wave of cellular electrical activity resulting in simultaneous stimulation of multiple body activities and functions. There are various types and extents of seizures often resulting in a short period of unconsciousness followed by improving stupor. Also referred to as "fits" and "fitting" in the U.K. and Australasia.

Esophagus Canal extending from the throat to the stomach.

Espohagitis Inflammation of the lining of the esophagus. Causes include gastric reflux infection and irritations.

Febrile Seizure Event in infancy or childhood, usually occurring between three months and five years of age, associated with fever but without evidence of intra-cranial infection or defined cause. Febrile seizures are to be distinguished from epilepsy, which is characterized by recurrent seizures, and those caused by brain infections such as meningitis.

Fibrillation Spontaneous contraction of individual muscle fibers. Also called atrial fibrillation and ventricular fibrillation.

Fire Priority Dispatch System™ (FPDS) The National Academy's set of fire protocols and quality assurance support system for the fire dispatch community.

First-Party Caller Person calling for emergency medical help who is also the patient or victim.

Focal Refers to a specific, singular location or region of the body.

Four Commandments The dispatch equivalent of vital signs that are always required to be determined and relayed to responding crews; they are considered to be the most basic standard of care and practice by EMDs.

Foreseeability From a medical-legal perspective, the determination of liability for accident or injury based on a consequence's predictability or foreseeable risk.

Fracture Broken bone. Divided into simple (closed) and compound (open) injuries, they may also be classed by the type of break that the bone sustains: comminuted, greenstick, impacted, linear, oblique, spiral, or transverse.

Frostbite Condition caused from cold exposure resulting in pale, gray, numb, bloodless, or cold skin. In deep frostbite, tissues feel woody or stony.

Frostnip Mild form of cold injury that occurs without loss of tissue.

Gallbladder Disease Pear-shaped sac, near the right lobe of the liver, which holds bile. During digestion of fats, it contracts, secreting bile into the duodenum. Obstruction of the system may lead to jaundice and pain. Severe, steady pain often results from passage of gallstones through its duct ot the bowel.

Gap Theory EMD-caused gaps in conversation during interrogation or advice that causes the caller to insert demands or make uncooperative statements. It is theorized these gaps create a lack of caller confidence in the EMD.

Gastritis Inflammation of the lining of the stomach. Symptoms include loss of appetite, nausea, vomiting, and discomfort after eating which usually subside after the cause has been removed. Types include: acute, chronic, atrophic, hemorrhagic, and hypertrophic.

Gastroenteritis Inflammation of the stomach and intestinal tract usually caused by a virus; called "stomach flu" or "bug" by lay persons.

Glucose Sugar found in foods, especially fruits, and a major source of energy in body fluids. Glucose, when eaten or produced by the digestion of carbohydrates, is taken into the blood from the intestine. Excess glucose in circulation is stored in the liver and muscles as glycogen and converted to glucose and released as needed.

Grand Mal Grand mal seizures are characterized by unconsciousness and various involuntary, skeletal muscle activities, followed by a period (post-ictal) of urinary incontinence and unresponsiveness, then confusion, and increasing awareness. Recently replaced by the term generalized tonic-clonic seizure.

Hazardous Materials Gas, liquid, or material that, even in small quantities, poses a threat to life, health, or property.

HAZMAT See Hazardous Materials.

HCFA Health Care Finance Administration

Heat Cramps Any cramp in the arm, leg, or stomach due to decreased water and salt in the body. It usually occurs after vigorous physical exertion in very hot weather or under other conditions that cause heavy sweating and loss of body fluids and salts.

Heat Exhaustion Non-life-threatening condition caused from heat exposure resulting in flu-like symptoms, paleness, sweating, nausea, or vomiting.

Heat Stroke Possible life-threatening condition caused from heat exposure resulting in red, dry skin accompanied by a decreased level of consciousness.

Heimlich Maneuver An abdominally-applied pressure process for relieving an airway obstruction caused by a foreign body invented by Cincinnati esophageal surgeon, Dr. Henry Heimlich, in 1970.

Hematoma Swelling caused by a pocket or collection of blood outside of the blood vessel.

Hemophilia Group of hereditary bleeding disorders in which there is a lack of one of the factors needed to clot blood. Hemophilia A involves the main factors needed to clot blood. Hemophilia B, also known as Christmas disease, is similar to but less severe than Hemophilia A. Hemophilia C, also called Rosenthal's syndrome, is also similar to but less severe than Hemophilia A.

Hemorrhage Abnormal internal or external discharge of blood.

Hiatal Hernia Kind of diaphragmatic hernia. A protrusion of a portion of the stomach upward through the diaphragm. Symptoms usually include heartburn after meals, when lying down, and on exertion. There may be vomiting and dull pain below the sternum that radiates to the shoulder.

Hits When a dispatcher "leads" a caller until getting an answer which falls into one of the dispatcher's "expected" categories. This type of fishing for irrelevant information is common for dispatchers not operating under a specific protocol structure.

Hives Swollen eruptions of very itchy bumps or spots on the skin usually caused by allergies.

Horizontal Dispatch Dispatcher configuration where several dispatchers divide individual responsibilities between call interrogation and unit "radio" dispatch functions. Also called tandem or team dispatching.

HOT Lights-and-siren emergency unit driving response mode.

Hyperbaric Oxygen Chamber Giving oxygen at high atmospheric pressure. It is done in pressure chambers that permit the delivery of pure oxygen and air at pressures up to five times normal. Hyperbaric oxygenation is used to treat carbon monoxide poisoning, air embolism, smoke inhalation, cyanide poisoning, decompression sickness, and infected wounds.

Hypertension Vascular condition of increased blood pressure. More commonly known as high blood pressure.

Hyperventilation Syndrome of increased inspiration and expiration of air as a result of increase in rate and/or depth of respiration usually accompanied by marked anxiety, numbness in both hands, lips, and earlobes, commonly accompanied by chest pain and a feeling of impending doom. Although it is benign, it is never assumed to exist in patients 35 years of age or older.

Hypothermia Condition caused from cold exposure resulting in sluggishness, a decreased level of consciousness, paleness, or cyanosis (blue or gray).

Hypovolemia Diminished blood volume usually caused by hemorrhage or severe dehydration.

Hypoxia Decreased oxygen in the cells. Symptoms include cyanosis, tachycardia, and altered levels of consciousness. The tissues most sensitive to hypoxia are the brain, heart, and liver.

Hysteria State of tension or excitement in a person or group, marked by unmanageable fear and short-term loss of control over the emotions.

Hysteria Threshold Point at which a person changes from hysterical behavior to calm cooperative action. This threshold varies from individual to individual and may be reached by repetitive persistence. Passage across it is often very noticable.

IAEMD International Academy of Emergency Medical Dispatch. See National Academy of Emergency Medical Dispatch.

Idiopathic Any primary disease with no understood apparent cause.

Immunity Exemption from duties the law generally requires others to perform.

Implied Indicated by deduction, inference, or necessary consequence.

Implied consent The assumption that, in a true emergency where a patient who is unresponsive or unable to make a rational decision is at significant risk of death, disability, or deterioration of condition, that patient would agree to emergency treatment.

Incontinent Inability to control urination or defecation; common in the aged and during seizures.

Informed consent Consent given only after full disclosure of what is being consented to; where a patient must be told the nature and risks of a medical procedure before the caregiver can validly claim exemption from liability for battery or from responsibility for medical complications.

Ingestion Accidental intake of a potentially harmful substance.

Insulin Naturally occurring hormone released by the pancreas in response to increased levels of sugar in the blood. The hormone acts to regulate the body's use of sugar and some of the processes involved with utilizing fats, carbohydrates, and proteins as fuel. Insulin lowers blood sugar levels and promotes transport and entry of sugar into the muscle cells and other tissues.

Jacksonian Seizure activity that begins in a localized muscle mass and moves or enlarges to include additional muscles without involving the whole body. Named after John Hughlings Jackson, British physician, 1835-1911.

JAMA Journal of the American Medical Association.

JEMS Journal of Emergency Medical Services.

JNAEMD Journal of the National Academy of Emergency Medical Dispatch now known as the National EMD Journal.

Ketoacidosis When the body burns its own tissue (fat, muscle, etc.). The ketoacids produced (acetones) are toxic (poisonous) to the patient making him increasingly ill. This is rarely a prehospital medical emergency.

Key Questions Systematized interrogation questions constituting the secondary survey of the EMD. Must be written in full sentence form and address the four objectives of pre-arrival evaluation.

Kidney Infection (pyelonephritis)

Kidney Stones Precipitation of solidified minerals, infectious concretions, or cholesterol-like material within the kidney that can block urine flow while inside the kidney or after being dislodged into the ureteral tube leading to the bladder; often results in excruciating back or groin pain once inside the ureter.

KQ See Key Questions.

Kussmal Breathing Deep, rapid respirations with sighing. It occurs in diabetic ketoacidosis.

Labor Time and processes that occur during childbirth from the beginning of cervical dilatation to the delivery of the placenta.

Laceration Tear or cut through the skin into the flesh.

Law Sets forth general medical and medical dispatch principles in an interesting and catchy form. In general medicine, they are referred to as "the pearls."

Liability Refers to the legal responsibility, obligation, or duty of an individual or organization to do, or refrain from doing, something. If found legally responsible for damages associated with an indicent in litigation, that individual or agency is considered liable.

Litigation The process of legally setteling a dispute; a judicial contest aiming to determine and enforce legal rights. A dispute is in "litigation" (or being "litigated") when is has become the subject of a formal court action or lawsuit.

Life Status Questionable Existence of any information suggesting a patient is unconscious, breathing abnormally, or in cardiac arrest.

Low Back Syndrome A chronically recurrent form a back pain often resulting from vertebral disc degeneration that irritates a major nerve root emanating from the spinal cord; can prevent a patient from walking or significant movement when acute.

Mass Casualty Incident Emergency medical problem that by its volume or circumstances overwhelms or threatens to overwhelm the capabilities of the local emergency medical services system.

Maximal Response Traditional public safety practice of sending the highest available response (manpower and unit) in hot mode.

Maximal Response Disease Referring to maximal response as an obsolete and dangerous practice; an abnormal practice.

Medical Control Process of ensuring that actions taken on behalf of ill or injured people are medically appropriate.

Medical Director Physician responsible for management and accountability for the medical care aspects of an emergency medical dispatch program including: the medical monitoring oversight of the training of the EMD personnel; approval and medical control of the operational medical priority dispatch system, evaluation of the medical care and pre-arrival instructions rendered by the EMD personnel; direct participation in the EMD system evaluation, quality assurance, and quality improvement process and mechanisms; and, responsibility for the medical decisions and care rendered by the EMD and EMD program.

Medical Miranda See Secondary Emergency Notification of Dispatch.

Medical Priority Dispatch System™
Medicallyapproved, unified system used by medical dispatch centers to dispatch appropriate aid to medical emergencies, which includes: 1. systematized caller interrogation; 2. systematized pre-arrival instructions; and 3. protocols which match the dispatcher's evaluation of the injury or illness type and severity with vehicle response mode and configuration. Includes a program of total quality management and a

standards maintaining process. The system was created by Dr. Jeff J. Clawson and is now maintained by the Academy's College of Fellows.

Meningitis Infection or inflammation of the membranes covering the brain and spinal cord. Symptoms include fever, headache, stiff neck and back, nausea, and skin rash. Commonly caused by bacterial infection with Streptococcus pneumoniae. May be caused by other bacteria, chemical irritation, or viruses including coxsackieviruses, echoviruses, and mumps.

MI See Myocardial Infarction.

Migraine Recurrent severe headache usually beginning with disordered vision and followed by vomiting and photophobia.

Miscarriage Post-delivery of a fetus or products of conception (tissue) during the first or second trimester of pregnancy.

MPDS See Medical Priority Dispatch System™.

Multigravida Woman who has been pregnant (and delivered) more than once.

Myocardial Infarction Insufficient blood supply to an area of the heart muscle usually as a result of occlusion of a coronary artery.

NAED See National Academies of Emergency Dispatch.

NAEMD See National Academy of Emergency Medical Dispatch.

NAEFD See National Academy of Emergency Fire Dispatch.

NAEMSP National Association of Emergency Medical Service Physicians.

NAEPD See National Academy of Emergency Police Dispatch.

National Academies of Emergency Dispatch The new umbrella, not-for-profit international organization which encompasses both the NAEMD, NAEFD, and the NAEPD. It sets the standards for the three disciplines of public safety dispatch including basic Emergency Telecommunications.

National Academy of Emergency Fire Dispatch Not-for-profit international organization which sets standards and requirements for EFD, certifies EFDs internationally, and evaluates, improves, and maintains the Fire Priority Dispatch System™ as a unified standard.

National Academy of Emergency Medical Dispatch Not-for-profit international organization which sets standards and requirements for EMD, certifies EMDs internationally, and evaluates, improves, and maintains the Medical Priority Dispatch System™ as a unified standard.

National Academy of Emergency Police Dispatch Not-for-profit international organization which sets standards and requirements for EPD, certifies EPDs internationally, and evaluates, improves, and maintains the Police Priority Dispatch System™ as a unified standard.

National EMD Journal Official journal of the National Academy of EMD, formerly JNAEMD.

National Health Service (NHS)

Negligence Failure to provide the degree of care (as defined by community or national standards) normally associated with a set of circumstances requiring that care. To establish negligence the plaintiff must prove four elements: duty to act, breach of that duty, damage (or injury), and a clear cause-and-effect relationship between the injury and breach of duty.

NEMDJ National EMD Journal; formerly the Journal of the NAEMD.

NHAAP National Heart Attack Alert Program (U.S.); a division of the National Institutes of Health.

NHS National Health Services (U.K.)

NHTSA National Highway Traffic Safety Administration (U.S.)

NIH National Institutes of Health (U.S.)

Off-Line Medical Control See Medical Director.

OMEGA Response A response level outlined in the protocol for special referral and response, such as forwarding the call to a poison control center, nurse advice, or ombudsman program.

Orbital Fracture Break in the portion of the skull which encases the eyeball.

Overdose Intentional intake of a potentially harmful substance.

PAI See Pre-Arrival Instructions.

Pancreas Fish-shaped, grayish-pink gland about five inches long that stretches across the posterior portion of the abdomen, behind the stomach. It releases insulin, glucagon, somastatin, and enzymes of digestion.

PANDA Parents Against Negligent Dispatch Agencies, an organization dedicated to changing the standards of many other communication centers who don't provide pre-arrival instructions.

PDI See Post-Dispatch Instructions.

Pelvic Inflammatory Disease Disease of the female pelvic organs, usually caused by bacteria. Symptoms include fever, vaginal discharge, pain in the lower abdomen, bleeding, and painful sexual intercourse. Also known as PID.

Peptic Ulcer Disease Loss of mucous membrane in any part of the digestive system, often caused by bacteria, allowing unprotected tissue to come in contact with gastric fluid. A duodenal ulcer is the most common type if of peptic ulcer. Also known as gastric ulcer.

Pericarditis Inflammation of the pericardium. Symptoms include chest pain, dry cough, dyspnea, fever, and palpitations.

Perineum Genital area.

Petit Mal Generalized non-convulsive seizure hallmarked by momentary suppression of awareness with immobility and blank stare.

Placenta A temporary blood-rich structure in the uterus through which the fetus receives oxygen and nutrients, and eliminates carbon dioxide and metabolic wastes.

Placenta Abruptio Parting of the placenta from the uterus before birth, often resulting in severe bleeding.

Placenta Previa Condition in which the placenta is placed abnormally in the uterus so that it partly or completely covers the opening of the cervix. It is the most common cause of painless but serious bleeding in the third trimester of pregnancy.

Plaintiff Person who brings suit in a court (opposed to defendant).

Pleura Two-layered membrane surrounding the lung. The visceral pleura adheres to the surface of the lung. The parietal pleura lines the chest wall. The two pleura are separated from each other by a serous fluid.

Pleurisy Inflammation of the pleura. Symptoms include dyspnea and sharp, localized pain when breathing or moving. Causes include injury, cancer, pneumonia, pulmonary embolus, and tuberculosis.

Pneumonia Inflammation (infection) of the lungs, commonly caused by bacteria (Diplococcus pneumoniae). Symptoms include fever, headache, cough, and chest pain.

Pneumothorax Accumulation of air in the chest cavity usually due to a wound penetrating the chest wall or a laceration of the lung.

Police Priority Dispatch System™ (PPDS)

Post-Dispatch Instructions Case-specific advice, warnings, and treatments relayed by trained EMDs through callers after dispatching field responders.

Post-Ictal Period immediately following the convulsive phase of a seizure, often characterized by combativeness, confusion, incontinence, and sleepiness.

Pre-Arrival Instructions Medically approved, scripted instructions given by trained EMDs to callers that help provide necessary assistance to the victim and control of the situation prior to the arrival of EMS personnel. Pre-Arrival Instructions are read word-for-word by the EMD to the fullest extent possible.

Pre-Eclampsia Toxemia of pregnancy with headache, increasing hypertension, and edema of the feet. Although the condition resolves once the pregnancy is completed, it can deteriorate to eclampsia during the pregnancy.

Primary Survey Information gathered during the Case Entry protocol. It includes the location and telephone number of the caller, and the four commandments. It is the equivalent of the filed provider's "initial assessment."

Primigravida First-time pregnancy.

Priority Symptoms Spectrum of a patient signs and symptoms which are commonly life-threatening and must be assessed quickly. Includes abnormal breathing, unconsciousness, chest pain in people of cardiac disease-susceptible age, and serious hemorrhage.

Proposal For Change A formal document that is filled out and submitted to the Academy representing a request for improvement to the MPDS; prior to submission the content of the request is evaluated and approved by the MDRC, Steering Committee, and Medical Director and supported by actual cases, data, or studies.

ProQA™ Computer software based on the MPDS protocols utilizing expert system logic and quality assurance data collection; an acronym for professional quality assurance.

Psychomotor Seizure Complex type of seizure characterized by abnormal patient activity. Patients often appear to act animal-like.

Pulmonary Edema Effusion of fluid into the lungs resulting in difficulty breathing.

Pulmonary Embolus Pulmonary artery blockage due to air, fat, thrombus, or tissue. This condition often causes sudden, unexplained shortness of breath and chest pain.

Pyelonephritis Bacterial infection of the filtration tissue of the kidney that results in back pain, chill, fever, and frequent urination generally requiring antibiotic treatment.

QA See Quality Assurance.

QA Quality Assurance Officer.

QI See Quality Improvement.

Qualified Ambulance Officer See Emergency Medical Technician.

Quality Assurance Organized method of auditing and evaluating care provided within EMS systems.

Quality Improvement Concept of a continual cycle of evaluation and improvement based on the findings of quality assurance.

Re-Freak Event A predictable event during the course of a call when the caller reacts to seeing, or being reminded of, the patient's state of distress. It is much more likely to occur when the patient is a relative or a loved one.

Repetitive Persistence Hysteria-controlling technique where the EMD, by repeating in identical phrasing of the same calming message or request, can help most callers regain self-control and become able to provide answers to interrogation or deliver pre-arrival care.

Respiratory Arrest Cessation of breathing (but not heart activity initially).

Response Mode Type of emergency driving techniques such as lights-and-siren (HOT) versus routine driving (COLD).

Rule A definitive action statement. Conveys specifically *how* axioms are used and provides many of the do's and don'ts of priority dispatch. The rules contained within a particular protocol are to be considered always true in the medical dispatch environment, without exception.

Ruptured Abdominal Aneurysm Dilation of the abdominal aortic blood vessel to the point that it breaks or tears. Once ruptured, can cause immediate shock and death.

Schizophrenia A form of mental psychosis in which the patient cannot always discern reality from fantasy and may hear voices or experience visions that can affect behavior. In one popularly depicted sub-form, results in a patient exhibiting more than one personality.

SCUBA Self-contained, underwater breathing apparatus for divers.

Second-Party Caller Person calling for emergency medical help who is in close proximity to the patient or victim.

Secondary Emergency Notification of Dispatch™ Protocol regarding the relay to dispatch of initial medical information including the four commandments that is issued to law enforcement and other field personnel to extend the effects of priority dispatch to these second-party professionals at the scene. Also known as Medical Miranda in the U.S.

Seizure See Epileptic Seizures.

SEND™ Secondary Emergency Notification of Dispatch™ protocol.

Severe Respiratory Distress Condition of a patient who is turning blue, is experiencing retractive breathing (fighting for air), or extreme breathing difficulty, or who is described as making "funny noises."

Shock Clinical syndrome exhibiting varying degrees of inadequate tissue perfusion to the body. Types include anaphylactic (systemic allergic reaction), cardiogenic (poor tissue perfusion as a result of decreased cardiac output), hypovolemic (decreased circulation from a reduction in blood volume), metabolic (a buildup of toxic waste product in the body due to organ failure), neurogenic (vasodilation below a level of disruption of the spinal cord), psychogenic (fainting), and septic (vasodilation associated with the bacterial toxins of overwhelming infection).

SHUNT Protocol connection in the Medical Priority Dispatch System™ facilitating identification and categorization of a chief complaint when a diagnosis or nondescript complaint is first provided by the caller.

Sick Person From a dispatch perspective, a patient with a non-categorizable chief complaint who does not have an identifiable priority symptom.

Side-cycling "Lateral," inventive deviation from the usual vertically listed key question objectives. Also known as lateral questioning, it is a form of ad-libbing and by definition is not condsidered correct interrogation enhancement.

Signs Any objective abnormality indicative of disease or injury.

Spock Principle An ethical view that places actions protecting the good of the many higher than that of protecting the few or even the one as quoted by Mr. Spock in the film "The Wrath of Khan."

Status Epilepticus Repeated seizures occurring without intervals of consciousness. Causes include meningitis, hypoglycemia, brain injury, fever, or poisoning.

Sternum Bone in the front of the chest to which the ribs attach. Also called the breastbone.

Stroke Disruption of blood flow to the brain or part of the brain due to blood clot or hemorrhage. Hemorrhage also causes increased pressure within the skull. Clots are spontaneous or traumatic. Paralysis or weakness of one side, trouble speaking, altered level of consciousness, and respiratory changes are all common symptoms. Also called "brain attack."

Subarachnoid Area underneath the middle membrane which encases the brain and spinal cord.

Subdural Hematoma Mass of blood (hematoma), often clotted, that has collected under the dura, which is one of the three membranes that line the brain and spinal cord. Although usually associated with trauma, a subdural hematoma may be seen for spontaneous reasons, particularly in the acloholic population.

Subdural Hemorrhage Bleeding between the dura mater and arachnoid, associated with injury to the underlying brain tissue. This type of bleeding (venous) may not be apparent for days or weeks after an injury, because of the slow buildup of pressure due to hemorrhage. Signs and symptoms include altered levels of consciousness, headache, and slurred speech.

Substernal Beneath the sternum or breastbone.

Suffixes Code-type differentiator letters found at the end of the full Response Code on some of the protocols (i.e. 27-D-3s or 27-D-3p).

Symptoms Any subjective abnormality in body function indicative of disease, illness or injury, such as headache, dizziness, nausea as described by the patient.

Syncope Fainting. May be caused by emotional stress, pooling of blood in the legs, heavy sweating, or sudden change in temperature or body position. This condition may also result from any of a number of cardio-pulmonary disorders.

Tachypnea Rapid breathing rate over 20 a minute (not the same as hyperventilation; see Hyperventilation Syndrome).

TDD Telecommunication Device for the Deaf

Temporal Lobe Outer lower region of the brain.

Third-Party Caller Person calling for emergency medical help who is removed from or not in close proximity to the patient or victim.

Thoracic Aortic Aneurysm Dilation of the main aortic blood vessel in the chest cavity. Rupture can cause shock or death.

Tiered Response Multi-level response availability for emergency medical assistance. Can include ambulance care, the closest basic-level first responder, and progressing to more advanced assistance based on need.

Toxic Poisonous or dangerous.

Transient Ishcemic Attack Temporary cerebrovascular event caused by a transient blockage of a cerebral blood vessel. The symptoms depend on where and how much of the brain is affected. The episode is most often brief, lasting a few minutes; rarely symptoms continue for several hours. Also known as TIA.

Trauma Physical injury or wound caused by an external force through accident or violence.

Treatment Sequence Protocols Earlier outdated name for pre-arrival instructions written as algorithmic scripts that are learned and read to the caller during life-threatening emergencies. These instructions include airway control, Heimlich maneuver, CPR, and childbirth.

Triage Assigning victims of a mass casualty incident a priority for care and transport based on the degree of injury and an individual's relative salvageability in a given situation. From the French, meaning, "to sort."

USDOT United States Department of Transportation. Includes the National Highway Traffic Safety Administration.

Vertibral Disk Disease

Vertical Dispatch Dispatcher configuration where a single dispatcher is responsible for a given geographical area requiring the dispatcher to handle all functions of interrogation, unit "radio" dispatch, and pre-arrival instructions for each call. Also called solitary dispatching.

Vitreous Humor Clear, jelly like substance contained in a thin membrane filling the space behind the lens of the eye. Also known as vitreous body.

Wake Effect Cause of a vehicle collision due to the passage of an emergency vehicle but does not actually involve the emergency vehicle itself.

Willful Misconduct Improperly conducting oneself on purpose, without regard to the consequences of that lack of appropriate behavior or action.

Medical Dispatch Case Evaluation Record

Case #: _____ Date: _____ Time: _____ How Obtained: **911 / E911 / Other**

Dispatcher(s): _____ Dispatcher ID:_____

Complaint description: _____ Shift:_____

Caller is: ☐ The patient *(1st party)* ☐ With patient *(2nd party)* ☐ Remote from patient *(3rd party)* ☐ Referring agency *(4th party)*

CASE ENTRY (EQ) INFORMATION ASKED *(Primary Survey)*

	Yes	Obvious	No		Yes	Obvious	No	Insig
1. Address asked?	☐	☐	☐	Address *verified*?	☐	☐	☐	
2. Callback number asked?	☐	☐	☐	Callback number *verified*?	☐	☐	☐	
3. "What's the problem…" asked?	☐	☐	☐	Asked Correctly?	☐	☐	☐	☐
3a. "Are you with the patient now?" asked?	☐	☐	☐	Asked Correctly?	☐	☐	☐	☐
3b. "How many people are hurt?" asked?	☐	☐	☐	Asked Correctly?	☐	☐	☐	☐
3c. "Is s/he still choking now?" asked?	☐	☐	☐	Asked Correctly?	☐	☐	☐	☐
4. "How old is s/he?" asked? _____	☐	☐	☐	Asked Correctly?	☐	☐	☐	☐
4a. "Tell me approximately…" stated?	☐	☐	☐					
5. "Is s/he conscious?" asked?	☐	☐	☐	Asked Correctly?	☐	☐	☐	☐
6. "Is s/he breathing?" asked?	☐	☐	☐	Asked Correctly?	☐	☐	☐	☐
6a. "You go check…" stated?	☐	☐	☐					
Gender of patient asked?	☐	☐	☐	Number of freelance questions asked _____				

☐ Check if any questions asked, were asked **out of order**   ** ECC Score: Beginning _____ End _____

CHIEF COMPLAINT SELECTION

Chief Complaint Protocol Selected: _____ ☐ Correct ☐ Incorrect Should have selected: _____

KEY QUESTIONS *(Secondary Survey)*

KQ asked?	Yes	Obvious	No	N/A	Insig	Asked Incorrect?	KQ asked?	Yes	Obvious	No	N/A	Insig	Asked Incorrect?
KQ _____	☐	☐	☐	☐	☐	☐	KQ _____	☐	☐	☐	☐	☐	☐
KQ _____	☐	☐	☐	☐	☐	☐	KQ _____	☐	☐	☐	☐	☐	☐
KQ _____	☐	☐	☐	☐	☐	☐	KQ _____	☐	☐	☐	☐	☐	☐
KQ _____	☐	☐	☐	☐	☐	☐	KQ _____	☐	☐	☐	☐	☐	☐
KQ _____	☐	☐	☐	☐	☐	☐	KQ _____	☐	☐	☐	☐	☐	☐
KQ _____	☐	☐	☐	☐	☐	☐	KQ _____	☐	☐	☐	☐	☐	☐
KQ _____	☐	☐	☐	☐	☐	☐	Number of freelance questions asked _____						

☐ Check if any questions asked, were asked **out of order**   ** ECC Score: Beginning _____ End _____

DISPATCH LIFE SUPPORT INSTRUCTIONS *(Pre-Arrival & Post-Dispatch Instructions)*

	Yes	No	N/A		Yes	No	N/A
Appropriate to give Pre-Arrival Instructions?	☐	☐		*Appropriate* to give Post-Dispatch Instructions?	☐	☐	
Possible to give Pre-Arrival Instructions?	☐	☐	☐	*Possible* to give Post-Dispatch Instructions?	☐	☐	☐
(If yes) Were PAIs/PDIs given?	☐	☐	☐	*(If yes)* Were PDIs given?	☐	☐	☐
(If yes) Were they given correctly? **(C, M, D, J, A)** _____				*(If yes)* Were they given correctly? **(C, M, D, J, A)** _____			

[C]orrect **[M]**inor Mo**[D]**erate Ma**[J]**or **[A]**bsolute   ** ECC Score: Beginning _____ End _____

FINAL DISPATCH CODE DETERMINATION

Dispatch Code Assigned: _____ - _____ - _____ - _____   Dispatch Code As Reviewed: _____ - _____ - _____ - _____

TOTAL COMPLIANCE SCORE

Case Entry	_____
Chief Complaint Selection	_____
Key Questions	_____
Dispatch Life Support Instructions	_____
Final Coding	_____
Sub-total	_____ /5 = **TOTAL COMPLIANCE SCORE =**

**CUSTOMER SERVICE SCORE

COMMENTS

	N/A	Minor	Incorrect	Score
1. Displayed Service Attitude	-0	-3	-10	_____
2. Used Correct Volume/Tone	-0	-3	-10	_____
3. Displayed Compassion	-0	-3	-10	_____
4. Avoided Gaps	-0	-3	-10	_____
5. Explained Actions	-0	-3	-10	_____
6. Provided Reassurance	-0	-3	-10	_____
7. Created Expectations	-0		-10	_____
8. Used Prohibited Behavior	-0		-100	_____
9. Provided Calming Techniques		N/A	No	
Case Entry		-0	-20	_____
Key Questions		-0	-20	_____
DLS Instructions		-0	-20	_____

If additional space is needed, attach a 2nd sheet of paper.

Review Date: _____ Reviewer: _____

Manager/Supervisor: _____

TOTAL CUSTOMER SERVICE SCORE = [   ] Calltaker: _____

SCORING CALCULATIONS

CASE ENTRY

100 Points Possible

25 points off if the address was not asked (Case Entry Question 1)
25 points off if the address was not verified (Case Entry Question 1)
25 points off if the callback number was not asked (Case Entry Question 2)
25 points off if the callback number was not verified (Case Entry Question 2)
33 points off if age was not asked (Case Entry Question 4)
33 points off if conscious was not asked (Case Entry Question 5)
33 points off if breathing was not asked (Case Entry Question 6)
20 points off if Case Entry Statement 4a or Case Entry Statement 6a was not stated when appropriate
20 points off if a question was asked incorrectly
20 points off for each freelance question asked
10 points off if any question asked was asked out of order
10 points off if gender was not asked (if not obvious)

CHIEF COMPLAINT

100 Points Possible

33 points off if Case Entry Question 3 was not asked
20 points off if Case Entry Question 3 was asked incorrectly
10 points off for each appropriate conditional question that was not asked (Case Entry Questions 3a, 3b, and 3c)
 5 points off for each appropriate conditional question that was asked incorrectly (3a, 3b, and 3c)
67 points off if the calltaker chose an incorrect Chief Complaint Protocol

KEY QUESTIONS

100 Points Possible

Note: The weight of each Key Question is based on 100 points divided by the total number of applicable (appropriate) questions
Full value of the Key Question off when the question was not asked (not attempted)
1/2 value of the question off when the question was asked incorrectly
10 points off if the Key Questions were not asked in order (of questions that were asked)
20 points off for each freelance question asked

DISPATCH LIFE SUPPORT

100 Points Possible

Note: If PAIs are possible and appropriate, score PAIs/PDIs as a single DLS (Dispatch Life Support) score and use the PAI section to score compliance. If PAIs are not possible, score only PDIs in the PDI section.
100 points off for ABSOLUTE deviation
50 points off for MAJOR deviation
25 points off for MODERATE deviation
10 points off for MINOR deviation
(See: NAEMD EMD-Q Scoring Standards for a complete description of DLS Scoring Calculations)

FINAL CODING

100 Points Possible

100 points off if the calltaker did not shunt to the correct Chief Complaint Protocol (when a shunt was required)
60 points off if the Level was incorrect (the Determinant Descriptor is always incorrect if the Level is incorrect)
20 points off if the Determinant Descriptor was incorrect (the Level is correct)
20 points off if the calltaker assigned an incorrect suffix or failed to assign a suffix when appropriate

TOTAL SCORE

Total possible compliance score is 100%
Add the scores of each of the five scoring categories. Divide sum by 5 to determine the final compliance percentage score.

CUSTOMER SERVICE

100 Points Possible

For Customer Service Standards 1 – 7
10 points off if not provided correctly
For Customer Service Standards 1 – 6
3 points off if provided with minor discrepancy
For Customer Service Standard 8
100 points off for use of any prohibited behavior

For Customer Service Standard 9 (Calming Techniques)
Case Entry	20 points off if not used and ECC Score >1
Key Questions	20 points off if not used and ECC Score >1
DLS Instructions	20 points off if not used and ECC Score >1

MPDS v11.1 SS7 (NAE) – 1 Mar. 2003

NA◆ED National Academies of Emergency Dispatch

Field Feedback Report

Reported by:_____ Agency: _____

Date:_____ Time: _____ Run #: _____ Unit(s): _____

Dispatchers: _____ and _____

Response Team: _____ and _____

Problem Encountered: _____

_____

_____

_____

_____

_____

_____

_____

_____

_____

Specific Protocol referred to: _____ #: _____

Operating procedure referred to: _____ #: _____

══════════════════════ For QIU Use Only ══════════════════════

Received at Quality Improvement Unit (Date): _____ By: _____

Investigation Outcome: _____

_____

_____

_____

_____

_____

_____

_____

_____

_____

_____

_____

_____

_____

Case Review Completed (Date): _____ Compliance %: _____ Correct Response Code: _____

Reported to: _____ at: _____

ED-Q's signature: _____ Date: _____

Version 3.0 – 03-2002